Multi-Detector CT Imaging Handbook

Multi-Detector CT Imaging

Principles, Head, Neck, and Vascular Systems

Multi-Detector CT Imaging Handbook

Multi-Detector CT Imaging: Principles, Head, Neck, and Vascular Systems

Multi-Detector CT Imaging: Abdomen, Pelvis, and CAD Applications

Multi-Detector CT Imaging

Principles, Head, Neck, and Vascular Systems

edited by

Luca Saba • Jasjit S. Suri

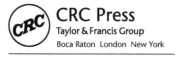

CRC Press
Taylor & Francis Group
Boca Raton London New York

CRC Press is an imprint of the
Taylor & Francis Group, an **informa** business

CRC Press
Taylor & Francis Group
6000 Broken Sound Parkway NW, Suite 300
Boca Raton, FL 33487-2742

First issued in paperback 2017

© 2014 by Taylor & Francis Group, LLC
CRC Press is an imprint of Taylor & Francis Group, an Informa business

No claim to original U.S. Government works

ISBN-13: 978-1-4398-9380-7 (hbk)
ISBN-13: 978-1-138-07648-8 (pbk)

Library of Congress Cataloging-in-Publication Data

Multi-detector CT imaging : principles, head, neck, and vascular systems / editors, Luca Saba and Jasjit S. Suri.
    p. ; cm.
  Includes bibliographical references and index.
  ISBN 978-1-4398-9380-7 (alk. paper)
  I. Saba, Luca. II. Suri, Jasjit S.
  [DNLM: 1. Multidetector Computed Tomography--methods. 2. Brain Diseases--radiography. 3. Neck--radiography. 4. Vascular Diseases--radiography. WN 206]

616.07'5722--dc23   2012048761

Visit the Taylor & Francis Web site at
http://www.taylorandfrancis.com

and the CRC Press Web site at
http://www.crcpress.com

Luca Saba dedicates this book to his parents

Giovanni Saba and Raffaela Polla for their love.

Jasjit S. Suri dedicates this book to his children

Harman Suri and Neha Suri for their love.

Contents

Section I General Principles

Section II Neck–Brain

Section III   Cardiovascular System

Section IV   Thorax and Mediastinum

Foreword

Medical imaging, and computed tomography (CT) in particular, have revolutionized medical care over the past four decades in ways unimaginable prior to the introduction of CT. The impact of CT extends over virtually every clinical field and region of the body, and through all aspects of care including screening, diagnosis and problem solving, monitoring disease progression and treatment responses, and directing minimally invasive procedural interventions. It is no wonder then, with the critical role CT plays, and with the rapid innovations in computer technology, that advances in the capabilities and complexity of CT imaging continue to evolve. An up-to-date complete and authoritative educational and reference volume covering the entire spectrum of CT is a difficult task to accomplish and lacking in the radiology literature. *Multi-Detector CT Imaging*, edited by Dr. Luca Saba and Dr. Jasjit Suri, excels in meeting this need.

Drs. Saba and Suri have brought together an outstanding collection of international authors recognized worldwide as leaders in their fields. Their extensive clinical experience and practical knowledge are logically presented, well organized, and brilliantly visualized. The two books in this set are amazingly complete in content, depth, and quality, yet read easily as an educational introduction or as a reference source.

The value of these books will be appreciated by readers in many ways. They cover all aspects of CT imaging, with technical principles and postprocessing methodologies comprehensibly presented, and extensive clinical specialty chapters easily searchable for specific information without need of an index. The value goes far beyond just a "how-to" or an encyclopedia of findings, however. The authors have uniformly put techniques, clinical findings, pathologic disease presentations, and clinical implications of imaging findings in practical perspective. The organization of the chapters is a wonderful progression that actually follows how the radiologist approaches unknown cases. Most chapters start with a review of imaging techniques for the organ or disease process. This is often followed with a practical discussion reviewing the spectrum of abnormal CT findings and their significance and differential diagnosis, followed subsequently by thorough material organized around understanding disease processes. Helpful correlative material with MRI and PET imaging is frequently presented to illustrate how these modalities complement each other.

This resource is a remarkable tool that will be of value to imaging professionals from every clinical vantage point and will serve well those experienced with CT or those using it to first learn about CT. I personally look forward to using this resource and having it available for our trainees, not only as an essential educational tool, but knowing that it will stimulate our community to further push the frontiers of CT imaging.

Richard L. Baron, MD
Dean for Clinical Practice
Professor of Radiology
University of Chicago Pritzker School of Medicine

Preface

The introduction of multi-detector row computed tomography (CT) in the early 1990s resulted in a fundamental and far-reaching improvement of CT imaging. For the first time, volumes of data could be acquired without misregistration of anatomical details, which indicated the development of 3D image processing techniques. In the last 20 years, CT technology has further improved with the introduction of systems up to 320-detector rows and with the development of dual-source and multispectral technology.

From these developments, the diagnostic potential of CT has impressively improved with an exceptional spatial resolution and the possibility to analyze with an exquisite level of detail several kinds of pathology. Thanks to the development of CT perfusion technique, functional brain imaging as well as liver imaging is now possible.

The purpose of this book is to cover clinical and engineering benefits in the diagnosis of human pathologies. It discusses the protocols and potential of advanced computed tomography scanners, explaining easily, but with an adequate level of detail, the role and potential of CT.

Acknowledgments

It is not possible to overstate our gratitude to the many individuals who helped to produce this book. In particular, Luca Saba would like to thank Professors Giorgio Mallarini and Giancarlo Caddeo, who first taught him the principles of computed tomography. Dr. Saba also thanks Stefano Marcia, Paolo Siotto, and Giovanni Argiolas and his many colleagues, residents, students, and friends for their continuous exchanges during these years. A special thanks also to Carlo Nicola de Cecco for his help. Finally, Dr. Saba would like to acknowledge the patience and understanding displayed by Tiziana throughout his work. Without her continuous encouragement, this book would not have been completed.

Jasjit S. Suri acknowledges Dr. Luca Saba for his continuous dedication in the field of computer tomography imaging and his willingness to participate in successfully launching this project. Dr. Suri also thanks his family, Malvika, Harman, and Neha, who are always a source of shine and laughter. Special thanks to all his friends and collaborators around the world who helped commercialize medical devices and healthcare imaging products over the course of years.

Both editors have received considerable support and cooperation from individuals at CRC/Taylor & Francis, particularly Michael Slaughter, Jessica Vakili, Joette Lynch, Michele Smith and from Dennis Troutman at diacriTech, each of whom helped to minimize the obstacles that the editors encountered.

Editors

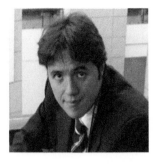

Luca Saba earned his MD from the University of Cagliari, Italy, in 2002. Today, he works in the University of Cagliari School of Medicine. His research fields are focused on multi-detector row computed tomography, magnetic resonance, ultrasound, neuroradiology, and diagnostics in vascular sciences.

His works, as lead author, have appeared in more than 100 high impact factor, peer-reviewed journals such as the *American Journal of Neuroradiology, European Radiology, European Journal of Radiology, Acta Radiologica, Cardiovascular and Interventional Radiology, Journal of Computer Assisted Tomography, American Journal of Roentgenology, Neuroradiology, Clinical Radiology, Journal of Cardiovascular Surgery*, and *Cerebrovascular Diseases*. He is a well-known speaker and has spoken over 45 times at national and international levels.

Dr. Saba has won 12 scientific and extracurricular awards during his career. He has presented more than 430 papers and posters at national and international congresses (RSNA, ESGAR, ECR, ISR, AOCR, AINR, JRS, SIRM, AINR). He has written eight book chapters, and he is currently serving as an editor of four books in the field of cardiovascular and neurodegenerative imaging.

He is a member of the Italian Society of Radiology, European Society of Radiology, Radiological Society of North America, American Roentgen Ray Society, and European Society of Neuroradiology.

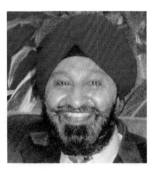

Jasjit S. Suri earned his MS in neurological MRI from the University of Illinois, a PhD in cardiac imaging from the University of Washington and an MBA from the Weatherhead School of Management, Case Western Reserve University. He has worked as scientist, manager, senior director, vice president, and chief technology officer at IBM, Siemens Medical, Philips Healthcare, Fisher, and Eigen Inc.

He has written over 400 publications, 60 patents, 4 FDA clearances, and more than 25 books in medical imaging and biotechnologies (diagnostic and therapeutic). Dr. Suri has had a leadership role in releasing products in the men's and women's market in the fields of cardiology, neurology, urology, vascular, ophthalmology, and breast cancer.

Dr. Suri has received the President's Gold Medal and Fellow of American Institute of Medical and Biological Engineering from the National Academy of Sciences. He has won over 50 awards during his career. Dr. Suri is also a strategic advisory board member for more than half a dozen industries and international journals focused on biomedical imaging and technologies.

Contributors

Michele Anzidei
Department of Radiological
    Sciences
Sapienza University of Rome
Rome, Italy

Philip A. Araoz
Mayo Clinic
Rochester, Minnesota

Irene Ariozzi
Department of Surgical Sciences
University of Parma University
    Hospital
Parma, Italy

Asim K. Bag
Department of Radiology
Neuroradiology Section
The University of Alabama at
    Birmingham
Birmingham, Alabama

Glenn Bauman
Schulich School of Medicine and
    Dentistry
Western University
and
London Regional Cancer
    Program
London Health Sciences Centre
London, Ontario, Canada

Luca Bertaccini
Department of Radiological
    Sciences
Sapienza University of Rome
Rome, Italy

Samuel Boynton
Department of Radiology
Mayo Clinic
Rochester, Minnesota

Carlo Catalano
Department of Radiological
    Sciences
Sapienza University of Rome
Rome, Italy

Irfan Celebi
Department of Radiology
Sisli Etfal Training and Research
    Hospital
Istanbul, Turkey

Philip R. Chapman
Neuroradiology Section
Department of Radiology
The University of Alabama at
    Birmingham
Birmingham, Alabama

Joel K. Curé
Neuroradiology Section
Department of Radiology
University of Alabama at
    Birmingham
Birmingham, Alabama

Christopher D. d'Esterre
Imaging Program
Lawson Health Research
    Institute
London, Ontario, Canada

Tobias De Zordo
Department of Radiology
Medical University Innsbruck
Innsbruck, Austria

Pier Luigi Di Paolo
Department of Neurology and
    Psychiatry
Sapienza University
Rome, Italy

Robert Donnino
Departments of Medicine and
    Radiology
NYU School of Medicine
and
Veterans Affairs New York
    Harbor Healthcare System
New York, New York

Shehanaz Ellika
Neuroradiology Section
Department of Radiology
Boston Children Hospital
Harvard Medical School
Boston, Massachusetts

Gudrun Feuchtner
Department of Radiology
Medical University Innsbruck
Innsbruck, Austria

Francesco Fraioli
Department of Radiological
    Sciences
Sapienza University of Rome
Rome, Italy

Jorge M. Fuentes-Orrego
Harvard Medical School
and
Division of Abdominal Imaging
    and Intervention
Radiology Department
Massachusetts General Hospital
Boston, Massachusetts

Jin Mo Goo
Department of Radiology
Seoul National University College
    of Medicine
Seoul, Korea

Kheng-Thye Ho
Mount Alvernia Hospital
Singapore

Angelika Hoffmann
Department of Radiology
University of Virginia
Charlottesville, Virginia

Werner Jaschke
Department of Radiology
Medical University Innsbruck
Innsbruck, Austria

Nikolaj K. G. Jensen
Western University
London, Ontario, Canada

Jeffrey P. Kanne
Section of Thoracic Imaging
University of Wisconsin
    School of Medicine and
    Public Health
Madison, Wisconsin

Ting-Yim Lee
Lawson Health Research Institute
and
Robarts Research Institute
and
Diagnostic Imaging
St. Joseph's Healthcare London
and
Medical Imaging
Schulich School of Medicine and
    Dentistry
Western University
London, Ontario, Canada

Christianne Leidecker
Siemens Healthcare
Malvern, Pennsylvania

Michael M. Lell
Department of Radiology
Erlangen University Hospital
University of
    Erlangen-Nuremberg
Erlangen, Germany

Carmelinda Manna
Department of Surgical Sciences
University of Parma University
    Hospital
Parma, Italy

Eugenio Marotta
Department of Radiological
    Sciences
Sapienza University of Rome
Rome, Italy

Kosuke Matsubara
Department of Quantum Medical
    Technology
Faculty of Health Sciences
Kanazawa University
Kanazawa, Japan

Alessandro Napoli
Department of Radiological
    Sciences
Sapienza University of Rome
Rome, Italy

Karoline Netzer
Department of Radiology
Medical University Innsbruck
Innsbruck, Austria

Yousef W. Nielsen
Department of Radiology
University Hospital at Herlev
Copenhagen, Denmark

Jonathan K. Park
David Geffen School of Medicine
    at UCLA
and
Ronald Reagan UCLA Medical
    Center
Los Angeles, California

Antonio Pavarani
Department of Surgical Sciences
University of Parma University
    Hospital
Parma, Italy

Rocío Pérez-Johnston
Harvard Medical School
and
Division of Abdominal Imaging
    and Intervention
Radiology Department
Massachusetts General Hospital
Boston, Massachusetts

Whitney Pope
David Geffen School of Medicine
    at UCLA
and
Ronald Reagan UCLA Medical
    Center
Los Angeles, California

Eytan Raz
Department of Radiology
New York University School of
    Medicine
New York, New York

and

Department of Neurology and
    Psychiatry
Sapienza University
Rome, Italy

**Ahmed Abdel Khalek Abdel
Razek**
Department of Diagnostic
    Radiology
Mansoura Faculty of Medicine
Mansoura, Egypt

Luca Saba
Department of Radiology
University of Cagliari
    School of Medicine
Cagliari, Italy

Dushyant V. Sahani
Harvard Medical School
and
Division of Abdominal Imaging
    and Intervention
Radiology Department
Massachusetts General Hospital
Boston, Massachusetts

Paul Schoenhagen
Cleveland Clinic Lerner College of
    Medicine
Case Western University
and
Imaging Institute and Heart &
    Vascular Institute
Cleveland Clinic
Cleveland, Ohio

Goffredo Serra
Department of Radiological
    Sciences
Sapienza University of Rome
Rome, Italy

Aaron So
Imaging Program
Lawson Health Research Institute
and
Diagnostic Imaging
St. Joseph's Healthcare London
London, Ontario, Canada

Monvadi B. Srichai
Medstar Georgetown University
    Hospital
and
Medstar Heart Institute
Washington, DC

Errol E. Stewart
Imaging Program
Lawson Health Research Institute
and
Diagnostic Imaging
St. Joseph's Healthcare London
London, Ontario, Canada

Zhonghua Sun
Department of Imaging
  and Applied Physics
Curtin University
Perth, Australia

Jasjit S. Suri
Division of Diagnosis and
  Monitoring
AtheroPoint™ LLC.
Roseville, California

and

Department of Biomedical
  Engineering
Idaho State University
Pocatello, Idaho

Nicola Sverzellati
Department of Surgical
  Sciences
University of Parma University
  Hospital
Parma, Italy

Ahmed M. Tawfik
Diagnostic and Interventional
  Radiology Department
Mansoura Faculty of Medicine
Mansoura, Egypt

and

Department of Diagnostic and
  Interventional Radiology
J. W. Goethe University Hospital
Frankfurt, Germany

Henrik S. Thomsen
Department of Radiology
University Hospital at Herlev
and
Department of Diagnostic Sciences,
  Faculty of Health Sciences
University of Copenhagen
Copenhagen, Denmark

Surjith Vattoth
Department of Radiology
Neuroradiology Section
University of Alabama at Birmingham
Birmingham, Alabama

Thomas J. Vogl
Department of Diagnostic and
  Interventional Radiology
J. W. Goethe University Hospital
Frankfurt, Germany

Max Wintermark
Department of Radiology
University of Virginia
Charlottesville, Virginia

Eugene Wong
Schulich School of Medicine and
  Dentistry
Western University
and
London Regional Cancer Program
London Health Sciences Centre
London, Ontario, Canada

Timothy Pok Chi Yeung
Schulich School of Medicine and
  Dentistry
Western University
and
London Regional Cancer Program
London Health Sciences Centre
London, Ontario, Canada

Eleonora Zambrini
Department of Surgical Sciences
University of Parma University
  Hospital
Parma, Italy

Section I

General Principles

1

Technical Principles of Computed Tomography

Michael M. Lell and Christianne Leidecker

CONTENTS

1.1 Introduction

Computed tomography (CT) was introduced in the early 1970s with the first commercial scanner available in 1972 from EMI Laboratories (Hayes, UK). Since then, it has revolutionized diagnostic imaging. CT combined a computer to a medical imaging device, heralding a new era of digital imaging, and was the first technology to acquire and display cross-sectional x-ray images.

The first CT scanner, developed by the English engineer G.N. Hounsfield, was introduced as a pure head scanner with a conventional x-ray tube and a dual-row detector system moving incrementally around the patient. It was able to acquire 12 slices, each 13 mm thick, and reconstruct the images with a matrix of 80×80 pixels in approximately 35 minutes. Today, the whole brain can be visualized with high quality from a 10-second scan.

Although the performance of CT scanners increased with the progress in engineering, it was the introduction of helical (or spiral) CT in the early 1990s [1,2] that constituted a fundamental evolutionary step in the development and ongoing refinement of CT imaging techniques. Theoretically proposed several years before [3,4], spiral CT requires the continuous rotation of the x-ray tube and the detector. This was enabled through the introduction of slip-ring technology, with continuous power transmission to and data extraction off the rotating gantry (Figure 1.1). Spiral CT enabled the acquisition of volume data, thus avoiding misregistration or double registration of anatomical details. Additionally, longitudinal resolution could be improved through overlapping image reconstruction, since images can be reconstructed at any position along the patient axis (longitudinal axis, z-axis).

The introduction of multislice CT in 1998 constituted a milestone with regard to increased scan speed, improved z-axis spatial resolution, and better use of the available x-ray power. With single-slice spiral CT, the main drawbacks are insufficient volume coverage within one breath-hold time and reduced longitudinal spatial resolution because of wide collimation. Isotropic resolution, that is, equal resolution in all three spatial directions, could be achieved for only very limited scan ranges in single-slice spiral CT [5]. Four-slice CT systems, made available by all major CT manufacturers in 1998 [6,7], allowed for increased volume coverage in shorter scan times and improved longitudinal resolution. Despite promising advances, clinical challenges and limitations remained for four-slice CT systems. True isotropic resolution for routine applications could not be achieved for many applications requiring extended scan ranges, since wider collimated slices (4×2.5 mm or 4×3.75 mm) had to be chosen to complete the scan within a reasonable time frame. Although four-slice

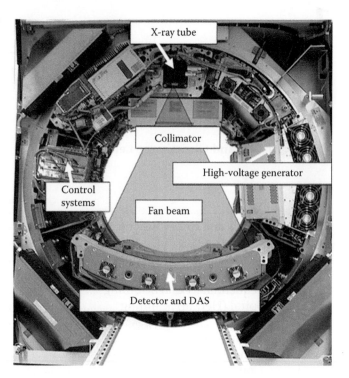

FIGURE 1.1
Basic components of a third-generation computed tomography system: unlike first-generation systems with a collimated pencil beam or second-generation systems with a small fan beam, the fan beam of a third-generation scanner covers the whole object and a pure rotational motion of the tube–detector unit can be performed instead of translation and rotation. DAS = data acquisition system.

CT systems with rotation times as short as 0.5 second enabled venturing into the realms of cardiac imaging [8,9], reliable imaging of patients with higher heart rates was not possible because of limited temporal resolution. In addition, insufficient longitudinal resolution and associated partial volume artifacts limited the imaging of stents or severely calcified arteries [10].

As a next step, the introduction of 16-slice CT systems enabled routine acquisition of large anatomical volumes with isotropic submillimeter spatial resolution. With further reduced rotation times and larger volume coverage, examination times could be significantly reduced for standard protocols or, alternatively, scan ranges could be significantly extended.

The routine acquisition of volume data became the basis for advanced applications such as CT angiography (CTA), which allows noninvasive assessment of vascular disease. Volume data was the prerequisite for the development of three-dimensional (3D) image-processing techniques such as multiplanar reformats (MPRs), curved multiplanar reformats (CPRs), maximum intensity projections (MIPs), shaded surface displays (SSDs), volume rendering techniques (VRTs), and image registration techniques, which are an indispensable tool in image evaluation today [11].

In 2004, the first generation of 64-slice CT systems was introduced. Two different scanner concepts were proposed by different vendors. The first was the so-called "volume concept" that aimed at a further increase in volume coverage speed by using 64 detector rows instead of 16 without changing the physical parameters of the scanner compared to the respective 16-slice version. The second was the "resolution concept," which uses 32 physical detector rows in combination with a refined z-sampling technique. Double z-sampling is enabled by a periodic motion of the focal spot in the z-direction with the goal to simultaneously acquire 64 overlapping slices with pitch-independent increase of longitudinal resolution and reduction of spiral artifacts. Along with increased volume coverage, temporal resolution was improved with gantry rotation times of 0.33 second. For the first time, CT had the potential to robustly image the heart even at higher heart rates, thereby significantly reducing the number of patients with unevaluable coronary segments and facilitating the successful integration of coronary CTA into routine clinical algorithms.

The "slice war" continued and today's high-end single-source scanners can acquire up to 256 slices with an isotropic resolution down to 0.3 mm. Rotation times are as low as 0.27 second with a corresponding temporal resolution of 135 ms. The "volume CT" concept utilizes 320 detectors at 0.5 mm thickness and a coverage of 16 cm at isocenter.

Dual-source CT (DSCT) systems were introduced in 2005 [12]. As the name implies, the system uses two x-ray tubes and two corresponding detectors offset by 90° (Figure 1.2). With a DSCT system, temporal resolution equals a quarter of the gantry rotation time, independent of the patient's heart rate. Hence, one of the key benefits of DSCT scanners lies in cardiac imaging. Alternatively, the simultaneous operation of both tubes provides higher power reserves for fast imaging in obese

patients, or the x-ray tubes can be operated at different tube voltages and/or different prefiltration, allowing dual energy acquisitions. Potential applications of dual-energy CT (DECT) include tissue characterization, calcium quantification, and quantification of the local blood volume in contrast-enhanced scans. In the meantime, second-generation DSCT scanners are available; wider detectors with 128 slices, further increased rotation speed, and new high-pitch scan modes enable further improvements in cardiac CT and DECT along with a significant dose reduction potential.

1.2 Basic Physics and Image Reconstruction

The fundamental principle in CT imaging lies in measuring the two-dimensional (2D) distribution of x-ray attenuation coefficient μ. The linear attenuation coefficient μ is characteristic for the material and the energy of the photons. Assuming a primary x-ray photon intensity I_0, μ determines the measured photon intensity I behind an object of thickness d. For the simple case of monoenergetic photons and a homogeneous object, this is given by a simple exponential relationship:

$$I = I_0 e^{-\mu d} \tag{1.1}$$

With μ being characteristic of the attenuating material, it is therefore possible to distinguish materials with different attenuation coefficients. In CT, the goal is to obtain the distribution of attenuation coefficients for any given slice, $\mu(x, y)$. For an image with n^2 pixels and thus a 2D distribution of attenuation coefficients with n^2 values, one needs at least n^2 independently measured intensities I in Equation 1.1. I_0 is usually known from a calibration measurement using rays outside the actual field of measurement (FOM), as the attenuation of air is negligible. A typical image matrix size today is 512^2, and thus, a minimum of $512^2 = 262{,}144$ independent projection values are needed. (In CT, any single measurement along a given direction is called a projection. Each projection consists of the sum of the attenuation coefficients of all materials along one ray.) If one tries to solve this problem iteratively, as it was the case in the early days of CT, this would result in a linear equation system of 512^2 equations with 512^2 unknown parameters.

Hence, one soon turns to the more practical approach of filtered back projection (FBP). This numerical approach is still the standard today and is the basis for CT reconstruction algorithms used in all scanners. As the name implies, a filter or convolution kernel is applied in the process, which determines the image characteristics by balancing resolution and noise. For example, "sharp"

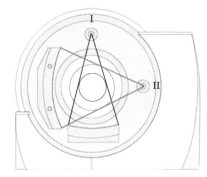

FIGURE 1.2
Schematic illustration of a dual-source CT (DSCT) system using two tubes and two corresponding detectors offset by 90° or 95°: the systems available commercially have one detector (I) that is restricted to a smaller, central field of view (26 or 33 cm, blue circle) and one detector (II) that covers the entire scan field of view (green circle).

kernels increase resolution and noise, whereas "soft" kernels decrease them. Resolution and noise are therefore inherently linked for such reconstruction approaches.

For practical purposes, the value displayed in CT images is not the attenuation coefficient itself but the so-called CT value or CT number (CT#), which is given in Hounsfield unit (HU). It is defined as

$$CT\# = \left[\frac{(\mu - \mu_{water})}{\mu_{water}} \right] \times 1000 \text{ HU} \qquad (1.2)$$

where μ_{water} is the attenuation coefficient of water. The reason for introducing the CT value lies in the fact that the attenuation coefficient is a rather inconvenient measure, as it depends on the x-ray spectrum used. It immediately follows that μ_{water} in Equation 1.2 is specific for the selected tube voltage and needs to be determined by calibration measurements for each voltage setting available. From Equation 1.2, it is also clear that the CT value of water is 0 for any given measurement and that of air (with negligible, meaning no, attenuation) is –1000 HU.

The typical x-ray spectrum used in CT imaging, however, is a polychromatic one. Hence, the spectrum changes as photons are attenuated on the x-ray's path through the material and the assumption of a monoenergetic mean energy in Equation 1.1 is violated. This effect is usually ignored in initial image reconstruction for all materials except water and results in beam hardening artifacts.

A more detailed overview of CT systems and image reconstruction techniques may be found in works by Flohr et al. [13,14].

1.2.1 Technology

The basic components of a CT system include the gantry, the x-ray source or tube, a high-powered generator, detector and detector electronics, data transmission systems (slip rings), and a computer system for image reconstruction and manipulation. The overall performance depends on each one of these key components.

Today's CT scanners use the so-called "rotate/rotate" geometry, where the x-ray tube and the detector are mounted onto a gantry that rotates around the patient. The detector arc typically contains 700 or more detector elements, which cover a FOM of usually 50–70 cm. For multislice systems, several such detector rows exist. The x-ray attenuation of the object is measured for each individual detector element. The measurements acquired at the same angular position of the system form a projection or view. Typically, 1000 projections are measured during a full rotation.

With rotation times in the millisecond range, the gantry has to withstand high gravitational forces (~28 G for 0.33 second rotation time). Of particular importance is the stability of the focal spot associated with the generation of x-rays as well as the corresponding detector position to ensure the high precision of measurements and eventually image resolution in the submillimeter domain. However, rotation times of less than 0.25 second (mechanical forces > 45 G) appear to be beyond today's mechanical limits.

With fast data acquisition times, today's x-ray tube/generator combinations are required to deliver peak power in the range of 60–100 kW. The typical x-ray spectra available in CT imaging today use a range of user-selectable voltage settings, usually in discrete steps ranging from 70 to 150 kV. As a typical example, systems might offer four settings at 80, 100, 120, and 140 kV. The range is due to different requirements by different clinical applications for optimal image quality and/or best possible signal-to-noise ratio at lowest dose. A conventional tube design includes an anode plate of typically 160–220 mm diameter that rotates in a vacuum housing. A cathode-generated electron beam is accelerated in vacuum toward the anode, and on hitting the anode the kinetic energy of the electrons is transformed into heat and x-ray photons. The resolution of the system depends on the size and stability of the focal spot at the anode. Typical dimensions are nominal sizes of 1.0–1.2 mm (large) and 0.3–0.6 mm (small) focal spots. The anode in most (diagnostic) x-ray tubes consists mainly of tungsten, mostly because of its high atomic number ($Z = 74$) and extremely high melting point, both required for efficient x-ray production and heat resistance, respectively. The heat storage capacity of the tube, hence, determines the performance level: the bigger the anode plate, the larger the heat storage capacity and the more scan seconds delivered until the anode plate reaches its temperature limit. An alternative design is the rotating envelope tube [15], where the anode plate constitutes an outer wall of the rotating tube housing. Efficient anode cooling via thermal conduction occurs owing to direct contact with the cooling oil. A permanent electromagnetic deflection of the electron beam is needed to position and shape the focal spot on the anode due to the central rotating cathode. This is also used for the double z-sampling technology mentioned earlier [13].

All state-of-the-art CT systems use solid-state detectors. Materials currently in use have comparable performance ensuring efficient x-ray detection. Suitable detector materials have a high atomic number and short afterglow time to enable the fast gantry rotation speeds and data acquisition. Typical materials are cadmium tungstate, gadolinium oxide, or gadolinium oxisulfide with suitable dopings. In course of the measurement, the absorbed x-rays are converted into visible light, which is then detected by a photodiode. The resulting electrical current is amplified and converted into a digital signal.

1.2.2 Data Rates and Data Transmission

With increasing number of detector rows and decreasing gantry rotation times, the data transmission systems of multislice CT scanners must be capable of handling significant data rates. With a typical 64-slice CT system, data rates of 180–200 MB/s are reached. This constitutes a challenge both for data transmission off the gantry and for subsequent image reconstruction systems, in particular, if real-time data processing is required. Contactless transmission technology is the state of the art used for data transfer, either laser transmission or electromagnetic transmission with a coupling between a rotating transmission ring antenna and a stationary receiving antenna. In image reconstruction, images are reconstructed at a rate of up to 40 images per second for a 512×512 matrix.

1.3 Scan Modes and Scan Parameters

The two basic modes of CT data acquisition are sequential (axial) and spiral (helical) scanning.

1.3.1 Sequential (Axial) Scanning

In sequential or axial scanning, a given scan volume is covered in a so-called "step-and-shoot" mode. Data are acquired during a full rotation and the patient table is moved between two individual acquisitions to a new z-position. A detailed theoretical description of the performance of sequential scan modes can be found in work by Hsieh [16]. As a key characteristic, the number of images acquired during a sequential scan corresponds to that of active detector slices. By combining detector signals of the adjacent sections during image reconstruction, the number of images per scan can be reduced and the image slice width can be increased. As an example, a scan with 4×1 mm collimation can be viewed at four images with 1 mm slice width, two images with 2 mm slice width, or alternatively one single image with 4 mm slice width. Realizing a thicker slice width by summation of several thin sections is beneficial for examinations that require, on the one hand, narrow collimation to avoid partial volume artifacts and, on the other hand, low image noise to detect low contrast details, such as examinations of the posterior fossa of the skull or the cervical spine.

With the advent of multislice CT, sequential scanning is used only for a few clinical applications, such as head CT, high-spatial-resolution lung CT, perfusion CT, and interventional applications. Recently, the technique experienced a revival in cardiac scanning.

1.3.2 Spiral (Helical) Scanning

Spiral or helical scanning is characterized by continuous gantry rotation and continuous data acquisition while the patient table moves at a constant speed (Figure 1.3). With multislice CT systems, it has become the method of choice for most applications. A main difference to sequential CT and at the same time a significant advantage is the possibility of freely and retrospectively choosing image positions and reconstruction increments. While in sequential CT, scan and image position are directly coupled, this restriction is no longer valid in spiral CT.

1.3.3 Pitch

An important parameter to characterize a spiral scan is the pitch p. According to International Electrotechnical Commission specifications (IEC 60601-2-44 Amd.1), the pitch p is given by table feed per rotation divided by the total width of the collimated beam. The pitch illustrates whether data acquisition occurs with gaps ($p > 1$) or with overlap ($p < 1$) in the longitudinal scan direction. For general radiology applications, clinically useful pitch values range from 0.5 to 2. Exceptions occur in the special case of electrocardiogram (ECG)-gated cardiac scanning, where very low pitch values of 0.2–0.4 are applied to ensure gapless volume coverage of the heart during each phase of the cardiac cycle, and in high-pitch scanning with DSCT systems, where pitch values as high as 3.4 can be used.

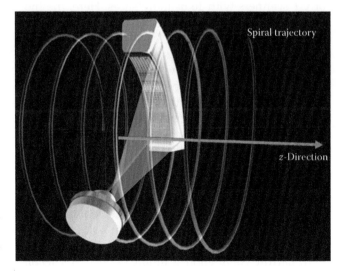

FIGURE 1.3
Principle of spiral (helical) CT scanning: the patient table moves continuously through the gantry while data are acquired during multiple rotations. Thus, the path of the x-ray tube and detector relative to the patient corresponds to a helix. To reconstruct an image at a specified image position, data needs to be interpolated in the z-direction to estimate a complete CT dataset at that position.

1.3.4 Collimated and Effective Slice Width

The continuous data acquisition during table movement results in a helical trajectory of the measured data points. Although the actual image reconstruction is, in principle, the same as in sequential CT, an additional interpolation step is required to reconstruct an image at a specified z-position. This interpolation in the longitudinal direction is used to generate a consistent planar dataset from the spiral data for an arbitrary image position.

The basic interpolation algorithms used are the 180-MLI and 360-MLI (multislice linear interpolation) approaches [17,18] or z-filter techniques [19]. In a z-filter reconstruction, all direct and complementary rays (i.e., rays in the same direction acquired half a rotation earlier or later) within a selectable distance from the image plane contribute to the image. Images with different slice widths can be retrospectively reconstructed from the same CT raw data by adjusting this distance and the corresponding weighting functions. Hence, z-filtering allows the user to trade off z-axis resolution with image noise (which directly correlates with required dose).

In spiral CT, the slice profile changes to a more bell-shaped curve as opposed to the trapezoidal shape in axial scanning. Interpolation algorithms determine the effective slice width, which now determines z-axis resolution as opposed to the collimated beam width in axial scanning.

1.3.5 Cone-Beam Problem in Multislice CT

Modified reconstruction approaches that account for the cone-beam geometry of measured rays are required for CT scanners with 16 or more slices. Here, the individual "fan beams" are tilted by the cone angle with respect to a plane perpendicular to the z-axis. The cone angle is largest for the slices at the outer edges of the detector, and it increases with increasing number of detector rows (assuming their width is kept constant). Of the introduced reconstruction approaches, an option is the 3D FBP reconstruction. Here, one accounts for the cone-beam geometry by back projecting the individual projections into a 3D volume along the lines of measurement [20]. An alternative reconstruction approach is to split the 3D reconstruction task into a series of conventional 2D reconstructions, each of them on tilted intermediate image planes. One such implementation is the adaptive multiple plane reconstruction [21].

Regardless of the specific reconstruction algorithm used, narrow collimation scanning is generally recommended. Even if the pitch has to be increased for equivalent volume coverage, partial volume artifacts can be better suppressed when data are acquired at narrow collimations. Hence, just like in single-slice spiral CT narrow collimation scanning is the key to reduce artifacts and to improve image quality.

1.3.6 Double z-Sampling

As a means to improve spatial resolution in the longitudinal direction, the concept of double z-sampling was introduced in 2003 [13]. By continuous electromagnetic deflection of an electron beam in a rotating envelope x-ray tube, the focal spot is alternated between two different positions on the anode plate, improving data sampling along the z-axis. Two subsequent readings are shifted by half a collimated slice width in the patient's longitudinal direction. As a consequence, spatial resolution in the longitudinal direction is increased. The first system using this technology, a 64–multi-detector CT (MDCT) system (Somatom Sensation 64; Siemens, Germany), combined two 32-slice readings to one 64-slice projection with a sampling distance of 0.3 mm at the isocenter (Figure 1.4). Thus, objects that are less than 0.4 mm in diameter can be routinely resolved at any pitch. Last but not least, a further benefit of double z-sampling lies in the suppression of spiral "windmill" artifacts.

1.3.7 Special Considerations: Cardiovascular CT

Imaging of the heart was enabled by ECG-synchronized data acquisition. Feasibility was proved with four-slice CT systems; using optimized image reconstruction techniques, a temporal resolution of ≤250 ms could be achieved with 0.5 second of gantry rotation time. This proved sufficient for adequate visualization of the coronary arteries at low heart rates [10].

However, it required the technological advances implemented in 64-slice scanners to potentially provide sufficient robustness for a successful integration of coronary CTA into routine clinical algorithms [22]. Temporal resolution is significantly improved because of the reduction of gantry rotation times to 0.33 second,

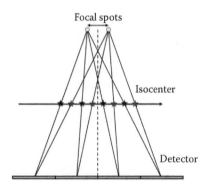

FIGURE 1.4
z-Flying focal spot technique: the electron beam is electromagnetically deflected between two positions on the anode plate. Two subsequent measurements shifted by half the collimated slice width at the isocenter can be combined, thus performing 64-slice acquisition with 32 detector element rows.

whereas increased volume coverage at submillimeter collimation enables high-resolution imaging of the coronary arteries. Today high-end single-source scanners offer rotation times as low as 0.27 second and can acquire up to 320 slices with an isotropic submillimeter resolution.

For ECG-synchronized examinations of the heart, either ECG-triggered sequential scanning or ECG-gated spiral scanning can be used. In ECG-triggered sequential scanning, the heart is covered by subsequent sequential scans in a step-and-shoot technique. In between the individual scans, the table moves to the next z-position. Owing to the time necessary for table motion, typically every second heartbeat is used for data acquisition (Figure 1.5).

With retrospective ECG gating, the heart is covered continuously in a spiral scan. The patient's ECG signal is recorded simultaneously to data acquisition to allow for a retrospective selection of the data segments used for image reconstruction. Only scan data acquired in a predefined cardiac phase, usually the diastolic phase, are used for image reconstruction. The data segments contributing to an image start with a user-defined offset relative to the onset of the R waves, similar to ECG-triggered axial scanning (Figure 1.6).

Temporal resolution is one key parameter in cardiac CT imaging. In a single-segment reconstruction, consecutive data from the same heart period are used to generate an image. At low heart rates, a single-segment reconstruction yields the best compromise between temporal resolution and volume coverage with thin slices. Temporal resolution can be improved by using scan data of subsequent heart cycles for image formation in a multisegment reconstruction. With increased number of segments higher temporal resolution is achieved but at the expense of slower volume coverage. Additionally, depending on the relationship between the rotation time and the patient's heart rate, temporal resolution is generally not constant: there are "sweet spots," heart rates with optimal temporal resolution and heart rates for which temporal resolution cannot be improved beyond half the gantry rotation time. Multisegment approaches rely on complete periodicity of heart motion, and they have limitations in patients with arrhythmia or patients with changing heart rates. In general, the reliability of obtaining good image quality with multisegment reconstruction decreases with increasing number of segments.

1.4 New Developments and Advances in CT

The technical advances in MDCT have been accompanied by a substantial enhancement of the clinical potential of CT. It seems, however, that adding even more detector rows will no longer directly translate

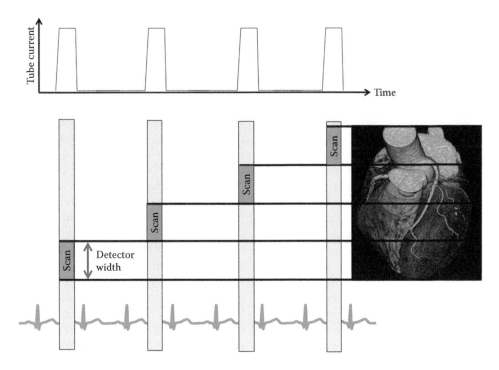

FIGURE 1.5
Axial or step-and-shoot mode: a series of axial scans at different z-positions is performed at a predefined temporal offset from the R wave. Every second RR interval is used for table movement.

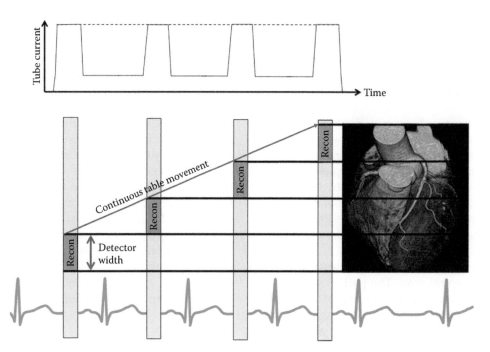

FIGURE 1.6
Electrocardiogram (ECG)-gated spiral scanning: as the table moves continuously at a low pitch, continuous spiral scan data of the heart are acquired. The patient's ECG signal is recorded as a function of time and is used to retrospectively identify scan data acquired in a defined cardiac phase to be used for image reconstruction. Tube current can be kept constant (dotted line) over the cardiac cycle or decreased during those phases that are not used for image reconstruction (solid line) to reduce dose.

into clinical benefit. Hence, recent advances in CT have focused on remaining limitations such as insufficient temporal resolution for cardiac CT or limited scan range to dynamic examinations of entire organs. Scanners with large area detectors and DSCT systems represent the two-system concepts at the moment.

1.4.1 CT Systems with Area Detector

The first commercially available system with an area detector was introduced in 2007. It consisted of a scanner with 320×0.5 mm collimation and 0.35 second gantry rotation time. CT scanners with area detectors are optimized for the acquisition of sequential scan data covering entire organs, such as the heart [23], the kidneys, or the brain [24] with zero table feed. The resulting reconstructed scan volume is cone shaped. Hence, with a detector collimation of 320×0.5 mm a coverage of 16 cm in the longitudinal direction is feasible at the isocenter, whereas coverage is 11.7 cm at a distance of 160 mm from the isocenter. By appending axial scans shifted in the z-direction, also called "stitching," larger scan volumes in the z-direction can be covered at the expense of overlap scanning. Single-step cardiac CTA and dynamic or perfusion CT are good indications for this technology [23,25,26].

Increased x-ray scatter due to larger detector z-coverage, however, poses a challenge in particular for perfusion scanning. Scattered radiation may cause hypodense

artifacts as well as affect CT-number stability. Ultimately, scatter-induced noise may reduce the contrast-to-noise ratio (CNR) in the images.

1.4.2 DSCT

In DSCT, two acquisition systems are mounted into one gantry with an angular offset of 90°–95° (Figure 1.2). Each acquisition system provides overlapping 0.6 mm slices using z-flying focal spot technique (Figure 1.4). Whereas one system covers the full FOM (FOM = 50 cm in diameter), the other is restricted to a central FOM (26–33 cm). We can acquire 64 or 128 overlapping 0.6 mm slices with double z-sampling, the shortest gantry rotation time being 0.33–0.28 second. DSCT provides higher temporal resolution without the necessity of faster gantry rotation. Generally 180° of scan data is used for image reconstruction in cardiac CT; this can be separated into two 90° data segments that are simultaneously acquired by the two acquisition systems of DSCT systems in the same phase of the patient's cardiac cycle and at the same anatomical level. Therefore, the total data acquisition time per image is reduced to a quarter of the gantry rotation time. For a rotation time of 0.28 second, the resulting temporal resolution is 75 ms, independent of the patient's heart rate.

Sampling gaps that lead to severe image artifacts occur if the pitch is increased beyond $p = 1.5$ in single-source

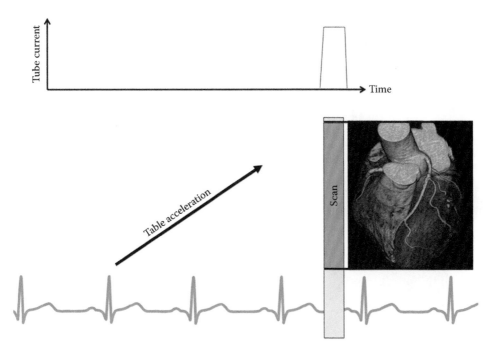

FIGURE 1.7
ECG-triggered high-pitch spiral dual-source CT (DSCT): the patient table is accelerated and reaches the scan volume at a predefined cardiac phase. At this z-position, data acquisition is started and the entire heart is covered in a fraction of a heartbeat. The blue box indicates the total scan time, which is typically 0.25–0.27 second. The images are reconstructed at slightly different phases of the cardiac cycle. Each of the images is reconstructed using data of a quarter rotation from each x-ray tube, resulting in a temporal resolution of 75 ms per image.

MDCT. DSCT systems can fill these gaps with data from the second measurement system a quarter rotation later, which allows to increase the pitch up to $p = 3.4$ (Figure 1.7). It is important to notice that no redundant data are acquired, each individual image has a temporal resolution of a quarter of the rotation time, and data acquisition is limited to an FOM of 33 cm in diameter. Scan speeds up to 450 mm/s can be achieved, sufficient to cover the heart in a single heartbeat [27–33]. The patient's ECG is used to trigger both table motion and data acquisition. Standard, that is, non-ECG-gated, scanning uses the high speed for the examination of larger anatomical ranges in very short scan times, for example, when the patient has limited ability to cooperate, such as in pediatric radiology [34].

1.4.3 Dual-Energy CT

In DSCT systems, both x-ray tubes can be operated at different tube voltage and current settings, allowing the nearly simultaneous acquisition of DECT data, thus overcoming the limitations of single-source DECT proposed more than 30 years ago [35–37]. DECT proved to be beneficial in a variety of clinical indications, including tissue characterization in abdominal imaging (small indeterminate hepatic or renal lesions, adrenal gland lesions, renal calculi, etc.), cardiovascular imaging (differentiation of iodine and calcium for bone-free CTA, follow-up of patients with endovascular

aneurysm repair, etc.), musculoskeletal imaging (calcium or uric acid quantification, calculation of pseudomonochromatic images for metal artifact reduction), and quantification of the local blood volume in contrast-enhanced scans [30–32,38–41].

Nowadays DECT data can also be acquired with high-end single-source CT systems, using either dual-layer detector panels or rapid kV-switching technology. Dual-layer detector systems involve placement of two layers of detector elements on top of each other. The upper detector layer predominantly absorbs lower-energy photons and the second detector layer absorbs higher-energy photons. Although it is not commercially available, this approach suffers disadvantages in that the spectral separation is inferior to dual-energy approaches relying on two different kV settings. With rapid kV-switching techniques used in single-source CT systems, the tube voltage alternates hundreds of times per second between two kV settings during the acquisition. The nearly simultaneous acquisition of both low- and high-energy data avoids registration problems owing to organ motion or contrast agent dynamics. However, the method is restricted to relatively slow rotation times (0.6–1 second) as a sufficient number of projections (>600) need to be acquired at each kV setting. Furthermore, current tube technology allows switching the voltage between consecutive readings, but not the tube current. Hence, a fixed tube current is required—at both low and high kV settings.

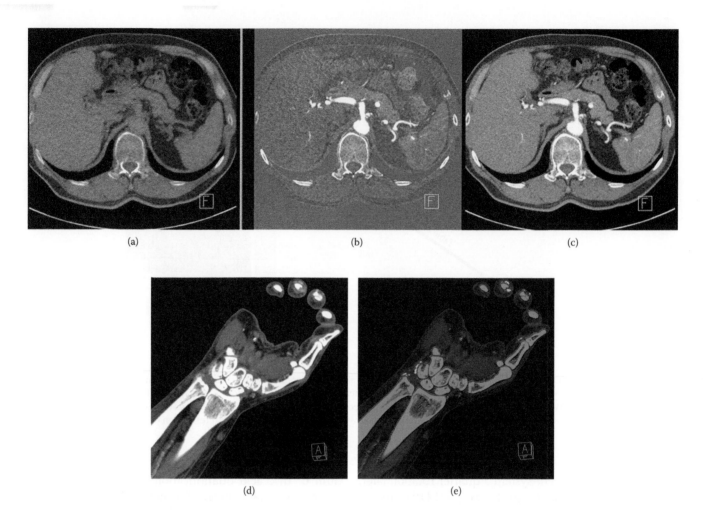

FIGURE 1.8
Three different visualizations of contrast-enhanced abdominal CT with dual energy: (a) virtual non-enhanced, (b) iodine map, and (c) combined 120-kV-equivalent contrast-enhanced CT. (d) Patient with a history of gout. (e) Differentiation of calcium (blue) and urate (green) deposition on color-coded DECT image.

DECT can obtain information on the chemical composition of tissue based on differences in the photoabsorption process; the dominant attenuation process at low photon energies; and Compton scattering, dominating at higher photon energies. Photoabsorption is very weak for hydrogen, but strong for iodine/contrast material. The relative strength of photoabsorption with respect to Compton scattering can be determined by DECT. Data analysis is based on material decomposition (Figure 1.8).

1.4.4 Iterative Reconstruction Algorithms

As mentioned in Section 1.2, FBP is a practical and efficient approach to image reconstruction, where spatial resolution is directly correlated with increased image noise. Iterative reconstruction techniques, well established in positron emission tomography (PET) and single photon emission CT) data reconstruction, have been only recently reinvigorated in CT as a method to improve image quality, enhance image resolution, and lower image noise [42].

A decisive benefit of iterative reconstruction constitutes the ability to decouple spatial resolution and image noise to a certain degree. In general, a correction loop is introduced in the image reconstruction process. After an initial image has been reconstructed from the measured projection data, synthetic projections are calculated that exactly represent the reconstructed image. The deviation between measured and calculated projections is used to reconstruct a correction image and refresh the original image in an iterative loop. Each time the image is updated, nonlinear image-processing algorithms are used to stabilize the solution. They maintain or enhance spatial resolution at higher object contrasts and reduce image noise in low-contrast areas. The repeated calculation of corrections reduces image artifacts, and image resolution can be increased by carefully modeling the measurement system during forward projection in a model-based iterative reconstruction [42].

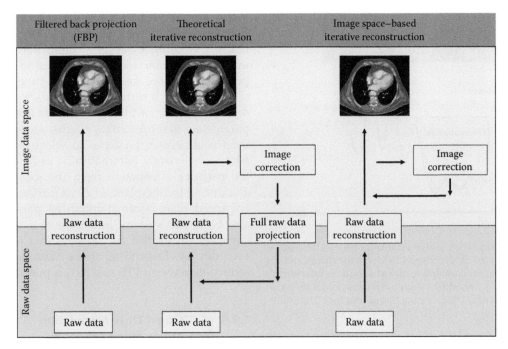

FIGURE 1.9
Image reconstruction: iterative correction loops are introduced to reduce noise and artifacts. Theoretical iterative reconstruction most accurately improves image quality but is computationally demanding. Image space-based iterative reconstruction skips the full raw data projection in the correction loop and is computationally less demanding. Variants and combinations of these techniques have been introduced in multi-detector CT (MDCT) reconstruction software.

In the meantime, several implementations of iterative reconstruction methods have been introduced commercially by the major vendors (Figure 1.9).

1.5 Radiation Dose Reduction

With CT being the imaging modality of choice in many situations, radiation exposure is of concern for both patients and physicians. To reduce the dose for an individual examination, the most important principle after critical review of the indication is to adhere to ALARA (as low as reasonably achievable). Besides adjusting the techniques to the diagnostic question, one can make use of many different techniques to reduce radiation exposure.

1.5.1 Tube Current Reduction

The most important lever to reduce radiation exposure is to adapt dose to the patient size and weight [43,44]. This is of particular importance in pediatric imaging. Not only patient habitus but also the imaging study itself has impact on radiation exposure: imaging the liver requires less noise—and therefore higher radiation exposure—to detect and differentiate small lesions, as compared to imaging the lung. More noise can be accepted in imaging the paranasal sinuses in the evaluation of sinusitis as compared to tumor staging. The acceptable level of noise is difficult to determine and is user dependent. Iterative reconstruction techniques compensate for higher noise to allow dose reduction of 50% in abdominal [45] and 25%–80% in chest CT [46–49].

1.5.2 Anatomical Tube Current Modulation

More straightforward than manually selecting patient-individual tube current settings by adjusting the x-ray tube current are techniques that use automatic anatomical tube current modulation (automatic exposure control [AEC]). AEC modifies the tube output in the through-plane (z-axis) direction to maintain adequate dose when scanning body regions with different attenuation, for instance, chest and abdomen. In addition, angular tube current modulation can be performed during each rotation of the gantry to compensate for strongly varying x-ray attenuations in asymmetrical body regions such as the shoulders and pelvis. The variation of the tube output is either predefined by analysis of the localizer scan (topogram, scout view) or determined online by evaluating the signal of a detector row online. In practice, a reference (either reference exposure or other types of image quality metrics) is selected, which will be applied if the patient's attenuation matches the stored standard reference. If the patient's attenuation deviates, the tube output will be adapted accordingly (Figure 1.10). Some

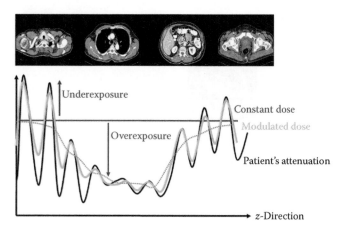

FIGURE 1.10
Anatomical dose modulation: with constant tube current, the thoracic inlet and the pelvis are underexposed, whereas the thorax and the abdomen are overexposed. Adapting the radiation dose to a patient's attenuation can be achieved by the online modulation of tube current, ensuring consistent image quality throughout the scan volume.

algorithms try to adapt the tube current such as to maintain constant image noise in all examined body parts, whereas others allow for a weaker increase of the tube current with increasing body size, trying to match the radiologist's perception. The potential for dose reduction is significant with the use of anatomical dose modulation approaches; values of 20%–68% without degrading image quality and depending on the body region have been reported [50–52]. However, the effects of AEC are limited with larger detector z-coverage, because the detector can cover different anatomical regions (i.e., transition from liver to lung or from shoulder to neck), each requiring individual tube current settings.

A variant of automatic anatomical tube current modulation designed to specifically reduce radiation exposure to selected organs is the organ-based tube current modulation. Thus, radiation exposure can be reduced for targeted organs such as eye lenses or the female breast. Therefore, the x-ray tube current is reduced in a selectable angular range, for example, when the x-ray tube moves directly in front of the female breast. The tube current has to be correspondingly increased when the x-ray tube is on the opposite side, to maintain image quality. Overall radiation dose is not reduced in this case, but distributed differently in the scan plane. Local radiation dose to the breast or to the thyroid gland can be reduced by 20%–35% without loss of image quality [53].

1.5.3 Adaptation of the X-Ray Tube Voltage

Not only the tube current, but also tube voltage may be adapted to patient size for further reduction of radiation exposure. Decreased tube voltage results in reduced dose and higher image noise, but attenuation values of iodine are also significantly higher. As a consequence, a specified CNR considered adequate for diagnosis can be reached by using lower tube voltage settings, especially in CTA. Since tube voltage is not linear to dose, in clinical practice it will not simply suffice to change tube voltage settings; rather, a simultaneous adjustment of tube current is required. It is therefore difficult to manually adjust parameters, and tube voltage adjustment has rarely been used routinely. Approaches to select tube voltage and adapt tube current automatically, using information on the patient's attenuation from the localizer scan, and accounting for the planned examination type (e.g., non-enhanced scan, contrast-enhanced parenchymal scan, and CTA) and system limitations (e.g., maximum tube current), are needed to translate this technology into everyday use. Depending on the examination type, dose reduction between 10% and 30% is possible [54,55].

1.5.4 ECG-Gated Dose Modulation for Cardiac Spiral CT

In spiral acquisition mode, data are acquired continuously over multiple heart phases while the patient's table moves at low pitch values. Although it thus provides the ability to retrospectively select the phase of the cardiac cycle during which images are reconstructed, and to maximize image quality, the penalty is increased radiation exposure. Dose reduction is facilitated through ECG-pulsing techniques, where tube current is modulated during the complete spiral CT scan: the tube current is maintained at 100% of the desired level only during a predefined phase of interest of the heart cycle. During the rest of the time the current is substantially reduced. This method is based on the continuous monitoring of the ECG and an algorithm that predicts when the desired ECG phase will start (Figure 1.6).

1.5.5 ECG-Triggered CT

ECG-triggered sequential CT, also known as step-and-shoot mode, is the recommended acquisition mode [56]. It is a very dose-efficient way of ECG-synchronized scanning because only the very minimum of scan data needed for image reconstruction is acquired during the previously selected heart phase (Figure 1.5). The patient's ECG signal is monitored during examination, and axial scans are started with a predefined temporal offset relative to the R waves. Although advanced algorithms can detect extrasystoles and skip them for data acquisition (Figure 1.11), the method reaches its limitations in patients with severe arrhythmia, since ECG-triggered axial scanning depends on a reliable prediction of the patient's next cardiac cycle by using the mean length of the preceding cardiac cycles.

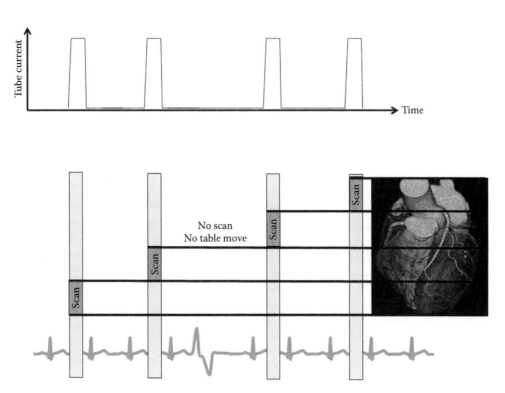

FIGURE 1.11
Axial scanning depends on a regular and predictable heart rate; advanced algorithms additionally allow flexible reaction to arrhythmia occurring during the scan.

A dedicated low-dose cardiac scanning mode is available on DSCT systems. Using fast scan speed (pitch values of up to 3.4 in combination with large detector coverage and fast gantry rotation), the heart can be scanned within 250–270 ms in ECG-triggered (high-pitch) spiral mode. No redundant data are acquired; thus, dose is reduced to a minimum [57]. Image quality depends on a low and regular heart rate to precisely predict the optimal scan start.

1.5.6 Dynamically Adjustable Collimation

Spiral CT reconstruction algorithms require scan data beyond the user-defined scan boundaries in the z-direction (through-plane direction). This is known as overranging. Over-ranging depends on the detector width and pitch value; with increasing number of slices, broader detectors, and higher pitch, overranging can contribute considerably to a patient's exposure. To reduce radiation exposure from overranging, dynamically adjustable prepatient collimators that allow independent control of both tube collimator blades have been introduced. The collimator blades open and close asymmetrically at the beginning and at the end of each spiral scan. Estimated reductions in effective dose were 16% for the head, 10% for the chest and liver, 6% for the abdomen and pelvis, and 4% and 55% for coronary CTA at pitch values of 0.2 and 3.4 [58,59].

1.6 Contrast Delivery and Safety

CT examinations can be divided into nonenhanced and contrast-enhanced studies. Contrast-enhanced studies may be angiography type (CTA-type) or parenchyma type. Whereas for CTA-type studies maximum contrast is warranted in the vessels of interest, parenchyma-type studies aim to maximize contrast between specific organs and lesions. The type of study significantly influences both contrast material application and scanning strategy.

1.6.1 Contrast Material

Most modern CT contrast agents for intravenous use are nonionic derivates of a tri-iodinated benzene ring. They are monomers that dissolve but do not dissociate in water (low-osmolar contrast media [LOCM]) or dimers that consist of two benzene rings (iso-osmolar contrast media [IOCM]). LOCM with an iodine concentration of 300 mg I/mL have typical osmolality values of 521–672 mosmol/kg H_2O at 37°C, whereas IOCM with an iodine concentration of 320 mg I/mL have an osmolality value of 290 mosmol/kg H_2O at 37°C. The viscosity values are 4.5–6.3 mPas at 37°C for LOCM and 11.8 mPas at 37°C for IOCM (ACR Manual on Contrast Media, version 7, 2010).

Contrast media (CM) are well tolerated with a low rate of adverse events (0.2%–0.7%) and serious events occurring in 0.01%–0.02% cases. The actual incidence is difficult to determine because similar symptoms may be caused by concomitant medication, anxiety, or other factors on the one hand and underreporting may occur on the other hand. Side effects are usually classified as mild (nausea, mild vomiting, urticaria, itching), moderate (severe vomiting, marked urticaria, bronchospasm, facial/laryngeal edema, vasovagal attack), and severe (hypotensive shock, cardiac arrest, respiratory arrest, convulsion). Moderate and severe reactions require immediate medical treatment and transfer to the emergency department or intensive care unit. First-line emergency drugs and instruments that should be in the examination suite are oxygen, adrenaline (1:1000), H1-receptor antagonist, atropine, β2-agonist inhaler, i.v. fluids (saline 0.9% or Ringers solution), diazepam, sphygmomanometer, and a bag valve mask (ESUR Guidelines on Contrast Media, version 7.0, 2008). A structured report for adverse event documentation is highly recommended.

For patients at increased risk of CM reaction, alternative imaging modalities without the need of iodinated CM should be considered. A different iodinated CM should be used in patients with previous reactions. Although clinical evidence of the effectiveness of premedication is limited, there is consensus that steroids and H1-antihistamine are the most relevant agents. The administration of steroids less than 4–6 hours before contrast injection seems to be ineffective. Oral administration of steroids is preferable in all patients except those with enteral malabsorption. In our institution, 30 mg prednisolone or 32 mg methylprednisolone is given p.o. 12 hours and 2 hours, and H1- and H2-antihistamine is given i.v. before CM injection in elective patients.

The other issue with CM is contrast-induced nephopathy (CIN). Different definitions of CIN exist; the most common definition is increase of serum creatinine > 25% or 0.5 mg/dL (44 mmol/L) within 3 days after CM injection without other reasons. Patients with estimated glomerular filtration rate (eGFR) less than 60 mL/min/1.73 m^2 (i.a. application) and eGFR less than 45 mL/min/1.73 m^2 (i.v. application), particularly if secondary to diabetic nephropathy, dehydration, congestive heart failure (NYHA 3–4) and low left ventricular ejection fraction, gout, age > 70 years, and concurrent administration of nephrotoxic medication (i.e., NSAR), are at higher risk of CIN. eGFR in men ($eGFR_{(m)}$) is estimated according to the Cockroft formula (140-age [years] × body weight [kg])/(72 × serum kreatinine [mg/dL]). For eGFR in females ($eGFR_{(f)}$), a conversion factor ($eGFR_{(f)}$ = $eGFR_{(m)}$ × 0.85) is introduced to compensate for different muscle mass. Patients at risk should be hydrated (p.o. or i.v.) at least 4–6 hours before and 24 hours after the examination (100 mL NaCl 0.9%/h), LOCM or IOCM should be used, and nephrotoxic concomitant medication should be stopped 24 hours before the examination.

High CM volume, repeated CM application, loop diuretics, and mannitol should be avoided.

If contrast-enhanced CT is necessary, because the critical questions cannot be answered with alternative imaging without the need of iodinated CM injection, we propose the following regime:

Elective examinations, in-house patients:

100 mL/h NaCl 0.9% 6–12 hours prior until 12 hours after the examination

Elective examinations, outpatients:

1000 mL fluids p.o. 12 hours prior and 12 hours after the examination and 300 mL/h NaCl 0.9% (i.v.) 2 hours prior to 4 hours after the examination

Emergency:

100 mL/h NaCl 0.9% as soon as possible prior until 6–12 hours after the examination

Serum creatinine levels should be monitored after CM application to monitor any change in renal function.

According to the updated European Society of Urogenital Radiology CM guidelines, the biguanide metformin can be continued in patients with chronic kidney disease (CKD) stages 1 and 2 (eGFR ≥ 60 mL/min/1.73 m^2) and also in patients with CKD 3 and eGFR greater than or equal to 45 mL/min/1.73 m^2 and i.v. CM injection, all other should stop metformin 48 hours before and restart metformin 48 hours after CM if renal function has not deteriorated. In the emergency situation, metformin should be stopped and restarted 48 hours after CM if serum creatinine/eGFR is unchanged from the preimaging level [60].

1.6.2 Contrast Material Injection in CTA

Short scan times require a short and compact CM bolus. To deliver an appropriate amount of iodine injection, rates of 4–6 mL/s are preferable. The utilization of the contrast bolus can be increased if it is followed by a saline bolus. Flushing of the veins also reduces streak artifacts due to beam hardening, especially at the thoracic inlet. With modern MDCT systems scan time is in the order of seconds, depending on the scan range and scanning technique, ranging from about 250–270 ms for high-pitch cardiac CTA [29] to approximately 10–20 seconds for thoracoabdominal CTA. Therefore, the scan time can be much shorter than the contrast injection time. The most important variable is the iodine delivery rate: the higher the iodine delivery rate, the higher the enhancement. If the injection rate is kept constant, higher concentrated CM (i.e., 350–400 mgI/mL) result in higher vascular enhancement and an earlier enhancement peak [61]. If the injection rate of less concentrated CM (i.e., 300 mgI/mL) is increased to keep the iodine delivery rate constant, the enhancement will be similar [62]. With multiphasic injection protocols it is possible to tailor vascular enhancement pattern to the specific needs [63,64], especially when using older CT systems with longer acquisition times; but with modern scanners this is necessary only in limited indications, for example, CTA of the lower extremities.

1.6.3 Saline Bolus

A significant amount of CM usually is trapped within the venous system. This CM is not only lost for imaging but may also be the source of streak artifacts. "Pushing" the CM bolus with 0.9% NaCl reduces CM bolus dissipation and reduces trapping of highly concentrated CM in the subclavian vein. In coronary CTA some radiologists prefer to clear the right ventricle (RV) to facilitate evaluation of the right coronary artery, whereas others prefer to have mild enhancement to improve morphologic and functional analysis of the RV (Figure 1.12). Up-to-date power injectors, which are a prerequisite for optimal CTA, have two pistons or reservoirs to supply CM and saline; many of them also have the "split-bolus" feature to mix CM and saline (e.g., 20%–30% CM, 70%–80% saline).

1.6.4 Bolus Tracking

Individual contrast timing (bolus tracking or test bolus injection) is mandatory to achieve optimal image quality. To individualize contrast timing, automatic bolus tracking techniques are provided by all vendors. This technique is fast, easy to use, and requires only a single contrast injection. The operator places a region of interest (ROI) within the target vessel and defines a threshold value at which the examination should start. An additional delay between the trigger time and the data acquisition may be necessary for table movement, switching of the scan mode, and patient instruction. The

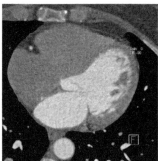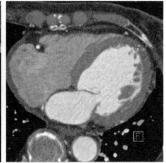

FIGURE 1.12
Saline bolus following contrast media (CM) bolus to "clear" the veins and right ventricle (left); split bolus (20% CM, 80% saline) to differentiate myocardium and blood pool of the right atrium and ventricle.

disadvantages of this technique are that a large target vessel for monitoring contrast arrival is required, calcified plaque can interfere with bolus detection, and there is an additional delay for table movement and patient instructions.

1.6.5 Test Bolus

Test bolus injection is the alternative to bolus tracking to assess individual circulation time. Again an ROI is positioned in the vessel of interest and a small amount of CM (10–20 mL) followed by a saline bolus is injected. Repetitive low-dose scans without table movement are performed to measure the bolus arrival and peak enhancement. Like with bolus tracking, an empirically determined start delay (i.e., 10–15 seconds for aortic CTA in case of peripheral i.v. line and 5 seconds in case of central i.v. line in a patient with normal cardiac output) can be used for the start of the monitoring scans to reduce radiation exposure. The major advantage of the test bolus technique is that it provides information about the enhancement of both arterial and venous systems. The enhancement peak of the full CM bolus will be later than that of the test bolus [65], but the shape of the test bolus curve, or time-attenuation curve (TAC), can be used to predict the TAC of the full bolus accurately. Furthermore, in organs where venous enhancement may be critical for diagnosis (i.e., carotid artery or renal artery) venous TAC can be determined by placing a second ROI in the vein (Figure 1.13).

Table movement and patient instructions can be performed prior to the optimal image acquisition window, which provides adequate time for the patient to respond. The necessity of an additional injection of CM (10%–20% increase of total amount) is unfavorable.

1.6.6 Parenchymal Imaging

CM delivery and timing is less critical in parenchymal imaging than that in CTA. Flow rates greater than 2.5–3 mL/s do not have a significant effect on organ enhancement [61], and within a wide range of cardiac output a delay of 70 seconds results in sufficient portal venous CM distribution within the liver. Bolus tracking or test bolus techniques can also be used for parenchymal imaging to optimize contrast enhancement, but this is rarely done because of additional radiation exposure and time demand. Most institutions use fixed delays.

1.7 Data Visualization

All modern MDCT systems can be operated in thin-slice collimation mode producing isotropic image data. Often, thin-slice data are reconstructed for visualization

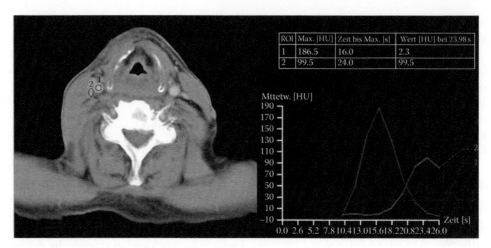

FIGURE 1.13
Test bolus measurement to determine contrast arrival time in common carotid artery and internal jugular vein for optimizing scan delay.

on 3D server–client systems and thick slices for standard image interpretation and image distribution throughout the hospitals. To optimize longitudinal (or z-axis) resolution, overlapping image reconstruction should be performed. The reconstruction increment (RI) can be arbitrarily chosen, independent of detector collimation, and 75% of slice width may be a good compromise. The RI denotes the spatial (or temporal) relation of two adjacent images. In-plane spatial resolution is influenced by the reconstruction algorithm or convolution kernel; soft kernels reduce image noise, allow for smooth surfaces with rendering techniques, and improve the perception of low-contrast objects. Sharper kernels improve edge definition, reduce blooming effects, and improve the perception of high-contrast objects at the expense of higher image noise. Image reconstruction is usually performed with a 512^2 matrix, the image matrix, and the reconstructed field of view (FOV) determines the pixel size. The third dimension is determined by the RI. Image matrix, FOV, and RI therefore define the voxel size, which must not be confounded with spatial resolution. The spatial resolution is mainly determined by the CT system geometry, detector aperture, and convolution kernel. Typical spatial resolution is 8–12 lp/cm, which corresponds to an object size of 0.4–0.6 mm [12] with soft tissue kernels; dedicated filter grids and sharp kernels can increase the spatial resolution to 20 lp/cm, which corresponds to an object size of 0.25 mm [66].

1.7.1 Image Post-Processing Techniques

Basic 3D tools like interactive multiplanar reformats, (thin) MIPs, and VRTs are widely available on the scanner console and reading stations. Except MPR, all other methods suppress data to a certain level to enhance special image details.

1.7.1.1 MPR

MPR creates views in arbitrary planes without loss of information. Individually adapted image planes are frequently used in cardiovascular and body imaging, as well as in the planning of interventional procedures. No image manipulation is required, but only 2D views are generated. To decrease image noise especially in low-dose CT, the slice thickness of MPR should be increased. MPR is the method of choice for precise measurements and may be combined with another visualization technique to display 3D anatomy.

A variant of MPR is CPR. CPR provides a 2D image that is created by sampling CT volume data along a predefined track. This technique is employed to display tortuous structures, for example, the coronary arteries (Figure 1.14); manual definition of such curved planes is time consuming and error prone, but algorithms that automatically track vessels are becoming widely available and increasingly accurate.

1.7.1.2 MIP

MIP images are created by displaying only the highest attenuation value from the data along a track through a data volume. Full-volume MIP is only rarely used, because soft tissues are not well represented. Thin-slab MIP images, where the slab thickness of data displayed with the MIP algorithm can be individually adapted, are more frequently used, especially in chest imaging for lung nodule detection. MIP is not suitable for the evaluation of stenosis in cases of dense calcification or stents, but a thin-slab MIP can provide an excellent road map of the vessel course for further evaluation with MPR. MIP is also not ideal to look for intraluminal thrombus or emboli, because the low-attenuating clot may be masked by surrounding contrast material (Figure 1.15).

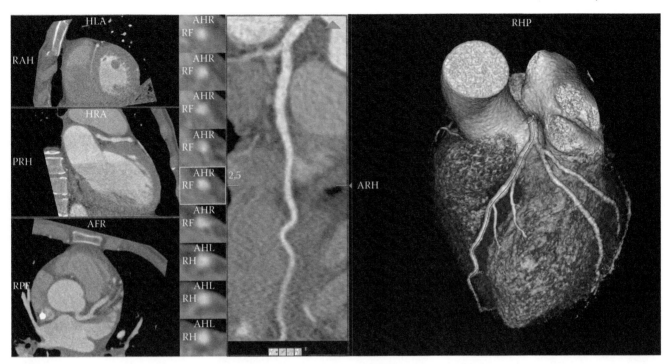

FIGURE 1.14
Visualization techniques: multiplanar reformats (MPR) (left) demonstrates only some parts of tortuous vessels. CPR (middle) displays a complete vessel within one image, and cross-sectional images perpendicular to vessel orientation (left to CPR) can be displayed to measure vessel lumen and wall thickness. The centerline of CPR is marked on a volume-rendered image (right).

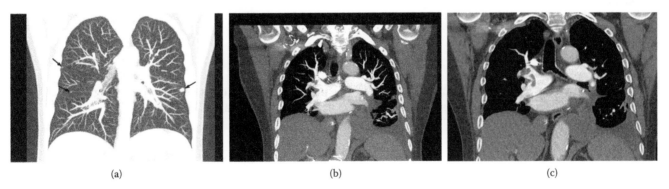

(a) (b) (c)

FIGURE 1.15
Thin maximum intensity projection (MIP): (a) lung nodule detection is enhanced with thin MIP (slab thickness of 10 mm). (b) Patient with pulmonary embolism. Emboli are partly hidden on thin-slab MIP, compared to (c) MPR.

1.7.1.3 Surface Rendering and Volume Rendering

SSD, or surface rendering, is an algorithm that provides a good 3D impression of the surface of an object. In a first step the surface of an object is separated from other structures, usually by thresholding. In a second step, a shading procedure is performed to create light intensity in a given 3D model, simulating surface reflections and shadowing from an artificial light source to enhance depth perception. VRT has supplanted SSD in basically all indications.

VRT is a visualization technique that creates a 3D impression and provides densitometric information. Visualization of CT data is based on transfer functions (TFs) that map measured intensities to colors and opacities [67]. Separation of different tissue types can be performed by applying multiple trapezoids, which can be color encoded, but color is assigned arbitrarily and does not correlate with the linear progression of gray-scale values on conventional CT images. Decreasing the upslope of the trapezoid is comparable to increasing

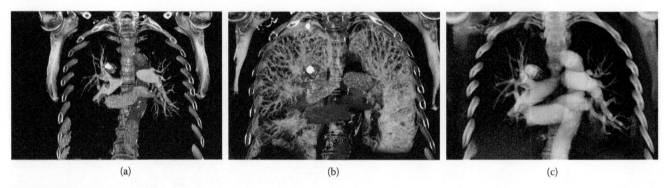

(a)   (b)   (c)

FIGURE 1.16
Volume rendering: the same patient as in Figure 1.15 is shown. Anatomical structures can be highlighted or suppressed; the depiction of emboli is dependent on parameter settings (a–c: different opacity and trapezoid settings).

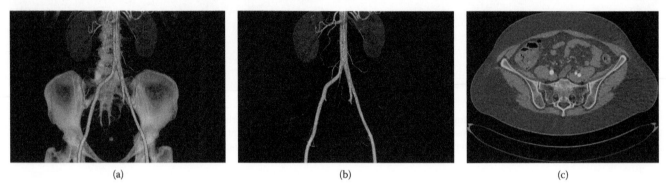

(a)   (b)   (c)

FIGURE 1.17
Bone segmentation to highlight abdominopelvic arteries: (a) volume rendering (VR), (b) VR without bones, and (c) segmented bone and patient table (green).

the window width on grayscale images. The definition of the trapezoid strongly affects the final image (Figure 1.16).

1.7.1.4 Segmentation

Segmentation can be performed manually or (semi) automatically. Segmentation algorithms are often based on the principle of region growing. Placing one or more seed points initiates the segmentation of the target structure. From these seed points, more and more neighboring voxels that fulfill predefined criteria are included in the segmentation [68]; the segmentation can be optimized using a priori knowledge. To refine the boundary of the segmented structures, morphologic dilation operations may be applied. A particular problem of threshold-based segmentation algorithms are areas with close contact of two tissue types with comparable attenuation, such as bone and contrast-enhanced vessels (Figure 1.17). Segmentation

techniques are also used for planning liver surgery and interventional procedures [69–72].

1.7.1.5 Bone Subtraction CTA

For bone subtraction CTA (BSCTA), a nonenhanced CT (NECT) dataset and a contrast-enhanced spiral CT dataset are required. Pixels in the NECT dataset with a CT value above a certain threshold are defined as bone and used to iteratively register the NECT to the CTA dataset. After registration, an initial bone mask is defined in the NECT volume by thresholding. The bone mask is tentatively expanded in three dimensions by morphological dilation, and the bone voxels are set to a HU value of −1024. BSCTA is a robust method of bone elimination, not requiring user interaction (Figure 1.18). Although patient movement between the two scans can be compensated for in cranial CTA, movements can result in incomplete bone or calcification removal in other regions unless additional registration steps or

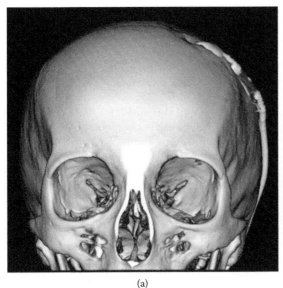
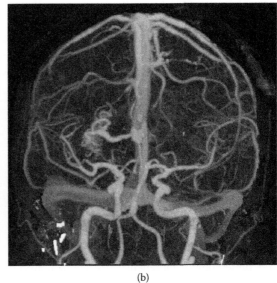

(a)   (b)

FIGURE 1.18
Bone subtraction CT angiography (CTA) in a patient with arteriovenous malformation: (a) A nonenhanced (low-dose) CT can be used to create a three-dimensional bone model, which can be registered with a CTA to automatically suppress bone while maintaining soft tissues and vessels (b) (maximum intensity projection).

preprocessing is performed [73–78]. BSCTA can also be applied successfully in peripheral CTA [79].

An alternative to BSCTA is DECT, where simultaneous data acquisition at two energy levels is performed (see earlier) and calcium can be easily differentiated from iodine by the different absorptions at 140 kV and 80/100 kV [40].

References

1. Crawford CR, King KF. Computed tomography scanning with simultaneous patient translation. *Med Phys* 1990;17:967–982.
2. Kalender WA, Seissler W, Klotz E, Vock P. Spiral volumetric CT with single-breath-hold technique, continuous transport, and continuous scanner rotation. *Radiology* 1990;176:181–183.
3. Mori I. Computerized tomographic apparatus utilizing a radiation source. U.S. Patent 4630202, 1986.
4. Nishimura H, Miyazaki O. CT system for specially scanning subject on a moveable bed synchronized to x-ray tube revolution. U.S. Patent 4789929, 1988.
5. Kalender WA. Thin-section three-dimensional spiral CT: Is isotropic imaging possible? *Radiology* 1995;197: 578–580.
6. Hu H, He HD, Foley WD, Fox SH. Four multidetector-row helical CT: Image quality and volume coverage speed. *Radiology* 2000;215:55–62.
7. Klingenbeck-Regn K, Schaller S, Flohr T, Ohnesorge B, Kopp AF, Baum U. Subsecond multi-slice computed tomography: Basics and applications. *Eur J Radiol* 1999;31:110–124.
8. Kachelriess M, Ulzheimer S, Kalender WA. ECG-correlated image reconstruction from subsecond multi-slice spiral CT scans of the heart. *Med Phys* 2000;27: 1881–1902.
9. Ohnesorge B, Flohr T, Becker C et al. Cardiac imaging by means of electrocardiographically gated multisection spiral CT: Initial experience. *Radiology* 2000;217:564–571.
10. Nieman K, Oudkerk M, Rensing BJ et al. Coronary angiography with multi-slice computed tomography. *Lancet* 2001;357:599–603.
11. Lell MM, Anders K, Uder M et al. New techniques in CT angiography. *Radiographics* 2006;26 Suppl 1:S45–S62.
12. Flohr TG, McCollough CH, Bruder H et al. First performance evaluation of a dual-source CT (DSCT) system. *Eur Radiol* 2006;16:256–268.
13. Flohr TG, Stierstorfer K, Ulzheimer S, Bruder H, Primak AN, McCollough CH. Image reconstruction and image quality evaluation for a 64-slice CT scanner with z-flying focal spot. *Med Phys* 2005;32:2536–2547.
14. Flohr TG, Schaller S, Stierstorfer K, Bruder H, Ohnesorge BM, Schoepf UJ. Multi-detector row CT systems and image-reconstruction techniques. *Radiology* 2005;235: 756–773.
15. Schardt P, Deuringer J, Freudenberger J et al. New x-ray tube performance in computed tomography by introducing the rotating envelope tube technology. *Med Phys* 2004;31:2699–2706.
16. Hsieh J. Investigation of the slice sensitivity profile for step-and-shoot mode multi-slice computed tomography. *Med Phys* 2001;28:491–500.
17. Hsieh J. Analytical models for multi-slice helical CT performance parameters. *Med Phys* 2003;30:169–178.
18. Hu H. Multi-slice helical CT: Scan and reconstruction. *Med Phys* 1999;26:5–18.
19. Taguchi K, Aradate H. Algorithm for image reconstruction in multi-slice helical CT. *Med Phys* 1998;25:550–561.

20. Feldkamp LA, Davis LC, Kress JW. Practical cone-beam algorithm. *J Opt Soc Am A* 1984;1:612–619.

21. Flohr T, Stierstorfer K, Bruder H, Simon J, Polacin A, Schaller S. Image reconstruction and image quality evaluation for a 16-slice CT scanner. *Med Phys* 2003; 30:832–845.

22. Mark DB, Berman DS, Budoff MJ et al. ACCF/ACR/AHA/NASCI/SAIP/SCAI/SCCT 2010 expert consensus document on coronary computed tomographic angiography: A report of the American College of Cardiology Foundation Task Force on Expert Consensus Documents. *Circulation* 2010;121:2509–2543.

23. Dewey M, Zimmermann E, Deissenrieder F et al. Noninvasive coronary angiography by 320-row computed tomography with lower radiation exposure and maintained diagnostic accuracy: Comparison of results with cardiac catheterization in a head-to-head pilot investigation. *Circulation* 2009;120:867–875.

24. Diekmann S, Siebert E, Juran R et al. Dose exposure of patients undergoing comprehensive stroke imaging by multidetector-row CT: Comparison of 320-detector row and 64-detector row CT scanners. *AJNR Am J Neuroradiol* 2010;31:1003–1009.

25. George RT, Arbab-Zadeh A, Cerci RJ et al. Diagnostic performance of combined noninvasive coronary angiography and myocardial perfusion imaging using 320-MDCT: The CT angiography and perfusion methods of the CORE320 multicenter multinational diagnostic study. *AJR Am J Roentgenol* 2011;197:829–837.

26. Klingebiel R, Siebert E, Diekmann S et al. 4-D imaging in cerebrovascular disorders by using 320-slice CT: Feasibility and preliminary clinical experience. *Acad Radiol* 2009;16:123–129.

27. Achenbach S, Marwan M, Schepis T et al. High-pitch spiral acquisition: A new scan mode for coronary CT angiography. *J Cardiovasc Comput Tomogr* 2009;3:117–121.

28. Hausleiter J, Bischoff B, Hein F et al. Feasibility of dual-source cardiac CT angiography with high-pitch scan protocols. *J Cardiovasc Comput Tomogr* 2009;3:236–242.

29. Lell M, Marwan M, Schepis T et al. Prospectively ECG-triggered high-pitch spiral acquisition for coronary CT angiography using dual source CT: Technique and initial experience. *Eur Radiol* 2009;19:2576–2583.

30. Johnson TR, Krauss B, Sedlmair M et al. Material differentiation by dual energy CT: Initial experience. *Eur Radiol* 2007;17:1510–1517.

31. Primak AN, Fletcher JG, Vrtiska TJ et al. Noninvasive differentiation of uric acid versus non-uric acid kidney stones using dual-energy CT. *Acad Radiol* 2007;14:1441–1447.

32. Scheffel H, Stolzmann P, Frauenfelder T et al. Dual-energy contrast-enhanced computed tomography for the detection of urinary stone disease. *Invest Radiol* 2007;42:823–829.

33. Ertel D, Lell MM, Harig F, Flohr T, Schmidt B, Kalender WA. Cardiac spiral dual-source CT with high pitch: A feasibility study. *Eur Radiol* 2009;19:2357–2362.

34. Lell MM, May M, Deak P et al. High-pitch spiral computed tomography: Effect on image quality and radiation dose in pediatric chest computed tomography. *Invest Radiol* 2011;46:116–123.

35. Alvarez RE, Macovski A. Energy-selective reconstructions in X-ray computerized tomography. *Phys Med Biol* 1976;21:733–744.

36. Avrin DE, Macovski A, Zatz LE. Clinical application of Compton and photo-electric reconstruction in computed tomography: Preliminary results. *Invest Radiol* 1978;13:217–222.

37. Kalender WA, Perman WH, Vetter JR, Klotz E. Evaluation of a prototype dual-energy computed tomographic apparatus. I. Phantom studies. *Med Phys* 1986;13:334–339.

38. Glazebrook KN, Guimaraes LS, Murthy NS et al. Identification of intraarticular and periarticular uric acid crystals with dual-energy CT: Initial evaluation. *Radiology* 2011;261:516–524.

39. Graser A, Becker CR, Staehler M et al. Single-phase dual-energy CT allows for characterization of renal masses as benign or malignant. *Invest Radiol* 2010;45:399–405.

40. Lell MM, Kramer M, Klotz E, Villablanca P, Ruehm SG. Carotid computed tomography angiography with automated bone suppression: A comparative study between dual energy and bone subtraction techniques. *Invest Radiol* 2009;44:322–328.

41. Lu GM, Wu SY, Yeh BM, Zhang LJ. Dual-energy computed tomography in pulmonary embolism. *Br J Radiol* 2010; 83:707–718.

42. Thibault JB, Sauer KD, Bouman CA, Hsieh J. A three-dimensional statistical approach to improved image quality for multislice helical CT. *Med Phys* 2007;34:4526–4544.

43. Donnelly LF, Emery KH, Brody AS et al. Minimizing radiation dose for pediatric body applications of single-detector helical CT: Strategies at a large Children's Hospital. *AJR Am J Roentgenol* 2001;176:303–306.

44. Wildberger JE, Mahnken AH, Schmitz-Rode T et al. Individually adapted examination protocols for reduction of radiation exposure in chest CT. *Invest Radiol* 2001;36:604–611.

45. May MS, Wust W, Brand M et al. Dose reduction in abdominal computed tomography: Intraindividual comparison of image quality of full-dose standard and half-dose iterative reconstructions with dual-source computed tomography. *Invest Radiol* 2011; 46:465–470.

46. Katsura M, Matsuda I, Akahane M et al. Model-based iterative reconstruction technique for radiation dose reduction in chest CT: Comparison with the adaptive statistical iterative reconstruction technique. *Eur Radiol* 2012;22:1613–1623.

47. Leipsic J, Nguyen G, Brown J, Sin D, Mayo JR. A prospective evaluation of dose reduction and image quality in chest CT using adaptive statistical iterative reconstruction. *AJR Am J Roentgenol* 195:1095–1099.

48. Pontana F, Duhamel A, Pagniez J et al. Chest computed tomography using iterative reconstruction vs filtered back projection (Part 2): Image quality of low-dose CT examinations in 80 patients. *Eur Radiol* 21:636–643.

49. Prakash P, Kalra MK, Digumarthy SR et al. Radiation dose reduction with chest computed tomography using adaptive statistical iterative reconstruction technique: Initial experience. *J Comput Assist Tomogr* 2010;34:40–45.

50. Greess H, Lutze J, Nomayr A et al. Dose reduction in subsecond multislice spiral CT examination of children by online tube current modulation. *Eur Radiol* 2004;14:995–999.

51. Greess H, Wolf H, Suess C, Kalender WA, Bautz W, Baum U. [Automatic exposure control to reduce the dose in subsecond multislice spiral CT: Phantom measurements and clinical results]. *Rofo* 2004;176:862–869.

52. Mulkens TH, Bellinck P, Baeyaert M et al. Use of an automatic exposure control mechanism for dose optimization in multi-detector row CT examinations: Clinical evaluation. *Radiology* 2005;237:213–223.

53. Ketelsen D, Buchgeister M, Fenchel M et al. Automated computed tomography dose-saving algorithm to protect radiosensitive tissues: Estimation of radiation exposure and image quality considerations. *Invest Radiol* 2012;47:148–152.

54. Winklehner A, Goetti R, Baumueller S et al. Automated attenuation-based tube potential selection for thoracoabdominal computed tomography angiography: Improved dose effectiveness. *Invest Radiol* 2011;46:767–773.

55. Eller A, May MS, Scharf M et al. Attenuation-based automatic kilovolt selection in abdominal computed tomography: Effects on radiation exposure and image quality. *Invest Radiol* 2012;47:559–565.

56. Neefjes LA, Dharampal AS, Rossi A et al. Image quality and radiation exposure using different low-dose scan protocols in dual-source CT coronary angiography: Randomized study. *Radiology* 261:779–786.

57. Achenbach S, Marwan M, Ropers D et al. Coronary computed tomography angiography with a consistent dose below 1 mSv using prospectively electrocardiogram-triggered high-pitch spiral acquisition. *Eur Heart J* 2010;31:340–346.

58. Christner JA, Zavaletta VA, Eusemann CD, Walz-Flannigan AI, McCollough CH. Dose reduction in helical CT: Dynamically adjustable z-axis X-ray beam collimation. *AJR Am J Roentgenol* 2010;194:W49–W55.

59. Deak PD, Langner O, Lell M, Kalender WA. Effects of adaptive section collimation on patient radiation dose in multisection spiral CT. *Radiology* 2009;252:140–147.

60. Stacul F, van der Molen AJ, Reimer P et al. Contrast induced nephropathy: Updated ESUR Contrast Media Safety Committee guidelines. *Eur Radiol* 2011;21: 2527–2541.

61. Bae KT. Intravenous contrast medium administration and scan timing at CT: Considerations and approaches. *Radiology* 2010;256:32–61.

62. Muhlenbruch G, Behrendt FF, Eddahabi MA et al. Which Iodine concentration in chest CT?—A prospective study in 300 patients. *Eur Radiol* 2008;18:2826–2832.

63. Fleischmann D, Rubin GD, Bankier AA, Hittmair K. Improved uniformity of aortic enhancement with customized contrast medium injection protocols at CT angiography. *Radiology* 2000;214:363–371.

64. Fleischmann D. Use of high concentration contrast media: principles and rationale-vascular district. *Eur J Radiol* 2003;45 Suppl 1:S88–S93.

65. Fleischmann D. Present and future trends in multiple detector-row CT applications: CT angiography. *Eur Radiol* 2002;12 Suppl 2:S11–S15.

66. Flohr TG, Stierstorfer K, Suss C, Schmidt B, Primak AN, McCollough CH. Novel ultrahigh resolution data acquisition and image reconstruction for multi-detector row CT. *Med Phys* 2007;34:1712–1723.

67. Calhoun PS, Kuszyk BS, Heath DG, Carley JC, Fishman EK. Three-dimensional volume rendering of spiral CT data: Theory and method. *Radiographics* 1999;19:745–764.

68. Udupa JK. Three-dimensional visualization and analysis methodologies: A current perspective. *Radiographics* 1999;19:783–806.

69. Hame Y, Pollari M. Semi-automatic liver tumor segmentation with hidden Markov measure field model and non-parametric distribution estimation. *Med Image Anal* 2012;16:140–149.

70. Schumann C, Bieberstein J, Braunewell S, Niethammer M, Peitgen HO. Visualization support for the planning of hepatic needle placement. *Int J Comput Assist Radiol Surg* 2012;7:191–197.

71. Linguraru MG, Pura JA, Chowdhury AS, Summers RM. Multi-organ segmentation from multi-phase abdominal CT via 4D graphs using enhancement, shape and location optimization. *Med Image Comput Comput Assist Interv* 2010;13:89–96.

72. Heimann T, van Ginneken B, Styner MA et al. Comparison and evaluation of methods for liver segmentation from CT datasets. *IEEE Trans Med Imaging* 2009;28:1251–1265.

73. Lell MM, Ruehm SG, Kramer M et al. Cranial computed tomography angiography with automated bone subtraction: A feasibility study. *Invest Radiol* 2009;44:38–43.

74. Loeckx D, Coudyzer W, Maes F et al. Nonrigid registration for subtraction CT angiography applied to the carotids and cranial arteries. *Acad Radiol* 2007;14:1562–1576.

75. Lell MM, Ditt H, Panknin C et al. Bone-subtraction CT angiography: Evaluation of two different fully automated image-registration procedures for interscan motion compensation. *AJNR Am J Neuroradiol* 2007;28:1362–1368.

76. Tomandl BF, Hammen T, Klotz E, Ditt H, Stemper B, Lell M. Bone-subtraction CT angiography for the evaluation of intracranial aneurysms. *AJNR Am J Neuroradiol* 2006;27:55–59.

77. Lell M, Anders K, Klotz E, Ditt H, Bautz W, Tomandl BF. Clinical evaluation of bone-subtraction CT angiography (BSCTA) in head and neck imaging. *Eur Radiol* 2006;16:889–897.

78. van Straten M, Venema HW, Streekstra GJ, Majoie CB, den Heeten GJ, Grimbergen CA. Removal of bone in CT angiography of the cervical arteries by piecewise matched mask bone elimination. *Med Phys* 2004;31:2924–2933.

79. Lee IJ, Chung JW, Hong H et al. Subtraction CT angiography of the lower extremities: Single volume subtraction versus multi-segmented volume subtraction. *Acad Radiol* 2011;18:902–909.

2

CT Perfusion: Principles, Implementations, and Clinical Applications

Aaron So, Errol E. Stewart, Christopher D. d'Esterre, Timothy Pok Chi Yeung, Glenn Bauman, Nikolaj K. G. Jensen, Eugene Wong, and Ting-Yim Lee

CONTENTS

2.1 Introduction

Shortly after the introduction of computed tomography (CT) in 1970s, a seminal paper by Leon Axel demonstrated the use of dynamic contrast-enhanced (DCE) CT to measure tissue blood flow (perfusion) [1]. This perfusion imaging capability has since transformed CT from an anatomic-oriented imaging modality into a functional one, allowing comprehensive assessment of structural and physiologic abnormalities in a single sitting. Initially, CT perfusion (CTP) was mainly confined to research rather than clinical studies due to the requirement of rapid image acquisition. With the advent of multirow detectors [2,3] and faster speed of gantry rotation [4] in clinical CT scanners, CTP has gained popularity over the past decade as a diagnostic tool for stroke [5–7], tumor [8–11], and more recently coronary artery disease (CAD) [12–15]. Having these diagnostic capabilities coupled with the operational advantages of low cost, accessibility, and high throughput of CT, it is expected that CTP will play a more and more important role on patient management.

All CTP methodologies require intravenous (IV) bolus administration of iodinated contrast medium and are dependent on the excellent linear relationship between x-ray attenuation and concentration of contrast material in tissue and blood. The first-pass bolus tracking perfusion analysis techniques are based on one of the three theories: indicator-dilution, Fick principle, and deconvolution. In this chapter, we aim to review the fundamental basis of each CTP method, followed by the technical considerations for implementations. Preclinical validations and clinical applications of deconvolution-based CTP methodology are also presented.

2.2 Basic Model and Terminology

For ease of discussion, let us first consider the schematic in Figure 2.1, which represents a unit mass of tissue. The inlet and outlet orifices represent an input artery (arteriole) and a draining vein (venule) of the tissue. "Blood flow" (*F*) through the tissue, or perfusion, is defined as the volume of blood that is moving through the vasculature of the tissue per unit time. It is expressed in units of $mL/min^{-1}/g^{-1}$. In CTP, perfusion is usually modeled as a plug of fluid (plug flow) through the vasculature, in which the flow velocity profile across the cross section of the vessels is constant. Additionally, "blood volume" (V) is defined as the volume of blood within the vasculature in the tissue that is flowing (nonstatic). It is expressed in mL/g^{-1}. In reality, there are numerous small

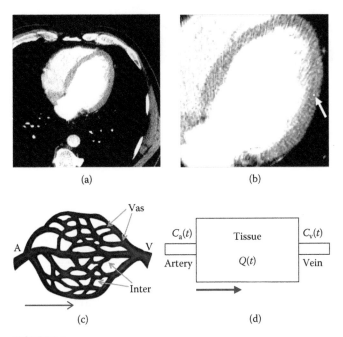

FIGURE 2.1

(a) Contrast-enhanced CT image of a patient's heart. (b) A voxel of interest in the myocardium. (c) Schematic of the vasculature of a tissue within the voxel shown in Figure 2.1b. The red arrow denotes the direction of blood flow through the capillaries from arteriole (A) to venule (V). (d) A simple model represents the vasculature in Figure 2.1c. The tissue region consists of the capillaries (intravascular space, vas) and the surrounding interstitium (interstitial space, inter). The relationship between the concentration of contrast medium in the input artery ($C_a(t)$) and draining vein ($C_v(t)$) and the mass of contrast in tissue ($Q(t)$) is governed by Fick principle. The exchange of contrast between the intravascular and interstitial spaces is described by the tracer kinetic models shown in Figures 2.5 and 2.6.

capillaries interconnecting with each other rather than a single capillary tube in the tissue (Figure 2.1c and d). Thus, upon arrival at the arterial inlet, contrast solutes can take different paths to reach the venous exit. As such, there exists a distribution of transit times, which can be described by a frequency or probability density function of transit time through a vascular bed, $h(t)$, as shown in Figure 2.2a. The integral of the probability density function, $H(t)$, describes the fraction of contrast solutes that has left the tissue at time t (Figure 2.2b). The total amount of contrast solutes that has left the tissue should increase with time and eventually reach the plateau at unity. This can be explained by the fact that all contrast solutes introduced into the tissue will eventually leave the tissue in due time, and the total amount of contrast leaving the tissue cannot exceed the amount that is introduced into the tissue. It follows that the residual function, $R(t)$, which describes the fraction of contrast solutes, remains in the tissue at time t, is equal to $1 - H(t)$ (Figure 2.2c), with the area under curve (AUC) of $R(t)$ equals the "mean transit time" (MTT)—the average time required for the contrast solutes to travel from the arterial inlet to the venous outlet of the tissue (Figure 2.2d) [16,17].

During a single capillary transit, contrast solutes can diffuse across the permeable endothelium (consists of a single cell layer) to the surrounding interstitial (extravascular) space. One exception is the healthy brain tissue, where the blood–brain barrier (BBB), consisting of tight junctions between endothelial cells, surrounding basement membrane, and astrocytic foot processes, restricts most of the diffusions taking place [18]. The transport of contrast solutes from the intravascular to interstitial space is driven entirely by passive diffusion (concentration gradient between the two spaces). The "extraction fraction," E, describes the fraction of contrast solutes diffused from the intravascular to interstitial space during

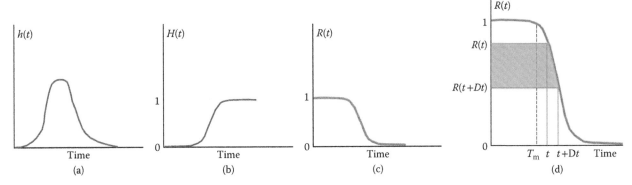

FIGURE 2.2

(a) The frequency function, $h(t)$, describes the distribution of transit time through a vasculature bed in tissue after a bolus injection of contrast. (b) Integral of the frequency function in Figure 2.2a, $H(t)$, describes the fraction of contrast that has left the system as a function of time. (c) The total amount of contrast remains in the tissue as a function of time is given by $1 - H(t)$, or $R(t)$. (d) Beyond the minimum transit time, T_m, the fraction of contrast that leaves the tissue between t and $t + \Delta t$ is equal to the difference of $R(t + \Delta t)$ and $R(t)$ (blue section). This fraction of contrast medium has a transit time of Δt. It follows that the total area under $R(t)$ is equivalent to the mean transit time (MTT).

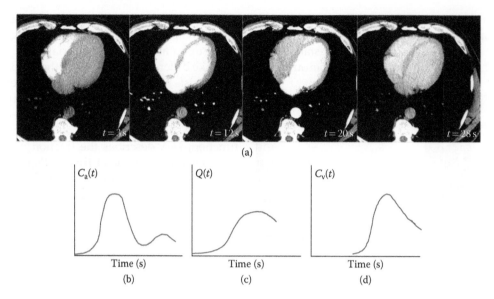

FIGURE 2.3
(a) DCE CT images of the same patient's heart in Figure 2.1 at different time points. Iodinated contrast medium circulated in the heart chambers and aorta during the time of imaging. The time postbolus injection of contrast of each image is shown in the bottom right corner. Schematics of typical arterial, tissue, and venous TDC measured from DCE CT images are shown in Figure 2.3b, c, and d, respectively.

a single passage from the arterial to venous ends of the capillaries [19]. E can be represented by the following equation:

$$E = 1 - e^{-\frac{PS}{F}} \qquad (2.1)$$

where PS is "permeability surface area product"—the product of permeability and the total surface area of capillary endothelium in a unit mass of tissue and hence is the total diffusional flux across all capillaries [19]. It is measured in units of $mL/min^{-1}/g^{-1}$.

After the introduction of a bolus of iodinated contrast material, repeated rapid CT scanning is acquired at the same location to allow determination of time-density curves (TDCs). Figure 2.3 illustrates the typical shape of arterial ($C_a(t)$), tissue ($Q(t)$), and venous ($C_v(t)$) TDCs acquired from DCE CT scanning. Several methods that are commonly used for analyzing these TDCs to derive perfusion values are reviewed in Sections 2.2.1 through 2.2.5.

2.2.1 Indicator-Dilution Method

Indictor-dilution method was originally proposed over a century ago to measure blood velocity (circulation time) and cardiac output [20]. It was then shown that this technique could also be used to measure tissue blood flow (perfusion) [16,21]. This technique is based on the fact that after administration into the circulation, the degree at which tracer molecules (e.g., CT contrast medium, radiolabeled particles, or dye) are mixed with blood (i.e., dilution) is dependent on

blood flow. The indicator-dilution method has since been modified to measure blood flow in tissue using dynamic CT scanning [1,22]. The basis of the method is briefly reviewed here. If a voxel of interest in a CT image is devoid of major blood vessels, the concentration of contrast medium in the tissue in this voxel at time t, $C_t(t)$, should be lower than that in the vascular space, $C_a(t)$, by the fraction f:

$$C_t(t) = f \cdot C_a(t) \qquad (2.2)$$

where f is defined as

$$f = \frac{V_b}{V_b + V_e + V_{cell}} \qquad (2.3)$$

with V_b, V_e, and V_{cell} being the distribution volumes of contrast medium in the vascular space, interstitial space, and cell(s), respectively. Equations 2.2 and 2.3 suggest that f is essentially the blood volume in tissue, which can be estimated by dividing the AUC of the tissue TDC to the AUC of the arterial TDC.

$$V = \frac{AUC_{tissue}}{AUC_{artery}} \qquad (2.4a)$$

$$AUC_{tissue} = \int_0^T C_t(t) \, dt \qquad (2.4b)$$

$$AUC_{artery} = \int_0^T C_a(t) \, dt \qquad (2.4c)$$

Once the blood volume in tissue is determined, perfusion can be calculated as the ratio of V to the MTT according to the central volume principle [16].

$$F = \frac{V}{\text{MTT}} \qquad (2.5)$$

MTT cannot be measured directly but can be estimated from either deconvolution [23] or the center of gravity [22] of the arterial and tissue TDCs:

$$\text{MTT} = C \cdot \left[<\text{tissue}> - <\text{artery}> \right] \qquad (2.6a)$$

$$= C \cdot \left[\frac{\int_0^T t \cdot C_t(t)\,dt}{\int_0^T C_t(t)\,dt} - \frac{\int_0^T t \cdot C_a(t)\,dt}{\int_0^T C_a(t)\,dt} \right] \qquad (2.6b)$$

where <tissue> and <artery> represent the centers of gravity of these two TDCs and the center of gravity of each curve is calculated as the first moment of the curve (which can be viewed as a quantitative measure of the shape of the curve) as in Equation 2.6b; C is a combined correction factor to account for the difference between large vessel (vein or artery) and small vessel (tissue) hematocrit, the difference between contrast arrival times at the measured artery (true input artery to the region of interest [ROI]) and tissue, and the variations in transit times through the ROI to the difference in the first moments of tissue and artery TDCs (<tissue> − <artery>) [22]. Although the indicator-dilution method is mathematically more simple than the deconvolution method, this technique has a few major limitations. First, the method relies heavily on the accuracy of blood volume estimate. For healthy brain tissue, contrast medium remains in the intravascular space throughout the capillary transit. However, in abnormal brain tissue where the BBB is no longer intact [24,25], and in other tissues such as the heart and liver [19], extravascular leakage of contrast may occur, which will lead to overestimation of blood volume and hence blood flow. Second, the correction factor, C, assumes a certain geometry/topology of the vasculature (or transit time distribution) that makes the method model dependent after all.

2.2.2 Maximal Slope Method

The relationship between tissue blood flow, the amount (mass) of contrast medium that remains in the tissue, and the concentration of contrast medium at the input artery and draining vein can be described using the Fick principle. If we denote $C_a(t)$ and $C_v(t)$ as the contrast concentration in the arterial inlet and venous outlet of the tissue at time t, respectively, and F is the tissue blood flow (perfusion) during the time of study, the influx and efflux rates of contrast are given by $F \cdot C_a(t)$ and $F \cdot C_v(t)$,

respectively. Under the assumption of conservation of mass, the following relationship holds:

$$\frac{dQ(t)}{dt} = F \cdot C_a(t) - F \cdot C_v(t) \qquad (2.7)$$

where $Q(t)$ is the mass of contrast in the tissue at time t. Equation 2.7 states that the rate of change of the mass of contrast in the tissue is equal to the difference in the influx and efflux rates of contrast. Integrating equation 2.7 yields

$$Q(t) = F \cdot \int_0^T [C_a(t) - C_v(t)] \cdot dt \qquad (2.8)$$

Equation 2.8 states that the accumulated mass of contrast in the tissue over the duration of acquisition, from 0 to T, is equal to the product of flow and the time integral of the difference in the arterial and venous concentration of contrast medium. One simplification that would make solving Equation 2.8 easier is to assume no venous outflow of contrast in tissue during the time of study ($C_v(t) = 0$). If the no venous outflow assumption is valid, Equation 2.8 is simplified to [26]

$$Q(t) = F \cdot \int_0^T C_a(t) \cdot dt \qquad (2.9)$$

By taking the differentiation on both sides of Equation 2.9 yields

$$\frac{dQ(t)}{dt} = F \cdot C_a(t) \qquad (2.10)$$

Equation 2.10 suggests the rate of contrast accumulation in tissue will be maximal when the arterial concentration of contrast reaches maximum.

$$\left. \frac{dQ(t)}{dt} \right|_{\max} = F \cdot C_a(t) \big|_{\max}$$

$$F = \left. \frac{\frac{dQ(t)}{dt}}{C_a(t)} \right|_{\max} \qquad (2.11)$$

It follows that F can be estimated by dividing the maximal slope of $Q(t)$ by the maximal arterial concentration (peak value of arterial TDC). This is known as the maximal slope method.

The advantage of the maximal slope method is its computational simplicity. Additionally, only the upslope of the TDCs used for perfusion analysis implies acquisition of the entire bolus curves is not necessary, which can reduce radiation exposure to the patients. However, the assumption of no venous outflow may not be valid in all disease states. To make the no venous outflow assumption more valid in practice, the bolus injection rate has to be very fast, usually >10 mL/s^{-1} [27,28], which is not always practical in clinical settings. As such, the assumption could be violated in real situations, which may lead to significant underestimation of the true perfusion value. An alternative solution to fast injection rate is to inject a less amount of contrast material but at a slower rate. However, this will lead to a poorer signal-to-noise ratio (SNR) of the TDC, which in turn will affect the accuracy of perfusion estimates.

2.2.3 Deconvolution Method

The deconvolution method takes a different approach and handles the contrast enhancement tissue/organ from perfusion as a time-invariant linear system problem. For reference, we will first briefly review the characteristics of such a system.

Figure 2.4 illustrates an output signal in response to an impulse signal presented to such a system. Both the input and the output signals are plotted as signal intensity versus time. An impulse signal is instantaneous and transient and can be represented by a Dirac delta function, which is defined as infinite at $t = 0$ but with an area of unity (for simplicity, we will say that impulse has a magnitude of unity) and zero elsewhere (i.e., $t > 0$) (Figure 2.4a). The output signal consists of a single step of finite width followed by an exponential tail (Figure 2.4b). The step

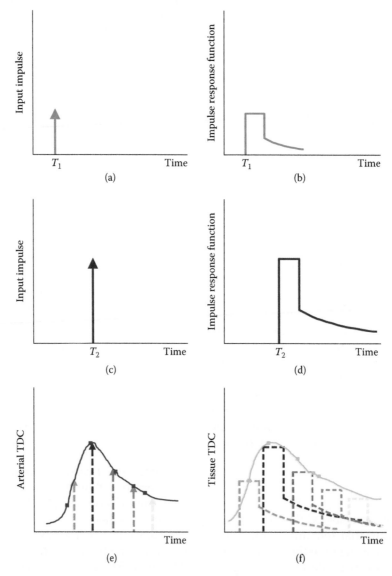

FIGURE 2.4

(a) An impulse signal to a time-invariant linear system and (b) the corresponding IRF. (c) A second impulse signal with twice the magnitude as the first impulse introduced to the system at a later time, and (d) the corresponding IRF to the second impulse. (e) An arterial TDC measured from DCE CT scanning can be interpreted as a superimposition of sequential impulses with different magnitudes at different times. (f) The corresponding tissue TDC can be viewed as a superimposition of the IRFs scaled by the magnitude and shifted in time to match those of the impulse signals.

has the height as the area underneath the impulse signal, which is unity, providing there is no signal lost in the linear system. Here, the width of the step corresponds to the minimum time required by the contrast to traverse the vasculature, whereas the tail describes the gradual decline of the signal over time from the washout of contrast from the tissue region (for intravascular contrast it would be washout from the vasculature). Now, consider a second impulse with twice the magnitude as the first impulse is introduced at a later time, the corresponding output signal would have a step that is twice as high and delayed with respect to the first output signal by the time interval between the two impulses (Figure 2.4c and d).

The output signal in response to a unit area impulse is also called the impulse response function (IRF), which provides useful information about the characteristic of the time-invariant linear system and allows one to infer how the system will respond to different stimuli. In CTP, the arterial TDC, $C_a(t)$, acquired with an arterial ROI in an artery from dynamic images obtained by continuous rapid CT scanning after contrast injection, can be viewed as a superimposition of sequential impulse signals with different magnitudes at different times (Figure 2.4e). Similarly, the corresponding tissue TDC, $Q(t)$, is a superimposition of the IRFs scaled by the magnitude of corresponding impulse signal and shift in time to match that of the impulse signal, both of these information are provided by the arterial TDC (Figure 2.4f). The superimposition of the same IRF using information from arterial TDC is equivalent to the mathematical operation of convolution between the IRF and $C_a(t)$. Thus, the concentration of contrast medium in tissue at a given time t is controlled by three factors: local blood flow (F), concentration of contrast material in the input artery ($C_a(t)$), and the physiological properties of local vasculature (i.e., blood volume and permeability) as encapsulated in the IRF. The mathematical expression of this statement is [16]

$$
\begin{aligned}
Q(t) &= F \cdot C_a(t) \otimes R(t) \\
&= C_a(t) \otimes F \cdot R(t) \\
&= \int_0^t C_a(\tau) \cdot [F \cdot R(t-\tau)] \mathrm{d}\tau
\end{aligned}
\tag{2.12}
$$

where $\otimes$ is the convolution integral and $R(t)$ is the IRF. Deconvolution is the opposite mathematical operation to convolution that can be used to "remove" the effect of arterial concentration of contrast on the tissue TDC to arrive at the flow-scaled IRF, $F \cdot R(t)$, the height of which is equal to perfusion as $R(t)$ has a height of unity by definition.

Deconvolution can be executed using a number of algorithms; one example is linear least square regression with single value decomposition [29,30]. Deconvolution can be performed without model assumption for the IRF; however, the deconvolution process is highly sensitive to noise in the arterial and tissue TDCs [31,32]. In presence of noise, deconvolution could result in a flow scaled IRF whose form has no physiologic meaning but could still reproduce the measured tissue TDC after convolution with the measured arterial TDC. In practice, it is preferred to perform model-based deconvolution where the IRF is modeled with a few tissue parameters such as blood flow and volume and permeability surface product, and the deconvolution process is equivalent to estimation of this set of limited number of parameters. With this approach, the initial guess of $F \cdot R(t)$ constructed from the initial estimates of the model parameters is convolved by the measured arterial TDC to obtain a synthesized tissue TDC. The difference between the measured and synthesized tissue TDCs will be taken into consideration in the generation of the next set of model parameter estimates. This process is iteratively repeated until the difference between the measured and synthesized tissue TDCs is minimized.

In Section 2.2.4, the tracer kinetic models that are most frequently employed for the modeling of the IRF are briefly reviewed. The complexity of each model depends on the degree of assumption made to facilitate the solving of the governing mathematical equations of the model. It should be noted that regardless of the choice of model, there is always a compromise between mathematical complexity of the model and the practical limits set by the data (i.e., limited temporal and spatial resolution and SNR).

2.2.4 Tracer Kinetic Models

2.2.4.1 Modified Kety Model

As x-ray contrast agents are hydrophilic and metabolically inert, they are normally excluded from the intracellular space and not metabolized within the intravascular and interstitial space. As such, a two-compartment model can be used to describe the intravascular-interstitial exchange of contrast solutes through the permeable capillary endothelium [33–36]. This model assumes instantaneous mixing of contrast solutes upon arrival in the intravascular and interstitial spaces. In other words, the contrast concentration within these compartments changes only temporally not spatially. The rate of change of the amount of contrast material in the interstitial compartment can be described by the following equation:

$$
V_e \frac{\mathrm{d}C_e(t)}{\mathrm{d}t} = k_1 \cdot C_b(t) - k_2 \cdot C_e(t)
\tag{2.13a}
$$

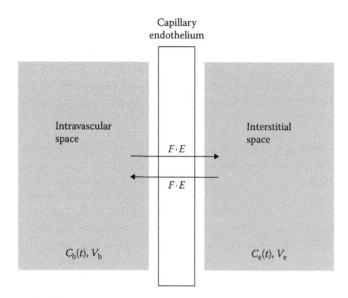

FIGURE 2.5
Diagram of a modified Kety (two-compartment) model used to describe the tracer kinetics in a tissue. The model assumes instantaneous mixing of contrast solutes upon arrival in blood and interstitium. Therefore, the concentration of contrast in the blood, C_b, and interstitium, C_e, are dependent on time t only. The governing rate constants of the forward and backward diffusion of contrast medium between these spaces are $F \cdot E$.

where V_e is the distribution volume of contrast solutes in the interstitial space, $C_e(t)$ and $C_b(t)$ are the concentration of contrast solutes in the interstitial and intravascular spaces, respectively. As contrast is assumed to be mixed instantaneously upon arrival, $C_b(t)$ is essentially equal to $C_a(t)$ as defined in Section 2.2.2. The variable k_1 is the forward transfer constant of contrast solutes from the intravascular to interstitial space and has a unit of min^{-1}, and similarly, k_2 is the backward transfer constant in min^{-1} from the interstitial to intravascular space. It has been shown that both k_1 and k_2 are equal to the product of flow and extraction fraction of the contrast solutes, or $F \cdot E$ [37]. A schematic of this model is provided in Figure 2.5. It should be emphasized that the vascular space represents all capillaries while the interstitial space represents the total interstitium outside all capillaries within a tissue. Equation 2.13a can be rewritten as follows:

$$\frac{dC_e(t)}{dt} = \frac{F \cdot E}{V_e}[C_a(t) - C_e(t)] \tag{2.13b}$$

The solution to Equation 2.13b is given by

$$C_e(t) = \frac{F \cdot E}{V_e} \cdot \int_0^t C_a(u) \cdot e^{-\frac{F \cdot E}{V_e}(t-u)} du \tag{2.14}$$

Because the mass of contrast in tissue measured by CT, $Q(t)$, is contributed by the contrasts in both the interstitial and the intravascular spaces

$$Q(t) = C_e(t) \cdot V_e + C_a(t) \cdot V_b$$
$$= F \cdot E \cdot \int_0^t C_a(u) \cdot e^{-\frac{F \cdot E}{V_e}(t-u)} du + C_a(t) \cdot V_b \tag{2.15}$$

where V_b is the distribution volume of contrast in the intravascular space. According to the definition of convolution, Equation 2.15 can be rewritten as follows:

$$Q(t) = C_a(t) \otimes [F \cdot E \cdot e^{-\frac{F \cdot E}{V_e}t} + V_b \cdot \delta(t)] \tag{2.16}$$

where $\delta(t)$ is the Dirac delta function defined in Section 2.2.3. The convolution of $C_a(t)$ with $\delta(t)$ yields $C_a(t)$, as the integration of $\delta(t)$ is equal to unity. By comparing Equations 2.12 and 2.16, the flow-scaled IRF ($F \cdot R(t)$) of the two-compartment model has the following form:

$$F \cdot R(t) = V_b \tag{2.17a}$$

when $t = 0$

$$= F \cdot E \cdot e^{-\frac{F \cdot E}{V_e}t} \tag{2.17b}$$

when $t > 0$

Given the dynamic CT measurements of $C_a(t)$ and $Q(t)$, the parameters $F \cdot E$, V_b, and V_e can be estimated using nonlinear regression methods [38]. The advantage of compartmental modeling is its mathematical simplicity. The major drawback of this approach is that F and E cannot be estimated separately as they are determined together as a transport constant (k_1 and k_2). By assuming both the intravascular and interstitial spaces are well-stirred compartments, all the information relating to the convective transport of contrast solutes along the capillaries is lost. To estimate F, a constant value of E has to be assumed. This is a limitation as E is likely to be different among different tissue types (e.g., normal vs. ischemic vs. infarcted).

2.2.4.2 Patlak Model

The Patlak model is based on the modified Kety model discussed in Section 2.2.4.1, but with an additional assumption that the efflux of contrast solutes from the interstitial space back to the intravascular space is negligible [35,36]. This assumption implies the contrast distribution volume in the interstitial space (V_e) is very much larger relative to the backward transfer constant ($k_2 = F \cdot E$). Under this assumption, the ratio of $F \cdot E$ to V_e is close to zero, and the exponential term in Equation 2.16, $e^{-F \cdot E / V_e}$, is roughly equal to unity. The flow-scaled IRF, $F \cdot R(t)$, becomes

$$F \cdot R(t) = F \cdot E \cdot H(t) + V_b \cdot \delta(t) \tag{2.18}$$

where $H(t)$ is the Heaviside unit step function and is equal to zero at $t \leq 0$ and unity at $t > 0$. The unit step function, which by definition is zero at $t = 0$, is added in this equation to ensure the diffusion process, as governed by the forward transfer rate constant ($k_1 = F \cdot E$), does not start before the arrival of contrast solutes. Equation 2.15 then becomes

$$Q(t) = F \cdot E \int_0^t C_a(u) \, du + C_a(t) \cdot V_b \qquad (2.19)$$

By dividing both sides by $C_a(t)$, Equation 2.19 can be rewritten as follows:

$$\frac{Q(t)}{C_a(t)} = F \cdot E \cdot \frac{\int_0^t C_a(u) \, du}{C_a(t)} + V_b \qquad (2.20)$$

Equation 2.20 is a linear equation in the form of $y = mx + b$, where m and b are the slope and intercept, respectively. Thus, if $\dfrac{Q(t)}{C_a(t)}$ is plotted against $\dfrac{\int_0^t C_a(u) \, du}{C_a(t)}$, a straight line is produced with its slope equal to $F \cdot E$ and intercept equal to V_b. This method is known as the Patlak graphical plot. This approach can be interpreted as a mathematical transformation to "stretch" the measured tissue TDC into a straight-line plot. Unfortunately, the limitation of the modified Kety model also applies to the Patlak model, which is the fact that F and E cannot be determined separately. Another problem with the Patlak graphical method is that the no backward diffusion assumption may not be applicable in all situations.

2.2.4.3 Johnson and Wilson Model

Compared to the two-compartment (Kety) model, the Johnson and Wilson (J&W) model is a more realistic model to describe the kinetic behavior of contrast solutes in a single capillary transit. The J&W model is a distributed parameter model, which assumes a spatially nonuniform concentration gradient from the arterial to venous ends in the intravascular space to account for the potential loss of contrast solutes in blood via diffusion through the capillary endothelium [39]. Radial gradient of contrast concentration within the capillaries is neglected because convective (blood flow) transport of contrast in the axial direction is much larger than radial diffusion. In contrast to the intravascular space, the surrounding interstitial space is regarded as a compartment. This assumption is valid because capillaries in tissue are randomly oriented (Figure 2.1c); contrast solutes essentially diffuse into the interstitial space from all directions, which mimics a well-mixed compartment. From conservation of the mass of tracer (contrast) in both the intravascular and interstitial spaces, the J&W

model leads to the following two equations describing the tracer transports during a single capillary transit:

$$\pi r^2 \frac{\partial C_b(x,t)}{\partial t} + \pi r^2 v \frac{\partial C_b(x,t)}{\partial x} = 2\pi r P \big(C_e(t) - C_b(x,t) \big) \qquad (2.21a)$$

$$V_e \frac{\partial C_e(t)}{\partial t} = \int_0^l 2\pi r P \big(C_b(x,t) - C_e(x,t) \big) \, dx \qquad (2.21b)$$

where r is the radius of the capillary; $C_b(x,t)$ is the concentration of contrast material within the capillary at time t and distance x relative to the arterial inlet; $C_e(t)$ is the concentration within the interstitial space at time t; v is the flow velocity of tracer; P is the permeability coefficient of the endothelial wall to the contrast; V_e is the distribution volume of contrast in the interstitial space; and l is the axial length of the capillary. A schematic of the J&W model is provided in Figure 2.6. Equation 2.21a describes the convective transport in the axial direction while equation 2.21b describes the diffusive transport of the contrast solutes between capillaries (intravascular) and interstitial space. As the total diffusional flux of contrast solutes is best described using

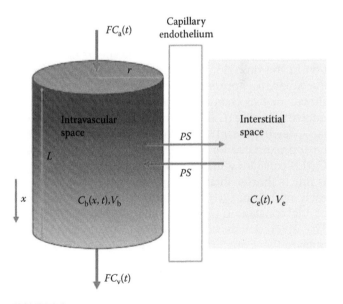

FIGURE 2.6
Diagram of a distributed parameter model (Johnson and Wilson model) used to describe the tracer kinetics in a tissue. According to the model, there is a concentration gradient of contrast medium in the capillaries along the flow direction as a result of potential diffusion across the endothelium into the interstitial space. Thus, $C_b(t)$ is a function of both the position in the capillaries (x) and time (t). The concentration gradient in the radical direction is assumed to be negligible. Diffusion of contrast across the capillary endothelium is governed by PS. The interstitial space is still considered as a compartment where contrast medium is instantaneously mixed with interstitium upon arrival.

the product of permeability coefficient (P) and the total surface area (S) of capillary endothelium, the preceding equations can be rewritten as follows:

$$\frac{\partial C_b(x,t)}{\partial t} + \frac{FL}{V_b}\frac{\partial C_b(x,t)}{\partial x} = \frac{PS}{V_b}[C_e(t) - C_b(x,t)] \quad (2.22a)$$

$$V_e\frac{dC_e(t)}{dt} = \frac{PS}{L}\int_0^L [C_b(x,t) - C_e(t)]dx \quad (2.22b)$$

Equations 2.22a and 2.22b are subject to the following initial and boundary conditions:

$$C_b(x, t = 0) = C_e(t = 0) = 0$$

$$C_b(x = 0, t > 0) = C_a(t) \quad (2.23)$$

The above initial and boundary conditions are justified by the fact that contrast concentration at $t = 0$ should be zero. Additionally, the concentration of contrast at the arterial end of the capillary is equal to the arterial concentration. Given the dynamic CT measurements of $C_a(t)$ and $Q(t)$, Laplace transform can be used to determine the solution of these equations, which satisfied the preceding boundary and initial conditions. As such, solutions to these differential equations only exist in the frequency domain, which significantly hamper the use of this tracer model [37]. It has been shown that a solution in the time domain can be derived by employing the adiabatic approximation, which assumes a much slower rate of change of contrast concentration in the interstitial space ($C_e(t)$) relative to that in the intravascular space ($C_b(x, t)$) [37]. With this assumption, $C_e(t)$ can be approximated by a sequence of discrete steps where $C_e(t)$ is constant within the duration of each step, which is much shorter than the capillary transit time. Within each discrete of $C_e(t)$, $C_b(x, t)$ can be expressed in terms of the constant $C_e(t)$ by solving Equation 2.22a [37]. The other details of the adiabatic approximation are outside the scope of this book chapter and are omitted here. The $F \cdot R(t)$ derived from the adiabatic solution has the following form:

$$F \cdot R(t) = \begin{cases} F & 0 < t < \text{MTT} \\ F \cdot E \cdot e^{-\frac{FE}{V_e}(t - T_c)} & t \geq \text{MTT} \end{cases} \quad (2.24)$$

According to the J&W model, there exists a finite transit time for contrast solutes to travel from the arterial to venous ends of the capillaries. As such, all contrast solutes should remain in the tissue within the MTT and is reflected by the plateau of the flow-scaled

residual function. At $t = \text{MTT}$, $F \cdot R(t)$ immediately drops to a value of $F \cdot E$, as a portion $(1 - E)$ of contrast solutes begins to leave the tissue through the venous end and the fraction (E) diffused into the interstitial space is what remains in the tissue. The extracted contrast in the tissue follows a mono-exponential decay for $t > \text{MTT}$, corresponding to the slower efflux from interstitial to vascular spaces and subsequent washout by blood flow [37].

2.2.5 Practical Issues of Tracer Kinetic Modeling

In a CTP study, the measured TDC may be affected by several factors. The potential effect of each factor on modeling of the IRF is reviewed in this section.

2.2.5.1 Recirculation of Contrast Medium

Recirculation refers to the reentry of contrast material to the organ/tissue of interest after previously leaving it and passing through the systematic circulation. Recirculation can occur as soon as 20–25 seconds after a bolus injection of contrast at 4 mL/s^{-1} (assuming 50 mL of contrast is administered and a normal resting heart rate and cardiac output of the patient). Thus, the effect of recirculation should be addressed in most CTP studies. Let us denote $C_a(t)_{fp}$ and $C_a(t)_r$ as the first-pass and recirculation components of an arterial TDC, respectively. Similarly, $Q(t)_{fp}$ and $Q(t)_r$ are the first-pass and recirculation components of a tissue TDC, respectively. With these definitions, $C_a(t)$ and $Q(t)$ are the summation of the two respective components.

$$C_a(t) = C_a^{fp}(t) + C_a^r(t) \quad (2.25a)$$

$$Q(t) = Q^{fp}(t) + Q^r(t) \quad (2.25b)$$

According to the convolution equation (Equation 2.12):

$$Q^{fp}(t) = C_a^{fp}(t) \otimes [F \cdot R(t)] \quad (2.26a)$$

$$Q^r(t) = C_a^r(t) \otimes [F \cdot R(t)] \quad (2.26b)$$

Substituting Equations 2.26a and 2.26b in Equation 2.25b, and according to the distributive property of convolution, we have

$$\begin{aligned} Q(t) &= Q^{fp}(t) + Q^r(t) \\ &= C_a^{fp}(t) \otimes [F \cdot R(t)] + C_a^r(t) \otimes [F \cdot R(t)] \quad (2.27) \\ &= [C_a^{fp}(t) + C_a^r(t)] \otimes [F \cdot R(t)] \end{aligned}$$

The preceding equation demonstrates that the $F \cdot R(t)$ can still be estimated from the measured arterial and tissue TDCs, with both containing the first-pass and recirculation phases, using the deconvolution approach. Therefore, there is no need to correct for recirculation in the measured TDCs. Although the preceding derivation can be easily generalized to include more than one recirculation component, the effect of second or third recirculation component is expected to be negligible compared to the first recirculation component.

2.2.5.2 Dispersion in True Arterial TDC Relative to Measured Arterial TDC

Dispersion refers to the "spreading" of the arterial TDC at the true input site to a tissue region relative to the measurement site. An arterial TDC is normally acquired at a distance upstream to the tissue region to avoid significant partial volume effect owing to the small size of the local input artery (will be discussed in Section 2.3.5.1). In the presence of dispersion, the true and measured arterial TDCs satisfy the following relationship:

$$C_a(t) = C_a^m(t) \cdot h(t) \tag{2.28}$$

where $h(t)$, as introduced in Section 2.1, is the probability function or transit time spectrum that describes the various times required by individual contrast solute to travel from the measurement site to the actual arterial input site following a bolus injection. Substituting Equation 2.28 in Equation 2.12, and based on the associative property of convolution, yields

$$Q(t) = [C_a^m(t) \cdot h(t)] \otimes F \cdot R(t)$$
$$= C_a^m(t) \otimes [h(t) \otimes F \cdot R(t)] \tag{2.29}$$

Equation 2.29 states that deconvolution of the measured arterial and tissue TDCs returns a flow-scaled residual function convolved with the arterial dispersion transit time spectrum. Previous phantom experiments suggested that the arterial TDC has negligible dispersion effect input curve if the measurement site is within 90 cm of the input site [37]. Thus, $h(t)$ can be approximated by a Dirac delta function, and Equation 2.29 is essentially identical to Equation 2.12. Hence, no dispersion correction is required for the arterial TDC as long as the measurement site is reasonably close to the true input site.

2.2.5.3 Delay of Tissue TDC Relative to Measured Arterial TDC

Because an arterial TDC is measured at a distance from the actual input site to a tissue region, there will be a slight time delay in the arrival of contrast in tissue relative to the measured arterial TDC. Such delay can be accounted for by making modifications to the equation for the IRF of each kinetics model. Let us denote $C_a^m(t)$

as the measured arterial TDC and T_o is the delay time relative to the measurement site.

$$C_a(t) = C_a^m(t - T_o) \tag{2.30}$$

Note that $(t - T_o)$ results in a positive time shift of the measured arterial TDC (as the true arterial TDC should lag behind the measured arterial TDC). Substituting Equation 2.30 in Equation 2.12 yields

$$Q(t) = C_a(t) \cdot F \cdot R(t) = C_a^m(t - T_o) \cdot F \cdot R(t)$$
$$= F \cdot \int_0^t C_a(t - T_o) \cdot R(t - \tau) d\tau$$
$$= F \cdot \int_0^t C_a(t) \cdot R(t - T_o - \tau) d\tau \tag{2.31}$$
$$= C_a^m(t) \otimes F \cdot R(t - T_o)$$

Equation 2.31 confirms that if there is a time delay between the measured and the true arterial input curves, the arrival of contrast in the tissue region will be delayed by the same amount of time. As such, the flow-scaled residual function for each of the preceding models can be modified accordingly to account for the delayed arrival of contrast in the tissue region relative to the measured arterial TDC.

For the modified Kety model, $F \cdot R(t)$ in Equation 2.17 is modified to

$$F \cdot R(t - T_o) = F \cdot E \cdot e^{-\frac{FE}{V_e}(t - T_o)} + V_b \cdot \delta(t - T_o) \tag{2.32}$$

For the Patlak model, $F \cdot R(t)$ in Equation 2.18 is modified to

$$F \cdot R(t - T_o) = F \cdot E \cdot H(t - T_o) + V_b \cdot \delta(t - T_o) \tag{2.33}$$

For the J&W model, $F \cdot R(t)$ in Equation 2.24 is changed to

$$F \cdot R(t - T_o) = \begin{cases} 0 & 0 \leq t < T \\ F & T_o \leq t \leq T_o + \text{MTT} \\ F \cdot E \cdot e^{-\frac{FE}{V_e}(t - T_o - \text{MTT})} & t > T_o + \text{MTT} \end{cases} \tag{2.34}$$

2.2.5.4 Dual Hepatic Artery and Portal Vein Input to the Liver

The liver receives approximately two-thirds of its blood supply from the portal vein and the remaining one-third from the common and proper hepatic arteries [40,41]. The portal vein input, $C_p(t)$, can be directly measured if one of the CT slices includes the portal vein in the scan field of view, while the hepatic artery input, $C_h(t)$, can be approximated by the aortic input at the level of the liver. If we denote α and $(1 - \alpha)$ as the fraction of total blood flow to liver tissue that arises from the hepatic artery (i.e., hepatic arterial fraction) and portal vein, respectively, then $C_a(t)$ can be expressed as the weighted sum of $C_h(t)$ and $C_p(t)$ [42]:

$$C_a(t) = \propto \cdot C_h(t) + (1-\alpha) \cdot C_p(t) \qquad (2.35)$$

By replacing $C_a(t)$ in Equation 2.12 with that expressed in Equation 2.35, hepatic arterial fraction can be estimated together with other physiologic parameters using the compartment or J&W model.

2.3 Implementations

After reviewing the theoretical basis of CTP, in this section, an overview of the technical implementations is provided. Discussion will focus on image acquisition and postprocessing, image artifacts commonly seen in CTP studies, typical radiation dose levels of CTP studies, and potential dose reduction techniques for CTP.

2.3.1 Contrast Administration

2.3.1.1 Contrast Medium

Some commonly used nonionic radiographic contrast agents for CTP imaging include Visipaque (Iodixanol, Amersham Health), Omnipaque (Iohexol, GE Healthcare), and Isovue (Iopamidol, Bracco Diagnostic). The typical molecular weight of these agents is about 760 g/mol^{-1} (dalton). The osmolality (solute concentration) of these contrast agents are considered to be low (290–796 mOsm/kg^{-1}) compared to blood plasma. Iodine concentration is available in the range of 140–370 mg iodine/mL, but concentration above 300 should be used for most CTP studies to ensure a good contrast-to-noise ratio of the dynamic images. As the viscosity of contrast media is lower at higher temperature, contrast agent should be warmed to be about the same body temperature (35°C–37°C) before administered to the patient.

2.3.1.2 Contrast Injection Rate

Contrast is usually injected into one of the antecubital veins (e.g., basilica vein) with an injection pump through a 18-gauge cannula taped in place. With a fixed volume of contrast medium, a faster injection rate increases the rate of iodine delivery, which leads to a faster accumulation of contrast material in the aorta and hence a

higher arterial enhancement [43]. A faster injection rate also shortens the injection duration and the time to and duration of peak enhancement. The typical bolus injection rate of contrast for CTP is 4–7 mL/s^{-1} [13,14,44–46]. As discussed in Section 2.2.2, a much faster bolus injection is required to satisfy the assumption of no venous outflow if the maximal slope method is used for estimating perfusion. However, an increase in the injection rate greater than 10 mL/s^{-1} is not likely to improve the enhancement further owing to the inherent mixing of contrast medium in the central blood compartment and retrograde reflux, which restricts fast propagation of contrast to the target region [47,48].

If a dual injector is used, a bolus of saline flash of 20–30 mL can be applied following the bolus injection of contrast to push the tail of the iodinated contrast medium into the left ventricle, thus increasing the efficiency of contrast delivery and level of contrast enhancement [47,49]. It can also minimize dispersion and improve the bolus geometry [50]. For CT myocardial perfusion (MP) studies, saline flush may also reduce streak artifacts from the highly attenuating contrast material in the right heart chamber, which may significantly distort the TDC measurement in the interventricular septal wall [51].

2.3.1.3 Contrast Concentration

At a fixed injection rate and volume of contrast medium, a higher concentration delivers a larger dose of iodine, which results in a higher degree of peak contrast enhancement [43]. Therefore, contrast agents with high iodine concentration (320–370 mgI/mL^{-1}) should be used to achieve the highest peak enhancement of the arterial and tissue TDCs to facilitate perfusion map calculation. For MP studies, a more diluted contrast concentration is sometimes preferred to reduce the beam hardening effect arising from the substantial amount of attenuating contrast medium in the left and right heart chambers during the first-pass phase (will be discussed in Section 2.3.5.3). However, iodine concentration below 300 mgI/mL^{-1} is not recommended to avoid suboptimal contrast-to-noise ratio in the images and TDCs.

2.3.1.4 Contrast Volume

Contrast medium is diluted during its passage through circulation. Heavy patients will dilute contrast more due to the fact that those patients have larger blood volume compared to less heavy patients. Thus, the volume of contrast agent used in CTP examinations should be tailored to the patient's body weight. The typical dosage applied at our institution is 0.7 mL/kg^{-1} up to a maximum of 60 mL.

2.3.2 Scanning Parameters

CT scanning parameters play an important role and should be carefully selected as they can greatly affect contrast enhancement and noise level in DCE CT images and hence the diagnostic accuracy of a CTP study. Radiation dose is also dependent on the scanning parameters chosen.

2.3.2.1 Tube Voltage

The optimal setting of tube voltage is different between different CTP applications. Ideally, CTP imaging should be performed at the lowest tube voltage available (80 kV), at this kilovolt setting the mean photon energy is closer to the k-edge of iodine (~33 keV) increasing the contrast-to-noise ratio of the TDCs due, in part, to greater photoelectric effect [52]. Thus, the standard protocol for brain perfusion studies employs 80 kV for dynamic scanning. For liver perfusion studies, however, a higher tube voltage (100 or 120 kV) should be used instead to compensate for the much larger cross section of the abdomen compared to the head, as photons at lower energies will likely be absorbed by the large patient's body and not be able to reach the detector and results in a poor SNR of the perfusion images while still subjecting the patient to radiation. For MP studies, 140 kV is preferred to minimize the beam hardening effect arising from the photoelectric absorption of low-energy photons when they pass through the heart chambers filled with the highly attenuating contrast medium (will be discussed in Section 2.3.5.3).

2.3.2.2 Tube Current

The choice of tube current (in mA) or tube current-seconds (the product of tube current and gantry rotation speed, in mA/s) should be adjusted according to the patient body size or expected attenuation and the radiosensitivity of the organ/tissue of interest. For example, the head has a relatively lower radiosensitivity [53]; therefore, a higher mA/s (200 mA/s) can be used in brain perfusion studies to compensate for the high x-ray attenuation by the skull. On the contrary, lower mA/s should be used for cardiac and liver perfusion studies due to the higher radiosensitivity and less attenuation of the chest (breast tissue) and abdomen regions [53]. At our institution, 30 and 50 mA/s are usually applied for the cardiac and liver perfusion studies, respectively. Although radiation dose reduction is in proportion to reduction in mA/s, image noise increases by 40% if the mA/s is reduced by half (noise $\propto \dfrac{1}{\sqrt{mA/s}}$) [54]. Therefore, the choice of mA/s should lead to a good balance between image quality and radiation dose level. Compared to filtered back projection (FBP), iterative reconstruction (IR)

may permit scanning at a lower mA (or mA/s) without the penalty of increased image noise and will be discussed in more detail in Section 2.3.6.3.

2.3.2.3 Gantry Rotation Speed

Gantry rotation speed controls the temporal resolution of a CT image. CTP demands high temporal resolution to account for the fast circulation of contrast in the input artery and tissue region. A 1-second gantry period is generally sufficient for most except cardiac CTP applications. Dynamic images of the heart should be acquired using the fastest gantry speed available (e.g., 0.25–0.35 ms for single-source CT) to minimize cardiac motion artifact. The tube current should be adjusted according to the gantry speed to ensure a reasonable photon flux level (mA/s) for a specific perfusion protocol as discussed in Section 2.3.2.2.

2.3.2.4 Scan Duration

Scan duration defines the amount of dynamic data acquired for perfusion analysis. Ideally, the acquisition time should be long enough to cover the entire first pass of contrast in tissue if no estimation of the permeability surface area product (PS) of the microvasculature is required. For this type of study, acquisition of 45 seconds is usually sufficient for a contrast injection rate of 4 mL/s^{-1} or higher. If the PS parameter is required, a longer scanning time is necessary for the reliable estimation of that parameter. Extending the scanning time, however, increases the patient's radiation exposure. One solution is to employ an additional second-phase acquisition at a delay time after the completion of the first-phase acquisition. Therefore, images in the second phase can be acquired at a much lower temporal frequency (e.g., 15 second interval) for 2 minutes. This setup is justified by the fact that exchange of contrast material between the interstitial and intravascular spaces is much slower at this phase [37], hence high sampling frequency is not necessary.

2.3.2.5 Scan Coverage

The volume of organ included in a quantitative (cine) CTP study is restricted by the CT scanner detector width. To avoid potential side effects from multiple injections of contrast, scanner with a large detector width is preferred as it allows whole organ CTP imaging with a single bolus injection of contrast. For scanners offering smaller detector width, the axial coverage can be doubled for each bolus by using a table "goggling" or "shuttling" technique, in which the scanner table moves back and forth between two adjacent cine sections, at the expense of a reduced temporal resolution of data acquisition in each cine section (the acquisition time interval could increase from 1 second to 2–3 seconds) [55].

2.3.3 Image Reconstruction

This section reviews some of the image reconstruction issues that may affect the CTP analysis.

2.3.3.1 Full-Scan Reconstruction

DCE CT images should be reconstructed using projections acquired from a full gantry rotation (360°) to avoid "half-scan" artifact [56,57]. Compared with full-scan reconstruction, half-scan reconstruction (180° + beam fan angle) offers a higher temporal resolution but requires the scanned object to remain "stationary" during the imaging time to work optimally. In a CTP study, contrast medium is circulating fast through the organ/tissue, leading to rapid changes of the scanned object between projection views. As a result, the missing projections cannot be accurately estimated from the measured half-scan projections, which result in shifts in CT number between consecutive half-scan images. Although shading artifacts induced from half-scan reconstruction are unlikely to cause misdiagnosis because human pathologies rarely resemble their appearances, the unpredictable changes in CT number may severely affect the measurement of arterial and tissue TDCs and hence perfusion estimation. As such, full-scan reconstruction should be used in all CTP studies, albeit with a slight degradation in temporal resolution of the images [56].

2.3.3.2 Reconstruction Kernel

Reconstruction kernel is the "filter" applied to the measured projections before back projection is executed. The kernel should be carefully selected as it can greatly affect the quality of perfusion images. The sharper (high-pass) filters that enhance or preserve the higher spatial frequencies would also amplify the noise in the image. Conversely, the smoother (low-pass) filters reduce image noise albeit at a reduced spatial resolution [58]. Generally speaking, a "standard" filter used for routine scanning provides a fine balance between image noise and resolution for most CTP applications.

2.3.4 Postprocessing Image Analysis

Following data acquisition, reconstructed source images (SI) are transferred from the scanner console to a stand-alone workstation for processing into parametric functional maps with a commercial software package. Some software packages use the indicator-dilution and maximal slope methods while others employ deconvolution methods outlined in Section 2.2.3. Parametric map calculation can be a manual or fully automated process. An input arterial TDC and venous TDC are selected by identifying a subset of pixels within an input artery and a draining vein either manually or automatically. The venous TDC is required especially for brain perfusion studies to correct for the partial volume averaging effect (see Section 2.3.5.1). Some software packages also incorporate correction for delay as well as beam hardening correction and image registration algorithms in the postprocessing workflow to minimize the effect of beam hardening and/or patient-related motion before yielding quantitative parametric maps of tissue blood flow (F), blood volume (V), MTT, and PS. A user interface of one commercial software package (CT Perfusion, GE Healthcare) is shown in Figure 2.7 for illustration.

2.3.5 Image Artifacts

CT systems are prone to many forms of image artifact, which is loosely defined as the discrepancy between the reconstructed values in the image and the true attenuation coefficients of the object. We restrict our discussion here to the most commonly seen artifacts in CTP imaging that may have significant impact on the quantitative perfusion measurement.

2.3.5.1 Partial Volume Effect

Partial volume effect due to the limited in-plane spatial resolution of CT can result in significant underestimation of the arterial TDC derived from a small artery. In a brain perfusion study, the arterial input curve measured from either the anterior cerebral artery or the middle cerebral artery (MCA) is underestimated as a result of partial volume averaging with the surrounding brain tissue. Such discrepancy in the arterial input curve can be estimated and corrected by obtaining a venous TDC from the posterior superior sagittal sinus, the draining vein of the brain. Because veins have larger lumens than arteries, they are not affected by partial volume averaging as is the case with arterial TDCs in CT images. Therefore, by comparing the AUC of the venous TDC to that of the arterial TDC, a correction factor for partial volume averaging in the arterial TDC can be derived. For other perfusion studies in the thorax such as MP measurement and abdomen, the partial volume effect in arterial input curve can be avoided by obtaining the curve from the nearby aorta that has a much larger cross-sectional area (Figure 2.8). As stated in Section 2.2.5.2, the dispersion effect of an arterial TDC should be negligible if the measurement site is within a short distance of the actual input site [37].

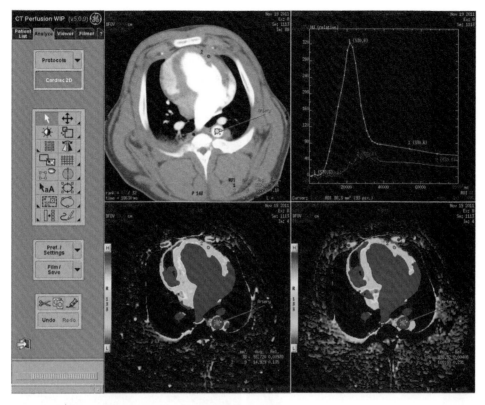

FIGURE 2.7
User interface of a commercial CT perfusion software package (CT Perfusion, GE Healthcare). An arterial TDC is selected either manually or automatically from a series of DCE CT image (top left panel) for the deconvolution analysis with the tissue TDC in each voxel (or small neighboring group of voxels) (top right). Absolute tissue blood flow (bottom right), blood volume (bottom left), mean transit time (MTT), and permeability surface area product (PS) are calculated and displayed as colored functional maps. Regions of interest can be drawn on these maps by the user to obtain quantitative values of the functional parameters.

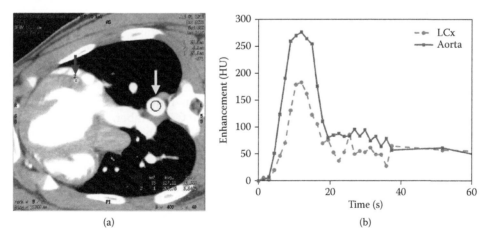

(a)   (b)

FIGURE 2.8
Comparison of the arterial TDC measured from a small branch of the left circumflex (LCx) artery (red arrow, a) with that acquired from the aorta (yellow arrow, a). The TDC measured from LCx was significantly underestimated due to partial volume averaging. In contrast, the aortic TDC was less affected by the partial volume effect due to the much larger cross-sectional area of the aorta (b).

2.3.5.2 Patient Motion

Patient-related motion is a major source of image artifact in a CTP study. For brain perfusion studies, the patient's head is normally held with a plastic head holder mounted to the scanner table to minimize the head movement during the acquisition. The holder can reduce but not completely eliminate head movement in some cases. Figure 2.9 shows how the arterial and tissue TDCs can be affected by the head movement despite the use of such a head holder. Thus, it is crucial that the patient is instructed

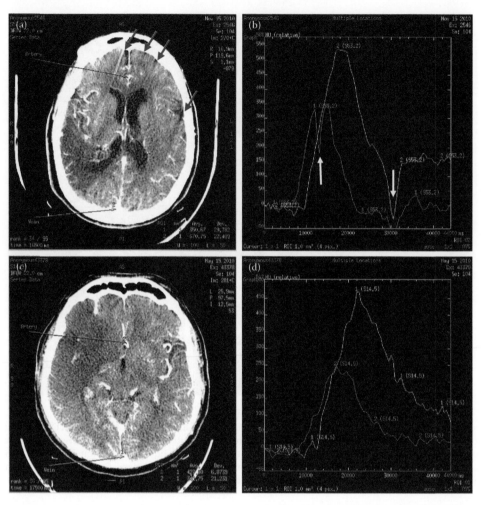

FIGURE 2.9
(a) Movement of the patient's head during acquisition induced significant artifacts (red arrows) in the DCE CT images. (b) The arterial and venous TDCs were significantly affected and exhibited large dips (yellow arrows). (c) CTP study of another patient whose head was minimally moved during scanning. No motion artifact was seen in the DCE CT images. (d) The corresponding arterial and venous TDCs did not show the dips seen in Figure 2.9b.

to keep his/her head still during the study. For liver and MP studies, the patient's breathing motion poses a major challenge (Figure 2.10). Although the first-phase acquisition is restricted to 30 seconds, some patients may still have problem holding their breaths for this short period of time. Residual lung and diaphragm movements may significantly deform the adjacent heart and liver, respectively, which make postreconstruction image registration a more difficult task. For MP studies, the involuntary cardiac motion presents additional challenge but cardiac motion can be largely minimized by employing either prospective or retrospective gating with the electrocardiogram (ECG) recorded in synchrony with the dynamic acquisition [59].

2.3.5.3 Beam Hardening

The root cause of beam hardening is the polychromatic nature of x-ray photons used in CT and the energy dependency of x-ray attenuation [60]. If not corrected,

the beam hardening effect can induce unpredictable shift in CT number, leading to tissue enhancement (or lack of enhancement) that is unrelated to perfusion status and hence misdiagnosis of physiologic ischemia [60]. Beam hardening affects mostly CT MP studies owing to the presence of substantial amount of contrast medium in the heart chambers in the scan field of view. Figure 2.11 demonstrates the pattern of myocardial enhancement in the presence of beam hardening in two patients who have very different conditions of CAD. Beam hardening correction can be achieved using either a projection-based or an image-based method. For the projection-based approach, beam hardening errors in each measured projection is first estimated based on the ideal linear relationship of projection and path length when beam hardening is absent. The discrepancy in each projection is then corrected before FBP. For the image-based correction method [61–63], a reconstructed image is first forward-projected to retrieve the measured

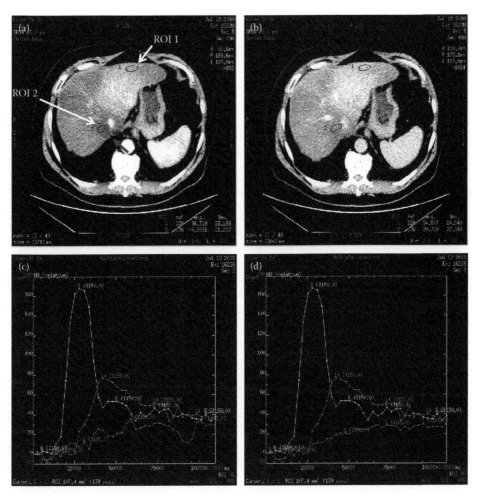

FIGURE 2.10

DCE CT images of a patient's liver at two different time points (a, b). Breathing motion was evident by the change in shape of the liver between the two images and the dark shading artifact induced in the first image (red arrow in Figure 2.10a). ROI 2 was more affected by the breathing motion than ROI 1. The tissue TDC in ROI 2 showed a larger fluctuation (pink curve, c) than that in ROI 1 (pink curve, d). Image registration was required to correct for the breathing motion artifact before perfusion analysis was performed.

projection in each view. The same correction procedures as the projection-based method are then executed. More recently, the effectiveness of dual-energy (spectrum, kV) CT for beam hardening correction in CTP has been investigated [64]. Dual-energy CT can generate synthesized monochromatic images that mimic those acquired from a single-energy (keV) x-ray beam and free of beam hardening [65]. As such, monochromatic images could improve the accuracy of CTP measurement of tissue blood flow. A recent study has suggested that the overestimation of MP in conventional single-energy (spectrum) CT due to beam hardening can be greatly reduced with dual-energy CT [64].

2.3.6 Radiation Dose and Reduction Methods

Owing to the need of sequential scanning of the tissue/ organ of interest over time, a quantitative CTP study delivers a higher radiation dose than most x-ray imaging applications. The typical effective dose of a quantitative CTP study, using the scanning parameters suggested in Section 3.2, ranges from 5 to 20 mSv (estimated from the dose-length product reported on a CT scanner console [53]). These dose levels are generally higher compared with other imaging techniques that provide quantitative perfusion measurement (e.g., MP) such as positron emission tomography (PET) and MRI [66]. The higher radiation dose does not facilitate repeated CTP studies for diagnostic and therapeutic purposes. For instance, repeated measurement of MP at rest and maximal pharmacologic stress to assess the functional significance of a coronary stenosis. Another scenario is repeated perfusion measurement before and after revascularization of an occluded coronary artery to evaluate the success of reperfusion to the downstream myocardium. In Section 2.3.6.1, potential dose reduction techniques that can be implemented for a CTP study are briefly reviewed.

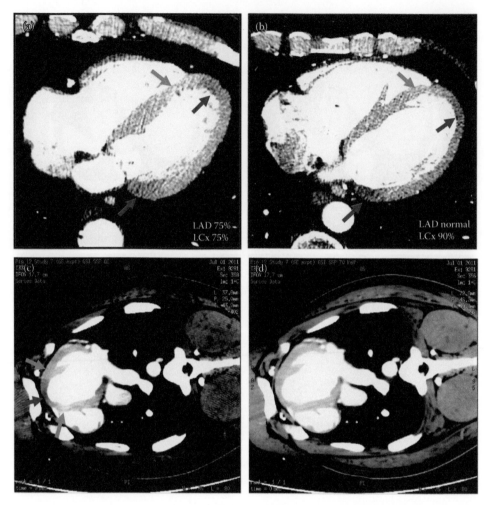

FIGURE 2.11
(a, b) Contrast-enhanced cardiac images of two CAD patients whose coronary conditions were very different (degree of luminal narrowing in each artery was labeled in the images) but exhibited similar pattern of beam hardening artifacts. In particular, hypo- (red arrows) and hyper-enhancement (green arrows) were seen in the apical and septal walls, respectively, that were unrelated to the severity of stenosis in the feeding coronary arteries. The window width and level of both images were 120/80. (c) Similar appearance of beam hardening artifact was seen in the average map of a nonischemic pig's heart acquired with conventional single energy (spectrum, kV) CT scanning. (d) Beam hardening effect was minimized in the corresponding average map acquired with dual-energy CT scanning. Contrast enhancement became more uniform throughout the nonischemic myocardium. The window width and level in Figure 2.11c and 2.11d are 35/80 and 75/80, respectively.

2.3.6.1 Reduction in Imaging Frequency

A larger number of images acquired from dynamic CT scanning provides more data points for the arterial and tissue TDCs and hence a more accurate estimate of absolute perfusion. From the patient's perspective, however, the increased radiation dose associated with the longer radiation exposure time is of concern. One simple dose reduction method is to decrease the image acquisition frequency. It has been previously shown that by increasing the sampling intervals from 1 to 3 seconds, there were no significant changes in the measurement of cerebral blood flow (CBF), cerebral blood volume (CBV), and MTT. The same parameters were overestimated only when the sampling interval exceeded 4 seconds [44,67]. These findings suggest that radiation dose can be reduced

by >60% without affecting the accuracy of quantitative CTP measurement [68]. However, a recent pilot study on 45 patients with colorectal cancer suggests the same increase in sampling interval results in significant overestimation of blood flow and underestimation of MTT in leaky tissue such as tumor [69]. Therefore, further investigations are needed to confirm whether this dose reduction approach is also applicable for tumor perfusion studies.

2.3.6.2 Prospective ECG Triggering (for Cardiac Application)

With the older CT scanners, the heart has to be scanned continuously for the entire duration of a CT MP study; following acquisition mid-diastolic cardiac images are retrospectively reconstructed to minimize the effect of cardiac motion for perfusion analysis. As such, patients are unnecessarily exposed for the most part of the study. Most clinical CT scanners today have the capability of performing CT MP imaging with prospective ECG triggering, in which the x-ray tube is turned on only at mid-diastolic phases and remains either completely turned off or operated at a very low tube current (mA) at other phases [59]. A recent prospective multicenter trial confirmed that the quality of the coronary CT angiography (CCTA) images acquired using the prospective triggering protocol was not different from that of the retrospective gating protocol, while radiation dose was significantly reduced by >70% [70].

2.3.6.3 Iterative Reconstruction

IR is currently a hot research topic in the CT community although it is not a new concept. IR is computationally intensive and its application for CT was hampered in the past due to the limited computer power available. Conversely, analytic reconstruction (FBP) is a fast algorithm, which is helped by several simplified assumptions of the system optics and has been the standard technique for CT image reconstruction over the past few decades. One of the disadvantages of FBP is its high sensitivity to noise in projections, which restricts the use of low mA/s for scanning. On the contrary, IR can provide a more effective image noise reduction than FBP, which may suit the need of quantitative CTP imaging. With the improvement in computer power in recent years, all major CT vendors have developed IR algorithms to facilitate low-dose CT acquisition. Some examples include adaptive statistical IR (ASIR) [71], model-based IR (MBIR) (GE Healthcare) [72], IR in image space (IRIS) [73], sinogram affirmed IR (SAFIRE) (Siemens Healthcare) [74], and adaptive iterative dose reduction (AIDR, Toshiba) [75]. Although these algorithms work slightly differently from each other, initial data have shown that these algorithms can effectively minimize image noise in low-dose CT scanning. As such, IR could be implemented to develop an ultra low-dose CTP protocol. The algorithm of ASIR (GE Healthcare) is briefly reviewed here for illustration: ASIR uses a FBP reconstructed image as the initial guess of the distribution of linear attenuation coefficients within the scanned subject. The initial FBP image is forward-projected to produce synthesized projection in each view, which is then compared with the ideal projection, which is the measured projection with Poisson noise removed using a statistical model. Reconstructed images are then refined by iteratively updating image voxels to optimize an objective function of the deviations of the synthesized from the measured set of projections.

2.3.6.4 Sparse-View Reconstruction

Sparse-view reconstruction (SVR) tackles radiation dose reduction in a different way than IR. In addition to

decreasing the x-ray tube current, one can also reduce radiation dose by reducing the number of projection views acquired. The number of projections acquired per gantry rotation with a clinical CT scanner is roughly 1000. When the projection views are sparsely sampled, FBP, which requires densely sampled projection views, can result in prominent streak artifacts. Current research is focused on developing algorithms that can accurately interpolate additional projection views from measured data for general beam configurations and geometries of scanned object [76,77]. The potential combined use of IR and SVR could ultimately reduce the effective dose of a whole organ quantitative CTP study to a sub millisievert level.

2.3.6.5 Advanced Postreconstruction Image Processing

In addition to the aforementioned novel image reconstruction techniques, advanced postreconstruction image processing algorithms such as principal component analysis (PCA) [78,79] and anisotropic diffusion (AD) [80] may also be used to further suppress image noise to facilitate low-dose CTP applications. PCA finds common temporal patterns (principal components) in all tissue TDCs from the entire tissue ROI by analyzing the variations of each TDC from the mean curve of all tissue TDCs. These variations will reflect the temporal behavior of TDCs after contrast injection and random noise. Each tissue TDC can be reconstituted by summation of the principal components found. By retaining only components that reproduce variations in keeping with the expected rapid first pass of contrast and discarding those that do not, random noise in the reconstituted tissue TDCs can be minimized. On the contrary, AD improves the signal-to-noise ratio of a tissue TDC by averaging nearby TDCs (e.g., within a 5×5 or 10×10 pixel block) that share common temporal patterns only (instead of averaging all the TDCs within that block). Both PCA and AD can work compatibly with IR as they perform TDC smoothing in different ways. While IR works in projections, PCA and AD smooth TDCs temporally and spatially, respectively, in reconstructed images.

Figure 2.12 demonstrates the potential use of prospective ECG triggering, ASIR, and PCA for ultra low-dose quantitative CT measurement of MP. CT MP imaging was performed on a normal porcine heart with a conventional high-dose protocol (cine with retrospective ECG gating and 28 mA/s) and repeated with a low-dose protocol (prospective ECG triggering and 7 mA/s). Dynamic images acquired with the high-dose protocol were reconstructed with FBP (Figure 2.12a) and those acquired with the low-dose protocol were reconstructed independently using FBP (Figure 2.12b) and ASIR with PCA (Figure 2.12c). For both CTP studies, a double bolus of contrast medium was deliberately administered

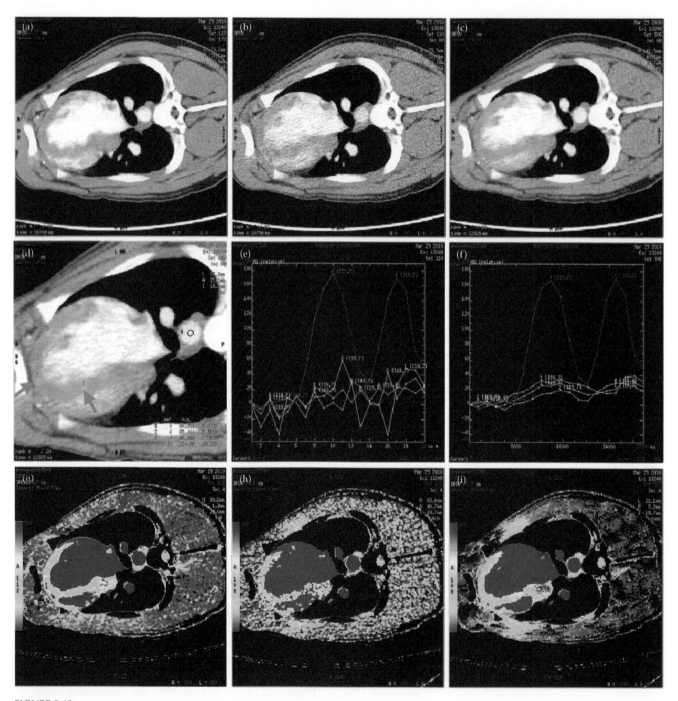

FIGURE 2.12

DCE CT images of a pig's heart acquired with the (a) high-dose (retrospective ECG gating and 32 mA/s) with FBP protocol, (b) low-dose (prospective ECG triggering and 7mA/s) with FBP protocol, and (c) low-dose with ASIR and PCA protocol. (d) Three ROIs in the myocardium from which the TDCs were measured. (e) Myocardial TDCs measured from the low-dose FBP images. (f) The corresponding myocardial TDCs from the low-dose ASIR and PCA images. MP maps correspond to (g) high-dose FBP, (h) low-dose FBP, and (i) low-dose ASIR and PCA.

instead of the conventional single-bolus protocol. Excessive image noise in the low-dose FBP image resulted in significant fluctuation in the tissue TDCs and the two bolus peaks could not be resolved (Figure 2.12e) The quality of the associated perfusion map was degraded by the high noise level in the TDCs, as reflected by the large fluctuation of perfusion values in the myocardium (Figure 2.12h). In contrast, image noise in the low-dose ASIR image was much reduced and the two bolus peaks in each tissue TDC were clearly resolved (Figure 2.12f). The associated perfusion map (Figure 2.12i) manifested a comparable quality with the perfusion map of the high-dose protocol (Figure 2.12g), with an estimated effective dose 16 times lower (15.9 vs. 1.0 mSv for 4-cm coverage).

2.4 Preclinical Validations

Quantitative CTP measurement of tissue blood flow has been successfully validated in animals against radiolabeled or fluorescent microspheres, which is regarded as the gold standard method for quantifying absolute perfusion, and in human against PET, which is the corresponding reference standard method in vivo. In this section, we reviewed a few preclinical validation studies with different animal models performed at our institution for one model-based (J&W model) deconvolution CTP technique.

2.4.1 Liver Perfusion

2.4.1.1 Validation Techniques of Hepatic Blood Flow

The validation of hepatic blood flow is difficult mainly because of the dual blood supply of the liver and the inaccessibility of the portal system [81]. Proposed methods such as radiolabeled microsphere and [15O] water PET have their own sets of challenges. [15O] water PET is limited by availability, cost, and limited spatial resolution to accurately

resolve the portal vein [82]. Radiolabeled microsphere cannot measure portal vein blood flow (PVBF) directly. Microspheres injected into the arterial bloodstream are lodged in capillary beds of the lungs; hence, the technique can only directly measure regional and total $H_A BF$. The PVBF can be indirectly estimated by summing all the flow in splanchnic organs that drain into the portal vein, but not regional PVBF [83]. Since a suitable method to validate regional measurement of $H_T BF$ is yet to be determined, we used $H_A BF$ measured with the microsphere technique to validate our CTP measurements and Monte Carlo simulations to determine the reliability of parameter estimates.

2.4.1.2 Microspheres Method and Monte Carlo Simulations

$H_A BF$ measured with CTP was compared against that measured using the ex vivo method of radiolabeled microsphere technique in 7 animals at 16 days posttumor detection [84]. To achieve a range in $H_A BF$, three arterial $P_a CO_2$ levels, normocapnia, hypercapnia, and hypocapnia were used [84]. Example parametric maps for $H_A BF$, $H_T BF$, $H_T BV$, PS, and T_0 are shown in Figure 2.13. Under steady

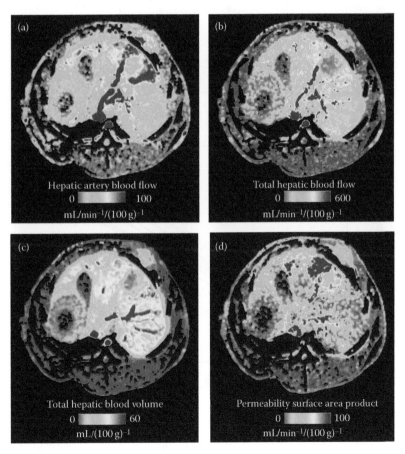

FIGURE 2.13

Parametric maps of the liver generated under normocapnia. (a) Hepatic artery blood flow ($H_A BF$) map. (b) Total hepatic blood flow ($H_T BF$) map. (c) Total hepatic blood volume ($H_T BV$) map. (d) Permeability surface area (PS) map. The tumor is visible in all of the maps. However, the $H_A BF$ map delineates the tumor rim from the tumor core most clearly. It also suggests that the tumor has increased arterial blood supply than normal liver.

state normocapnic condition, the microsphere H_ABF were 51.9 ± 4.2, 40.7 ± 4.9, and 99.7 ± 6.0 mL/min^{-1}/(100 g)$^{-1}$ while CTP H_ABF were 50.0 ± 5.7, 37.1 ± 4.5, and 99.8 ± 6.8 mL/min^{-1}/(100 g)$^{-1}$ in normal liver, tumor core, and rim, respectively. An analysis of variance (ANOVA) showed no significant differences between CTP and microsphere H_ABF measurements, $p > .05$. The Bland–Altman plot comparing CTP and microsphere H_ABF measurements gives a mean difference of -0.13 mL/min^{-1}/(100 g)$^{-1}$, which is not significantly different from zero (Figure 2.14a). The limits of agreement, the region in which 95% of the differences lie are from -29.21 to 28.95 mL/min^{-1}/(100 g)$^{-1}$. A plot of CTP versus microsphere H_ABF measurements

in all rabbits and under all capnic conditions is shown in Figure 2.14b. To account for multiple measurements in the same rabbit, the generalized estimating equation method was used instead of a regular regression analysis [85]. The average slope of the individual linear regression of H_ABF measurements from a single rabbit was 0.92 ± 0.05, which was significantly different from a value of zero ($p < .05$), but not significantly different from the line of identity ($p > .05$). This indicates that there was a significant correlation between the CTP and microsphere H_ABF measurements. The average intercept, 4.62 ± 2.69 mL/min^{-1}/(100 g)$^{-1}$, was not significantly different from zero, $p > .05$. The average R^2 was 0.81 ± 0.05 (range 0.64–0.96).

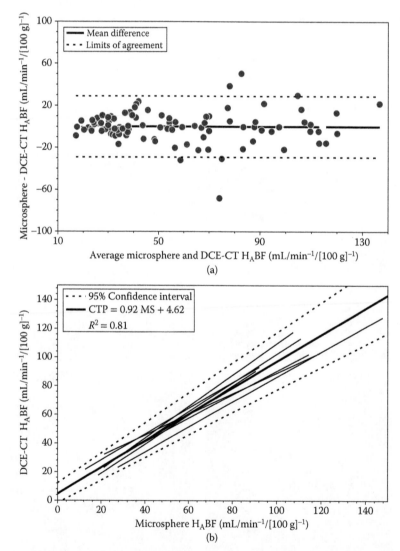

FIGURE 2.14

(a) Bland–Altman plot comparing DCE CT and microsphere H_ABF measurements. The mean difference (solid line) between the two methods is -0.13 mL/min^{-1}/(100 g)$^{-1}$. The limits of agreement (dotted lines), that is, the boundaries of the region in which 95% of the differences lie, are -29.21 and 28.95 mL/min^{-1}/(100 g)$^{-1}$. (b) Plot of DCE CT versus microsphere H_ABF measurements in all rabbits under all capnic conditions. The thin solid lines are the individual linear regression lines for each rabbit and the thick solid line is the average of all the individual rabbit regression lines (slope = 0.92 ± 0.05, intercept = 4.62 ± 2.69 mL/min^{-1}/(100 g)$^{-1}$). The dotted lines represent the 95% confidence interval for the average slope and intercept.

Monte Carlo simulations were used to determine the reliability of parameter estimates. The simulations were performed using procedures described by St. Lawrence and Lee [37]. The simulation was performed using parameter values that represent the normal tissue, tumor rim, and core obtained under normal condition [84]. The Monte Carlo simulations showed that our perfusion model (J&W model) is well suited for the separation of tissue blood flow (F) and extraction fraction (E) while the compartment model cannot. The simulation showed that H_TBF in the normal tissue and tumor rim were equivalent in reproducibility (determined using the coefficient of variation [CV]), while the tumor core was the most sensitive to noise (Figure 2.15). The higher CV of tumor core parameter estimates was due to lower H_TBF and corresponding low SNR. In general, the CVs derived from the Monte

Carlo simulation at a noise level of SD = 4 were comparable to those in the CTP study. The simulation showed that PS had the poorest CV among all the parameters for each tissue type.

2.4.2 Brain Perfusion

Fluorescent microspheres have been used for the past 30 years for validating regional CBF measurement methods [86]. Cenic et al. validated CTP-derived CBF measurements, using this ex vivo microsphere technique [87]. Specifically, closely spaced (<1 minute apart) measurements of the deconvolution-based dynamic CTP-CBF and microsphere-based CBF were determined in a healthy rabbit model [87]. A strong correlation was found between the CTP and fluorescent microsphere measurements of CBF (Figure 2.16). The mean CBF obtained from the CTP and microsphere techniques for $n = 39$ measurements was 73.3 ± 31.5 mL/min^{-1}/(100 g)$^{-1}$ and 74.3 ± 31.6 mL/min^{-1}/(100 g)$^{-1}$, respectively. This correlation compares well with the findings from others who have validated their dynamic CTP and stable xenon-CT techniques with microsphere measurements [88,89].

2.4.3 Myocardial Perfusion

Previous animal studies have shown that CTP measurement of MP had excellent agreement with the microspheres' measurements [90–93]. However, some of those CTP measurements were not corrected for beam hardening [90,91], as a result, the comparison could only be performed in segments that were less affected by beam hardening artifacts. We compared the CTP

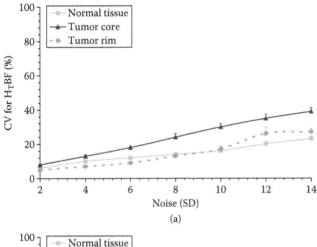

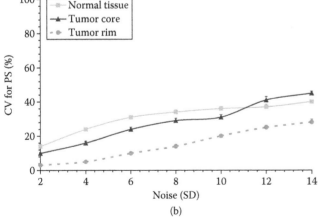

FIGURE 2.15
Monte Carlo simulation results on the precision of model parameter estimates at different noise conditions created by adding Gaussian noise with different standard deviation (SD) to the simulated tissue curve using the Monte Carlo method. The incremental noise resulted in SNR ranging from 2.4 to 17.2 in the normal tissue, 1.1 to 7.7 in the tumor core, and 2.9 to 20.4 in the tumor rim. Coefficient of variation (CV) was used to express the precision of each parameter estimate. (a) CV of H_TBF and (b) CV of PS in normal tissue, tumor core, and rim.

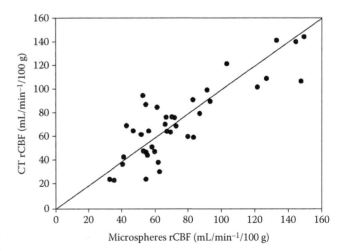

FIGURE 2.16
Dynamic CT measurement plotted against microsphere measurement of regional CBF (in mL/min^{-1}/100 g). $r = 0.837$, $p < .001$, slope of the regression line was close to unity (0.97 ± 0.03).

measurement of MP without and with beam hardening correction using an image-based algorithm against the radiolabeled microspheres' measurements in a pig model of acute myocardial infarction (MI), created by a transient (i.e., 1 hour) ligation of the distal left anterior descending (LAD) artery followed by reperfusion [92]. The pigs were monitored for 4 weeks after surgery

before radiolabeled microspheres were directly injected into the left atrial appendage after the last CT study at 4 weeks post. We demonstrated that the MP measurements without beam hardening correction had a larger scatter from the linear regression line (Figure 2.17a) compared with the measurements where BH correction was applied (Figure 2.17b). Our findings were corroborated

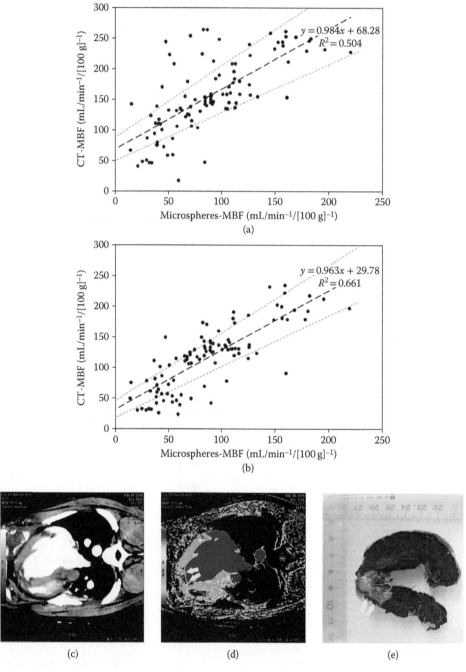

FIGURE 2.17
CTP measurement of myocardial perfusion without (a) and with (b) image-based beam hardening correction against the measurements by radiolabeled microspheres in a pig model of acute MI. Correlation between the CTP and microspheres' measurements was improved after beam hardening correction was applied. (c) Average map and (d) myocardial perfusion map with image-based BH correction in comparison with the TTC-stained heart tissue section (e). The "no flow" apical segment (yellow arrows in Figure 2.17d) in the beam hardening corrected perfusion map agreed well with the corresponding TTC finding, which confirmed infarction in the apical myocardium (yellow arrows in Figure 2.17e).

by another validation study that also demonstrated an improved correlation between CTP and microspheres after beam hardening correction was employed [93]. The MP map with beam hardening correction also agreed well with the finding of postmortem tissue staining with viability agent (2,3,5 triphenyltetrazolium chloride [TTC]). The apical myocardium that exhibited low/no flow in the MP map (Figure 2.17d) was unstained in the corresponding TTC-stained tissue section (Figure 2.17e) confirming infarction in this segment.

2.5 Clinical Applications

In this section, a general overview of the current or potential clinical application of CTP for a number of prevalent diseases is provided. Results from one model-based (J&W model) deconvolution CTP method is also shown for the purpose of illustration.

2.5.1 Acute Stroke

CT plays an important role in acute stroke diagnosis and prognosis. At our institution, a noncontrast CT (NCCT), from skull base to vertex, and CT angiography (CTA), from carotid bifurcation to vertex, are used for triage. In the case of a patient with cerebral ischemia, a two-phase CTP is administered. Herein we discuss multimodal CT applications for cerebral ischemia and hemorrhagic subtypes, with a focus on CTP imaging. Briefly, the current and potential uses of CTP in acute stroke include (1) quantifying total ischemia and defining infarct core and penumbra for acute ischemic stroke (AIS), (2) predicting hemorrhagic transformation (HT) of AIS, (3) predicting hematoma expansion volume in primary intracerebral hemorrhage (ICH), and (4) assessing ischemia associated with vasospasm in subarachnoid hemorrhage (SAH).

2.5.1.1 Acute Ischemic Stroke

2.5.1.1.1 Treatment Window

Cerebral ischemia makes up 80% of all stroke subtypes. Early restoration of blood flow using thrombolytic therapy is the most effective way to reverse stroke symptoms [94]. Until recently, the IV tissue plasminogen activator (tPA) therapeutic window was 3 hours from stroke onset [95]. This time constraint has limited its use to less than 7% of AIS patients as the risk of HT outweighed the clinical benefit beyond the 3-hour treatment window [96]. Several important studies have investigated

the use of tPA beyond the 3-hour treatment window, namely, the 2008 European Cooperative Acute Stroke Study (ECASS III), followed by a similar study in 2009 examining a broad range of subgroups of patients, both comparing groups given alteplase or placebo after the 3 hours postictus; observational studies investigating the Safe Implementation of Treatments in Stroke (SITS) through an Internet-based audit of the International Stroke Thrombolysis Registry (ISTR); and the Canadian Alteplase for Stroke Effectiveness Study (CASES), both comparing patients receiving alteplase before and after the 3-hour window [94,97–99]. Administration of IV-tPA within the 3–4.5 hours window was shown to be efficacious in ECASS III, a double-blind placebo-controlled trial, which represents a higher level of evidence than the nonrandomized uncontrolled SITS, ISTR, and CASES trials. Nevertheless, overall consensus that IV-tPA has proven benefits up to 4.5 hours from stroke onset was shown. Current alternatives to thrombolysis are the Mechanical Embolus Removal in Cerebral Ischemia device and Penumbra clot retrieval device, which can be used up to 8 hours poststroke onset, and are the only treatments available after the 4.5-hour IV-tPA treatment window [100,101]. Both devices have high reperfusion rates and low rates of intracranial hemorrhage; however, sample sizes of those trials were small, and proof of clinical benefit has not been firmly established [102].

A positive correlation exists between the size of the hyperacute parenchymal hypoattenuation on CT (defined as tissue that is nonviable, even if reperfusion occurs), incidence of HT, and subsequent clinical deterioration [103]. With this in mind, a major goal of acute neuroimaging for AIS is to eliminate the rigid temporal criterion used to decide if thrombolytic therapy is appropriate. Instead, a patient-specific criterion, based on the amount of nonviable tissue at the time of onset, is currently being explored by many investigators, using a number of imaging modalities.

2.5.1.1.2 Assessment of Early Ischemic Changes

Currently, the NCCT acquisition is the most common imaging modality used to make tPA administration decisions. Contraindications for tPA, as observed on NCCT, are (1) ICH and (2) any region of hypointensity, which likely reflects nonviable tissue, greater than 1/3 MCA territory [104,105]. Notwithstanding general acceptance of the above criteria, interobserver agreement for the criterion of 1/3 MCA territory involvement is rather poor [104]. The Alberta Stroke Program Early CT Score (ASPECTS) is a 10-point rating system for assessing the extent of early ischemic changes (EIC) on NCCT [106]. It is easy to implement, using two representative slices from the admission NCCT, and provides valuable information on predicting patient outcome after thrombolysis. When compared with the 1/3 MCA rule, ASPECTS has been shown to have an improved reliability and interobserver concurrence in identifying stroke patients unlikely to make an independent recovery despite thrombolytic treatment [105–107]. The Clot Burden Score and the Boston Acute Stroke Imaging Scale are also used for the successful assessment of EIC [108]. In spite of their clinical usefulness, through the semiquantification of EIC, the ability of these diagnostic tests to localize embolisms, predict outcome, determine HT risk, and even correctly assess EIC is unsatisfactory [109,110].

Assessment of CTP maps using ASPECTS has been explored by several investigators [7,111,112]. There was consensus that, compared to NCCT-ASPECTS, CBV-ASPECTS was a better predictor of clinical outcome at 24 hours and could be considered an early predictor of fatal stroke [7,111–113]. Moreover, one study suggested that CTP-ASPECTS was able to identify the amount of potentially salvageable ischemic tissue [111].

Recently, CTA-SI have been shown to corroborate final infarct volumes from diffusion-weighted imaging, even when reperfusion occurs [114]. This method of ischemic tissue delineation is appealing for clinicians as CTA provides whole brain coverage [115]. Yet, many CTA-SI lesions have been shown to overestimate the infarct core, by including tissue at risk [116].

2.5.1.1.3 Perfusion Parameter Thresholds for Infarction

Using CTP, hemodynamic thresholds from multiple parameters could be utilized to define the acute infarct core. Since absolute CTP parameter values may depend on the details of the processing (or deconvolution)

algorithm, using relative thresholds have been proposed as an alternative. Schaefer et al. had success with defining infarction using normalized (to contralateral hemisphere) CTP CBF values [117]. It is critical that the contralateral ROI contains a similar distribution of gray and white matter, as both tissue types have different CBF and CBV values [118]. Similarly, absolute thresholds obtained from ROIs with a mix of gray and white matter tissue may present a problem, as both tissue types have different CBF and CBV. To circumvent this issue, two studies by Murphy et al. determined individual gray and white matter threshold values for infarct core [119,120]. The goal of these studies was to determine which hemodynamic parameter (derived by delay-sensitive deconvolution algorithm) best differentiated between regions of ischemic tissue that recovered upon recanalization (penumbra and oligemia) and regions of ischemic tissue that infarcted, as confirmed on 5–7 day NCCT. Logistic regression was applied to patients who recanalized by 24 hours postonset, to determine a CBF × CBV product (interaction) threshold for both tissue types. The CBF × CBV product values of 31.3 and 8.14 for gray and white matter, in that order, were the most sensitive (97% and 95%) and specific (97% and 94%) among all other parameters (Figure 2.18).

2.5.1.2 Secondary Hemorrhage Risk

The risk of hemorrhage secondary to ischemic stroke often precludes treatment with thrombolysis, as it occurs in 2.2%–44.0% of AIS patients and is the single most important risk factor to consider in deciding

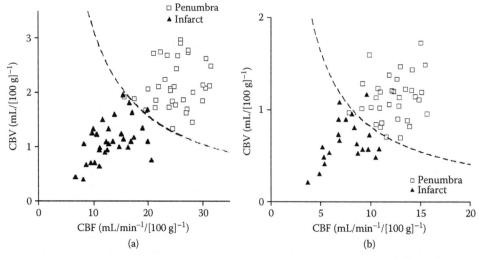

FIGURE 2.18

Scatter plots show mean CBV versus mean CBF in penumbra and infarct regions in patients with acute stroke and confirmed recanalization at 24 hours. Gray matter and white matter regions are left (a) and right (b) graphs, respectively. Dashed line is defined by equation derived from logistic regression (CBF·CBV = 8.14, white matter; CBF·CBV = 31.3, gray matter) that offers the optimal sensitivity and specificity for infarction. By definition, all points above this line are classified as penumbras by the model, while all points below the line are classified as infarcts.

whether thrombolytic therapy should be given [121]. AIS-related hemorrhage is divided into parenchymal hemorrhage (PH) and hemorrhagic infarction (HI), the former increasing mortality risk by 10-fold [122]. While more severe hemorrhage is undoubtedly associated with worse outcome, there is controversy whether less severe forms of hemorrhage are clinically important. Some investigators believe non-PH HT may represent a clinically irrelevant epiphenomenon, with different pathogenesis [123]. If this is the case, the ability to predict PH, the symptomatic hemorrhage subtype, at the acute stroke phase is critical to guide early treatment. Several groups have explored the use of biomarkers as well as CT and MRI imaging in an attempt to predict secondary hemorrhage; however, low sensitivity and specificity have limited their use in acute triage. The authors recently determined whether BBB PS at admission differed between patients with ($n = 23$) and without ($n = 18$) subsequent hemorrhage [121]. Figure 2.19 depicts a patient with HI-2 and a patient with PH-1, according to the ECASS III criteria [97]. The mean PS for the HT group was 0.49 mL/min^{-1}/(100 g)$^{-1}$, which was significantly higher than that for the non-HT group, 0.09 mL/min^{-1}/(100 g)$^{-1}$. The optimal PS cutoff to predict HT during the acute stroke phase was 0.23 mL/min^{-1}/(100 g)$^{-1}$, which had a 77% sensitivity

and 94% specificity. Unfortunately, higher PS values were not correlated with the more severe type of hemorrhage, PH-1 and PH-2 in this trial involving only a small number of patients. In a similar study examining acute BBB permeability in 32 patients with AIS, Hom et al. were able to predict symptomatic HT and malignant edema (using a predefined lower threshold of 5 mL/min^{-1}/100 g^{-1}) with 100% sensitivity and 79% specificity [124]. However, only three patients developed symptomatic HT, a diagnosis that has since been refuted [125]. There is a need for a multicenter study to examine the use of the PS parameter during AIS triage.

2.5.1.3 Subarachnoid Hemorrhage

Delayed vasospasm is the leading cause of death from SAH [126]. Unfortunately, even for patients who undergo early aneurysm repair, the risk of morbidity and mortality due to vasospasm-related ischemia remains high [127]. Transcranial Doppler and CTA are both used for vasospasm identification; however, narrowing in small distal vessels cannot be detected with transcranial Doppler due to its limited spatial resolution and low sensitivity [128]. CTA is limited for evaluation of vessels near to a treated aneurysm because of streak artifacts from the surgical clip or coil pack [129]. Recently, CTP

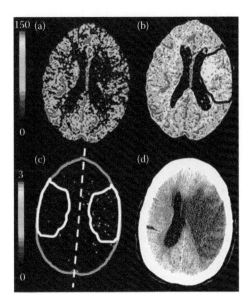
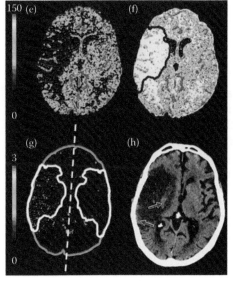

FIGURE 2.19
Panel 1: Patient with small leakage in ischemic region. (a) Admission CT perfusion–derived CBF map of 5-mm-thick brain section displayed with color scale from 0 (dark blue) to 150 (red) mL/min^{-1}/(100 g)$^{-1}$. (b) Corresponding CBF map shows ischemic ROI outlined with help of a yellow overlay of pixels with CBF of less than 25 mL/min^{-1}/(100 g)$^{-1}$. (c) PS map corresponding to Figure 2.19a shows superimposed ischemic ROI and mirrored ROI in contralateral hemisphere. (d) Corresponding delayed NCCT scan of same section shows infarct and HI (arrow). Panel 2: Patient with ischemic region lesion that is larger than that in panel 1. (e) Admission CT perfusion–derived CBF map of 5-mm-thick brain section displayed with color scale from 0 (dark blue) to 150 (red) mL/min^{-1}/(100 g)$^{-1}$. (f) Corresponding CBF map shows ischemic ROI outlined with help of a yellow overlay of pixels with CBF of less than 25 mL/min^{-1}/(100 g)$^{-1}$. (g) PS map corresponding to Figure 2.19e shows superimposed ischemic ROI and mirrored ROI in contralateral hemisphere. (h) Corresponding delayed NCCT scan of same section shows infarct and PH (arrows).

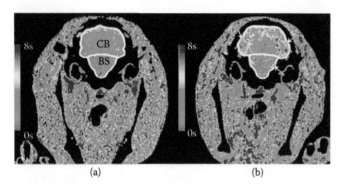

FIGURE 2.20
CTP MTT functional maps for an animal with moderate to severe delayed vasospasm. MTT increases from baseline (a) to day 4 (b) in the brain stem (BS) and cerebellum (CB). The white arrows in Figure 2.20b show areas of increased MTT.

has been used for assessing vasospasm. In 27 patients, Wintermark et al. showed that MTT was more sensitive than CBF or CBV for delayed vasospasm. Moreover, a study from our institution demonstrated a similar outcome in a rabbit model of SAH (Figure 2.20) [126]. Specifically, the prolongation of MTT predicted not only development of vasospasm but also early mortality. The administration of therapeutic vasodilators has also been assessed using CTP; intra-arterial nicardipine improved CBF and MTT within ischemic regions in patients with SAH-induced vasospasm [130]. Clearly, the CTP-derived hemodynamics and the anatomical information on vasospasm from CTA are invaluable in the management of SAH.

2.5.1.4 Primary Intracerebral Hemorrhage

Primary, nontraumatic ICH accounts for 10%–15% of strokes worldwide, with a 30-day mortality of 32%–50%, almost half of these deaths occurring during the acute stage [131]. ICH affects supra- and infratentorial areas of the brain as a result of ruptured vessels affected by hypertension, amyloid angiopathies, and use of anticoagulants. Conventional catheter angiography is the gold standard for identification of ICH etiology; however, CTA and NCCT imaging are now considered the modalities of choice for the acute investigation of ICH.

Total volume of extravasated blood and hematoma expansion are associated with poorer neurological outcome [132]. The cause of early hematoma expansion is unknown, but secondary vessel injury and perihematomal ischemia have been implicated [133]. Although CTP is rarely used for acute diagnosis of ICH, recent perfusion studies have attempted to find secondary ischemic changes in surrounding tissue, leading to edema and possibly worsening clinical outcome. Briefly, Rosand et al. revealed a gradient of perihematomal hypoperfusion, which may have been associated with ischemic

changes [134]. Subsequent findings by Fainardi et al. demonstrated that this centrifugal CBF distribution around the hematoma was not suggestive of ischemic penumbra destined to survive, but rather indicative of edema formation, a potential confounding factor in hematoma growth [135]. During the first 3 hours of symptom onset, early hematoma growth is seen in 18%–38% of patients with ICH, reducing to 11% thereafter [132]. Mitigating secondary bleeding is imperative when dealing with ICH. Reduction in blood pressure along with the administration of recombinant factor VIIa may relieve hematoma expansion; however, improvement in clinical outcome has not been shown, except in a small subset of patients [136,137].

Extravasation is demonstrated on acute CTA and postcontrast CT (PCCT) in 40%–50% of patients, which is associated with hematoma expansion and increased mortality [138]. Using a dual-phase CTP scan, the authors measured PS, the rate of contrast extravasation, within the CTA and PCCT foci of contrast leakage. Patients with/without extravasation had a percentage hematoma volume change of 28% and −1.5%, respectively. Hematoma expansion correlated with the rate of contrast extravasation given by the PS parameter. Average PS values were CTA foci (spot sign), 6.5 ± 1.60 mL/min^{-1}/(100 g)$^{-1}$; PCCT foci (postcontrast leakage), 0.95 ± 0.39 mL/min^{-1}/(100 g)$^{-1}$; hematoma without extravasation, 0.12 ± 0.39 mL/min^{-1}/(100 g)$^{-1}$ (Figure 2.21). Thus, PS is a useful CTP parameter to objectively assess early hematoma expansion, rather than the qualitative assessment of CT scans. CTP studies may play an important part in the management of ICH.

2.5.2 Brain Tumor

Malignant gliomas, the most common primary intracranial tumors in adults, are World Health Organization (WHO) grade III and IV tumors that may arise from astrocytes, oligodendrocytes, and ependymal cells and give rise to astrocytomas, oligodendrogliomas, and ependymomas, respectively. Of these, grade IV glioma (glioblastoma multiforme) is the most common, and the standard of care for these tumors includes surgical resection followed by radiotherapy and concurrent and adjuvant temozolomide chemotherapy, and the median survival for these patients is around 14 months [139]. Conventional anatomical imaging techniques using contrast-enhanced CT and magnetic resonance (MR) are routinely used for guiding surgery and radiotherapy [140] and for assessing radiographic response [141].

Anatomical imaging provides information for delineating areas of increased contrast enhancement, but it does not provide physiologic and hemodynamic information regarding the vascularity of the tumor. BBB disruption is evident when brain tumors grow beyond a diameter of 1–2 mm [142]. Malignant gliomas are

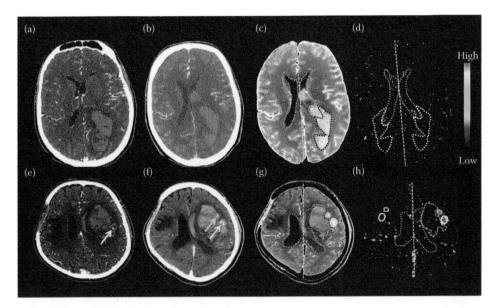

FIGURE 2.21
Panel 1: (a) CTA and (b) PCCT with no visible contrast extravasation within the hematoma. (c) Perfusion weighted image (PWI) and (d) PS map. A region of interest encircles the hematoma on the PWI. The hematoma region of interest is superimposed on the PS map, excluding overlap with ventricles, and is reflected about the midline. Panel 2: (e) CTA with the spot sign visible (yellow arrow). (f) PCCT shows PCL (green arrow) and the spot sign with extravasation (yellow arrow). (g) PWI and (h) PS map. Regions of interest encircle the contrast extravasation (spot sign and PCL) on the PWI and the entire hematoma, excluding extravasation and overlap with ventricles (intraventricular hemorrhage). Regions of interest are superimposed on the PS map and are reflected about the\ midline.

aggressive tumors that infiltrate the brain parenchyma by recruiting leaky and defective vascular networks through angiogenesis [142], which results in higher blood volume and permeability within the tumors [143]. For this reason, there is a growing interest in using perfusion imaging for assessing malignant gliomas. CTP is one of several perfusion imaging techniques that can be used to provide valuable information about brain tumors not available using conventional anatomical imaging. CBF, CBV, and PS measured with CTP have been shown to be higher in brain tumors than the normal brain (Figure 2.22) [144–148]. CTP has potential applications in preoperative grading of malignant gliomas, guiding biopsies to sample the most aggressive portion of the tumor, and assessing patient prognosis and response to treatment.

2.5.2.1 Histopathologic Grading

The WHO classification of brain tumors is currently the most widely used system for differentiating glioma grades. Grading of gliomas is based on histopathologic assessment of cellularity, pleomorphism, mitotic rate, and the presence of endothelial proliferation and necrosis [149]. The presence of vascular proliferation and necrosis are characteristic of high-grade glioma and can potentially be interrogated by vascular imaging techniques. In particular, gliomas can be very heterogeneous tumors in which low-grade, high-grade, and necrotic regions may be present within the same tumor volume [150]. Histopathologic assessment and grading are typically based on a limited number of tissue samples obtained by stereotactic biopsy or surgical resection. Thus, inaccurate grading may occur as a result of limited sampling of tissue. CTP studies–derived CBV and PS can be used to differentiate low- versus high-grade gliomas (C-statistic = 0.930 and 0.927, respectively), while PS can also differentiate WHO grade III gliomas from grade IV gliomas (C-statistic = 0.926) [151–153]. Thus, perfusion studies may be a valuable adjunct to histopathologic sampling and using CBV and PS could potentially help guide stereotactic biopsy to sample the most aggressive part of the tumor.

2.5.2.2 Prognosis

CTP can also provide prognostic information. Perfusion parameters have demonstrated significant associations with more aggressive phenotypes in gliomas. Specifically, CBV demonstrated a significant correlation with microvascular density in newly diagnosed and recurrent malignant gliomas [154,155]. Patients with a higher relative CBV were also associated with a shorter time to progression than those with a lower relative CBV [156]. Voxel-based analysis of CBV acquired at weeks 1 and 3 posttreatment initiation showed strong correlations with 6-month progression-free survival, 1-year survival, and overall survival, which could not be predicted

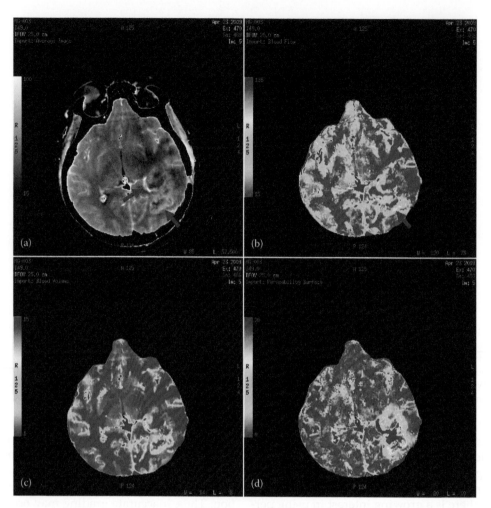

FIGURE 2.22
Representative images of (a) an averaged CT image and maps of (b) cerebral blood flow, (c) cerebral blood volume, and (d) permeability-surface area product of a patient's brain. Red arrows indicate the location of the glioma.

by conventional radiographic assessment [157,158]. Furthermore, PS has been correlated with microvascular cellular proliferation and the expressions of proangiogenic genes [154,159]. The volume of vascular leakage was shown to be a strong predictor of overall survival, while the average vascular permeability was a predictor of time to progression in malignant gliomas [160]. Evidence from these studies suggests that perfusion imaging using CT or MR can identify tumor regions that have a more aggressive phenotype and that perfusion parameters may be used as prognostic markers of survival.

2.5.2.3 Assessment of Treatment Response

Radiographic response assessment is traditionally based on changes in the size of the contrast-enhancing lesion that is visible on CT or MR. However, posttreatment changes in contrast enhancement could be induced by treatments (e.g., use of steroids and antiangiogenic agents and treatment-induced necrosis), nontumoral

processes (e.g., postsurgical changes, inflammation, and ischemia), and tumor progression [141]. For these reasons, differentiating recurrent or progressive tumors from other underlying causes of contrast enhancement is a challenge to radiographic assessment. Jain et al. showed that recurrent tumors had a higher CBF, CBV, and PS than treatment-induced necrosis [8,161]. Relative CBV could distinguish treatment-induced necrosis from recurrence with a 81.5% and 90% sensitivity and specificity, respectively, while PS had a sensitivity and specificity of 81.5% and 81.8%, respectively [161].

The addition of antiangiogenic agents (e.g., bevacizumab) to the treatment of malignant gliomas can complicate the assessment of radiographic response. Since some antiangiogenic agents could reduce vascular permeability, a rapid decrease in contrast enhancement shortly after the administration of antiangiogenic agent may not reflect true antitumor effect [141]. Perfusion imaging techniques have potential applications in assessing response to antiangiogenic therapies. Using

CTP, a significant reduction in tumor perfusion could be observed in a number of cancers treated with antiangiogenic agents [11,162,163]. In addition, reductions in perfusion parameters after antiangiogenic therapy were shown to be predictive of progression-free and overall survival in brain tumor patients [164,165].

2.5.3 Liver Tumor

Early stage liver tumors are often asymptomatic and therefore not diagnosed until resection is no longer an option due to nodal involvement, extrahepatic spread, tumor size, or preexisting liver disease. Patients with inoperable liver cancer will receive a number of noncurative therapies including chemotherapy, chemoembolization, ablation, or radiotherapy—all these therapies rely on medical imaging for treatment planning and monitoring.

CTP has been shown to be able to differentiate cancerous and normal tissue in both primary and metastatic tumors in a number of studies. Tumors cause elevation in arterial blood flow and permeability surface product and reduction in blood volume compared to normal tissue [45,166–168]. Cirrhosis is known to also cause elevated arterial blood flow especially in patients with Child C class disease [169,170], but does not elevate PS [171], which may aid in differentiating cancerous tissue from cirrhotic noncancerous tissue, which can be difficult using traditional triphasic contract-enhanced CT imaging. No studies have been published comparing tumor delineation from CTP to traditional anatomical imaging modalities in the liver, although many studies have shown the efficacy of CTP in early evaluation of treatment response of liver cancer and normal tissue complications. Examples of contrast-enhanced CT images and CTP functional maps (blood flow and arterial blood flow) are shown for two patients diagnosed with hepatocellular carcinoma (HCC) in Figure 2.23. Images shown for patient A were acquired 6 months postexternal beam radiotherapy (32 Gy in six fractions) and 9 months post-trans-arterial chemoembolization (TACE) and showed elevated total and arterial blood flow in most of the tumor, indicating existence of functioning vascular network. Patient B was treated with external beam radiotherapy 24 months prior to when the shown images were acquired, and no significant elevation of total or arterial blood flow is noticeable in the main lesion (yellow arrow); however, a smaller focus of elevated arterial and total blood flow is apparent posterior to main lesion (white arrows)—this lesion was clinically confirmed to be a metastasis.

2.5.3.1 Chemotherapy

Pretreatment tumor blood flow and blood volume have shown some promise in predicting early response to treatment with thalidomide in patients with HCC [172]. In patients with metastatic colorectal carcinoma, reduction rate in tumor blood flow has shown correlation with response evaluation criteria in solid tumors (RECIST) response criteria following a cycle of chemotherapy with XELOX, FOLFOX, or FOLFIRI [173]. Pretreatment tumor permeability surface product was found to correlate with RECIST response in colorectal carcinoma patients treated with oxaliplatin, capecitabine, and bevacizumab; however, no correlation was found with pretreatment or posttreatment blood flow or blood volume [174].

2.5.3.2 Chemoembolization

HCC patients with partial RECIST response following TACE display significant reduction in tumor blood flow, blood volume, and arterial blood flow, whereas patients with stable or progressive disease show increasing or unchanged tumor perfusion parameters [175]. Following TACE treatment of HCC parts of the tumor may remain viable; CTP has been shown to be capable of distinguishing these viable regions that present with continued elevated arterial and total blood flow compared to parenchyma and responding parts of the tumor [46].

2.5.3.3 Radiofrequency Ablation

Local recurrence rates following radiofrequency ablation of HCC range from 12% to 35% in published literature [176–178]. Significant focal arterial blood flow elevation was found to be indicative of local recurrence at the rim of the treated lesion and correlated with 18-FDG (fluorodeoxyglucose) PET [10].

2.5.3.4 Radiotherapy

CTP has yet to be tested as a predictor of tumor control following external beam radiotherapy or for assessment of local recurrence in the liver. Initial studies indicate that CTP can be used to monitor normal liver response following radiotherapy and predict reduction in organ dysfunction, specifically portal vein perfusion has been shown to be reduced in healthy liver by radiation [179] and reduction in portal vein perfusion has been shown to correlate with overall organ function measured through indocyanine green clearance [180].

2.5.4 Coronary Artery Disease

One important management goal for patients with chronic CAD and left ventricular dysfunction is to prevent the onset of acute MI, which has a poor short-term prognosis—the median 30-day mortality rate post-acute MI is 16% [181]. Additionally, acute MI may trigger complications including heart failure, arrhythmias,

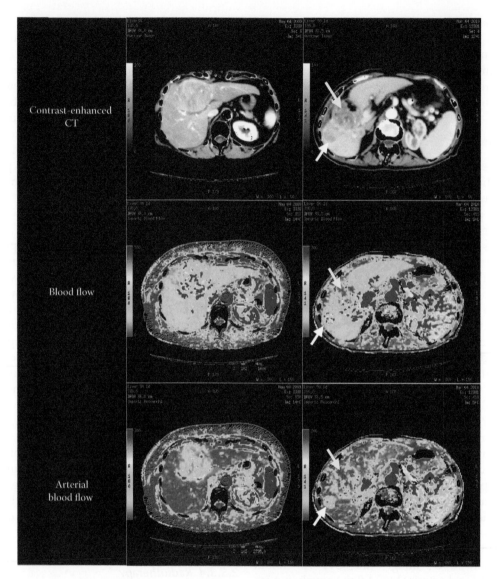

FIGURE 2.23
Patient A is 70 years old, diagnosed with hepatocellular carcinoma, clearly visible in all images. Patient B is 80 years old, diagnosed with recurrent hepatocellular carcinoma. The main lesion (indicated by yellow arrows) was treated with 3D conformal radiotherapy two years before recurrence in the right posterior liver adjacent to original tumor site (indicated with white arrows).

and secondary MI, leading to high hospital readmission rate [181] and poor survival rate [182]. Currently, patients with advanced multivessel or left main CAD can be treated with two types of interventions: coronary artery bypass grafting and percutaneous coronary intervention with bare-metal or drug-eluted stents. However, these procedures contribute a heavy economic burden to the health-care system [183,184]. Decision making on revascularization is further complicated by the high risks associated with these procedures including stroke, bleeding requiring transfusion, and vascular complications [185–187]. This emphasizes better diagnostic strategies are needed to reduce unnecessary interventions and demands on health-care resources. Currently, noninvasive imaging tests are focused on three aspects

to determine the need of intervention for CAD patients associated with chronic left ventricular dysfunction: (1) anatomic evaluation of stenosis severity, (2) functional assessment of myocardial ischemia, and (3) anatomic/functional identification of myocardial viability.

2.5.4.1 SPECT versus CTP for Assessing Myocardial Ischemia

SPECT stress testing has been the most commonly used technique to identify functional ischemia associated with CAD over the past decades [188]. Compelling evidence from the Clinical Outcomes Utilizing Revascularization and Aggressive Drug Evaluation (COURAGE) trial [189] and a large single-center trial involving over

10,000 patients [190] suggests that patients with a moderate to severe ischemia detected by SPECT has reduced mortality rate and infarction with revascularization. Although a meta-analysis on over 80 high-quality studies demonstrated that SPECT has a pooled sensitivity and specificity of 90% and 75% for identifying high-grade coronary stenosis [191], its sensitivity for detecting multivessel CAD is particularly poor [192]. SPECT, being a qualitative technique, requires comparison of abnormal to normal. As such, it tends to underestimate the true extent of multivessel CAD in which there is no normally perfused myocardium as reference for abnormally perfused segments to compare [193]. More recently, a few groups have shown that CTP can be a useful tool for measuring MP [13–15,194,195]. Specifically, a recent pilot study on 26 CAD patients performed at our hospital [13] demonstrated that, after proper correction of beam hardening, CTP measurement of MP reserve (MPR),

defined as the ratio of MP during maximal vasodilatory stress to that at rest, is in good agreement with perfusion deficit and coronary stenosis identified by SPECT and invasive coronary angiography (ICA), respectively. The advantage of quantitative CTP over qualitative SPECT was highlighted by a clinical case shown in Figure 2.24, in which all three coronary arteries of the CAD patient were ≥75% stenosed. While CTP demonstrated reversible ischemia in all three coronary territories, SPECT could only detect reversible ischemia in the RC territory.

2.5.4.2 Combined CTA and CTP for Anatomic and Functional Diagnosis of CAD

Over the past decade, CCTA has become a routine technique for evaluating CAD by direct anatomic visualization of stenosis similar to ICA but without the complications associated with catheterization due to the use

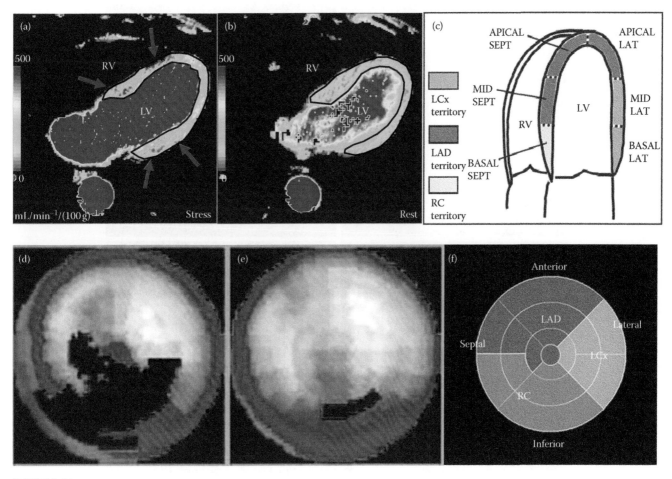

FIGURE 2.24
Quantitative CT myocardial perfusion (MP) maps at maximal vasodilatory stress (a) and at rest (b) of a patient who had a significant triple-vessel CAD, in which all the three coronary arteries were ≥75% stenosed. Reversible ischemia (red arrows in Figure 2.24a) was seen in all three coronary territories (schematic in Figure 2.24c) in the approximate horizontal long-axis CTP MP maps. Qualitative SPECT MIBI MP maps of the same patient at stress (d) and rest (e), displayed in the bulls-eye view, revealed reversible ischemia only in the right coronary territory (red arrows in Figure 2.24d and "RC" in Figure 2.24f). Qualitative perfusion analysis tends to underestimate the true extent of a triple-vessel CAD as there is no normally perfused myocardium for reference.

of noninvasive CT scanning [196,197]. Although multicenter trials have demonstrated high sensitivity and negative predictive value to detect high-grade stenosis as compared to the gold standard ICA, identification of high-grade stenosis by CCTA itself is not a reliable indicator of physiologic ischemia. Two recent clinical studies comparing CCTA with SPECT [198] and fractional flow reserve [199] demonstrated limited diagnostic accuracies, highlighting the inconsistent relationship between stenosis and functional myocardial ischemia. By acquiring additional CTP scans while the patient remains on the scanner table after the CCTA study, information regarding the functional significance of a specific coronary lesion can be revealed. Figure 2.25 shows a combined CTA-CTP examination of a CAD patient, whose LAD artery was subtotally occluded while the left circumflex (LCx) artery was absent of stenosis. Reversible ischemia was induced in the LAD territory downstream of the significant LAD

stenosis after maximal dipyridamole (vasodilator) stimuli, while in the adjacent LCx territory, there was a normal increase in MP from baseline after stress. In the aforementioned pilot study [13], CTP measurement of MPR with beam hardening correction exhibited a nonlinear inverse relationship with the severity of coronary stenosis identified by ICA (Figure 2.26a), suggesting the potential use of combined CTA-CTP anatomic and functional assessment of CAD. Furthermore, myocardial volume reserve (MVR), defined similarly as MPR but with respect to myocardial blood volume (MBV), can also be measured simultaneously with MP and MPR using a model-based deconvolution analysis method (Figure 2.26a). Logistic regression analysis suggested that MPR·MVR could be a better predictor than MPR or MVR alone for differentiating <50% from ≥50% coronary stenosis. This implies MVR may provide additional information regarding any physiologic change induced by coronary lesions above

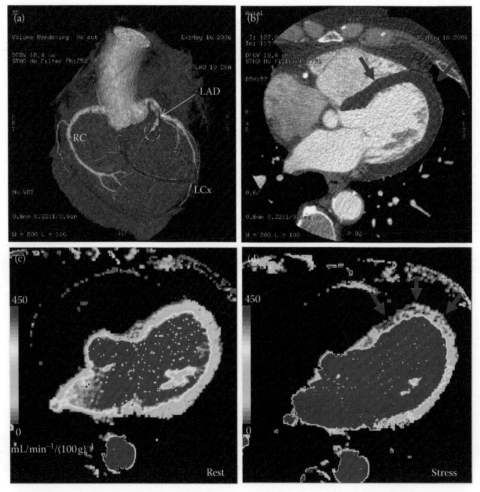

FIGURE 2.25

(a) Volume rendered CCTA image of a CAD patient and (b) the corresponding CCTA source image. Contour of the myocardium was highlighted with a green ROI, which was superimposed to the volume rendered CCTA image in Figure 2.25a. MP maps (c) at rest and (d) during maximal vasodilatory stress. Increase in MP from rest was significantly attenuated in the apical and septal wall (red arrows in Figure 2.25a and 2.25c), which was perfused by a subtotally occluded left anterior descending (LAD) artery (occlusion indicated by white dashed circle in Figure 2.25a), whereas there was over two times increase in MP from baseline in the lateral wall perfused by a nonstenosed left circumflex (LCx) artery.

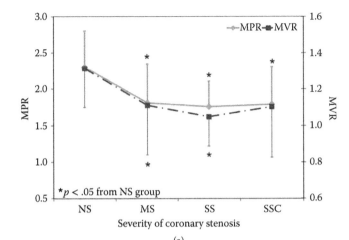

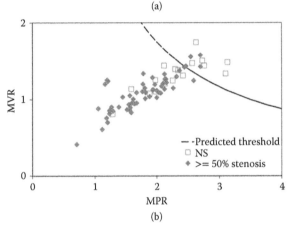

FIGURE 2.26
(a) CTP measurements of MPR and MVR exhibited an inverse relationship with the severity of coronary stenosis in 26 CAD patients. Error bars represent standard deviation of the mean values. (b) Scatter plot of MVR versus MPR of all coronary territories in the same group of CAD patients. The dashed line represents the threshold of MPR·MVR (3.5) determined by logistic regression for maximal separation between the nonstenosed (NS) and stenosed (MS, SS, SSC) coronary arteries.

and beyond that provided by the measurement of MP or MPR alone. The threshold of MPR·MVR that provides the optimal differentiation of <50% and ≥50% stenoses is shown in Figure 2.26b. Further investigations on the usefulness of MVR in addition to the MPR measurement are warranted.

2.5.4.3 Assessment of Myocardial Infarction

CT measurement of MP could also provide unique diagnostic information regarding the viability status of ischemic myocardium [200,201]. Because there is no technique enabling the direct visualization of the coronary microcirculation in vivo, MP measurement at rest and during maximal pharmacologic stress provides surrogate evaluation on the functional status of coronary microcirculation [202]. Absence of MP both at rest and during stress indicates the presence of microvascular

obstruction, which is a hallmark of infarction [203]. The superior spatial resolution of CTP allows accurate delineation of the infarct size (Figures 2.17d and 2.17e), which is closely related to the short- and long-term mortality risk associated with acute MI [204,205].

2.6 Conclusion

In this chapter, we reviewed the theoretical basis of various CTP methods, technical issues of CTP implementations, preclinical validations, and clinical applications of one model-based deconvolution CTP technique. Compared with the indicator-dilution and maximal slope approaches, the model-based deconvolution method provides a more robust and accurate estimation of blood flow and other physiologic parameters at the tissue level. Iodinated contrast material and scanning parameters should be carefully selected to ensure optimal quality of the DCE CT images for CTP analysis. Previous animal studies have demonstrated excellent agreement between CTP and gold standard microspheres for quantitative perfusion measurement. Initial clinical data supports CTP as a useful tool to prognose, diagnose, and guide therapy of common diseases including stroke, cancer, and CAD. Dose reduction techniques should be implemented to facilitate the application of CTP in these clinical settings.

References

1. Axel L. Cerebral blood flow determination by rapid-sequence computed tomography: Theoretical analysis. *Radiology* 1980; 137: 679–686.
2. Prokop M. New challenges in MDCT. *Eur Radiol* 2005; 15(Suppl 5): E35–E45.
3. Page M, Nandurkar D, Crossett MP, Stuckey SL, Lau KP, Kenning N, Troupis JM. Comparison of 4 cm z-axis and 16 cm z-axis multidetector CT perfusion. *Eur Radiol* 2010; 20: 1508–1514.
4. Flohr TG, Raupach R, Bruder H. Cardiac CT: How much can temporal resolution, spatial resolution, and volume coverage be improved? *J Cardiovasc Comput Tomogr* 2009; 3: 143–152.
5. Obach V, Oleaga L, Urra X, Macho J, Amaro S, Capurro S et al. Multimodal CT-assisted thrombolysis in patients with acute stroke: A cohort study. *Stroke* 2011; 42: 1129–1131.
6. Silvennoinen HM, Hamberg LM, Lindsberg PJ, Valanne L, Hunter GJ. CT perfusion identifies increased salvage of tissue in patients receiving intravenous recombinant tissue plasminogen activator within 3 hours of stroke onset. *AJNR Am J Neuroradiol* 2008; 29: 1118–1123.

7. Aviv RI, Mandelcorn J, Chakraborty S, Gladstone D, Malham S, Tomlinson G, Fox AJ, Symons S. Alberta stroke program early CT scoring of CT perfusion in early stroke visualization and assessment. *AJNR Am J Neuroradiol* 2007; 28: 1975–1980.

8. Jain R, Scarpace L, Ellika S, Schultz LR, Rock JP, Rosenblum ML, Patel SC, Lee TY, Mikkelsen T. First-pass perfusion computed tomography: Initial experience in differentiating recurrent brain tumors from radiation effects and radiation necrosis. *Neurosurgery* 2007; 61: 778–786; discussion 786–787.

9. Nakashige A, Horiguchi J, Tamura A, Asahara T, Shimamoto F, Ito K. Quantitative measurement of hepatic portal perfusion by multidetector row CT with compensation for respiratory misregistration. *Br J Radiol* 2004; 77: 728–734.

10. Meijerink MR, van Cruijsen H, Hoekman K, Kater M, van Schaik C, van Waesberghe JH, Giaccone G, Manoliu RA. The use of perfusion CT for the evaluation of therapy combining AZD2171 with gefitinib in cancer patients. *Eur Radiol* 2007; 17: 1700–1713.

11. Jiang T, Kambadakone A, Kulkarni NM, Zhu AX, Sahani DV. Monitoring response to antiangiogenic treatment and predicting outcomes in advanced hepatocellular carcinoma using image biomarkers, CT perfusion, tumor density, and tumor size (RECIST). *Invest Radiol* 2012; 47: 11–17.

12. George RT, Arbab-Zadeh A, Cerci RJ, Vavere AL, Kitagawa K, Dewey M et al. Diagnostic performance of combined noninvasive coronary angiography and myocardial perfusion imaging using 320-MDCT: The CT angiography and perfusion methods of the CORE320 multicenter multinational diagnostic study. *AJR Am J Roentgenol* 2011; 197: 829–837.

13. So A, Wisenberg G, Islam A, Amann J, Romano W, Brown J et al. Non-invasive assessment of functionally relevant coronary artery stenoses with quantitative CT perfusion: Preliminary clinical experiences. *Eur Radiol* 2012; 22: 39–50.

14. Bastarrika G, Ramos-Duran L, Rosenblum MA, Kang DK, Rowe GW, Schoepf UJ. Adenosine-stress dynamic myocardial CT perfusion imaging: Initial clinical experience. *Invest Radiol* 2010; 45: 306–313.

15. Ho KT, Chua KC, Klotz E, Panknin C. Stress and rest dynamic myocardial perfusion imaging by evaluation of complete time-attenuation curves with dual-source CT. *JACC Cardiovasc Imaging* 2010; 3: 811–820.

16. Meier P, Zierler KL. On the theory of the indicator-dilution method for measurement of blood flow and volume. *J Appl Physiol* 1954; 6: 731–744.

17. Bassingthwaighte JB, Knopp TJ, Anderson DU. Flow estimation by indicator dilution (bolus injection). *Circ Res* 1970; 27: 277–291.

18. Pardridge WM, Oldendorf WH, Cancilla P, Frank HJ. Blood-brain barrier: Interface between internal medicine and the brain. *Ann Intern Med* 1986; 105: 82–95.

19. Crone C. The permeability of capillaries in various organs as determined by use of the 'indicator diffusion' method. *Acta Physiol Scand* 1963; 58: 292–305.

20. Hamilton WF, Moore JW, Kinsman JM, Spurling RG. Simultaneous determination of the pulmonary and systemic circulation times in man and of a figure related to cardiac output. *Am J Physiol* 1928; 84: 338–344.

21. Stephenson JL. Theory of the measurement of blood flow by the dilution of an indicator. *Bull Math Biophys* 1948; 10: 117–121.

22. Gobbel GT, Cann CE, Fike JR. Measurement of regional cerebral blood flow using ultrafast computed tomography. Theoretical aspects. *Stroke* 1991; 22: 768–771.

23. Axel L. Tissue mean transit time from dynamic computed tomography by a simple deconvolution technique. *Invest Radiol* 1983; 18: 94–99.

24. Yang Y, Rosenberg GA. Blood-brain barrier breakdown in acute and chronic cerebrovascular disease. *Stroke* 2011; 42: 3323–3328.

25. de Vries HE, Kuiper J, de Boer AG, Van Berkel TJ, Breimer DD. The blood-brain barrier in neuroinflammatory diseases. *Pharmacol Rev* 1997; 49: 143–155.

26. Mullani NA, Gould KL. First-pass measurements of regional blood flow with external detectors. *J Nucl Med* 1983; 24: 577–581.

27. Miles KA. Measurement of tissue perfusion by dynamic computed tomography. *Br J Radiol* 1991; 64: 409–412.

28. Klotz E, Konig M. Perfusion measurements of the brain: Using dynamic CT for the quantitative assessment of cerebral ischemia in acute stroke. *Eur J Radiol* 1999; 30: 170–184.

29. Ostergaard L, Weisskoff RM, Chesler DA, Gyldensted C, Rosen BR. High resolution measurement of cerebral blood flow using intravascular tracer bolus passages. Part I: Mathematical approach and statistical analysis. *Magn Reson Med* 1996; 36: 715–725.

30. Wintermark M, Thiran JP, Maeder P, Schnyder P, Meuli R. Simultaneous measurement of regional cerebral blood flow by perfusion CT and stable xenon CT: A validation study. *AJNR Am J Neuroradiol* 2001; 22: 905–914.

31. Gamel J, Rousseau WF, Katholi CR, Mesel E. Pitfalls in digital computation of the impulse response of vascular beds from indicator-dilution curves. *Circ Res* 1973; 32: 516–523.

32. Ostergaard L, Sorensen AG, Kwong KK, Weisskoff RM, Gyldensted C, Rosen BR. High resolution measurement of cerebral blood flow using intravascular tracer bolus passages. Part II: Experimental comparison and preliminary results. *Magn Reson Med* 1996; 36: 726–736.

33. Groothuis DR, Lapin GD, Vriesendorp FJ, Mikhael MA, Patlak CS. A method to quantitatively measure transcapillary transport of iodinated compounds in canine brain tumors with computed tomography. *J Cereb Blood Flow Metab* 1991; 11: 939–948.

34. Groothuis DR, Vriesendorp FJ, Kupfer B, Warnke PC, Lapin GD, Kuruvilla A, Vick NA, Mikhael MA, Patlak CS. Quantitative measurements of capillary transport in human brain tumors by computed tomography. *Ann Neurol* 1991; 30: 581–588.

35. Patlak CS, Blasberg RG, Fenstermacher JD. Graphical evaluation of blood-to-brain transfer constants from multiple-time uptake data. *J Cereb Blood Flow Metab* 1983; 3: 1–7.

36. Patlak CS, Blasberg RG. Graphical evaluation of blood-to-brain transfer constants from multiple-time uptake data. Generalizations. *J Cereb Blood Flow Metab* 1985; 5: 584–590.

37. St Lawrence KS, Lee TY. An adiabatic approximation to the tissue homogeneity model for water exchange in the brain: I. Theoretical derivation. *J Cereb Blood Flow Metab* 1998; 18: 1365–1377.

38. Gill PE, Murray W, Wright MH. *Practical optimization.* London: Academic Press; 1981.

39. Johnson JA, Wilson TA. A model for capillary exchange. *Am J Physiol* 1966; 210: 1299–1303.

40. Richardson PD, Withrington PG. Liver blood flow. I. Intrinsic and nervous control of liver blood flow. *Gastroenterology* 1981; 81: 159–173.

41. Schenk WG Jr, Mcdonald JC, Mcdonald K, Drapanas T. Direct measurement of hepatic blood flow in surgical patients: With related observations on hepatic flow dynamics in experimental animals. *Ann Surg* 1962; 156: 463–471.

42. Stewart EE, Chen X, Hadway J, Lee TY. Correlation between hepatic tumor blood flow and glucose utilization in a rabbit liver tumor model. *Radiology* 2006; 239: 740–750.

43. Bae KT. Intravenous contrast medium administration and scan timing at CT: Considerations and approaches. *Radiology* 2010; 256: 32–61.

44. Wintermark M, Smith WS, Ko NU, Quist M, Schnyder P, Dillon WP. Dynamic perfusion CT: Optimizing the temporal resolution and contrast volume for calculation of perfusion CT parameters in stroke patients. *AJNR Am J Neuroradiol* 2004; 25: 720–729.

45. Sahani DV, Holalkere NS, Mueller PR, Zhu AX. Advanced hepatocellular carcinoma: CT perfusion of liver and tumor tissue—initial experience. *Radiology* 2007; 243: 736–743.

46. Ippolito D, Bonaffini PA, Ratti L, Antolini L, Corso R, Fazio F, Sironi S. Hepatocellular carcinoma treated with transarterial chemoembolization: Dynamic perfusion-CT in the assessment of residual tumor. *World J Gastroenterol* 2010; 16: 5993–6000.

47. Claussen CD, Banzer D, Pfretzschner C, Kalender WA, Schörner W. Bolus geometry and dynamics after intravenous contrast medium injection. *Radiology* 1984; 153: 365–368.

48. Miles KA. Perfusion CT for the assessment of tumour vascularity: Which protocol? *Br J Radiol* 2003; 76 Spec No 1: S36–S42.

49. Hopper KD, Mosher TJ, Kasales CJ, TenHave TR, Tully DA, Weaver JS. Thoracic spiral CT: Delivery of contrast material pushed with injectable saline solution in a power injector. *Radiology* 1997; 205: 269–271.

50. Schoellnast H, Tillich M, Deutschmann MJ, Deutschmann HA, Schaffler GJ, Portugaller HR. Aortoiliac enhancement during computed tomography angiography with reduced contrast material dose and saline solution flush: Influence on magnitude and uniformity of the contrast column. *Invest Radiol* 2004; 39: 20–26.

51. Haage P, Schmitz-Rode T, Hübner D, Piroth W, Günther RW. Reduction of contrast material dose and artifacts by a saline flush using a double power injector in helical CT of the thorax. *AJR Am J Roentgenol* 2000; 174: 1049–1053.

52. Coursey CA, Nelson RC, Boll DT, Paulson EK, Ho LM, Neville AM, Marin D, Gupta RT, Schindera ST. Dual-energy multidetector CT: How does it work, what can it tell us, and when can we use it in abdominopelvic imaging? *Radiographics* 2010; 30: 1037–1055.

53. McNitt-Gray MF. AAPM/RSNA physics tutorial for residents: Topics in CT. Radiation dose in CT. *Radiographics* 2002; 22: 1541–1553.

54. McCollough CH, Zink FE. Performance evaluation of a multi-slice CT system. *Med Phys* 1999; 26: 2223–2230.

55. Roberts HC, Roberts TP, Smith WS, Lee TJ, Fischbein NJ, Dillon WP. Multisection dynamic CT perfusion for acute cerebral ischemia: The "toggling-table" technique. *AJNR Am J Neuroradiol* 2001; 22: 1077–1080.

56. Primak AN, Dong Y, Dzyubak OP, Jorgensen SM, McCollough CH, Ritman EL. A technical solution to avoid partial scan artifacts in cardiac MDCT. *Med Phys* 2007; 34: 4726–4737.

57. Meinel JA, Hoffman E, Clough A, Wang G. Reduction of half-scan shading artifact based on full-scan correction. *Acad Radiol* 2006; 13: 55–62.

58. Eldevik K, Nordhoy W, Skretting A. Relationship between sharpness and noise in CT images reconstructed with different kernels. *Radiat Prot Dosimetry* 2010; 139: 430–433.

59. Lee TY, Chhem RK. Impact of new technologies on dose reduction in CT. *Eur J Radiol* 2010; 76: 28–35.

60. Brooks RA, Di Chiro G. Beam hardening in x-ray reconstructive tomography. *Phys Med Biol* 1976; 21: 390–398.

61. Joseph PM, Spital RD. A method for correcting bone induced artifacts in computed tomography scanners. *J Comput Assist Tomogr* 1978; 2: 100–108.

62. So A, Hsieh J, Li JY, Lee TY. Beam hardening correction in CT myocardial perfusion measurement. *Phys Med Biol* 2009; 54: 3031–3050.

63. Stenner P, Schmidt B, Allmendinger T, Flohr T, Kachelrie M. Dynamic iterative beam hardening correction (DIBHC) in myocardial perfusion imaging using contrast-enhanced computed tomography. *Invest Radiol* 2010; 45: 314–323.

64. . So A, Lee TY, Imai Y, Narayanan S, Hsieh J, Kramer J, Procknow K, Leipsic J, Labounty T, Min J. Quantitative myocardial perfusion imaging using rapid kVp switch dual-energy CT: Preliminary experience. *J Cardiovasc Comput Tomogr* 2011; 5: 430–442.

65. Alvarez RE, Macovski A. Energy-selective reconstructions in X-ray computerized tomography. *Phys Med Biol* 1976; 21: 733–744.

66. Einstein AJ, Moser KW, Thompson RC, Cerqueira MD, Henzlova MJ. Radiation dose to patients from cardiac diagnostic imaging. *Circulation* 2007; 116: 1290–1305.

67. Wiesmann M, Berg S, Bohner G, Klingebiel R, Schöpf V, Stoeckelhuber BM, Yousry I, Linn J, Missler U. Dose reduction in dynamic perfusion CT of the brain: Effects of the scan frequency on measurements of cerebral blood flow, cerebral blood volume, and mean transit time. *Eur Radiol* 2008; 18: 2967–2974.

68. Konstas AA, Goldmakher GV, Lee TY, Lev MH. Theoretic basis and technical implementations of CT perfusion in acute ischemic stroke, part 2: Technical implementations. *AJNR Am J Neuroradiol* 2009; 30: 885–892.

69. Goh V, Liaw J, Bartram CI, Halligan S. Effect of temporal interval between scan acquisitions on quantitative vascular parameters in colorectal cancer: Implications for helical volumetric perfusion CT techniques. *AJR Am J Roentgenol* 2008; 191: W288–W292.

70. Bischoff B, Hein F, Meyer T, Krebs M, Hadamitzky M, Martinoff S, Schömig A, Hausleiter J. Comparison of sequential and helical scanning for radiation dose and image quality: Results of the Prospective Multicenter Study on Radiation Dose Estimates of Cardiac CT Angiography (PROTECTION) I Study. *AJR Am J Roentgenol* 2010; 194: 1495–1499.

71. Thibault JB, Sauer KD, Bouman CA, Hsieh J. A three-dimensional statistical approach to improved image quality for multislice helical CT. *Med Phys* 2007; 34: 4526–4544.

72. Yu Z, Thibault JB, Bouman CA, Sauer KD, Hsieh J. Fast model-based X-ray CT reconstruction using spatially nonhomogeneous ICD optimization. *IEEE Trans Image Process* 2011; 20: 161–175.

73. Becker HC, Augart D, Karpitschka M, Ulzheimer S, Bamberg F, Morhard D, Neumaier K, Graser A, Johnson T, Reiser M. Radiation exposure and image quality of normal computed tomography brain images acquired with automated and organ-based tube current modulation multiband filtering and iterative reconstruction. *Invest Radiol* 2012; 47: 202–207.

74. Winklehner A, Karlo C, Puippe G, Schmidt B, Flohr T, Goetti R, Pfammatter T, Frauenfelder T, Alkadhi H. Raw data-based iterative reconstruction in body CTA: Evaluation of radiation dose saving potential. *Eur Radiol* 2011; 21: 2521–2526.

75. Gervaise A, Osemont B, Lecocq S, Noel A, Micard E, Felblinger J, Blum A. CT image quality improvement using adaptive iterative dose reduction with wide-volume acquisition on 320-detector CT. *Eur Radiol* 2012; 22: 295–301.

76. Chen GH, Tang J, Leng S. Prior image constrained compressed sensing (PICCS). *Proc Soc Photo Opt Instrum Eng* 2008; 6856: 685618.

77. Bian J, Siewerdsen JH, Han X, Sidky EY, Prince JL, Pelizzari CA, Pan X. Evaluation of sparse-view reconstruction from flat-panel-detector cone-beam CT. *Phys Med Biol* 2010; 55: 6575–6599.

78. Flury B. *Common principal components and related multivariate models*. New York: John Wiley & Sons; 1988.

79. Jolliffe I. *Principal component analysis*. New York: Springer; 2004.

80. Perona P, Malik J. Scale-space and edge detection using anisotropic diffusion. *IEEE Trans Pattern Anal Mach Intell* 1990; 12: 629–639.

81. Johnson DJ, Muhlbacher F, Wilmore DW. Measurement of hepatic blood flow. *J Surg Res* 1985; 39: 470–481.

82. Ziegler SI, Haberkorn U, Byrne H, Tong C, Kaja S, Richolt JA et al. Measurement of liver blood flow using oxygen-15 labelled water and dynamic positron emission tomography: Limitations of model description. *Eur J Nucl Med* 1996; 23: 169–177.

83. Materne R, Van Beers BE, Smith AM, Leconte I, Jamart J, Dehoux JP, Keyeux A, Horsmans Y. Non-invasive quantification of liver perfusion with dynamic computed tomography and a dual-input one-compartmental model. *Clin Sci (Lond)* 2000; 99: 517–525.

84. Stewart EE, Chen X, Hadway J, Lee TY. Hepatic perfusion in a tumor model using DCE-CT: An accuracy and precision study. *Phys Med Biol* 2008; 53: 4249–4267.

85. Zeger SL, Liang KY, Albert PS. Models for longitudinal data: A generalized estimating equation approach. *Biometrics* 1988; 44: 1049–1060.

86. Heymann MA, Payne BD, Hoffman JI, Rudolph AM. Blood flow measurements with radionuclide-labeled particles. *Prog Cardiovasc Dis* 1977; 20: 55–79.

87. Cenic A, Nabavi DG, Craen RA, Gelb AW, Lee TY. Dynamic CT measurement of cerebral blood flow: A validation study. *AJNR Am J Neuroradiol* 1999; 20: 63–73.

88. Gobbel GT, Cann CE, Iwamoto HS, Fike JR. Measurement of regional cerebral blood flow in the dog using ultrafast computed tomography. Experimental validation. *Stroke* 1991; 22: 772–779.

89. DeWitt DS, Fatouros PP, Wist AO, Stewart LM, Kontos HA, Hall JA, Kishore PR, Keenan RL, Marmarou A. Stable xenon versus radiolabeled microsphere cerebral blood flow measurements in baboons. *Stroke* 1989; 20: 1716–1723.

90. Wolfkiel CJ, Ferguson JL, Chomka EV, Law WR, Labin IN, Tenzer ML, Booker M, Brundage BH. Measurement of myocardial blood flow by ultrafast computed tomography. *Circulation* 1987; 76: 1262–1273.

91. George RT, Silva C, Cordeiro MA, DiPaula A, Thompson DR, McCarthy WF, Ichihara T, Lima JA, Lardo AC. Multidetector computed tomography myocardial perfusion imaging during adenosine stress. *J Am Coll Cardiol* 2006; 48: 153–160.

92. So A, Hsieh J, Li JY, Hadway J, Kong HF, Lee TY. Quantitative myocardial perfusion measurement using CT Perfusion: A validation study in a porcine model of reperfused acute myocardial infarction. *Int J Cardiovasc Imaging* 2012; 28: 1237–1248.

93. Kitagawa K, George RT, Arbab-Zadeh A, Lima JA, Lardo AC. Characterization and correction of beam-hardening artifacts during dynamic volume CT assessment of myocardial perfusion. *Radiology* 2010; 256: 111–118.

94. . Wahlgren N, Ahmed N, Dávalos A, Hacke W, Millán M, Muir K et al. Thrombolysis with alteplase 3–4.5 h after acute ischaemic stroke (SITS-ISTR): An observational study. *Lancet* 2008; 372: 1303–1309.

95. Hacke W, Kaste M, Fieschi C, Toni D, Lesaffre E, von Kummer R et al. Intravenous thrombolysis with recombinant tissue plasminogen activator for acute hemispheric stroke. The European Cooperative Acute Stroke Study (ECASS). *JAMA* 1995; 274: 1017–1025.

96. Schumacher HC, Bateman BT, Boden-Albala B, Berman MF, Mohr JP, Sacco RL, Pile-Spellman J. Use of thrombolysis in acute ischemic stroke: Analysis of the Nationwide Inpatient Sample 1999 to 2004. *Ann Emerg Med* 2007; 50: 99–107.

97. Hacke W, Kaste M, Bluhmki E, Brozman M, Dávalos A, Guidetti D. Thrombolysis with alteplase 3 to 4.5 hours after acute ischemic stroke. *N Engl J Med* 2008; 359: 1317–1329.

98. Bluhmki E, Chamorro A, Dávalos A, Machnig T, Sauce C, Wahlgren N, Wardlaw J, Hacke W. Stroke treatment with alteplase given 3.0–4.5 h after onset of acute ischaemic stroke (ECASS III): Additional outcomes and subgroup analysis of a randomised controlled trial. *Lancet Neurol* 2009; 8: 1095–1102.

99. Shobha N, Buchan AM, Hill MD. Thrombolysis at 3–4.5 hours after acute ischemic stroke onset—Evidence from the Canadian Alteplase for Stroke Effectiveness Study (CASES) registry. *Cerebrovasc Dis* 2011; 31: 223–228.

100. Gobin YP, Starkman S, Duckwiler GR, Grobelny T, Kidwell CS, Jahan R. MERCI 1: A phase 1 study of mechanical embolus removal in cerebral ischemia. *Stroke* 2004; 35: 2848–2854.

101. Tenser MS, Amar AP, Mack WJ. Mechanical thrombectomy for acute ischemic stroke using the MERCI retriever and penumbra aspiration systems. *World Neurosurg* 2011; 76: S16–S23.

102. Baker WL, Colby JA, Tongbram V, Talati R, Silverman IE, White CM, Kluger J, Coleman CI. Neurothrombectomy devices for the treatment of acute ischemic stroke: State of the evidence. *Ann Intern Med* 2011; 154: 243–252.

103. Larrue V, von Kummer RR, Müller A, Bluhmki E. Risk factors for severe hemorrhagic transformation in ischemic stroke patients treated with recombinant tissue plasminogen activator: A secondary analysis of the European-Australasian Acute Stroke Study (ECASS II). *Stroke* 2001; 32: 438–441.

104. Kalafut MA, Schriger DL, Saver JL, Starkman S. Detection of early CT signs of >1/3 middle cerebral artery infarctions: Interrater reliability and sensitivity of CT interpretation by physicians involved in acute stroke care. *Stroke* 2000; 31: 1667–1671.

105. Pexman JH, Barber PA, Hill MD, Sevick RJ, Demchuk AM, Hudon ME, Hu WY, Buchan AM. Use of the alberta stroke program early CT score (ASPECTS) for assessing CT scans in patients with acute stroke. *AJNR Am J Neuroradiol* 2001; 22: 1534–1542.

106. Barber PA, Demchuk AM, Zhang J, Buchan AM. Validity and reliability of a quantitative computed tomography score in predicting outcome of hyperacute stroke before thrombolytic therapy. ASPECTS study group. Alberta stroke programme early CT score. *Lancet* 2000; 355: 1670–1674.

107. Dzialowski I, Hill MD, Coutts SB, Demchuk AM, Kent DM, Wunderlich O, von Kummer R. Extent of early ischemic changes on computed tomography (CT) before thrombolysis: Prognostic value of the alberta stroke program early CT score in ECASS II. *Stroke* 2006; 37: 973–978.

108. Sillanpaa N, Saarinen JT, Rusanen H, Hakomaki J, Lahteela A, Numminen H, Elovaara I, Dastidar P, Soimakallio S. The clot burden score, the Boston Acute Stroke Imaging Scale, the cerebral blood volume ASPECTS, and two novel imaging parameters in the prediction of clinical outcome of ischemic stroke patients receiving intravenous thrombolytic therapy. *Neuroradiology* 2012; 54: 663–672.

109. Madden KP, Karanjia PN, Adams HP Jr, Clarke WR. Accuracy of initial stroke subtype diagnosis in the TOAST study. Trial of ORG 10172 in acute stroke treatment. *Neurology* 1995; 45: 1975–1979.

110. Wardlaw JM, Dorman PJ, Lewis SC, Sandercock PA. Can stroke physicians and neuroradiologists identify signs of early cerebral infarction on CT? *J Neurol Neurosurg Psychiatry* 1999; 67: 651–653.

111. Sillanpaa N, Saarinen JT, Rusanen H, Hakomaki J, Lahteela A, Numminen H, Elovaara I, Dastidar P, Soimakallio S. CT perfusion ASPECTS in the evaluation of acute ischemic stroke: Thrombolytic therapy perspective. *Cerebrovasc Dis Extra* 2011; 1: 6–16.

112. Kim JT, Park MS, Choi KH, Nam TS, Choi SM, Lee SH, Kim BC, Kim MK, Cho KH. The CBV-ASPECT Score as a predictor of fatal stroke in a hyperacute state. *Eur Neurol* 2010; 63: 357–363.

113. Lin K, Rapalino O, Law M, Babb JS, Siller KA, Pramanik BK. Accuracy of the alberta stroke program early CT score during the first 3 hours of middle cerebral artery stroke: Comparison of noncontrast CT, CT angiography source images, and CT perfusion. *AJNR Am J Neuroradiol* 2008; 29: 931–936.

114. Schramm P, Schellinger PD, Fiebach JB, Heiland S, Jansen O, Knauth M, Hacke W, Sartor K. Comparison of CT and CT angiography source images with diffusion-weighted imaging in patients with acute stroke within 6 hours after onset. *Stroke* 2002; 33: 2426–2432.

115. Sharma M, Fox AJ, Symons S, Jairath A, Aviv RI. CT angiographic source images: Flow- or volume-weighted? *AJNR Am J Neuroradiol* 2011; 32: 359–364.

116. Hill MD, Coutts SB, Pexman JH, Demchuk AM. CTA source images in acute stroke. *Stroke* 2003; 34: 835–837; author reply 835–837.

117. Schaefer PW, Roccatagliata L, Ledezma C, Hoh B, Schwamm LH, Koroshetz W, Gonzalez RG, Lev MH. First-pass quantitative CT perfusion identifies thresholds for salvageable penumbra in acute stroke patients treated with intra-arterial therapy. *AJNR Am J Neuroradiol* 2006; 27: 20–25.

118. Simon JE, Bristow MS, Lu H, Lauzon ML, Brown RA, Manjón JV et al. A novel method to derive separate gray and white matter cerebral blood flow measures from MR imaging of acute ischemic stroke patients. *J Cereb Blood Flow Metab* 2005; 25: 1236–1243.

119. Murphy BD, Fox AJ, Lee DH, Sahlas DJ, Black SE, Hogan MJ et al. White matter thresholds for ischemic penumbra and infarct core in patients with acute stroke: CT perfusion study. *Radiology* 2008; 247: 818–825.

120. Murphy BD, Fox AJ, Lee DH, Sahlas DJ, Black SE, Hogan MJ et al. Identification of penumbra and infarct in acute ischemic stroke using computed tomography perfusion-derived blood flow and blood volume measurements. *Stroke* 2006; 37: 1771–1777.

121. Aviv RI, d'Esterre CD, Murphy BD, Hopyan JJ, Buck B, Mallia G, Li V, Zhang L, Symons SP, Lee TY. Hemorrhagic transformation of ischemic stroke: Prediction with CT perfusion. *Radiology* 2009; 250: 867–877.

122. Berger C, Fiorelli M, Steiner T, Schäbitz WR, Bozzao L, Bluhmki E, Hacke W, von Kummer R. Hemorrhagic transformation of ischemic brain tissue: Asymptomatic or symptomatic? *Stroke* 2001; 32: 1330–1335.

123. Thomalla G, Sobesky J, Köhrmann M, Fiebach JB, Fiehler J, Zaro Weber O et al. Two tales: Hemorrhagic transformation but not parenchymal hemorrhage after thrombolysis is related to severity and duration of ischemia: MRI study of acute stroke patients treated with intravenous tissue plasminogen activator within 6 hours. *Stroke* 2007; 38: 313–318.

124. Hom J, Dankbaar JW, Soares BP, Schneider T, Cheng SC, Bredno J, Lau BC, Smith W, Dillon WP, Wintermark M. Blood-brain barrier permeability assessed by perfusion CT predicts symptomatic hemorrhagic transformation and malignant edema in acute ischemic stroke. *AJNR Am J Neuroradiol* 2011; 32: 41–48.

125. Lin K. Predicting transformation to type 2 parenchymal hematoma in acute ischemic stroke by CT permeability imaging. *AJNR Am J Neuroradiol* 2011; 32: E124; author reply E125.

126. Laslo AM, Eastwood JD, Pakkiri P, Chen F, Lee TY. CT perfusion-derived mean transit time predicts early mortality and delayed vasospasm after experimental subarachnoid hemorrhage. *AJNR Am J Neuroradiol* 2008; 29: 79–85.

127. Brilstra EH, Rinkel GJ, Algra A, van Gijn J. Rebleeding, secondary ischemia, and timing of operation in patients with subarachnoid hemorrhage. *Neurology* 2000; 55: 1656–1660.

128. Sloan MA, Haley EC Jr, Kassell NF, Henry ML, Stewart SR, Beskin RR, Sevilla EA, Torner JC. Sensitivity and specificity of transcranial Doppler ultrasonography in the diagnosis of vasospasm following subarachnoid hemorrhage. *Neurology* 1989; 39: 1514–1518.

129. Reilly C, Amidei C, Tolentino J, Jahromi BS, Macdonald RL. Clot volume and clearance rate as independent predictors of vasospasm after aneurysmal subarachnoid hemorrhage. *J Neurosurg* 2004; 101: 255–261.

130. Nogueira RG, Lev MH, Roccatagliata L, Hirsch JA, Gonzalez RG, Ogilvy CS, Halpern EF, Rordorf GA, Rabinov JD, Pryor JC. Intra-arterial nicardipine infusion improves CT perfusion-measured cerebral blood flow in patients with subarachnoid hemorrhage-induced vasospasm. *AJNR Am J Neuroradiol* 2009; 30: 160–164.

131. Sudlow CL, Warlow CP. Comparable studies of the incidence of stroke and its pathological types: Results from an international collaboration. International stroke incidence collaboration. *Stroke* 1997; 28: 491–499.

132. Broderick JP, Brott TG, Duldner JE, Tomsick T, Huster G. Volume of intracerebral hemorrhage. A powerful and easy-to-use predictor of 30-day mortality. *Stroke* 1993; 24: 987–993.

133. Kidwell CS, Saver JL, Mattiello J, Warach S, Liebeskind DS, Starkman S et al. Diffusion-perfusion MR evaluation of perihematomal injury in hyperacute intracerebral hemorrhage. *Neurology* 2001; 57: 1611–1617.

134. Rosand J, Eskey C, Chang Y, Gonzalez RG, Greenberg SM, Koroshetz WJ. Dynamic single-section CT demonstrates reduced cerebral blood flow in acute intracerebral hemorrhage. *Cerebrovasc Dis* 2002; 14: 214–220.

135. Fainardi E, Borrelli M, Saletti A, Schivalocchi R, Azzini C, Cavallo M, Ceruti S, Tamarozzi R, Chieregato A. CT perfusion mapping of hemodynamic disturbances associated to acute spontaneous intracerebral hemorrhage. *Neuroradiology* 2008; 50: 729–740.

136. Mayer SA, Brun NC, Begtrup K, Broderick J, Davis S, Diringer MN et al. Efficacy and safety of recombinant activated factor VII for acute intracerebral hemorrhage. *N Engl J Med* 2008; 358: 2127–2137.

137. Mayer SA, Davis SM, Skolnick BE, Brun NC, Begtrup K, Broderick JP et al. Can a subset of intracerebral hemorrhage patients benefit from hemostatic therapy with recombinant activated factor VII? *Stroke* 2009; 40: 833–840.

138. Kim J, Smith A, Hemphill JC 3rd, Smith WS, Lu Y, Dillon WP, Wintermark M. Contrast extravasation on CT predicts mortality in primary intracerebral hemorrhage. *AJNR Am J Neuroradiol* 2008; 29: 520–525.

139. Stupp R, Mason WP, van den Bent MJ, Weller M, Fisher B, Taphoorn MJ et al. Radiotherapy plus concomitant and adjuvant temozolomide for glioblastoma. *N Engl J Med* 2005; 352: 987–996.

140. Heiss WD, Raab P, Lanfermann H. Multimodality assessment of brain tumors and tumor recurrence. *J Nucl Med* 2011; 52: 1585–1600.

141. Wen PY, Macdonald DR, Reardon DA, Cloughesy TF, Sorensen AG, Galanis E et al. Updated response assessment criteria for high-grade gliomas: Response assessment in neuro-oncology working group. *J Clin Oncol* 2010; 28: 1963–1972.

142. Jain RK, di Tomaso E, Duda DG, Loeffler JS, Sorensen AG, Batchelor TT. Angiogenesis in brain tumours. *Nat Rev Neurosci* 2007; 8: 610–622.

143. Jain R. Perfusion CT imaging of brain tumors: An overview. *AJNR Am J Neuroradiol* 2011; 32: 1570–1577.

144. Aronen HJ, Gazit IE, Louis DN, Buchbinder BR, Pardo FS, Weisskoff RM et al. Cerebral blood volume maps of gliomas: Comparison with tumor grade and histologic findings. *Radiology* 1994; 191: 41–51.

145. Roberts HC, Roberts TP, Lee TY, Dillon WP. Dynamic, contrast-enhanced CT of human brain tumors: Quantitative assessment of blood volume, blood flow, and microvascular permeability: Report of two cases. *AJNR Am J Neuroradiol* 2002; 23: 828–832.

146. Jackson A, Kassner A, Annesley-Williams D, Reid H, Zhu XP, Li KL. Abnormalities in the recirculation phase of contrast agent bolus passage in cerebral gliomas: Comparison with relative blood volume and tumor grade. *AJNR Am J Neuroradiol* 2002; 23: 7–14.

147. Di Nallo AM, Vidiri A, Marzi S, Mirri A, Fabi A, Carapella CM, Pace A, Crecco M. Quantitative analysis of CT-perfusion parameters in the evaluation of brain gliomas and metastases. *J Exp Clin Cancer Res* 2009; 28: 38.

148. Yeung T, Wong E, Lee TY, Yartsev S, Bauman G. Inititial findings of perfusion and metabolic imaging of malignant glioma during radiotherapy. *Int J Radiat Oncol Bio Phys* 2010; 78(Suppl): S279.

149. Louis DN, Ohgaki H, Wiestler OD, Cavenee WK, Burger PC, Jouvet A, Scheithauer BW, Kleihues P. The 2007 WHO classification of tumours of the central nervous system. *Acta Neuropathol* 2007; 114: 97–109.

150. Paulus W, Peiffer J. Intratumoral histologic heterogeneity of gliomas. A quantitative study. *Cancer* 1989; 64: 442–447.

151. Ding B, Ling HW, Chen KM, Jiang H, Zhu YB. Comparison of cerebral blood volume and permeability in preoperative grading of intracranial glioma using CT perfusion imaging. *Neuroradiology* 2006; 48: 773–781.

152. Ellika SK, Jain R, Patel SC, Scarpace L, Schultz LR, Rock JP, Mikkelsen T. Role of perfusion CT in glioma grading and comparison with conventional MR imaging features. *AJNR Am J Neuroradiol* 2007; 28: 1981–1987.

153. Jain R, Ellika SK, Scarpace L, Schultz LR, Rock JP, Gutierrez J, Patel SC, Ewing J, Mikkelsen T. Quantitative estimation of permeability surface-area product in astroglial brain tumors using perfusion CT and correlation with histopathologic grade. *AJNR Am J Neuroradiol* 2008; 29: 694–700.

154. Jain R, Gutierrez J, Narang J, Scarpace L, Schultz LR, Lemke N, Patel SC, Mikkelsen T, Rock JP. In vivo correlation of tumor blood volume and permeability with histologic and molecular angiogenic markers in gliomas. *AJNR Am J Neuroradiol* 2011; 32: 388–394.

155. Hu LS, Eschbacher JM, Dueck AC, Heiserman JE, Liu S, Karis JP et al. Correlations between perfusion MR imaging cerebral blood volume, microvessel quantification, and clinical outcome using stereotactic analysis in recurrent high-grade glioma. *AJNR Am J Neuroradiol* 2012; 33: 69–76.

156. Law M, Young RJ, Babb JS, Peccerelli N, Chheang S, Gruber ML, Miller DC, Golfinos JG, Zagzag D, Johnson G. Gliomas: Predicting time to progression or survival with cerebral blood volume measurements at dynamic susceptibility-weighted contrast-enhanced perfusion MR imaging. *Radiology* 2008; 247: 490–498.

157. Galbán CJ, Chenevert TL, Meyer CR, Tsien C, Lawrence TS, Hamstra DA et al. The parametric response map is an imaging biomarker for early cancer treatment outcome. *Nat Med* 2009; 15: 572–576.

158. Galbán CJ, Chenevert TL, Meyer CR, Tsien C, Lawrence TS, Hamstra DA et al. Prospective analysis of parametric response map-derived MRI biomarkers: Identification of early and distinct glioma response patterns not predicted by standard radiographic assessment. *Clin Cancer Res* 2011; 17: 4751–4760.

159. Jain R, Poisson L, Narang J, Scarpace L, Rosenblum ML, Rempel S, Mikkelsen T. Correlation of perfusion parameters with genes related to angiogenesis regulation in glioblastoma: A feasibility study. *AJNR Am J Neuroradiol* 2012; 33: 1343–1348.

160. Cao Y, Nagesh V, Hamstra D, Tsien CI, Ross BD, Chenevert TL, Junck L, Lawrence TS. The extent and severity of vascular leakage as evidence of tumor aggressiveness in high-grade gliomas. *Cancer Res* 2006; 66: 8912–8917.

161. Jain R, Narang J, Schultz L, Scarpace L, Saksena S, Brown S, Rock JP, Rosenblum M, Gutierrez J, Mikkelsen T. Permeability estimates in histopathology-proved treatment-induced necrosis using perfusion CT: Can these add to other perfusion parameters in differentiating from recurrent/progressive tumors? *AJNR Am J Neuroradiol* 2011; 32: 658–663.

162. Ng CS, Charnsangavej C, Wei W, Yao JC. Perfusion CT findings in patients with metastatic carcinoid tumors undergoing bevacizumab and interferon therapy. *AJR Am J Roentgenol* 2011; 196: 569–576.

163. Vidiri A, Pace A, Fabi A, Maschio M, Latagliata GM, Anelli V, Piludu F, Carapella CM, Giovinazzo G, Marzi S. Early perfusion changes in patients with recurrent

164. Sorensen AG, Batchelor TT, Zhang WT, Chen PJ, Yeo P, Wang M et al. A "vascular normalization index" as potential mechanistic biomarker to predict survival after a single dose of cediranib in recurrent glioblastoma patients. *Cancer Res* 2009; 69: 5296–5300.

165. Sawlani RN, Raizer J, Horowitz SW, Shin W, Grimm SA, Chandler JP, Levy R, Getch C, Carroll TJ. Glioblastoma: A method for predicting response to antiangiogenic chemotherapy by using MR perfusion imaging—pilot study. *Radiology* 2010; 255: 622–628.

166. Koh TS, Thng CH, Lee PS, Hartono S, Rumpel H, Goh BC, Bisdas S. Hepatic metastases: In vivo assessment of perfusion parameters at dynamic contrast-enhanced MR imaging with dual-input two-compartment tracer kinetics model. *Radiology* 2008; 249: 307–320.

167. Guyennon A, Mihaila M, Palma J, Lombard-Bohas C, Chayvialle JA, Pilleul F. Perfusion characterization of liver metastases from endocrine tumors: Computed tomography perfusion. *World J Radiol* 2010; 2: 449–454.

168. Goetti R, Leschka S, Desbiolles L, Klotz E, Samaras P, von Boehmer L et al. Quantitative computed tomography liver perfusion imaging using dynamic spiral scanning with variable pitch: Feasibility and initial results in patients with cancer metastases. *Invest Radiol* 2010; 45: 419–426.

169. Hashimoto K, Murakami T, Dono K, Hori M, Kim T, Kudo M et al. Assessment of the severity of liver disease and fibrotic change: The usefulness of hepatic CT perfusion imaging. *Oncol Rep* 2006; 16: 677–683.

170. Motosugi U, Ichikawa T, Sou H, Morisaka H, Sano K, Araki T. Multi-organ perfusion CT in the abdomen using a 320-detector row CT scanner: Preliminary results of perfusion changes in the liver, spleen, and pancreas of cirrhotic patients. *Eur J Radiol* 2012; 81: 2533–2537.

171. Li JP, Zhao DL, Jiang HJ, Huang YH, Li DQ, Wan Y, Liu XD, Wang JE. Assessment of tumor vascularization with functional computed tomography perfusion imaging in patients with cirrhotic liver disease. *Hepatobiliary Pancreat Dis Int* 2011; 10: 43–49.

172. Petralia G, Fazio N, Bonello L, D'Andrea G, Radice D, Bellomi M. Perfusion computed tomography in patients with hepatocellular carcinoma treated with thalidomide: Initial experience. *J Comput Assist Tomogr* 2011; 35: 195–201.

173. Kim DH, Kim SH, Im SA, Han SW, Goo JM, Willmann JK et al. Intermodality comparison between 3D perfusion CT and 18F-FDG PET/CT imaging for predicting early tumor response in patients with liver metastasis after chemotherapy: Preliminary results of a prospective study. *Eur J Radiol* 2012; 81: 3542–3550.

174. Anzidei M, Napoli A, Zaccagna F, Cartocci G, Saba L, Menichini G et al. Liver metastases from colorectal cancer treated with conventional and antiangiogenetic chemotherapy: Evaluation with liver computed tomography perfusion and magnetic resonance diffusion-weighted imaging. *J Comput Assist Tomogr* 2011; 35: 690–696.

175. Chen G, Ma DQ, He W, Zhang BF, Zhao LQ. Computed tomography perfusion in evaluating the therapeutic effect of transarterial chemoembolization for hepatocellular carcinoma. *World J Gastroenterol* 2008; 14: 5738–5743.

176. Lam VW, Ng KK, Chok KS, Cheung TT, Yuen J, Tung H, Tso WK, Fan ST, Poon RT. Risk factors and prognostic factors of local recurrence after radiofrequency ablation of hepatocellular carcinoma. *J Am Coll Surg* 2008; 207: 20–29.

177. Hori T, Nagata K, Hasuike S, Onaga M, Motoda M, Moriuchi A et al. Risk factors for the local recurrence of hepatocellular carcinoma after a single session of percutaneous radiofrequency ablation. *J Gastroenterol* 2003; 38: 977–981.

178. Harrison LE, Koneru B, Baramipour P, Fisher A, Barone A, Wilson D, Dela Torre A, Cho KC, Contractor D, Korogodsky M. Locoregional recurrences are frequent after radiofrequency ablation for hepatocellular carcinoma. *J Am Coll Surg* 2003; 197: 759–764.

179. Cao Y, Platt JF, Francis IR, Balter JM, Pan C, Normolle D, Ben-Josef E, Haken RK, Lawrence TS. The prediction of radiation-induced liver dysfunction using a local dose and regional venous perfusion model. *Med Phys* 2007; 34: 604–612.

180. Cao Y, Pan C, Balter JM, Platt JF, Francis IR, Knol JA, Normolle D, Ben-Josef E, Ten Haken RK, Lawrence TS. Liver function after irradiation based on computed tomographic portal vein perfusion imaging. *Int J Radiat Oncol Biol Phys* 2008; 70: 154–160.

181. Krumholz HM, Merrill AR, Schone EM, Schreiner GC, Chen J, Bradley EH et al. Patterns of hospital performance in acute myocardial infarction and heart failure 30-day mortality and readmission. *Circ Cardiovasc Qual Outcomes* 2009; 2: 407–413.

182. Tillmanns H, Waas W, Voss R, Grempels E, Hölschermann H, Haberbosch W, Waldecker B. Gender differences in the outcome of cardiac interventions. *Herz* 2005; 30: 375–389.

183. Gurevich Y, McFarlane A, Morris K, Jokovic A, Peterson GM, Webster GK. Estimating the number of coronary artery bypass graft and percutaneous coronary intervention procedures in Canada: A comparison of cardiac registry and Canadian Institute for Health Information data sources. *Can J Cardiol* 2010; 26: e249–e253.

184. Wang X, Rokoss M, Dyub A, Gafni A, Lamy A. Cost comparison of four revascularisation procedures for the treatment of multivessel coronary artery disease. *J Med Econ* 2008; 11: 119–134.

185. Brener SJ, Ellis SG, Schneider J, Topol EJ. Frequency and long-term impact of myonecrosis after coronary stenting. *Eur Heart J* 2002; 23: 869–876.

186. Henriques JP, Remmelink M, Baan J Jr, van der Schaaf RJ, Vis MM, Koch KT et al. Safety and feasibility of elective high-risk percutaneous coronary intervention procedures with left ventricular support of the Impella Recover LP 2.5. *Am J Cardiol* 2006; 97: 990–992.

187. Sjauw KD, Konorza T, Erbel R, Danna PL, Viecca M, Minden HH et al. Supported high-risk percutaneous coronary intervention with the Impella 2.5 device the Europella registry. *J Am Coll Cardiol* 2009; 54: 2430–2434.

188. Shaw LJ, Marwick TH, Zoghbi WA, Hundley WG, Kramer CM, Achenbach S, Dilsizian V, Kern MJ, Chandrashekhar Y, Narula J. Why all the focus on cardiac imaging? *JACC Cardiovasc Imaging* 2010; 3: 789–794.

189. Shaw LJ, Berman DS, Maron DJ, Mancini GB, Hayes SW, Hartigan PM et al. Optimal medical therapy with or without percutaneous coronary intervention to reduce ischemic burden: Results from the Clinical outcomes utilizing revascularization and aggressive drug evaluation (COURAGE) trial nuclear substudy. *Circulation* 2008; 117: 1283–1291.

190. Hachamovitch R, Hayes SW, Friedman JD, Cohen I, Berman DS. Comparison of the short-term survival benefit associated with revascularization compared with medical therapy in patients with no prior coronary artery disease undergoing stress myocardial perfusion single photon emission computed tomography. *Circulation* 2003; 107: 2900–2907.

191. Kim C, Kwok YS, Heagerty P, Redberg R. Pharmacologic stress testing for coronary disease diagnosis: A meta-analysis. *Am Heart J* 2001; 142: 934–944.

192. Zaacks SM, Ali A, Parrillo JE, Barron JT. How well does radionuclide dipyridamole stress testing detect three-vessel coronary artery disease and ischemia in the region supplied by the most stenotic vessel? *Clin Nucl Med* 1999; 24: 35–41.

193. Beller GA, Ragosta M. Decision making in multivessel coronary disease: The need for physiological lesion assessment. *JACC Cardiovasc Interv* 2010; 3: 315–317.

194. Bastarrika G, Ramos-Duran L, Schoepf UJ, Rosenblum MA, Abro JA, Brothers RL, Zubieta JL, Chiaramida SA, Kang DK. Adenosine-stress dynamic myocardial volume perfusion imaging with second generation dual-source computed tomography: Concepts and first experiences. *J Cardiovasc Comput Tomogr* 2010; 4: 127–135.

195. Mahnken AH, Klotz E, Pietsch H, Schmidt B, Allmendinger T, Haberland U, Kalender WA, Flohr T. Quantitative whole heart stress perfusion CT imaging as noninvasive assessment of hemodynamics in coronary artery stenosis: Preliminary animal experience. *Invest Radiol* 2010; 45: 298–305.

196. Budoff MJ, Dowe D, Jollis JG, Gitter M, Sutherland J, Halamert E et al. Diagnostic performance of 64-multidetector row coronary computed tomographic angiography for evaluation of coronary artery stenosis in individuals without known coronary artery disease: Results from the prospective multicenter ACCURACY (Assessment by Coronary Computed Tomographic Angiography of Individuals Undergoing Invasive Coronary Angiography) trial. *J Am Coll Cardiol* 2008; 52: 1724–1732.

197. Meijboom WB, Meijs MF, Schuijf JD, Cramer MJ, Mollet NR, van Mieghem CA et al. Diagnostic accuracy of 64-slice computed tomography coronary angiography: A prospective, multicenter, multivendor study. *J Am Coll Cardiol* 2008; 52: 2135–2144.

198. van Werkhoven JM, Schuijf JD, Gaemperli O, Jukema JW, Boersma E, Wijns W et al. Prognostic value of multislice computed tomography and gated single-photon emission computed tomography in patients with suspected coronary artery disease. *J Am Coll Cardiol* 2009; 53: 623–632.

199. Gould KL. Does coronary flow trump coronary anatomy? *JACC Cardiovasc Imaging* 2009; 2: 1009–1023.

200. Hoffmann U, Millea R, Enzweiler C, Ferencik M, Gulick S, Titus J, Achenbach S, Kwait D, Sosnovik D, Brady TJ. Acute myocardial infarction: Contrast-enhanced multidetector row CT in a porcine model. *Radiology* 2004; 231: 697–701.

201. Rogers IS, Cury RC, Blankstein R, Shapiro MD, Nieman K, Hoffmann U, Brady TJ, Abbara S. Comparison of postprocessing techniques for the detection of perfusion defects by cardiac computed tomography in patients presenting with acute ST-segment elevation myocardial infarction. *J Cardiovasc Comput Tomogr* 2010; 4: 258–266.

202. Camici PG, Rimoldi OE. The clinical value of myocardial blood flow measurement. *J Nucl Med* 2009; 50: 1076–1087.

203. Ørn S, Manhenke C, Greve OJ, Larsen AI, Bonarjee VV, Edvardsen T, Dickstein K. Microvascular obstruction is a major determinant of infarct healing and subsequent left ventricular remodelling following primary percutaneous coronary intervention. *Eur Heart J* 2009; 30: 1978–1985.

204. Miller TD, Christian TF, Hopfenspirger MR, Hodge DO, Gersh BJ, Gibbons RJ. Infarct size after acute myocardial infarction measured by quantitative tomographic 99mTc sestamibi imaging predicts subsequent mortality. *Circulation* 1995; 92: 334–341.

205. Burns RJ, Gibbons RJ, Yi Q, Roberts RS, Miller TD, Schaer GL. The relationships of left ventricular ejection fraction, end-systolic volume index and infarct size to six-month mortality after hospital discharge following myocardial infarction treated by thrombolysis. *J Am Coll Cardiol* 2002; 39: 30–36.

3

Contrast Media in Computed Tomography Imaging

Yousef W. Nielsen and Henrik S. Thomsen

CONTENTS

FOCUS POINT

Iodine-based contrast media for radiography and computed tomography are generally safe even in large amounts. However, significant adverse reactions may occur. The risk can be reduced in particular by identifying patients at risk before the administration of the agent. When it occurs, one should be ready to treat the reaction immediately if possible.

3.1 Contrast Media

Contrast media (CM) are administered commonly during radiological procedures including fluoroscopy, computed tomography (CT), and magnetic resonance imaging (MRI) as well as sometimes during ultrasonography. Cardiac angiography and CT are the two examinations for which an overwhelming amount of CM is used. Whereas angiography always requires the use of CM, enhanced CT constitutes about two-thirds of the CT examinations. The mechanism of CM is to enhance differences between structures and fluids within the body tissues. This is more important for CT and radiography as the unenhanced soft-tissue discrimination with x-rays is poor compared to MRI and ultrasonography.

3.1.1 Iodinated Contrast Media

3.1.1.1 Chemistry

All modern iodine-based CM (I-CM) are 2,4,6-triiodinated benzene derivatives (Table 3.1). Positions 1, 3, and 5 in the benzene ring are occupied by moieties that act to either increase water solubility or protect the overall molecule from interactions with proteins. The CM are highly stable, which allows heat/autoclave sterilization of the final solutions in sealed bottles.

Osmolality is an important property of CM. In the ideal setting, the CM should match the physiological osmolality of approximately 300 mOsmol/kg-water. Relative to physiological osmolality, I-CM are divided into three groups: high-osmolar CM (HOCM), low-osmolar CM (LOCM), and iso-osmolar CM (IOCM) (Figure 3.1 and Table 3.2). An indication of osmolality of a given CM is provided by the contrast agent ratio, defined as the number of iodine atoms in the

TABLE 3.1

Iodine-Based Contrast Media

Contrast agent	Trade name	Structure
	Class	
HOCM—Ionic monomers		
Diatrizoate	Urografin	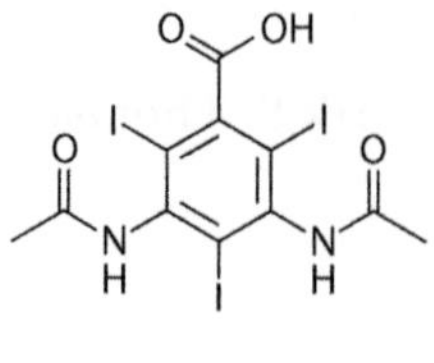
Iothalamate	Conray	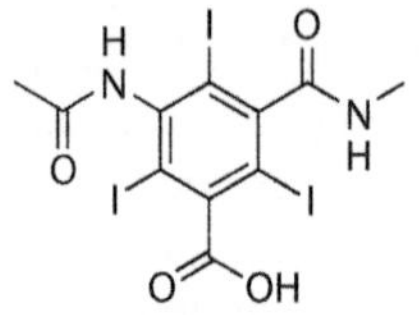
Ioxithalamate	Telebrix	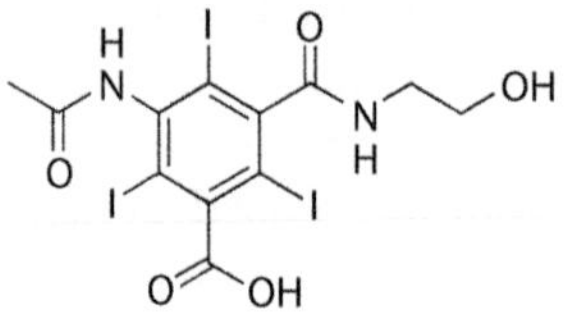
LOCM—Ionic dimer		
Ioxaglate	Hexabrix	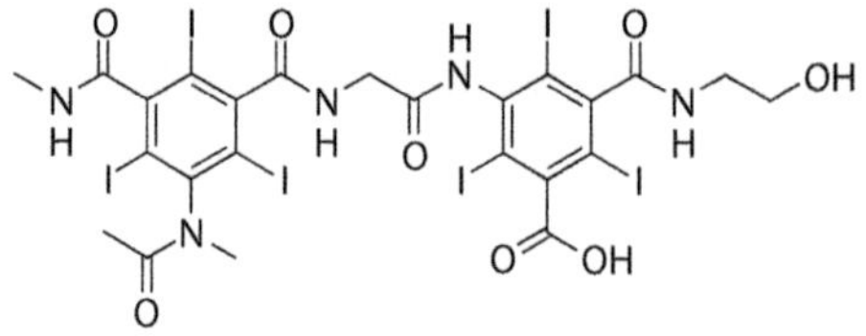
LOCM—Nonionic monomers		
Ioversol	Optiray	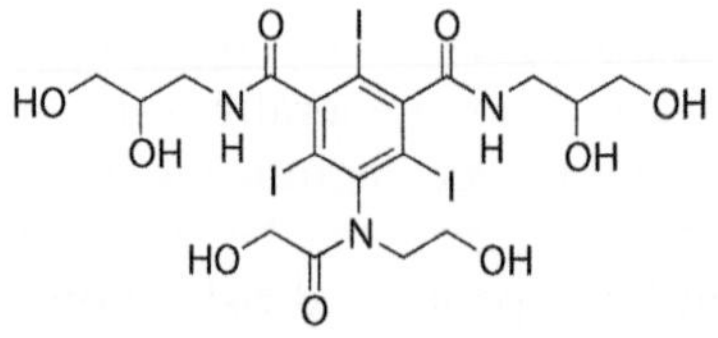
Iopromide	Ultravist	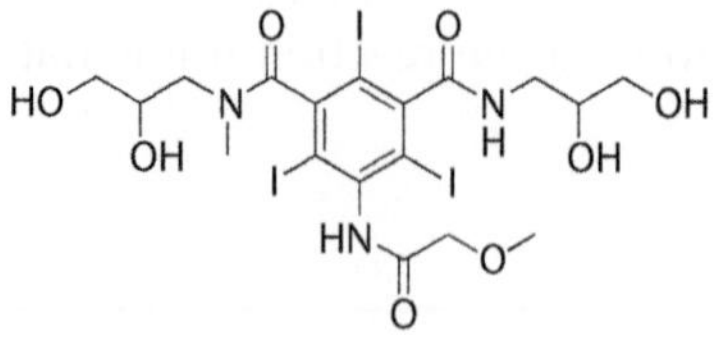
IOCM—Nonionic dimers		
Iotrolan	Isovist	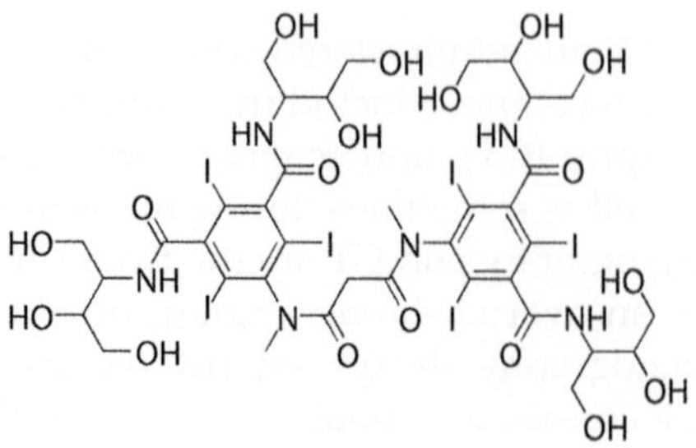

TABLE 3.1

Iodine-Based Contrast Media (*Continued*)

Class		
Contrast agent	**Trade name**	**Structure**
Iodixanol	Visipaque	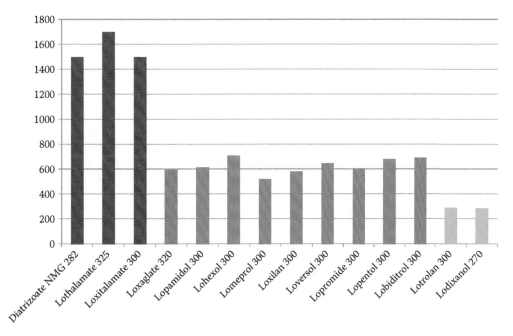

Note: Examples of chemical structure.

HOCM, high-osmolar contrast media; LOCM, low-osmolar contrast media; IOCM, iso-osmolar contrast media.

FIGURE 3.1

Osmolality (mOsmol/kg-water) of the various I-CM at a concentration about 300 mgI/mL.

TABLE 3.2

Classification of Iodine-Based Contrast Media

Contrast Agent	Trade Name	Structure	Charge	Class	Maximum (gI/mL)
Amidotrizoate	Urografin	Monomer	Ionic	HOCM	300
Iothalamate	Conray	Monomer	Ionic	HOCM	370
Ioxithalamate	Telebrix	Monomer	Ionic	HOCM	350
Ioxaglate	Hexabrix	Dimer	Ionic	LOCM	320
Iopamidol	Iopamiro	Monomer	Nonionic	LOCM	370
Iohexol	Omnipaque	Monomer	Nonionic	LOCM	350
Iomeprol	Iomeron	Monomer	Nonionic	LOCM	400
Iopentol	Imagopaque	Monomer	Nonionic	LOCM	300
Ioxilan	Oxilan	Monomer	Nonionic	LOCM	350
Ioversol	Optiray	Monomer	Nonionic	LOCM	350
Iopromide	Ultravist	Monomer	Nonionic	LOCM	370
Iotrolan	Isovist	Dimer	Nonionic	IOCM	320
Iodixanol	Visipaque	Dimer	Nonionic	IOCM	320

HOCM, high-osmolar contrast media; LOCM, low-osmolar contrast media; IOCM, iso-osmolar contrast media.

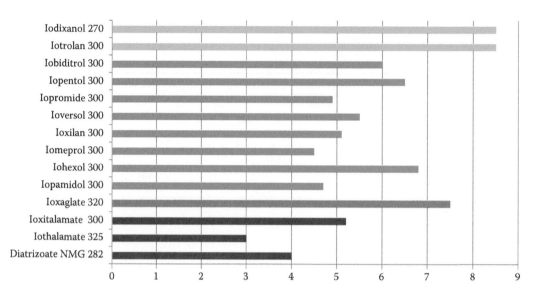

FIGURE 3.2
Viscosity (mPa·s) of the various I-CM at a concentration about 300 mgI/mL and at 37°C.

CM/the number of particles in the solution. Low ratio is associated with high osmolality. The number of iodine atoms differs between monomers and dimers. Monomeric iodinated CM contain one triiodinated aromatic ring, whereas dimeric CM contain two linked triiodinated aromatic rings. The number of particles in solution is one for nonionic CM and two for ionic CM. HOCM are ionic monomeric CM (ratio 3/2 = 1.5) with osmolality of approximately 2000 mOsmol/kg-water. These agents caused osmolality-related adverse reactions, such as vasodilatation, cell crenation, and pain on injection. HOCM are no longer used intravascularly in the Western world. LOCM are ionic dimeric CM and nonionic monomers (ratios 6/2 = 3 and 3/1 = 3, respectively). Today, the nonionic monomers are the most commonly used CM in contrast-enhanced CT. The slightly increased osmolality (~700–900 mOsmol/kg-water) of LOCM compared to blood may be beneficial to the kidneys as well as it does not cause more nonrenal adverse reactions than the iso-osmolar agents. The nonionic dimeric structure (ratio 6/1 = 6) allows one to formulate solutions with an osmolality similar to blood. By adding various electrolytes, the medium is kept at isotonic levels at all iodine concentrations. However, these agents cannot be formulated at high concentrations because of viscosity restraints. In relation to osmolality-related discomfort, IOCM may be preferable for peripheral runoffs, but with regard to acute renal and nonrenal as well as very late reactions, they do not differ from the nonionic LOCM. IOCM cause significantly more late adverse reactions (skin lesions) compared to LOCM. Production costs are markedly higher for IOCM.

Viscosity is another important property of CM; it increases with increasing concentration of the agent. There are significant differences among viscosities of commercially available I-CM, the nonionic dimer iodixanol being the most viscous of all (Figure 3.2). Viscosity should be low to allow for fast injection. Temperature affects viscosity strongly, and heating the CM before injection into the body may reduce viscosity markedly.

3.1.1.2 Pharmacokinetics

Pharmacokinetics follows a two-compartment model. The first compartment is the intravascular plasma, and the second is the interstitial space. I-CM do not enter cells to any significant extent; therefore, they are often referred to as extracellular CM. After injection, the agents are simultaneously diluted in the circulating plasma and begin to pass out into the interstitial space over capillary membranes. This process continues until there is transient equilibrium between CM in plasma and the interstitial space. From that moment, the opposite movement of CM (i.e., from interstitium to plasma) dominates as CM are removed from the blood by glomerular excretion. An important exception to the model is the brain where the intact blood–brain barrier hinders CM diffusion to the interstitial space. Pathologic conditions like a tumor or an abscess destroy the blood–brain barrier and CM will leak outside the intravascular compartment when such lesions are present (Figure 3.3).

Excretion of I-CM is almost completely by passive glomerular filtration in the kidneys without any tubular excretion or reabsorption. Less than 1% is excreted extrarenally (hepatobiliary, sweat, salvia, and tears) in patients with normal renal function [1]. The half-life is approximately 2 hours, and 98% is excreted within 24 hours in patients with normal renal function (>60 mL/min × 1.73 m^2). Furthermore, it has been shown that 75% of the administered dose is excreted in the urine within four hours [2]. In patients with severely reduced renal function, it may take days to weeks before all CM are out of the body. There is no absorption from the intact gastrointestinal (GI) tract after oral administration of iodinated CM. If given into intact body cavities, there is little absorption into the blood (intravasation). Presence of CM in the bladder after injection into a body cavity (other than the urinary tract) or oral intake confirms that the wall is no longer intact and that there is a lesion.

The pharmacokinetic profile of I-CM leads to characteristic phases of contrast enhancement (Figure 3.4). In liver and pancreas CT, arterial, portal venous, and late phases of enhancement are of importance [3]. During the arterial phase (20–30 seconds after injection), the contrast is predominantly in the arteries; little leaks into the interstitial space. Imaging in the portal venous and late phases is characterized by contrast in both the vascular and the interstitial compartments. Portal venous acquisitions are performed 70–90 seconds after injection. The nomenclature of contrast phases is different in genitourinary CT [4]. The corticomedullary phase, with preferential cortical enhancement, lasts from 25 to 70 seconds after injection. It is followed by the

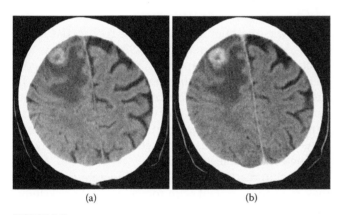

FIGURE 3.3
Contrast-enhanced CT of the brain in a patient with a tumor. Due to blood–brain barrier, the lesion enhances after contrast. (a) Unenhanced brain CT, (b) contrast-enhanced CT.

nephrographic phase with homogeneous parenchymal enhancement (80–180 seconds). Later acquisitions (>5 minutes after I-CM administration) are used to evaluate excretion, as contrast will be present in the renal pelvis and ureters at that time.

3.1.1.3 Adverse Reactions

The ideal contrast agent is physiologically inert. It enhances the appropriate lesions, causes no adverse reactions, and is excreted fast and unchanged. However, no such CM exist, and all agents cause adverse reactions. An adverse drug reaction is defined as "a response to a medical product which is noxious and which occurs in doses normally used in man for the prophylaxis, diagnosis or therapy of disease or for the restoration, correction, or modification of physiological function" [5]. Adverse reactions after administration of CM are divided into acute reactions (occurring within 60 minutes), late reactions (from one hour to seven days), and very late reactions (later than a week). Furthermore, it is relevant to divide acute reactions into nonrenal and renal reactions.

Adverse reactions can occur after extravascular contrast administration, but the overwhelming majority is seen after intravascular administration.

3.1.1.4 Nonrenal Adverse Reactions

3.1.1.4.1 Acute Reactions

These reactions are feared as they may be fatal and are unpredictable. The majority of nonrenal acute adverse reactions are considered idiosyncratic/pseudo-allergic reactions. They are not related to doses above a certain level; they can be seen even after 1 mL of I-CM. Chemotoxic reactions, on the contrary, are dose-related and dependent on the physicochemical properties of the CM (i.e., osmolality, viscosity, hydrophilicity, and protein binding). However, in the clinical setting, it is not easy to distinguish between the two types of reactions.

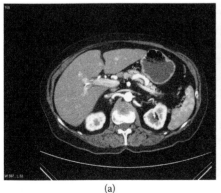 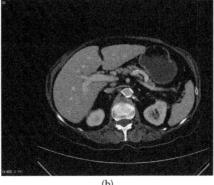 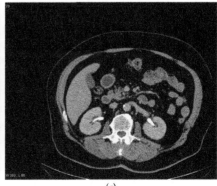

FIGURE 3.4
Contrast phases in CT. (a) Arterial phase, (b) portal venous phase, (c) late acquisition.

Acute reactions are classified as mild, moderate, or severe [6]. Mild reactions are nausea, mild vomiting, urticaria, and itching. Usually these reactions do not require treatment, but in a few cases, they may be the first signs of a severe reaction. Moderate reactions include severe vomiting, marked urticaria, bronchospasm, facial/laryngeal edema, and vasovagal attacks. The severe reactions are hypotensive shock, respiratory arrest, cardiac arrest, and convulsions [7]. Most of the acute reactions occur early. In a large study of over 330,000 patients, more than 70% of acute reactions occurred within five minutes of contrast injection [8]. Both ionic and nonionic monomeric agents were administered in this study.

The exact pathophysiological mechanisms of acute reactions are still to be determined. Some of the reactions are true allergic hypersensitivity reactions [9] while others are not. Positive allergic skin testing with I-CM has been reported in patients with previous reactions [9]. Subsequently, noncross reactors have been administered with other I-CM without problems. Immediate nonallergic reactions could be caused by direct chemotoxicity or by nonspecific release of histamine from mast cells.

A lot of effort has been made to identify factors of the acute nonrenal reactions. In this regard, the type of CM plays a role: acute reactions are approximately five times more common with the old ionic CM (HOCM) compared to newer nonionic CM (LOCM and IOCM). Incidences of severe reactions have been reported to be 0.22 and 0.04 in patients administered with ionic and nonionic CM, respectively [8]. Patient-related factors are also important when assessing the risk of acute reactions. Accordingly, patients with previous moderate to severe reactions are at increased risk. With ionic agents, the risk is increased 16%–35% [10,11]. If patients with previous reactions to ionic agents are administered with a nonionic agent, the risk of an acute reaction is reduced to 5% [12]. Asthma increases the risk of acute reactions by a factor of 5.8 (nonionic) to 8.5 (ionic) [8]. Other conditions like hay fever, eczema, and food allergy also increase the risk although to a lesser degree than asthma. Previous or ongoing treatment with interleukin-2 also increases the risk of acute reactions. There is no link between CM injection rate and acute adverse reactions [13].

The European Society of Urogenital Radiology [7] has issued guidelines to reduce the risk of acute reactions: nonionic agents should always be used. As most reactions occur early, all patients should be kept in the radiology department for 30 minutes after CM injection. A crash cart with appropriate drugs, tubes, fluids, and so on should be readily available in the room where the CM are administered. In patients with risk factors for acute reactions, other diagnostic tests, not requiring iodinated CM, should be considered (i.e., ultrasound or MRI). Use of a different I-CM in previous reactors is recommended. Even though evidence is sparse for nonionic agents, it can be considered to premedicate patients before contrast administration. The use of premedication varies considerably from country to country as premedication is done systematically in some countries whereas in other countries premedication is almost never done. Despite premedication, acute reactions can occur (breakthrough reactions). A suitable premedication regime is prednisolone 30 mg orally given 12 and 2 hours before contrast injection.

Following intravascular administration of I-CM, patients often experience warmth, flushing, and altered taste. The discomfort quickly resolves and is of no clinical significance. It is, however, relevant to inform the patients about the discomfort before injection.

Treatment of acute reactions falls beyond the scope of this chapter and the reader is referred to www.esur.org or the literature [14] for more details.

3.1.1.4.2 Late Reactions

Late adverse reactions to I-CM were recognized nearly three decades ago in the mid-1980s. Numerous late reactions have been reported. The long list includes skin rash, headache, itching, nausea, urticaria, fever, GI discomfort, arm pain, and dizziness. However, studies comparing late reactions after CT with/without contrast administration (nonionic agents) have shown skin reactions to be the only reactions seen more frequently following contrast injection [15,16].

Most skin reactions are mild or moderate. Some cases may require treatment with topical steroid or systemic antihistamine. Severe reactions are very rare. Most reactions occur within three days of CM administration and resolve within seven days. The clinical presentation is variable and findings may include maculopapular rash, urticaria, macular exanthema, angioedema, and scaling skin eruption.

Even though the pathogenesis behind late reactions is fully understood, it seems that many are type IV hypersensitivity reactions, that is, T-cell-mediated [17].

The frequency of late adverse reactions ranges from 1% to 3%. There seems to be no significant difference in the incidence of late reactions between ionic and nonionic monomeric agents [18,19] as well as between the various nonionic monomers [18]. However, the nonionic dimers iodixanol cause significantly more late reactions than the nonionic monomers [20,21].

Risk factors for late reactions to I-CM have been identified. Previous reactions to I-CM increase the risk by a factor of 2–3. Allergy (especially drug or contact allergy) approximately doubles the likelihood of a late reaction. Treatment with interleukin-2 is also a known risk factor.

Patients who have had a late reaction to I-CM are not at increased risk of a subsequent acute adverse reaction [22].

3.1.1.4.3 Very Late Reactions

Thyrotoxicosis is the important very late reaction that may occur after administration of I-CM. As these CM contain some free iodine, they can induce thyrotoxicosis in patients with either untreated Graves' disease or thyroid autonomy. Dietary iodine deficiency is an important risk factor for multinodar goiter and thyroid autonomy. Thus, the number of patients with increased risk of developing CM-induced thyrotoxicosis is greater in geographic areas of iodine deficiency (primarily European countries). In normal euthyroid patients, no changes in thyroid function parameters (TSH, T3/4) are seen following CM administration. In geriatric patients, CM-induced hyperthyroidism is more common, probably because of undiagnosed thyroid autonomous nodules in this patient group [23].

The incidence of CM-induced thyrotoxicosis is low, and it is sometimes difficult to identify the source of the iodine that caused thyrotoxicosis. In addition to CM, other sources of iodine excess include disinfectants, secretolytic agents, the iodine containing antiarrhythmic amiodarone, eye drops and ointments, seaweed, multivitamin preparations, skin ointments, toothpaste, and so on [24]. In unselected patients in areas of dietary iodine deficiency, the rate is <0.4% [25]. CM-induced hyperthyroidism is usually self-limiting. However, if clinically significant thyrotoxicosis occurs, it presents with signs and symptoms similar to thyrotoxicosis of other causes (i.e., weight loss, anxiety, palpations, and cardiac arrhythmias).

CM-induced thyrotoxicosis is not a concern in normal euthyroid patients. However, in elderly patients or patients with previous thyroid disease, the condition should be considered. I-CM should never be administered to patients with manifest hyperthyroidism; instead, alternative imaging modalities not requiring iodinated CM should be performed. Prophylactic treatment against CM-induced thyrotoxicosis may be given in selected high-risk patients by an endocrinologist. Furthermore, these patients require close monitoring by endocrinologists after iodinated CM [7].

As free iodine from CM may interfere with tracers used in thyroid scintigraphy and radioiodine treatment, two-month intervals are recommended between these nuclear medicine procedures and the time of iodinated CM injection [7].

3.1.1.5 Renal Adverse Reactions

Contrast medium-induced nephropathy (CIN) is defined as a condition in which impairment in renal function (an increase in serum creatinine by more than 25% or 44 µmol/L) occurs within three days of contrast medium administration in the absence of alternative etiology (Morcos et al. 1999).

CIN ranges in severity from asymptomatic, transient decrease in renal function to severe acute renal failure necessitating dialysis. However, most episodes of CIN are self-limited and resolve within 14 days [26].

The incidence of CIN varies between different studies, but it seems that the incidence is higher when the contrast medium is administered intra-arterially (above the renal arteries) compared to intravenous administration. CIN is rare among individuals with normal renal function (incidence <2%). The incidence of CIN is higher in patients with diabetic nephropathy following intra-arterial as well as intravenous administration of iodinated CM. In patients with a glomerular filtration rate between 20 and 60 mL/min × 1.73 m^2, the incidence is about 5% when I-CM are given intravenously for CT slightly higher in the lower end than in the upper end [27]. For patients with a glomerular filtration between 5 and 20 mL/min × 1.73 m^2, the incidence is unknown (but estimated to range between 10% and 15%), as such patients have never been recruited for CIN studies in relation to enhanced CT.

The exact pathophysiological mechanism of CIN is unclear. However, different mechanisms induced by CM have been proposed: hemodynamic effects leading to reduction in renal perfusion, local toxic effects in the tubuli, and endogenous biochemical disturbances [28].

A number of risk factors for CIN have been identified, the most important being preexisting renal failure particularly when caused by diabetic nephropathy [29,30]. Other risk factors are large doses of contrast medium/multiple injections, concurrent administration of nephrotoxic drugs (e.g., nonsteroidal anti-inflammatory drug [NSAID], aminoglycosides, and chemotherapy), dehydration, congestive heart failure, gout, and advanced age (>70 years). The type of iodinated CM is also important, because HOCM is more nephrotoxic than IOCM and LOCM [29,31].

As preexisting renal impairment is an important risk factor of CIN, it is necessary to have an easy and reliable predictor of renal function available. Serum creatinine provides such an estimate of renal function. However, renal function can be reduced significantly when serum creatinine is within the normal range. A more accurate measurement of renal function is provided by the estimated glomerular filtration rate (eGFR) [32]. eGFR is a better estimate of the renal function, but it also has its problems. Correct determination of the glomerular filtration is troublesome and time consuming and impossible to perform in all at-risk persons before enhanced CT. Currently, eGFR seems to be the most practical determination.

To avoid development of CIN during CT procedures (or other imaging procedures with intravascular CM administration), the following strategy is recommended by the European Society for Urogenital Radiology [7]: in patients with increased risk of CIN, eGFR (or serum creatinine) should be measured before the imaging procedure. In practice, this applies to patients with known eGFR reduction (<60 mL/min/1.73 m^2) and to patients with a history of renal disease, renal surgery, diabetes mellitus, hypertension, proteinuria, gout, or recent nephrotoxic drugs.

If eGFR is <45 mL/min/1.73 m^2 (or if one or more of the above-mentioned risk factors are present), one should consider an alternative imaging method not requiring iodinated CM given intravenously. Furthermore, nephrotoxic drugs should be stopped after consultation with the referring physician at least 24 hours before contrast medium administration. Importantly, hydration with intravenous normal saline (1 mL/kg body weight/h) six hours before and after the imaging procedure should be given. Alternative sodium bicarbonate can be given from one hour before the CM administration to six hours after the CM administration [33]. Both hydration regiments should be equally good. Hydration is so far the most effective preventive strategy against CIN [30]. For the enhancement during the imaging procedure, IOCM or LOCM should be administered and in the lowest dose giving a diagnostic result. It has been stated that the group of nonionic monomers (LOCM) are more nephrotoxic than the commercially available nonionic dimer iodixanol (IOCM). However, there is so far no conclusive evidence of a difference in the nephrotoxic potential between the various monomers and the dimer [26].

All CM can be removed by dialysis (hemo- or peritoneal dialysis). However, there is no evidence that dialysis protects against CIN. It is unnecessary to schedule CM injection with a hemodialysis session. In patients on continuous ambulatory peritoneal dialysis, it is not necessary to schedule additional hemodialysis sessions [7].

Special awareness relates to diabetic patients taking metformin. This drug is excreted unchanged in the urine. In case of renal failure, either preexisting or because of CIN, metformin may accumulate in the body and cause metabolic lactate acidosis. To avoid this serious condition, patients with eGFR <45 mL/min/1.73 m^2 who takes metformin and who are going to have the agent intravenously should stop taking the drug 48 hours before contrast medium administration and remain off for 48 hours after contrast medium administration. Metformin should only be restarted if serum creatinine is unchanged. Metformin does not cause renal damage.

3.1.1.5.1 Interaction

Measurements of clotting time and other coagulation factors can be falsely increased after the intravascular administration of CM. Therefore, clotting tests should be avoided for six hours or more after injection of CM. I-CM in the urine may also interfere with some of the protein assay techniques leading to false-positive results. Care must be exercised in interpreting tests for proteinuria for 24-hour after CM injection. I-CM may interfere with determination of bilirubin, copper, iron, phosphate, and proteins in the blood. Therefore, biochemical assays are better performed before CM injection or delayed for at least 24 hours afterward or longer in patients with renal impairment. Urgent laboratory tests shortly after CM injection should be carefully assessed.

3.1.2 Other Contrast Media

3.1.2.1 Barium Contrast Media

Barium CM have been used to image the GI tract in the past century. All barium CM are based on barium sulfate, a heavy insoluble material produced from barite. Barium sulfate is generally regarded as an inert compound that has no absorption or metabolization in the body. Thus, it is eliminated unchanged in the feces. Pure barium sulfate preparations are not suitable for GI imaging as they flocculate easily and produce poor mucosal coating. Additives that enhance mucosal coating are therefore added to barium sulfate in commercially available barium CM [34]. Barium CM are usually well tolerated but adverse events may occur.

Minor adverse events include constipation and abdominal discomfort. More serious adverse events occur if barium leaks into the peritoneal cavity, causing severe peritonitis. In many cases, this is a fatal event, if the patient recovers severe peritoneal adhesions might develop. Water-soluble iodinated agents (LOCM) should therefore be used in patients with suspected compromise of bowel wall integrity. Perforation with leakage of barium into the mediastinum or retroperitoneum is also a serious condition as fatal toxic shock may develop.

Aspiration of barium sulfate may lead to chemical pneumonia and respiratory failure. LOCM are better tolerated and should be used if there is risk of aspiration.

Hypersensitivity reactions to barium agents are extremely rare.

3.1.2.2 Gadolinium-Based Contrast Media

Chelates of the lanthanide metal gadolinium (Gd) are used for contrast-enhanced MRI studies. However, Gd-based CM have previously also been used for conventional angiography and CT imaging as the Gd atom attenuates x-rays better than iodine at the most frequently used kVs. It was believed that Gd-chelates were not nephrotoxic and could be used as an alternative to iodinated CM when performing CT in patients with renal insufficiency [35,36]. Such studies required high doses of Gd [37]. Today Gd-based agents are not used for radiography after the association between some of these agents and development of the devastating disease nephrogenic systemic fibrosis was identified. Furthermore, the nephrotoxic potential of Gd-chelates is now recognized [38].

3.1.2.3 Water

Oral administration of water can be used as natural CM in CT. It is of relevance for abdominal CT when bowel distension is desirable. Water acts as a negative CM because of its low value on the Hounsfield scale. Compared to oral administered barium, the use of water has two advantages. First of all, no adverse reactions are associated with water. Furthermore, the negative contrast effect in the bowel lumen allows for evaluation of the enhancement characteristics of the bowel wall after intravenous contrast. This is not possible if the lumen is filled with positive barium or I-CM.

Water is quickly resorbed from the small bowel. Therefore, little delay between water administration and CT scanning is advisable.

3.1.3 Contrast Media Administration

In CT, CM are most commonly administered intravenously but oral administration is also used in abdominal CT. Finally, I-CM are also given directly into cavities, for example, the bladder.

3.1.3.1 Routes of Administration

3.1.3.1.1 Intravenous Contrast Media Administration

When performing contrast-enhanced CT with intravenously injected agents, I-CM are used. Barium agents are not for intravenous use.

Before injection of CM, intravenous access must be established. In most cases, cannulation is performed in a superficial upper extremity vein. Cannulation in the antecubtital fossa is simple in the majority of patients. However, if there are difficulties in establishing access in this area, cannulation can be performed in any superficial vein. Correct placement of the intravenous cannula should be confirmed by injecting saline. When the intravenous line has been placed, it should be fixated properly to avoid displacement during the CT scan. If these safety measures are not followed, there is risk of CM extravasation (see Section 3.1.3.3). Usually it is not important if the CM injection is performed in the right or left upper extremity. If, however, CT angio/venography of the upper extremities is performed, the side of injection should be taken into consideration. Even though it is uncommon, intravenous contrast injection can be performed in the lower extremity veins. This may be relevant if it is difficult to gain intravenous access in the upper extremity. Lower extremity injection alters the contrast dynamics in the body, that is, contrast filling of the inferior vena cava precedes filling of the abdominal aorta. The difference is, however, of no significance when scanning is performed later than the arterial phase.

In modern CT, contrast injection is usually performed with automated power injectors. With such devices, injection rates and volumes can be accurately controlled. This is of major importance when performing multiphase acquisitions. If contrast injections are not performed in a reproducible manner, suboptimal studies will be the result (see Section 3.1.3.2). Maximum injection rates are related to the size of the used intravenous cannula. Large size cannulas (16–18G) have lower flow resistance and are preferred for studies requiring high injection rates, that is, CT angiography. With the exception of contrast-enhanced brain CT studies, manual contrast injection is rarely performed. I-CM can be injected using central venous catheters (CVCs). However, such injections require a meticulous sterile injection technique. CVCs may burst if high injection pressures are applied. Manual injection or low-pressure power injection (<1.8 mL/s) should be used when injecting CM in CVCs. It is advisable to consult the product summary of the specific CVC before injecting the contrast.

3.1.3.1.2 Oral Contrast Media Administration

The main reason to use oral CM during CT scans is to distend the small bowel, facilitating diagnosis in this area. Both positive and negative CM are used for this purpose. Positive agents (increase enhancement) include dilutions of barium and I-CM. The negative (decrease enhancement) "CM" is normal drinking water. Before oral administration of either barium or I-CM, the radiologist must obtain information about the patient's clinical condition. If acute surgical intervention is likely after the imaging procedure, barium agents should be avoided. Likewise, iodinated agents should be used in recently operated patients. These recommendations are similar to standard recommendations for fluoroscopic procedures.

I-CM do not cause any harm if leaked into the peritoneal cavity, whereas barium agents induce severe toxic peritonitis. Use of barium agents should be reserved for nonacute patients with an intact bowel wall.

Of special interest is the use of oral CM in CT colonography (CTC). This so-called fecal tagging procedure is used to reduce the problem of poor bowel cleansing. The patient is given small amounts of either I-CM or barium CM before the CTC examination. CM are then incorporated into the patient's fecal matter, which facilitates identification during the CTC procedure. With modern workstations, electronic cleansing techniques are applied to remove the high-attenuation fecal material from the colonic lumen making polyp detection easier.

Oral CM (water-soluble iodine) are advisable when performing CT of gastric bypass patients suspected of internal herniation [39]. In this case, oral CM aid the visualization of the complex postsurgery small bowel anatomy.

3.1.3.1.3 Other Routes of Contrast Media Administration

When administering CM by other than the intravenous and oral routes, iodinated CM are used. If the passage of CM into the vascular system seems possible, the same precautions as prior intravenous administration should be taken. Examples are rectal and intravesical administration, typically performed when postsurgical leakage is suspected. Another example is CT fistulography.

3.1.3.2 Bolus Timing Techniques

The technical quality of contrast-enhanced CT scans is heavily dependent on images being acquired in the correct contrast phases. If this is not the case, nondiagnostic or inconclusive scans are likely to occur. In modern multi-detector CT systems capable of acquiring large volumes of data in few seconds, bolus timing has become even more important. Thus, different bolus timing techniques have been developed to ensure that contrast-enhanced examinations can be performed in a reproducible manner. All these techniques refer to bolus timing after intravenous administration of CM. Administration of CM with automated power injectors is regarded mandatory for accurate bolus timing. In the context of different types of CT applications, bolus timing is most important in CT angiography. The arterial phase following intravenous CM injection is transient, allowing only a few seconds with arterial contrast, before venous and parenchymal enhancement begins (Figure 3.5). Scanning beyond the arterial phase has less time constraint, as the portal venous and delayed phases last longer than the arterial phase (see Section 3.1.1.2). Even in nonarterial phase CT, it is still advisable to use automated CM injection, as this secures

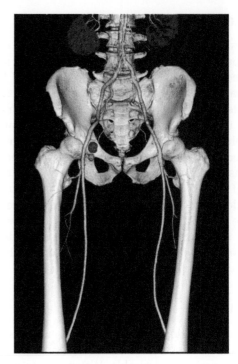

FIGURE 3.5
CT angiography. Patient showing a pseudoaneurysm originating from the right common femoral artery.

similar acquisitions between the patient and the individual, making comparison easier.

Important bolus timing techniques for CT angiography are automated bolus detection, test bolus techniques, and "best guess" strategies. It is necessary to use such strategies as the hemodynamics differ in each patient because of, for instance, low cardiac output or extensive atherosclerotic lesions. With the automated bolus detection technique, a small region of interest (ROI) is placed in a large artery in the anatomical area of interest (e.g., the pulmonary trunk in pulmonary CT angiography, or the ascending aorta for carotid CT angiography). Immediately after CM injection, fast repetitive acquisitions are performed in the ROI. As the contrast bolus reaches, the ROI attenuation increases, and when reaching a predefined level (e.g., 80 HU), image acquisition is started (Figure 3.6). With the test bolus technique, a small volume of CM is injected followed by fast repetitive acquisitions over the anatomical area of interest. The time point, at which contrast enhancement peaks, defines the arterial phase. Using this information, delay between contrast injection and image acquisition can be accurately set. It is important that the same injection rate is used for the test bolus and the subsequent contrast bolus injection. The most simple bolus timing strategy is the "best guess" technique, in which time from contrast injection to image acquisition is predefined after taking into account different patient-related factors (ischemic

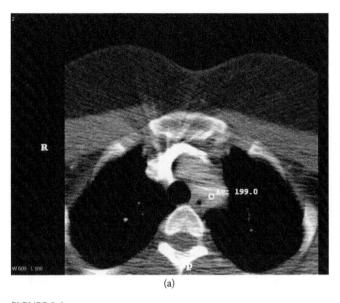

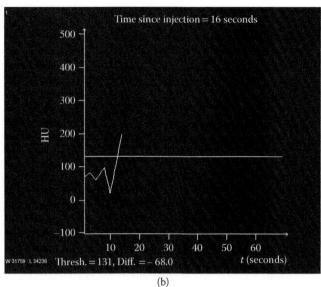

FIGURE 3.6
Automated bolus detection in CT angiography. (a) Axial scan showing the localizer (ROI) placed in the ascending aorta for carotid CT angiography, (b) graph showing automated bolus detection. Acquisition was initiated 16 seconds after injection, when the predefined threshold of 131 HU was reached.

heart disease, age, peripheral arterial disease, etc.). It is obviously not a very robust technique for CT angiography and therefore rarely used in modern multi-detector CT systems.

3.1.3.3 Contrast Media Extravasation

In most cases, extravasation of CM is a self-limiting event that resolves spontaneously within two to four days. However, severe cases may progress to tissue necrosis or even acute compartment syndrome [40]. It is therefore essential that care is taken to prevent CM extravasation. The incidence of CM extravasation is higher after mechanical bolus injection compared to hand injection [41]. Thus, most cases are seen following CT or MRI using automated power injectors. This section focuses on extravasation of I-CM in CT. Important aspects regarding pathogenesis, risk factors, clinical presentation, and treatment are presented.

The exact pathogenic mechanism leading to tissue damage after extravasation of I-CM is unclear. It is, however, clear that osmolality and volume of the extravasated CM play a role in development of tissue damage. High-osmolar agents induce more damage than low/iso-osmolar agents. Severe skin lesions are more common with extravasation of larger volumes (>15 mL) of CM [42,43].

Numerous risk factors have been identified. Patients unable to complain about pain at the injection area (i.e., infants, small children, and unconscious patients) are at increased risk of CM extravasation. Other risk factors include chemotherapy, arterial or venous insufficiency, atrophy of muscles, and subcutaneous fatty tissue. Chemotherapy is a risk factor as it might induce weakness of the vascular walls.

The incidence of CM extravasation in CT with automated power injectors is reported to be <1% [44]. However, no relation to injection rate, catheter location, or catheter size has been identified.

The clinical presentation of CM extravasation is variable. Usual symptoms are pain and discomfort at the injection area, but some cases are asymptomatic. Clinical findings are a red, swollen, and tender extravasation area. As stated earlier, most cases are minor and self-limiting. Severe cases can progress to tissue necrosis and/or compartment syndrome. It may be difficult to separate extravasation from local irritation and hypersensitivity reactions. A key point allowing differentiation is a well-placed catheter in nonextravasation reactions.

There is no consensus on treatment of CM extravasation. Conservative treatment with elevation of the limb along with topical application of warm or cold is used in the majority of cases [7]. Limb elevation reduces the hydrostatic pressure and thus reduces swelling. Topical application of warmth leads to vasodilatation, promoting resorption of extracellular fluid. On the contrary, application of cold leads to vasoconstriction and has an anti-inflammatory effect. More aggressive therapy with surgical suction or topical aspiration of the extravasated CM is controversial. If used at all, these methods should be reserved to the most severe cases.

References

1. Thomsen HS, Golman K, Hemmingsen L et al. Contrast medium induced nephropathy: animal experiments. *Front Eur Radiol* 1993; 9: 83–108.

2. Katzberg WR. Urography in the 21st century: new contrast media, renal handling, imaging characteristics, and nephrotoxicity. *Radiology* 1997; 204: 297–312.

3. Urban BA, McGhie PA, Fishman EK. Diagnostic pitfalls of arterial phase imaging of the upper abdomen. *AJR Am J Roentgenol* 2001; 174: 455–461.

4. Sheth S, Scatarige JC, Horton KM et al. Current concepts in the diagnosis and management of renal cell carcinoma: role of multidetector CT and three-dimensional CT. *Radiographics* 2001; 21: S237–S254.

5. Stenver DI. Pharmacovigilance: when to report adverse reactions. In: Thomsen HS, Webb JAW, eds. *Contrast Media. Safety Issues and ESUR Guidelines*. 2nd ed. Heidelberg: Springer Verlag; 2009: 21–23.

6. Bush WH, Swanson DP. Acute reactions to intravascular contrast media: types, risks factors, recognition and specific treatment. *AJR Am J Roentgenol* 1991; 157: 1153–1161.

7. European Society of Urogenital Radiology—ESUR. Guidelines on contrast media. Version 8. Available at: www.esur.org (accessed July 30, 2012).

8. Katayama H, Yamaguchi K, Kozuka T et al. Adverse reactions to ionic and nonionic contrast media. *Radiology* 1990; 175: 621–628.

9. Laroche D, Aimone-Gastin I, Dubois F et al. Mechanisms of severe, immediate reactions to iodinated contrast media. *Radiology* 1998; 209: 183–190.

10. Witten DM, Hirsch FD, Hartman GW. Acute reactions to urographic contrast medium. *AJR Am J Roentgenol* 1973; 119: 832–840.

11. Shehadi WH. Adverse reactions to intravascularly administered contrast media. *AJR Am J Roentgenol* 1975; 124: 145–152.

12. Siegle RL, Halvorsen RA, Dillon J et al. The use of iohexol in patients with previous reactions to ionic contrast material. *Invest Radiol* 1991; 26: 411–416.

13. Jacobs JE, Birnbaum BA, Langlotz CP. Contrast media reactions and extravasation: relationship to intravenous injection rates. *Radiology* 1998; 209: 411–416.

14. Thomsen HS. Management of acute adverse reactions to contrast media. In: Thomsen HS, Webb JAW, eds. *Contrast Media. Safety Issues and ESUR Guidelines*. 2nd ed. Heidelberg: Springer Verlag; 2009: 53–60.

15. Yasuda R, Munechika H. Delayed adverse reactions to nonionic monomeric contrast-enhanced media. *Invest Radiol* 1998; 33: 1–5.

16. Schild H. Delayed allergy-like reactions in patients: monomeric and dimeric contrast media compared with plain CT. *Eur Radiol* 1996; 6: 9–10.

17. Kanny G, Pichler WJ, Morisset M et al. T cell-mediated reactions to iodinated contrast media: evaluation by skin and lymphocyte activations tests. *J Allergy Clin Immunol* 2005; 115: 179–185.

18. Pedersen SH, Svaland MG, Reiss A-L et al. Late allergy-like reactions following vascular administration of radiography contrast media. *Acta Radiol* 1998; 39: 344–348.

19. McCullough M, Davies P, Richardson R. A large trial of intravenous Conray 325 and Nipoman 300 to assess immediate and delayed reactions. *Br J Radiol* 1989; 62: 260–265.

20. Sutton AGC, Finn P, Campbell PG et al. Early and late reactions following the use of iopamidol 340, iomeprol 350 and iodixanol 320 in cardiac catheterization. *J Invasive Cardiol* 2003; 15: 133–138.

21. Bellin MF, Stacul F, Webb JA et al. Late adverse reactions to intravascular iodine based contrast media: an update. *Eur Radiol* 2011; 21: 2305–2310.

22. Hosoya T, Yamaguchi K, Akutzu T et al. Delayed adverse reactions to iodinated contrast media and their risk factors. *Radiat Med* 2000; 18: 39–45.

23. Conn JJ, Sebastian MJ, Deam D et al. A prospective study of the effect of ionic contrast media on thyroid function. *Thyroid* 1996; 6: 107–110.

24. van der Molen AJ. Effects on thyroid function. In: Thomsen HS, Webb JAW, eds. *Contrast Media. Safety issues and ESUR Guidelines*. 2nd ed. Heidelberg: Springer Verlag; 2009: 139–145.

25. Hintze G, Blombach O, Fink H et al. Risk of iodine-induced thyrotoxicosis after coronary angiography: an investigation of 788 unselected subjects. *Eur J Endocrinol* 1999; 140: 264–267.

26. Thomsen HS. Contrast medium-induced nephropathy. In: Thomsen HS, Webb JAW, eds. *Contrast Media. Safety Issues and ESUR Guidelines*. 2nd ed. Heidelberg: Springer Verlag; 2009: 63–80.

27. Thomsen HS, Morcos SK. Risk of contrast-medium-induced nephropathy in high-risk patients undergoing MDCT—A pooled analysis of two randomized trials. *Eur Radiol* 2009; 19: 891–897.

28. Katzberg R. Contrast medium-induced nephrotoxicity: which pathways? *Radiology* 2005; 235: 752–755.

29. Rudnick MR, Goldfarb S, Wexler L et al. Nephrotoxicity of ionic and nonionic contrast media in 1196 patients: a randomized trial. *Kidney Int* 1995; 47: 254–261.

30. Morcos SK, Thomsen HS, Webb JAW. Contrast media induced nephrotoxicity: a consensus report. *Eur Radiol* 1999; 9: 1602–1613.

31. Morcos SK. Contrast media-induced nephrotoxicity—questions and answers. *Br J Radiol* 1998; 71: 357–365.

32. Levey AS, Bosch JP, Lewis JB et al. A more accurate method to estimate glomerular filtration rate from serum creatinine: a new prediction equation. *Ann Intern Med* 1999; 130: 461–470.

33. Stacul F, van der Molen AJ, Reimer P et al. Contrast induced nephropathy: updated ESUR Contrast Media Safety Committee guidelines. *Eur Radiol* 2011; 21: 2527–2541.

34. Morcos SK. Barium preparations: safety issues. In: Thomsen HS, Webb JAW, eds. *Contrast Media. Safety Issues and ESUR Guidelines*. 2nd ed. Heidelberg: Springer Verlag; 2009: 223–226.

35. Thomsen HS, Almén T, Morcos SK et al. Gadolinium-containing contrast media for radiographic examination: a position paper. *Eur Radiol* 2002; 12: 2600–2605.

36. Hoppe H, Spagnuolo S, Froehlich JM et al. Retrospective analysis of patients for development of nephrogenic systemic fibrosis following conventional angiography using gadolinium-based contrast agents. *Eur Radiol* 2010; 20: 595–603.

37. Strunk HM, Schild H. Actual clinical use of gadolinium-chelates for non-MRI applications. *Eur Radiol* 2004; 14: 1055–1062.

38. Elmståhl B, Nyman U, Leander P et al. Gadolinium contrast media are more nephrotoxic than iodine media. The importance of osmolality in direct renal artery injections. *Eur Radiol* 2006; 16: 2712–2720.

39. Lockhart ME, Tessler FN, Canon CL et al. Internal hernia after gastric bypass: sensitivity and specificity of seven CT sign with surgical correlation and controls. *AJR Am J Roentgenol* 2007; 188: 745–750.

40. Benson LS, Sathy MJ, Port RB. Forearm compartment syndrome due to automated injection of computed tomography contrast material. *J Orthop Trauma* 1996; 10: 433–436.

41. Jakobsen JÅ. Extravasation injury. In: Thomsen HS, Webb JAW, eds. *Contrast Media. Safety Issues and ESUR Guidelines.* 2nd ed. Heidelberg: Springer Verlag; 2009: 115–119.

42. Cohan RH, Ellis JH, Garner WL. Extravasation of radiographic contrast material: recognition, prevention, and treatment. *Radiology* 1996; 200; 593–604.

43. Cohan RH, Bullard MA, Ellis JH et al. Local reactions after injection of iodinated contrast material: detection, management, and outcome. *Acad Radiol* 1997; 4: 711–718.

44. Federle MP, Chang PJ, Confer S et al. Frequency and effects of extravasation of ionic and nonionic CT contrast media during rapid bolus injection. *Radiology* 1998; 206: 637–640.

4

Computed Tomography Angiography: Postprocessing Methods and Clinical Applications

Zhonghua Sun

CONTENTS

4.1 Introduction

Since the computed tomography (CT) scanner was first developed by the English engineer Godfrey Hounsfield in the early 1970s, it has been widely recognized as a very useful diagnostic imaging technique as it allows visualization of the cross-sectional views of the body structures. In the early 1990s, the introduction of helical or spiral CT scanners was considered a major breakthrough for CT technology. With spiral CT, the patient table is continuously moved and translated through the gantry while scan data are acquired simultaneously. Spiral CT scanning does not suffer from misregistration problems or loss of anatomic details since the scan is performed in a single breath-hold, thus enabling acquisition of volume data. Images could be reconstructed at any position along the patient's longitudinal axis, and overlapping image reconstruction could be generated (normally 50% overlap) to improve longitudinal resolution. Acquisition of volumetric data has become the very basis for applications such as CT angiography (CTA) [1].

The introduction of multislice CT (MSCT) is considered a major evolutionary leap in CT technology. By late 1998, all major CT manufacturers launched MSCT scanners capable of at least four slices per x-ray tube rotation. The MSCT scanner, with its cone-shaped beam and multiple slices per rotation, allows for acquisition of multiple slices during one gantry rotation. This difference, along with the reduced gantry rotation time in the MSCT scanners, leads to shorter scanning time, enables greater coverage of scanning volume per gantry rotation, and provides superior image quality [2].

The most important clinical benefit for MSCT lies in its ability to scan a given anatomic region within a given scan time with substantially reduced slice thickness, at many times increased longitudinal resolution when compared to single-slice CT. Thus, many clinical applications can be performed using very thin slice thickness (e.g., submillimeter slice thickness), resulting in isotropic volume data, thus improving the image quality of three-dimensional (3D) visualizations. The early generation of MSCT scanners enables simultaneous acquisition of four slices at a rotation time of 500 ms, which is four times faster than the traditional single-slice CT scanners, providing significant improvement of scan speed and longitudinal resolution [3,4]. Later technical developments such as 64-slice or more slice CT scanners allow for acquisition of large volume data in a very short time, with a rotation time down to 165 ms and with high spatial and temporal resolution [5–7]. The developments of MSCT have been widely recognized as revolutionary improvements in the medical imaging field, which eventually enable cardiovascular imaging to be performed with high diagnostic accuracy [8].

4.2 Computed Tomography Angiography

A significant advantage and development of spiral CT data acquisition is its application in 3D imaging of vascular structures with an intravenous injection of contrast medium. This application is referred to as CT angiography or CTA.

CTA is achieved with two essential requirements: volumetric data must be acquired with spiral CT scanning while contrast medium is delivered intravenously. CTA images can be captured when vessels are fully opacified to show either arterial or venous phase enhancement through acquisition of both datasets (arterial or venous phase, depending on the scan delay of contrast medium administration). CTA has been widely applied to a number of examinations investigating both normal vascular anatomy and abnormal changes, and it has been regarded as one of the most valuable applications in CT imaging. CTA produces angiography-like images noninvasively in a 3D format, thus it has replaced conventional angiography in many clinical applications. In particular, CTA techniques have proved useful in imaging the neurovasculature, thoracic and abdominal aorta, and peripheral vasculature, and in evaluating the vasculature of the abdominal viscera [9–11].

Diagnostic value of CTA has been significantly augmented with the use of MSCT techniques, owing to its improved resolution, allowing excellent visualization of both main artery and side arterial branches. MSCT angiography produces angiography-like images with high diagnostic accuracy, further enhancing the CTA applications. In particular, MSCT angiography has proved valuable in imaging the vascular tree for diagnosis

of a variety of cardiovascular diseases. Studies have shown that in many applications, MSCT angiography can be used as a reliable alternative to invasive angiography [11–18]. This is of clinical significance because the number of invasive angiographic examinations can be reduced or unnecessary invasive procedures can be avoided based on MSCT angiography findings.

4.3 Postprocessing Visualization Tools

Image postprocessing is an essential part of CTA. This process involves the generation and modification of 3D volume data that consist of a stack of individual two-dimensional (2D) axial images. MSCT angiography in imaging cardiovascular diseases is complemented by a series of 2D and 3D postprocessing visualizations, including multiplanar reformation (MPR), maximum-intensity projection (MIP), surface shaded display (SSD), volume rendering (VR), and virtual intravascular endoscopy (VIE). However, 2D axial CT images still remain as the standard reference in most situations as the initial visualization tool, whereas 2D and 3D reconstructed visualizations provide additional information to support clinical diagnosis. The reliable recognition of the diagnostic performance of these reconstructions will assist clinicians to choose the appropriate image visualization for the assessment of cardiovascular diseases and to efficiently use the MSCT imaging modality for clinical purposes. Each visualization tool is presented in Sections 4.3.1 through 4.3.6 in terms of the additional value each tool offers compared with 2D axial views.

4.3.1 Axial Image Slices

Transaxial images are the basic outcome of a CT scan and include all of the information that is contained within a CT scan. Thus, axial images should be reviewed in all cases, for example, by scrolling through them up and down, which gives a quick overview of the relevant cardiovascular structures, including pathological changes. The in-plane spatial resolution of original axial images determines the quality of reconstructed 2D and 3D images.

The matrix size for axial images in CT is generally 512×512 picture elements (pixels). Considered as part of a 3D image volume, an axial image is a layer of 512×512 voxels within that volume dataset. The voxel size in the image plane (x–y direction) is determined by the in-plane pixel size and, therefore, by the reconstructed field of view (FOV) during a CT scan. The size of the voxel in the longitudinal direction (z direction) is given by the slice width and the image increment, which is determined by the detector collimation. Typically, an FOV of 200–300 mm is chosen for image reconstruction in body imaging, resulting in 0.39–0.58 mm in-plane voxel size, whereas a narrowed FOV of 150–180 mm is chosen for image reconstruction in cardiac imaging, resulting in 0.29–0.35 mm in-plane voxel size. With 64-slice CT, a voxel size of 0.5 × 0.5 × 0.5 mm can be achieved in all three dimensions (*x*, *y*, and *z* directions) in axial CT images, thus enabling excellent visualization of cardiovascular structures, including the tiny coronary arteries (Figure 4.1).

4.3.2 Multiplanar Reformation

In MPR, a plane is defined in a 3D image volume, and all voxels on that plane are visualized in a planar image. MPR is a powerful tool to display and communicate complex anatomic and pathological information. It is most commonly reconstructed to improve understanding of the relationship among complex anatomical structures. However, it is crucial to have a fine

longitudinal resolution for MPR display to be useful, since resolution along the longitudinal axis with conventional CT has been an order of magnitude worse than transaxial resolution [19]. The choice of CT beam collimation has a direct impact on the quality of image postprocessing and on lesion detection. With the current MSCT scanners, high longitudinal resolution with a voxel size as small as 0.5 mm can be achieved in all three dimensions, resulting in excellent spatial resolution (longitudinal resolution). Consequently, the stair-step artifacts that used to be the main concern with single-detector row CT [20] and trade-off between slice thickness and image noise [21] that was present in early generation of MSCT scanners no longer exist in MPR images acquired with modern MSCT scanners (Figure 4.2).

Simple examples of MPR are coronal and sagittal views that are widely used in general radiology but of limited use in cardiac imaging as coronary arteries show complex course and they do not follow a straight path along the cardiac muscle. Thus, a number of MPR images are required to show the entire course of coronary arteries,

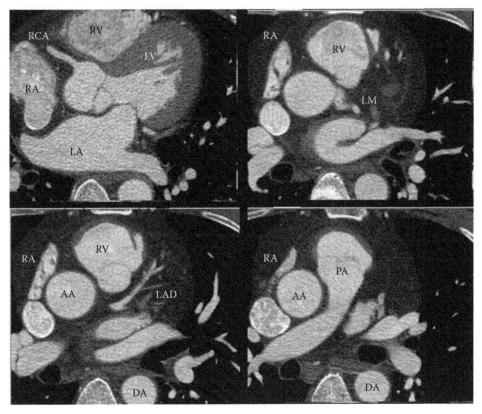

FIGURE 4.1
Axial images are acquired using a 64-slice computed tomography (CT) scanner with slice thickness of 0.625 mm at different anatomical levels of a coronary CT angiography examination in a patient suspected of coronary artery disease. Axial images include all of the information acquired in a CT scan and should be reviewed in any case, for example, by scrolling through them. AA, ascending aorta; PA, pulmonary artery; DA, descending aorta; SVC, superior vena cava; RA, right atrium; RV, right ventricle; LA, left atrium; LV, left ventricle; LM, left main stem; LAD, left anterior descending coronary artery; RCA, right coronary artery.

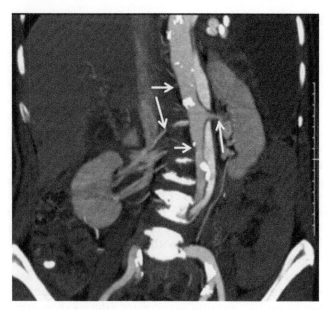

FIGURE 4.2
Coronal multiplanar reformatted image clearly shows aortic dissection with bilateral renal arteries arising from the false lumen (long arrows). Short arrows refer to the false lumen that has lower CT attenuation than that in the true lumen.

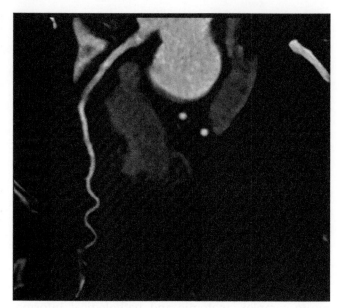

FIGURE 4.3
Curved planar reformatted image showing the entire right coronary artery tree.

since not all of the coronary segments can be displayed in a single MPR view. In contrast, curved MPR, also defined as curved planar reformation, is the most useful visualization tool for cardiac CT as MPR views are generated along the curved planes instead of straight planes. Thus, curved MPR allows capturing the course of tortuous coronary arteries along their entire length in a single image (Figure 4.3).

4.3.3 Surface Shaded Display

In SSD, user-selected upper and lower thresholds are used to define a specific range of Hounsfield unit (HU) to be displayed. As the aim of CTA is to show the contrast-enhanced arteries, the range of threshold is determined by measuring the region of interest in the arteries on sequential axial CT images, which normally ranges from 150 to 250 HU. Therefore, voxels lower than the selected threshold are invisible in final images (Figure 4.4). SSD is easy and quick to produce, as generation of SSD images depends on threshold selection; however, it only utilizes approximately 10% of the volume data, thus, not all of the information is used for final image display.

4.3.4 Maximum-Intensity Projection

MIP is considered as the most useful visualization tool in CTA as it provides angiography-like images non-invasively. The principle of MIP visualization is the

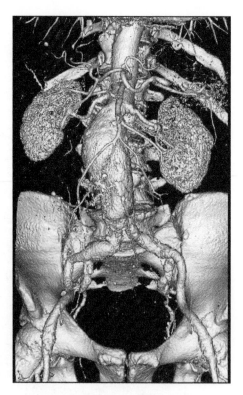

FIGURE 4.4
The 3D surface shaded display showing an infrarenal aortic aneurysm involving bilateral common iliac arteries.

demonstration of maximum CT number encountered in each ray. As a result of the projection, the pixels in the MIP image represent the maximum CT number encountered in each ray. MIP does not require selection of any

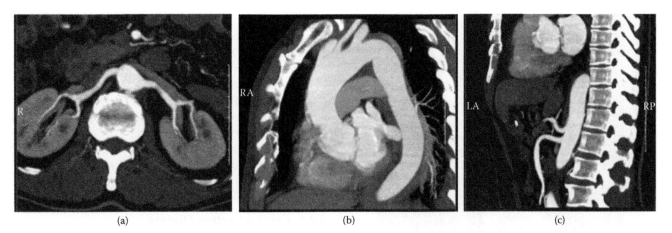

FIGURE 4.5
(a) An axial maximum-intensity projection (MIP) showing renal arteries arising from the abdominal aorta. (b) A sagittal MIP showing the thoracic aorta with three main branches arising from the aortic arch. (c) Another sagittal MIP showing the celiac axis and superior mesenteric artery arising from the abdominal aorta.

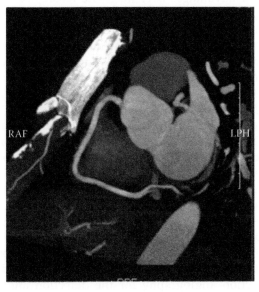

FIGURE 4.6
Thin-slab maximum-intensity projection showing the entire right coronary artery tree without any evidence of abnormal change.

thresholds as it displays only the brightest voxel along every ray of sight. As a result, all darker voxels in front of or behind a brighter voxel are not displayed. Contrast-enhanced blood vessels together with high-density structures such as calcifications or bones are clearly displayed on MIP images (Figure 4.5). However, MIP images do not provide depth information, which is the main drawback for visualization of complex anatomy. Thin-slab MIPs are introduced to overcome this short-coming. In particular, for visualization of the tortuous vessels such as coronary arteries, planes in parallel to a line connecting the coronary artery and those along the coronary artery should be used to visualize the course of coronary arteries (Figure 4.6).

4.3.5 Volume Rendering

In contrast to SSD and MIP, VR uses all of the information contained inside a volume dataset, thus allowing production of more meaningful images. By assigning a specific color and opacity value for every attenuation value of the CT data, groups of voxels are selected for display. A voxel-based intensity histogram is generated, and several parameters such as color, brightness, and opacity are assigned to each voxel according to its Hounsfield unit value. Similar to MIP projections, rays are cast through the 3D image volume. Unlike MIP projections, however, all voxels along a ray contribute to the resulting pixel in the VR image corresponding to their opacities. Therefore, 3D relationship between different structures can be easily displayed and appreciated on VR, as shown in Figure 4.7. VR requires extensive user interaction for accurate evaluation of complex anatomical structures. The transparency option of the software allows the viewer to see through the object maps with various structures displayed simultaneously.

4.3.6 Virtual Intravascular Endoscopy

As part of the VR, VIE provides unique intravascular views of the main aorta, arterial tree and any pathological changes, and their relationship to the artery branches. The CT data are prepared for VIE by removing the contrast-enhanced blood from the artery using a CT number thresholding technique (Figure 4.8). A CT number threshold range of arterial lumen is identified using selected region-of-interest measurements. The methodology of generation of VIE images has been described in detail in Reference 22. It should be emphasized that successful generation of VIE images depends on appropriate selection of threshold values and the quality of original 2D source images.

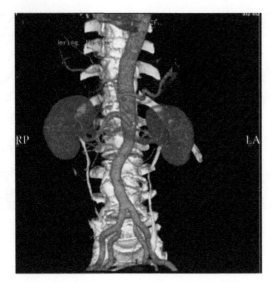

FIGURE 4.7
3D volume rendering clearly shows the abdominal aorta and arterial branches coded with pink color. Bones and ureters are assigned with white color.

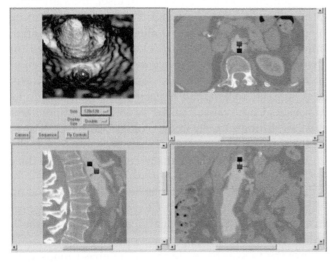

FIGURE 4.8
Virtual intravascular endoscopy view produced by applying a threshold measured at the level of superior mesenteric artery based on a CT number (200 HU) to remove the contrast-enhanced blood from the aorta.

4.4 Clinical Applications of Computed Tomography Angiography and Postprocessing Reconstructions

Imaging of the cardiovascular system has undergone rapid developments over the past decade because of advancements in CT imaging techniques, such as MSCT with evolution from early generation of 4-slice

to 64-slice, and the most recent model of 320-slice CT scanners [2–8]. With improved spatial and temporal resolution, MSCT angiography has proved to be superior to conventional angiography in the diagnosis of many cardiovascular diseases, thus it has been extensively used as the method of choice in the diagnostic applications of cardiovascular imaging. Sections 4.4.1 through 4.4.8 will present clinical applications of CTA in a number of common cardiovascular diseases, with a focus on the diagnostic value of various postprocessing reconstructions.

4.4.1 Cerebral Artery Disease

CTA has been increasingly used as the first-line diagnostic tool for the detection of intracranial aneurysms; its diagnostic value has been significantly improved with the development of MSCT scanners [23,24]. It has superior advantages over magnetic resonance angiography, which are shown by high spatial resolution, fast scanning, and uncomplicated feature. Reliable quantification of intracranial arterial stenosis is also possible in patients with severe vessel kinking; and more accurate reading and interpretation of results can be achieved with the aid of visualization tools such as MPR, MIP, and VR (Figure 4.9) [25].

Studies performed with 64-slice CT have shown that CTA has a similar diagnostic accuracy as that of conventional angiography in the evaluation of patients suspected of having intracranial aneurysms [26,27]. However, CTA has disadvantages in the detection of small intracranial aneurysms (<3 mm) and aneurysms near the skull base because of the influence of overprojecting bone structures. Subtracted 3D CTA has been developed to allow bone-free visualization of aneurysms, and it compares favorably with digital subtraction angiography for the detection and characterization of intracranial aneurysms (Figure 4.10) [28–31]. Automatic segmentation or subtraction of bone or plaque using dual-energy CT has been shown to be feasible and promising, producing highly sensitive results [32]. Dual-energy CT is recommended as a valuable additional tool for head and neck CTA studies because it is fully automatic and involves no user interaction.

4.4.2 Carotid Artery Stenosis

It is estimated that 80% of all strokes that occur annually in the advanced countries are ischemic, and about 30% of these are caused by thromboemboli arising from atherosclerotic lesions leading to an abnormal narrowing (stenosis) at the carotid artery bifurcation [33,34]. Therefore, a leading indicator for assessing stroke risk

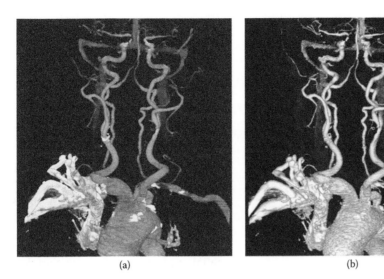

FIGURE 4.9
(a) 2D maximum-intensity projection and (b) 3D volume rendering images showing normal carotid arteries arising from the aortic arch with visualization of cerebral branches.

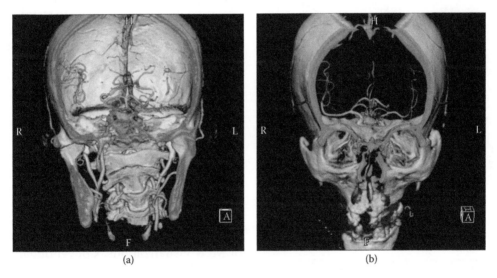

FIGURE 4.10
(a) 3D CT angiography (CTA) showing the circle of Willis with bony structures. (b) Subtracted CTA with some bone structures removed clearly shows the artery branches in the circle of Willis.

for patients with symptoms of minor ischemic stroke is the degree of stenosis of the carotid artery. Several studies have shown that degree of carotid artery stenosis is a critical parameter in the evaluation of stroke risk, because the risk of ischemic stroke distal to the carotid stenosis increases with the degree of stenosis and can be markedly reduced with endarterectomy [35–37].

Intra-arterial catheter angiography still remains the gold standard for detection of the degree of carotid artery stenosis [38]; however, it is not only an invasive investigation but is also associated with complications. Numerous less-invasive imaging techniques are

increasingly used in the evaluation of carotid artery stenosis, such as MSCT angiography, magnetic resonance angiography, and duplex ultrasound. It is important to evaluate the performance of these less-invasive modalities and determine which modality could be used as an alternative to invasive angiography in the diagnosis of carotid artery stenosis.

A moderate to high diagnostic value has been reported with the use of MSCT angiography in the detection of carotid artery stenosis [25,39]. In addition to routine 2D and 3D reconstructions (Figure 4.11), intraluminal views provided by VIE allow the identification of carotid plaques (Figure 4.12) and the appearance of

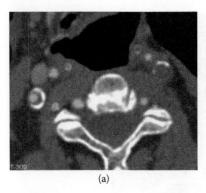
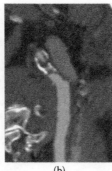

(a)   (b)

FIGURE 4.11
(a) 2D axial image showing a significant stenosis in the right internal carotid artery because of atherosclerotic plaques. (b) Sagittal multiplanar reformation confirms the significant stenosis with presence of thrombus.

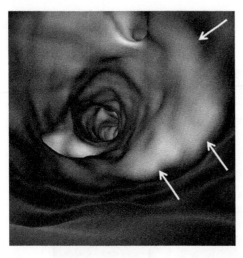

FIGURE 4.12
Virtual intravascular endoscopy showing narrowed arterial lumen caused by the plaques (arrows).

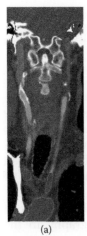
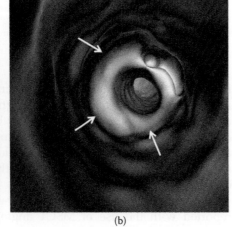

(a)   (b)

FIGURE 4.13
(a) A carotid stent implanted to treat right carotid stenosis as shown in the coronal multiplanar reformation. (b) Virtual intravascular endoscopy showing the intraluminal views of carotid stent with patent lumen (arrows).

carotid stent (Figure 4.13). The interference of blooming artifacts from severe calcified plaques at the carotid artery results in inaccurate assessment of the degree of carotid artery stenosis. This is the main limitation of MSCT angiography in the diagnosis of carotid artery stenosis.

4.4.3 Coronary Artery Disease

Coronary artery disease (CAD) is the leading cause of death in advanced countries and its prevalence is increasing among developing countries [40,41]. Traditionally, diagnosis of CAD is performed by invasive coronary angiography, which is recognized as the gold standard technique, since it has superior spatial and temporal resolution leading to excellent diagnostic accuracy. However, it is an invasive and expensive procedure associated with a small but distinct procedure-related morbidity (1.5%) and mortality (0.2%) [42]. Furthermore, invasive coronary angiography usually requires patients to stay for a short period in the hospital after the examination, and this causes discomfort for the patients. The diagnosis and management of CAD is increasingly dependent on noninvasive imaging modalities. Over the past decades, MSCT coronary angiography has undergone rapid developments, and it has been increasingly used in the diagnosis of CAD as an effective alternative to invasive coronary angiography [15,16].

The imaging of the coronary artery is technically challenging because of its small diameter, which ranges from 3–5 mm in the main segments to 1 mm in the distal segments. Moreover, the coronary artery follows a circular path around the myocardium, which then puts a strong demand on the requirement of MPR visualizations. Conventional 2D axial views are unable to visualize the entire coronary artery that consists of the proximal, middle, and distal segments, as well as side branches. In contrast, MPR, such as curved MPR, is most commonly used to show the entire coronary tree and detection of pathological changes, such as the presence of plaques (Figure 4.14). MIP offers excellent angiography-like views of the coronary artery tree and easily identifies coronary plaques (Figure 4.15), whereas VR uses entire volume data to present 3D views of the coronary artery tree in relation to the cardiac chambers (Figure 4.16).

VIE provides unique intraluminal views of the coronary artery wall and the pathological changes caused by plaques. VIE images clearly show the intraluminal appearance of different types of plaques [43], thus VIE does provide useful information about coronary wall changes when compared to conventional visualization tools (Figure 4.17). Although VIE is not recommended as a routine visualization, it can serve as a complementary

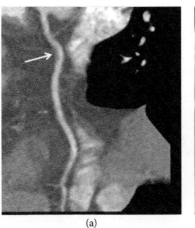
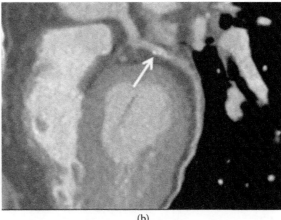

(a)   (b)

FIGURE 4.14
Curved MPR showing a noncalcified plaque in the proximal segment of right coronary artery (arrow) resulting in 50% lumen stenosis.
(b) A calcified plaque is detected in the left anterior descending artery without significant stenosis (arrow).

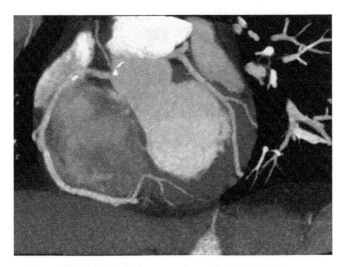
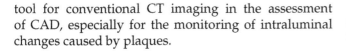

FIGURE 4.15
Coronary maximum-intensity projection showing a calcified plaque in the proximal segment of right coronary artery.

tool for conventional CT imaging in the assessment of CAD, especially for the monitoring of intraluminal changes caused by plaques.

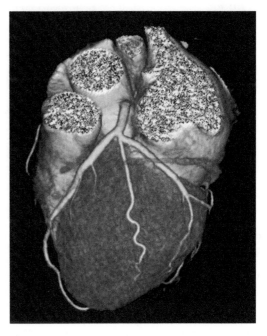

FIGURE 4.16
3D volume rendering showing excellent visualization of left coronary artery and side branches, without any motion artifacts.

4.4.4 Coronary Stenting

In recent years, CAD has been increasingly treated by coronary stent placement. Although stent implantation has been shown to greatly reduce restenosis after balloon angioplasty [44,45], in-stent restenosis can occur in 20%–35% of patients for bare metal stents, and 5%–10% for drug-eluting stents [46,47], as shown by intravascular ultrasound. MSCT angiography is increasingly used for imaging coronary stents and has been reported to have a high diagnostic

accuracy to visualize and detect coronary stent stenosis, especially with the latest 64-slice or more slice scanners [48,49].

Most stents are well visible on CT images. The CT density of natural tissues inside and around the coronary artery is much lower than that of the metal stent material. Intravenous contrast enhancement used in MSCT angiography leads to a lower concentration of contrast medium of the intracoronary lumen, thus making stents appear as bright structures on CT images.

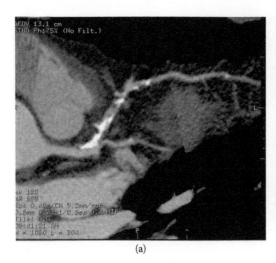

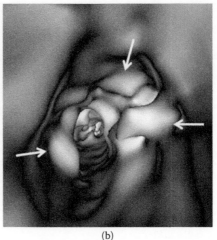

(a)   (b)

FIGURE 4.17
(a) Curved MPR showing extensively mixed type plaques present in the left anterior descending artery. (b) Corresponding virtual intravascular endoscopy showing irregular intraluminal appearance in the coronary wall because of atherosclerotic change (arrows).

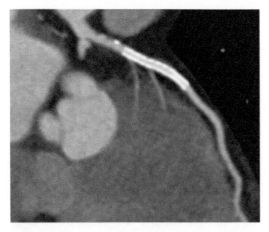

FIGURE 4.18
Curved MPR clearly shows the stent and coronary lumen within the stent in the proximal segment of left anterior descending artery without any sign of in-stent restenosis.

Various postprocessing techniques are used for evaluation of coronary stents, including MPR, MIP, and VR. Cross-sectional 2D axial and MPR images are best suited for evaluation of the coronary lumen within the stents (Figure 4.18). The anatomical location of coronary stents can be clearly visualized with MIP and VR (Figure 4.19). Coronary in-stent restenosis appears as an overall density that is lower than that of the adjacent coronary segments, and this is clearly visualized with 2D axial and MPR images (Figure 4.20). Reliable visualization of tissue within the stents requires high spatial resolution, and this is achieved with the latest 64-slice scanner, with the spatial resolution of 0.4–0.5 mm. Therefore, diagnostic accuracy has been significantly improved with 64-slice CT when compared to 4- and 16-slice scanners [48,49]. Selection of appropriate scanning protocols is

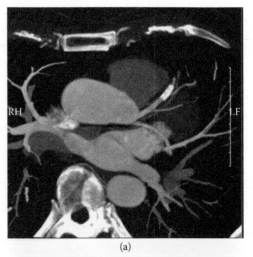

(a)

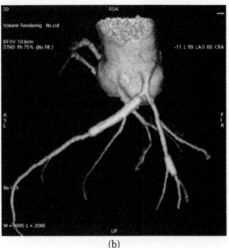

(b)

FIGURE 4.19
(a) 2D maximum-intensity projection showing the stent in the left anterior descending artery, although the intrastent lumen cannot be clearly visualized. (b) 3D volume rendering showing patent stents in the left anterior descending artery and left circumflex branches.

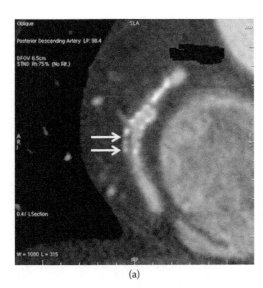 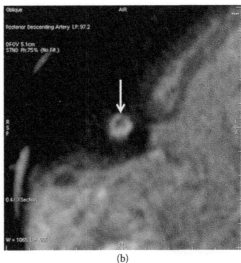

(a)   (b)

FIGURE 4.20

(a) In-stent restenosis at the right coronary stent revealed on curved MPR image as low-density attenuation (arrows) within the stent. (b) 2D cross-sectional view (arrow) confirming in-stent restenosis.

important in better visualization of the stent lumen with minimal artifacts [50].

4.4.5 Aortic Dissection

Aortic dissection is a life-threatening condition that occurs nearly three times as frequently as the rupture of abdominal aortic aneurysm (AAA) [51]. It is critical to make prompt diagnosis of aortic dissection, as this can decrease mortality and prolong survival rate. Currently, MSCT angiography is the method of choice for diagnosis of aortic dissection because of its high spatial and temporal resolution with nearly 100% sensitivity and specificity [52,53], and it has been reported to be more sensitive than invasive angiography for diagnosing aortic dissection [52,53].

In most of the cases, axial CT images supplemented by 2D and 3D reconstructions are able to identify the intimal flap that separates the true lumen from the false lumen (Figure 4.21). However, this may not be possible in all cases because of variable appearances corresponding to different types of aortic dissection [54,55]. Moreover, the 3D aortic arch is difficult to assess on an axial planes. VIE has been reported as a valuable tool for the assessment of aortic dissection, especially in the identification of intimal tear, indicating the advantages of VIE visualization in complex dissection cases [8,56]. In addition to the identification of the entry site, the extent of the entry site can be determined and further explored by VIE, and the assessment of vessel involvement can be confirmed (Figure 4.22). VIE can be used as a complementary tool to conventional CT visualizations for the accurate assessment of aortic dissection.

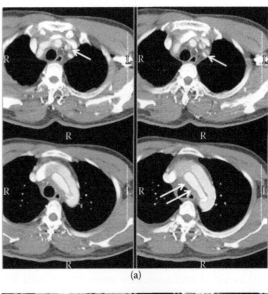

(a)

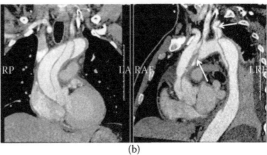

(b)

FIGURE 4.21

(a) A series of 2D axial images showing Stanford A aortic dissection involving the left common carotid and subclavian arteries (arrows in top row images) and aortic arch (arrows in bottom row images). (b) Coronal and sagittal multiplanar reformatted images confirm that aortic dissection originates in the ascending aorta and extends to the aortic arch, and in the descending aorta with involvement of arterial branches arising from the aorta (arrows).

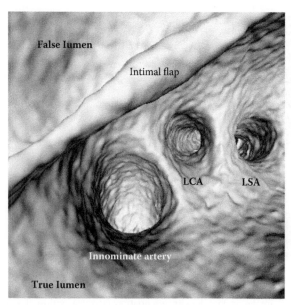

FIGURE 4.22
Virtual intravascular endoscopy (VIE) visualization showing both true and false lumens that are separated by an intimal flap. The three main artery branches are perfused by the true lumen, as shown on VIE view. LSA, left subclavian artery; LCA, left common carotid artery.

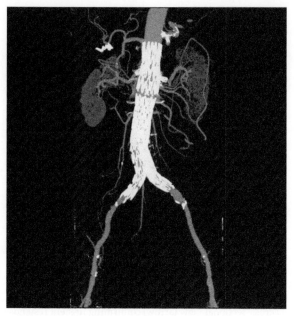

FIGURE 4.23
Coronal maximum-intensity projection image clearly shows the patency of renal arteries in a patient treated with suprarenal stent graft.

4.4.6 Abdominal Aortic Aneurysm and Endovascular Stent Grafts

Since its first introduction in clinical practice two decades ago, endovascular repair of AAA has been widely used and reported to be an effective alternative to conventional open surgery, especially in patients with comorbid medical conditions [57–59]. Unlike open surgical repair of AAA, successful completion of endovascular repair mainly depends on medical imaging, and spiral CTA has been confirmed to be the preferred modality in both preoperative planning and postoperative follow-up of endovascular stent graft repair [60,61].

Application of CTA-generated postprocessing and reconstructions has become a part of the clinical protocol, and this has been widely used as an effective alternative to conventional angiography for both preoperative planning and postoperative follow-up of endovascular stent grafts [11,61]. 3D CTA is commonly used as a routine imaging modality to obtain the essential measurements for planning aortic stent graft placement, to assess the patency of stent-covered renal and other visceral arteries, and to detect endoleaks for postoperative follow-up of stent grafts [23,62].

While 2D axial and MPR images are routinely used in clinical practice, various reconstructions, including MIP, VR, and VIE, have been reported to provide clinicians with additional information for evaluating the treatment outcomes of endovascular aneurysm repair [63–68]. MIP clearly shows the aortic stents and the arterial branches,

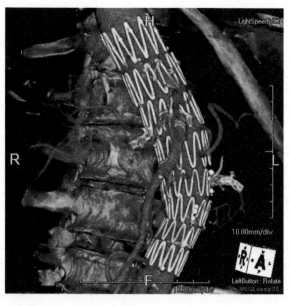

FIGURE 4.24
3D volume rendering in a patient treated with fenestrated stent graft showing blood vessels and bones that are assigned with red color and stent wires with white color.

and it is more accurate for measuring the stent graft migration than the conventional 2D images (Figure 4.23) [63], while VR is an efficient visualization tool for showing the 3D relationship between the stent graft and the arterial branches (Figure 4.24) [8,63,65]. The additional information provided by VIE is considered valuable for endovascular specialists to assess the outcomes of suprarenal and fenestrated stent grafts, which is shown by demonstrating the encroachment of stent wires to the renal artery ostia (Figure 4.25) and by identifying the appearance of fenestrated vessel stents in relation to the aortic artery branches (Figure 4.26) [23,62,66–68].

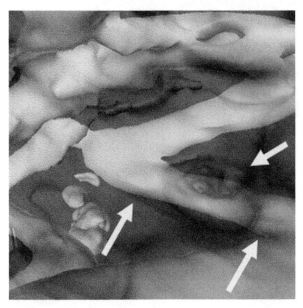

FIGURE 4.25
Virtual intravascular endoscopy showing that the left renal ostium is crossed by a single stent wire in a patient treated with suprarenal stent graft; short arrow indicates the renal artery ostium and long arrows refer to suprarenal stent wires.

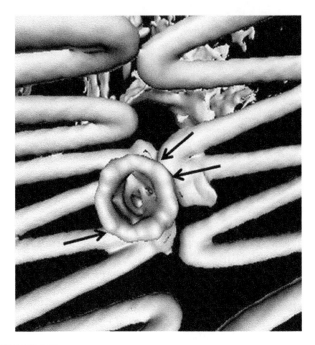

FIGURE 4.26
Virtual intravascular endoscopy (VIE) showing the fenestrated renal stents with normal circular appearance. An extended intra-aortic protrusion of the left renal stent is observed with VIE (arrows).

4.4.7 Pulmonary Embolism

With the rapid developments of CT techniques, CT pulmonary angiography (CTPA) was initially used as an adjunct and an alternative to other imaging modalities [69], and recently it is widely recognized as the method of choice for diagnosis of suspected pulmonary embolism (PE) because of its superior sensitivity and specificity to ventilation–perfusion isotope scanning [70,71]. Moreover, CTPA allows a quantitative assessment that correlates well with clinical severity and has good interobserver agreement.

For visualization of PE with CTPA, 2D axial and MPR images are the most commonly used visualization tools for detection of segmental and subsegmental embolism (Figure 4.27). The main disadvantage of these views is lack of direct intraluminal view of the thrombus or artery wall changes. This is overcome with use of VIE visualization because of its superior advantage of providing intraluminal views.

In contrast to conventional 2D or 3D extraluminal views, VIE allows for a unique display of the intraluminal thrombus (Figure 4.28), regardless of the location of thrombus in the main pulmonary artery or in the lobar or segmental branches. VIE is especially useful for the identification of the thrombus in segmental or subsegmental arteries, as embolism that is located at these side branches is sometimes difficult to detect with conventional visualizations (Figure 4.29). Combined with 2D views, VIE confirms the thrombus in distal pulmonary branches. While conventional 2D and 3D reconstructions from CTPA remain as the primary visualization tools to diagnose PE, VIE is recommended as a complementary tool to evaluate PE [14]. The potential applications of VIE in PE are to provide the quantitative assessment of thrombus changes after medical treatment and to identify intraluminal changes to the arterial wall because of thrombus and extent of PE.

4.4.8 Peripheral Arterial Disease

Peripheral arterial disease (PAD) is an important health problem with a high prevalence in the industrialized countries [72,73]. Conventional invasive angiography has been considered the gold standard technique in the assessment of PAD. However, its diagnostic value in many vascular regions has been challenged over the past decade with the rapid development of noninvasive imaging methods such as CTA. Diagnostic accuracy of CTA in PAD has been significantly enhanced with the development of MSCT scanning techniques, which enable scanning of long segments of the vascular tree during a single breath-hold with submillimeter section thickness [74–77].

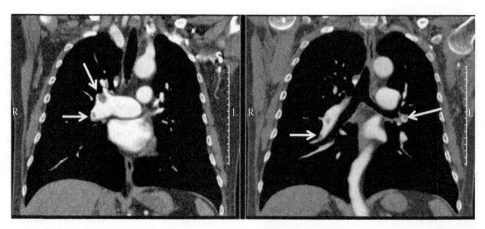

FIGURE 4.27
Coronal multiplanar reformation images showing that multiple emboli (arrows) are present in bilateral pulmonary arteries.

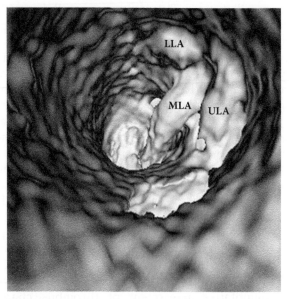

FIGURE 4.28
Virtual intravascular endoscopy visualization of multiple emboli in the left lobar arteries. ULA, upper lobar artery; MLA, middle (lingular) lobar artery; LLA, lower lobar artery.

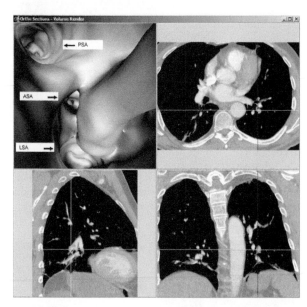

FIGURE 4.29
Virtual intravascular endoscopy (VIE) views of the left lower pulmonary segmental embolism involving two arterial branches. Left lateral and anterobasal segmental arteries become narrowed because of the presence of thrombus (top right VIE view), while the left posterobasal segmental artery is normal. Corresponding orthogonal views confirm the relationship between the thrombus and the segmental artery branches. ASA, anterobasal segmental artery; LSA, lateral basal segmental artery; PSA, posterobasal segmental artery.

3D image reconstructions from MSCT angiography have been widely used in the visualization of abdominal aorta and its distal branches, and MIP and VR are the most commonly used reconstruction methods (Figure 4.30). Studies have shown that 3D VR reconstructions compared favorably with MIP plus axial images alone with similar diagnostic value, although a combination of MIP and 2D axial images always showed a relatively higher accuracy than that obtained from axial alone, MPR alone, or semitransparent VR alone [78,79].

The diagnostic accuracy of MSCT angiography is affected to some extent in the presence of severe calcification in the peripheral arteries. It has been reported

that diagnostic performance of MSCT angiography was significantly different between the groups of patients with and without severe calcification in terms of specificity and accuracy, but not in terms of sensitivity [80]. Portugaller et al. [79] in their study concluded that MIP was the most commonly affected 3D imaging visualization compared to other 3D reconstructions for imaging calcified aortoiliac vessels (Figure 4.31). The combined view of MIP with axial CT or cross-sectional images

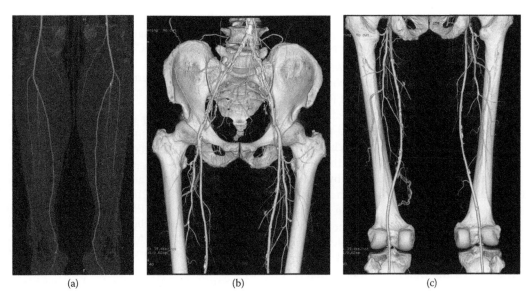

(a)　　　　　　　(b)　　　　　　　(c)

FIGURE 4.30
(a) Coronary maximum-intensity projection image acquired with 64-slice CT angiography clearly shows the femoral and tibial arteries as well as small arterial branches in the lower extremity. (b and c) 3D volume rendering images in another patient showing atherosclerotic plaques in the common iliac arteries, involving femoral arteries.

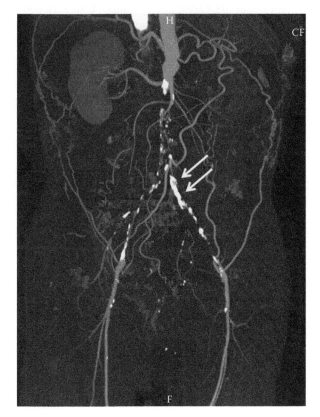

FIGURE 4.31
Coronal maximum-intensity projection showing an occluded aortic aneurysm with extensive calcification in the infrarenal aorta, extending to the common iliac arteries. Severely calcified plaques in the left common iliac artery (arrows) cause blooming artifacts, resulting in overestimation of the degree of lumen stenosis.

was reported to show an improved diagnostic performance of MSCT angiography in PAD with severe calcification.

4.5 Conclusion

There is sufficient evidence to confirm that MSCT angiography represents the most rapidly developed imaging modality in cardiovascular imaging, with satisfactory results having been achieved. The high diagnostic accuracy of MSCT angiography has made it an effective alternative to invasive angiography in the diagnosis of many cardiovascular diseases, such as detection of aortic dissection, PE, AAA, and peripheral vascular disease. In imaging other cardiovascular diseases, such as coronary stenting and CAD, further technical developments in both spatial and temporal resolution are required before MSCT angiography can be recommended as a reliable alternative to invasive coronary angiography. In particular, MSCT angiography serves as a reliable screening technique in patients with suspected CAD because of its very high negative predictive value, thus avoiding unnecessary invasive angiography examinations.

Various CT visualizations offer additional information compared with 2D axial images in both preoperative planning and posttreatment follow-up. Reliably recognizing the diagnostic value of each reconstruction is of paramount importance for clinicians to efficiently use the MSCT angiography as some of the postprocessing methods are time consuming. Although 2D axial and MIP images are routinely used in clinical practice, some forms of 2D and 3D reconstructions are recommended to assist clinical diagnosis; these include MPR, VR, and VIE visualization tools. MPR and VR are used for showing the relationship of arterial branches and pathological changes, such as plaques, stenosis, or occlusion. VIE is recommended for accurately assessing the intraluminal changes of the arterial wall caused by plaques, evaluating the intraluminal pathology such as thrombus or aortic dissection, and measuring the treatment outcomes of endovascular repair of aortic aneurysms in terms of the intraluminal appearances and stent protrusion. Selection of appropriate reconstructed visualization tools will enhance the diagnostic performance of MSCT angiography in cardiovascular diseases.

References

1. Rubin GD, Dake MD, Semba CP., Current status of three-dimensional spiral CT scanning for imaging the vasculature. *Radiol Clin North Am* 1995; 33: 51–70.

2. Fishman EK, Horton KM. The increasing impact of multidetector row computed tomography in clinical practice. *Eur J Radiol* 2007; 62(S): S1–S13.

3. Nieman K, Oudkerk M, Rensing BJ, van Ooijen P, Munne A, van geuns FRJ, de Feyter PJ. Coronary angiography with multi-slice computed tomography. *Lancet* 2001; 357: 599–603.

4. Achenbach S, Giesler T, Ropers D, Ulzheimer S, Derlien H, Schulte C, Wenkel E, Moshage W, Baultz W, Daniel WG et al. Detection of coronary artery stenoses by contrast-enhanced, retrospectively electrocardiographically-gated, multislice computed tomography. *Circulation* 2001; 103: 2535–2538.

5. Raff GL, Gallagher MJ, O'Neill WW, Goldstein JA. Diagnostic accuracy of non-invasive coronary angiography using 64-slice spiral computed tomography. *J Am Coll Cardiol* 2005; 46: 552–557.

6. Chao SP, Law WY, Kuo CJ, Hung HF, Cheng JJ, Lo HM, Shyu KG. The diagnostic accuracy of 256-row computed tomographic angiography compared with invasive coronary angiography in patients with suspected coronary artery disease. *Eur Heart J* 2010; 31:1916–1923.

7. Rybicki F, Otero H, Steigner M, Vorobiof G, Nallamshetty L, Mitsouras D, Ersoy H, Mather RT, Judy PF, Cai T et al. Initial evaluation of coronary images from 320-detector row computed tomography. *Int J Cardiovasc Imaging* 2008; 24: 535–546.

8. Sun Z. Multislice CT angiography in the diagnosis of cardiovascular disease: 3D visualisations. *Front Med* 2011; 5: 254–270.

9. Lell MM, Anders K, Uder M, Klotz E, Ditt H, Vega-Higuera F, Boskamp T, Bautz WA, Tomandl BF. New techniques in CT angiography. *Radiographics* 2006; 26:S45–S62.

10. Schoepf UJ, Zwerner PL, Savino G, Herzog C, Kerl JM, Costello P. Coronary CT angiography. *Radiology* 2007; 244: 48–63.

11. Sun Z. Helical CT angiography of abdominal aortic aneurysms treated with suprarenal stent grafting. *Cardiovasc Intervent Radiol* 2003; 26: 290–295.

12. Schoepf UJ, Goldhaber SZ, Costello P. Spiral computed tomography for acute pulmonary embolism. *Circulation* 2004; 109: 2160–2167.

13. Perrier A, Roy PM, Sanchez O, Le Gal G, Meyer G, Gourdier Al, Furber A, Revel MP, Howarth N, Davido A et al. Multidetector-row computed tomography in suspected pulmonary embolism. *N Engl J Med* 2005; 352: 1760–1768.

14. Sun Z, Al Dosari S, Ng C, al-Muntashari A, Almaliky S. Multislice CT virtual intravascular endoscopy for assessing pulmonary embolisms: A pictorial essay. *Korean J Radiol* 2010; 11: 222–230.

15. Sun Z, Ng KH. Multislice CT angiography in cardiac imaging. Part II: Clinical applications in coronary artery disease. *Singapore Med J* 2010; 51[4]: 282–289.

16. Sun Z, Lin CH, Davidson R, Dong C, Liao Y. Diagnostic value of 64-slice CT angiography in coronary artery disease: A systematic review. *Eur J Radiol* 2008; 67: 78–84.

17. Rydberg J, Kopecky KK, Lalka SG, Johnson MS, Dalsing MC, Persohn SA. Stent grafting of abdominal aortic aneurysms: Pre- and postoperative evaluation with multislice helical CT. *J Comput Assit Tomogr* 2001; 25[4]: 580–586.

18. Sun Z. Diagnostic accuracy of multislice CT angiography in peripheral vascular disease. *J Vasc Intervent Radiol* 2006; 17: 1915–1921.

19. Kalender WA, Polacin A. Physical performance characteristics of spiral CT scanning. *Med Phys* 1991; 18: 910–915.

20. Fleischmann D, Rubin GD, Paik DS, Yen SY, Hilfiker PR, Beaulieu CF, Napel S. Stair-step artifacts with single versus multiple detector-row helical CT. *Radiology* 2000; 216: 185–196.

21. Hu H, He HD, Foley WD, Fox SH. Four multidetector-row helical CT: Image quality and volume coverage speed. *Radiology* 2000; 215: 55–62.

22. Sun Z, Winder J, Kelly B, Ellis P, Hirst D. CT virtual intravascular endoscopy of abdominal aortic aneurysms treated with suprarenal endovascular stent grafting. *Abdom Imaging* 2003; 28: 580–587.

23. Al Shuhaimi A, Ababtain K, Sun Z. Diagnostic value of noninvasive imaging techniques in the detection of carotid artery stenosis: A systematic review. *Radiographer* 2009; 56: 14–18.

24. Chen CJ, Lee TH, Hsu HL, Tseng YC, Lin SK, Wang LJ, Wong YC. Multi-slice CT angiography in diagnosing total versus near occlusions of the internal carotid artery: Comparison with catheter angiography. *Stroke* 2004; 35(1): 83–88.

25. Lell M, Fellner C, Baum U, Hothorn T, Steiner R, Lang W, Bautz W, Fellner FA. Evaluation of carotid artery stenosis with multisection CT and MR imaging: Influence of imaging modality and postprocessing. *AJNR Am J Neuroradiol* 2007; 28(1): 104–110.

26. Agid R, Lee SK, Willinsky RA, Farb RI, terBrugge KG. Acute subarachnoid hemorrhage: Using 64-slice multidetector CT angiography to "triage" patients' treatment. *Neuroradiology* 2006; 48(11): 787–794.

27. Pozzi-Mucelli F, Bruni S, Doddi M, Calgaro A, Braini M, Cova M. Detection of intracranial aneurysms with 64 channel multidetector row computed tomography: Comparison with digital subtraction angiography. *Eur J Radiol* 2007; 64(1): 15–26.

28. Gratama van Andel HA, Venema HW, Streekstra GJ, van Straten M, Majoie CB, den Heeten GJ, Grimbergen CA. Removal of bone in CT angiography by multiscale matched mask bone elimination. *Med Phys* 2007; 34(10): 3711–3723.

29. Lell MM, Ditt H, Panknin C, Sayre JW, Klotz E, Ruehm SG, Villablanca JP. Cervical CT angiography comparing routine noncontrast and a late venous scan as masks for automated bone subtraction: Feasibility study and examination of the influence of patient motion on image quality. *Invest Radiol* 2008; 43(1): 27–32.

30. Lell MM, Ditt H, Panknin C, Sayre JW, Ruehm SG, Klotz E, Tomandl BF, Villablandca JP. Bone-subtraction CT angiography: Evaluation of two different fully automated image-registration procedures for interscan motion compensation. *AJNR Am J Neuroradiol* 2007; 28(7): 1362–1368.

31. Luo Z, Wang D, Sun X, Zhang T, Liu F, Dong D, Chan NK, Shen B. Comparison of the accuracy of subtraction CT angiography performed on 320-detector row volume CT with conventional CT angiography for diagnosis of intracranial aneurysms. *Eur J Radiol* 2012; 81(1): 118–122.

32. Thomas C, Korn A, Krauss B, Ketelsen D, Tsiflikas I, Reimann A, Brodoefel H, Claussen CD, Kopp AF, Ernemann U et al. Automatic bone and plaque removal using dual energy CT for head and neck angiography: Feasibility and initial performance evaluation. *Eur J Radiol* 2010; 76: 61–67.

33. Leys D. Atherosclerosis: A major health burden. *Cerebrovasc Dis* 2001; 11: 1–4.

34. al Rajeh SA, Awada A, Niazi G, Larbi E. Stroke in a Saudi Arabian national guard community. Analysis of 500 consecutive cases from a population-based hospital. *Stroke* 1993; 24: 1635–1639.

35. North American Symptomatic Carotid Endarterectomy Trial Collaborators. Beneficial effect of carotid endarterectomy in symptomatic patients with high-grade carotid stenosis. *N Engl J Med* 1991; 325: 445–453.

36. European Carotid Surgery Trialists' Collaborative Group. Randomised trial of endarterectomy for recently symptomatic carotid stenosis: Final results of the MRC European Carotid Surgery Trial (ECST). *Lancet* 1998; 351: 1379–1387.

37. Executive Committee for the Asymptomatic Carotid Atherosclerosis Study. Endarterectomy for asymptomatic carotid artery stenosis. *JAMA* 1995; 273: 1421–1428.

38. Borisch I, Horn M, Butz B, Zorger N, Draganski B, Hoelscher T, Bogdahn U, Link J. Preoperative evaluation of carotid artery stenosis: Comparison of contrast-enhanced MR angiography and duplex sonography with digital subtraction angiography. *Am J Neuroradiol* 2003; 24: 1117–1122.

39. Berg M, Zhang Z, Ikonen A, Sipola P, Kälviäinen R, Manninen H, Vanninen R. Multi-detector row CT angiography in the assessment of carotid artery disease in symptomatic patients: Comparison with rotational angiography and digital subtraction angiography. *Am J Neuroradiol* 2005; 26: 1022–1034.

40. Lloyd-Jones D, Adams RJ, Brown TM, Carnethon M, Dai S, DeSimone G, Ferguson TB, Ford E, Furie K, Gillespie C et al. Executive summary: Heart disease and stoke statistics: 2010 update: A report from the American Heart Association. *Circulation* 2010; 121: 948–954.

41. Gaziano TA, Bitton A, Anand S, Abrahams-Gessel S, Murphy A. Growing epidemic of coronary heart disease in low-and middle-income countries. *Curr Probl Cardiol* 2010; 35: 72–115.

42. Noto TJ Jr, Johnson LW, Krone R, Weaver WF, Clark DA, Kramer JR Jr, Vetrovec GW. Cardiac catheterization 1990: A report of the Registry of the Society for Cardiac Angiography and Interventions. (SCA&I). *Cathet Cardiovasc Diagn* 1991; 24: 75–83.

43. Sun Z, Dimpudus F, Nugroho J, Adipranoto J. CT virtual intravascular endoscopy assessment of coronary artery plaques: A preliminary study. *Eur J Radiol* 2010; 75: e112–e119.

44. Serruys PW, de Jaegere P, Keimeneij F, Macaya C, Rutsch W, Heyndrickx G, Emanuelsson H, Marco J, Legrand V, Materne P. A comparison of balloon-expandable-stent implantation with balloon angioplasty in patients with coronary artery disease. Benestent Study Group. *N Engl J Med* 1994; 331: 489–495.

45. Fischman DL, Leon MB, Baim DS, Schatz RA, Savage MP, Penn I, Detre K, Veltri L, Ricci D, Nobuyoshi M. A randomized comparison of coronary-stent placement and balloon angioplasty in the treatment of coronary artery disease. Stent Restenosis Study Investigators. *N Engl J Med* 1994; 331: 496–501.

46. Holmes DR Jr, Leon MB, Moses JW, Popma JJ, Cutlip D, Fitzgerald PJ, Brown C, Fischell T, Wong SC, Midei M et al. Analysis of 1-year clinical outcomes in the SIRIUS trial: A randomized trial of a sirolimus-eluting stent versus a standard stent in patients at high risk for coronary restenosis. *Circulation* 2004; 109: 634–640.

47. Morice MC, Colombo A, Meire B, Serruys P, Tamburino C, Guagliumi G, Sousa E, Stoll HP. Sirolimus- vs paclitaxel-eluting stents in de novo coronary artery lesions: The REALITY trial: A randomized controlled trial. *JAMA* 2006; 295: 895–904.

48. Sun Z, Davidson R, Lin CH. Multi-detector row CT angiography in the assessment of coronary in-stent restenosis: A systematic review. *Eur J Radiol* 2009; 69: 489–495.

49. Sun Z, Almutairi A. Diagnostic accuracy of 64 multi-slice CT angiography in the assessment of coronary in-stent restenosis: A meta-analysis. *Eur J Radiol* 2010; 73: 266–273.

50. Almutairi A, Sun Z, Ng C, Al-Safran ZA, Al-Mulla AA, Al-Jamaan AI. Optimal scanning protocols of 64-slice CT angiography in coronary artery stents: An in vitro phantom study. *Eur J Radiol* 2010; 74: 156–160.

51. Coady MA, Rizzo JA, Goldstein LJ, Elefteriades JA. Natural history, pathogenesis, and etiology of thoracic aortic aneurysms and dissections. *Cardiol Clin* 1999; 17: 615–635.

52. Castaner E, Andreu M, Gallardo X, Mata JM, Cabezuelo MA, Pallardo Y. CT in nontraumatic acute thoracic aortic disease: Typical and atypical features and complications. *Radiographics* 2003; 23: 93–110.

53. Sebastià C, Pallisa E, Quiroga S, Alvarez-Castells A, Dominguez R, Evangelista A. Aortic dissection: Diagnosis and follow-up with helical CT. *Radiographics* 1999; 19: 45–60.

54. Scaglione M, Salvolini L, Casciani E, Giovagnoni A, Mazzei MA, Volterrani L. The many faces of aortic dissections: Beware of unusual presentations. *Eur J Radiol* 2008; 65: 359–364.

55. Berger FH, van Lienden KP, Smithuis R, Nicolaou S, van Delden OM. Acute aortic syndrome and blunt traumatic aortic injury: Pictorial review of MDCT imaging. *Eur J Radiol* 2010; 74: 21–39.

56. Cao Y, Sun Z, Shang Y, Jiang B, Ma X. Aortic dissection: Identification of entry site with CT virtual intravascular endoscopy. *Biomed Imaging Interv J* 2010; 6(3): e22.1–e22.7.

57. Buth J, van Marrewijk CJ, Harris PL, Hop WC, Riambau V, Laheij RJ. Outcome of endovascular abdominal aortic aneurysm repair in patients with conditions considered unfit for an open procedure: A report on the EUROSTAR experience. *J Vasc Surg* 2002; 35: 211–221.

58. Cao P, Verzini F, Parlani G, Romano L, Rango PD, Pagliuca V, Iacono G. Clinical effect of abdominal aortic aneurysm endografting: 7-year concurrent comparison with open repair. *J Vasc Surg* 2004; 40: 841–848.

59. Prinssen M, Verhoeven EL, Buth J, Cuypers PW, vanSambeek MR, Balm R, Buskens E, Grobbee DE, Blankensteijn JD, Dutch Randomized Endovascular Aneurysm Management (DREAM) Trial Group. A randomized trial comparing conventional and endovascular repair of abdominal aortic aneurysms. *N Engl J Med* 2004; 14(351): 1607–1618.

60. Broeders IA, Blankensteijn JD, Olree M, Mali W, Eikelboom BC. Preoperative sizing of grafts for transfemoral endovascular aneurysm management: A prospective comparative study of spiral CT angiography, arterial angiography and conventional CT imaging. *J Endovasc Surg* 1997; 4: 252–261.

61. Armerding MD, Rubin GD, Beaulieu CF, Slonim SM, Olcott EW, Samuels SL, Jorgensen MJ, Semba CP, Jeffrey RB Jr, Dake MD. Aortic aneurysmal disease: Assessment of stent-grafted treatment-CT versus conventional angiography. *Radiology* 2000; 215: 138–146.

62. Sun Z, Winder RJ, Kelly BE, Ellis PK, Kennedy PT, Hirst DG. Diagnostic value of CT virtual intravascular endoscopy in aortic stent grafting. *J Endovasc Ther* 2004; 11: 13–25.

63. Sun Z. Three-dimensional visualization of suprarenal aortic tent-grafts: Evaluation of migration in midterm follow-up. *J Endovasc Ther* 2006; 1: 85–93.

64. Sun Z. 3D multislice CT angiography in post-aortic stent grafting: A pictorial essay. *Korean J Radiol* 2006; 7: 205–211.

65. Sun Z, Allen Y, Mwipatayi B, Hartley D, Lawrence-Brown M. Multislice CT angiography of fenestrated endovascular stent grafting of abdominal aortic aneurysms: A pictorial review of 2D/3D visualizations. *Korean J Radiol* 2009; 10: 285–293.

66. Sun Z, Allen Y, Nadkarni S, Wright R, Hartley D, Lawrence-Brown M. CT virtual intravascular endoscopy in the visualization of fenestrated endovascular grafts. *J Endovasc Ther* 2008; 15: 42–51.

67. Sun Z, Mwipatayi B, Allen Y, Hartley D, Lawrence-Brown M. Multislice CT virtual intravascular endoscopy in the evaluation of fenestrated stent graft repair of abdominal aortic aneurysms: A short-term follow-up. *ANZ J Surg* 2009; 79: 836–840.

68. Sun Z, Allen Y, Mwipatayi B, Hartley D, Lawrence-Brown M. Multislice CT angiography in the follow-up of fenestrated endovascular grafts: Effect of slice thickness on 2D and 3D visualization of the fenestrated stents. *J Endovasc Ther* 2008; 15: 417–426.

69. British Thoracic Society Standards of Care Committee Pulmonary Embolism Guideline Development Group. British thoracic society guidelines for the management of suspected acute pulmonary embolism. *Thorax* 2003; 58: 470–483.

70. Hayashino Y, Goto M, Noguchi Y, Fukui T. Ventilation-perfusion scanning and helical CT in suspected pulmonary embolism: Meta-analysis of diagnostic performance. *Radiology* 2005; 234: 740–748.

71. Guilabert JP, Manzur DN, Tarrasa MJ, Llorens ML, Braun P, Arques MP. Can multislice CT alone run out reliably pulmonary embolism? A prospective study. *Eur J Radiol* 2007; 62: 220–226.

72. Fowkes FG, Housley E, Cawood EH, Macintyre CC, Ruckley CV, Prescott RJ. Edinburgh Artery Study: Prevalence of asymptomatic and symptomatic peripheral arterial disease in the general population. *Int J Epidemiol* 1991; 20: 384–392.

73. Hiatt WR. Medical treatment of peripheral arterial disease and claudication. *N Engl J Med* 2001; 344: 1608–1621.

74. Martin ML, Tay KH, Flak B, Fry PD, Doyle DL, Taylor DC, Hsiang YN, Machan LS. Multidetector CT angiography of the aortoiliac system and lower extremities: A prospective comparison with intraarterial digital subtraction angiography. *AJR Am J Roentgenol* 2003; 180: 1085–1091.

75. Ofer A, Nitechi SS, Linn S, Epelman M, Fischer D, Karram T, Litmanovich D, Schwartz H, Hoffman A, Engel A. Multidetector CT angiography of peripheral vascular disease: A prospective comparison with intraarterial digital subtraction angiography. *AJR Am J Roentgenol* 2003; 180: 719–724.

76. Edwards AJ, Wells IP, Roobottom CA. Multidetector row CT angiography of the lower limb arteries: A prospective comparison of volume-rendered techniques and intra-arterial digital subtraction angiography. *Clin Radiol* 2005; 60: 85–95.

77. Willman JK, Baumert B, Schertler T, Wildermuth S, Pfammatter T, Verdun FR, Seifert B, Marincek B, Böhm T. Aortoiliac and lower extremity arteries assessed with 16-detector row CT angiography: Prospective comparison with digital subtraction angiography. *Radiology* 2005; 236: 1083–1093.

78. Portugaller HR, Schoellnast H, Hausegger KA, Tiesenhausen K, Amann W, Berghold A. Multislice CT angiography in peripheral arterial disease: A valuable tool in detecting significant arterial lumen narrowing? *Eur Radiol* 2004; 14: 1681–1687.

79. Portugaller HR, Schoellnast H, Tauss J, Tiesenhausen K, Hausegger K. Semitransparent volume-rendered CT angiography for lesion display in aortoiliac arterioslcerotic disease. *J Vasc Interv Radiol* 2003; 14: 1023–1030.

80. Ota H, Takase K, Igarashi K, Chiba Y, Haga K, Saito H, Takahashi S. MDCT compared with digital subtraction angiography for assessment of lower extremity arterial occlusive disease: Importance of reviewing cross-sectional images. *AJR Am J Roentgenol* 2004; 182: 201–209.

5

Radiation Dose in Computed Tomography

Kosuke Matsubara

CONTENTS

5.1 Introduction

Since the introduction of computed tomography (CT) for clinical use, it has proven to be a valuable diagnostic tool. The medical information derived from CT scans has contributed to saving many lives not only in developed countries but also in developing countries worldwide. Moreover, the evolution of CT from single-detector CT (SDCT) to multi-detector CT (MDCT) has greatly enhanced its value in medical diagnosis. As a result, although CT is used in only 17% of all radiological examinations, it contributed to nearly 49% of the individual patient dose from these examinations in the United States for the year 2006 [1]. It is thought that the dose to an individual from one CT examination does not cause radiation-induced biological effects, but the radiation dose for each CT procedure should be managed by appropriate methods.

When considering radiation dose in CT, it is important to understand that the absorbed dose distribution within each patient differs compared with other x-ray examinations (e.g., radiography and fluoroscopy). This is because the x-ray beam is narrow as a result of the collimator, and the exposure is controlled using an x-ray tube that is rotated around the patient. Hence, specific methods must be used for the evaluation of radiation doses in CT.

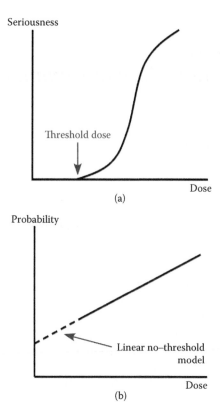

FIGURE 5.1
Biological effects induced by radiation exposure. (a) Deterministic effects. (b) Stochastic effects.

5.2 Why Is Radiation Dose Management Necessary in CT?

Biological effects induced by radiation exposure can be classified into two categories: deterministic and stochastic effects (Figure 5.1). The deterministic effects (harmful tissue reactions) are induced because of cell malfunctions after radiation exposure, and the stochastic effects (cancer and heritable effects) are induced because of reproductive or germ cell mutations after exposure [2].

Deterministic effects are induced following high doses above the threshold dose that causes 1% of tissue reactions [2]. In general, the dose level in each CT examination is far below the threshold dose for deterministic effects such as skin injury. However, these effects cannot be ruled out as patients undergo perfusion CT. A previous report described cases of temporary bandage-shaped hair loss after undergoing perfusion MDCT and cerebral angiographic examinations [3]. Therefore, the possibility of induction of such effects cannot be excluded if multiple radiological examinations are performed on the same patient. To prevent the induction

of deterministic effects, it is important to manage the patient dose for each type of examination including CT.

Whether threshold doses exist for the stochastic effects remain unclear. Epidemiological and experimental studies provide evidence of increasing cancer incidence with effective doses of more than 100 mSv, but there is no specific evidence for increased risk with effective doses of less than 100 mSv [2]. For radiation protection and management, the linear no-threshold (LNT) model, which is based on the assumption that the risk is directly proportional to the dose at all dose levels, is generally adopted because it does not underestimate the risk of cancer incidence. Although heritable diseases have been observed in experimental studies, there is no current evidence of heritable risks to humans. Radiation dose in CT is classified according to the examinations that use radiation at low-dose rates. Although the risk of cancer incidence from radiation exposure with low-dose rates is lower than that with high-dose rates, when a human is exposed to the same radiation dose, the International Commission on Radiological Protection (ICRP) recommends using a dose and dose-rate effectiveness factor (DDREF) of 2 [2], and the radiation dose for each CT examination should be managed according to the LNT model because the risk of cancer incidence from radiation exposure on CT examinations cannot be excluded completely.

TABLE 5.1

Tissue Weighting Factors Recommended in the ICRP Publication 103

Tissue	W_T	$\sum W_T$
Bone marrow (red), colon, lung, stomach, breast, remainder tissues[a]	0.12	0.72
Gonads	0.08	0.08
Bladder, esophagus, liver, thyroid	0.04	0.16
Bone surface, brain, salivary glands, skin	0.01	0.04
	Total	1.00

Source: Data from Valentin J (Editor), *Ann ICRP*, 37(2–4): 1–332, 2007.

[a] Remainder tissues: Adrenals, extrathoracic (ET) region, gall bladder, heart, kidneys, lymphatic nodes, muscle, oral mucosa, pancreas, prostate (male), small intestine, spleen, thymus, uterus/cervix (female).

5.3 Radiation Dose Levels

CT radiation dose levels in patients are expressed as follows.

5.3.1 Absorbed Dose

Absorbed dose is a measure of the energy deposited in a medium by ionizing radiation and is equal to the energy deposited per unit mass of medium, which is measured as joules per kilogram (J/kg) and represented by gray (Gy). When it is applied to patient dose measurement, the dose is averaged over the whole volume of each tissue or organ.

5.3.2 Equivalent Dose

Equivalent dose is used in radiation protection and is not measurable in practice. It accounts for the biological damage potential of different types of ionizing radiation. The equivalent dose is obtained by multiplying the absorbed dose for each organ or tissue by the radiation weighting factor (x-ray is defined as 1). It can be calculated from the following equation:

$$H_T = w_R D_T$$

where H_T is the equivalent dose (in sieverts, Sv), w_R is the radiation weighting factor, and D_T is the absorbed dose for each organ or tissue.

5.3.3 Effective Dose

Effective dose is also used in radiation protection and is not measurable in practice. It can compare the stochastic risk of a nonuniform exposure to ionizing radiation

with the risks caused by a uniform exposure of the whole body. The effective dose is obtained by calculating a weighted average of the whole-body equivalent dose to different body tissues with tissue weighting factors, which are designed to reflect the different radiosensitivities of the tissues. It can be calculated from the following equation:

$$E = \sum_T w_T H_T$$

where E is the effective dose (Sv) and w_T is the tissue weighting factor. The tissue weighting factors recommended in ICRP Publication 103 [2] are shown in Table 5.1.

The effective dose is defined and estimated in a reference person and provides a value that considers the given exposure conditions but not the characteristics of a specific individual [2]. Thus, the effective dose represents only a mean dose value for humans averaged over both sexes and all ages and cannot represent the dose value of particular individuals.

5.4 Which Dose Quantity Is Useful in CT?

It is possible to quantitatively compare how the patient local dose differs with various modalities, scanners, or scan parameters by measuring organ-absorbed or equivalent doses, and it is also possible to compare how the patient synthetic dose differs with the effective dose.

In typical CT procedures, organ-absorbed doses are confirmed to be less than 100 mGy. These values are far below the threshold dose for deterministic effects such as skin injury. Moreover, fetal doses below 100 mGy should not be considered a reason for terminating a pregnancy [6]. In other words, organ-absorbed or equivalent doses can be used as evaluation values for the deterministic effects.

On the other hand, the effective dose can be used as an evaluation value for stochastic effects. However, ICRP described how the effective dose is used in medical exposure, which is given as follows [2]:

- Comparison of the relative doses from different diagnostic procedures.
- Comparison of the use of similar technologies and procedures in different hospitals and countries and of the use of different technologies for the same medical examination.

Moreover, ICRP described that the assessment and interpretation of the effective dose from medical exposure of patients is problematic when organs and tissues receive only partial exposure or a very heterogeneous exposure.

Therefore, the effective dose is useful for comparing the patient dose among different scan parameters and for optimizing scan parameters in CT, but it should not be used for estimating risks, such as cancer incidence and mortality. In addition, it should be used carefully when organs and tissues receive high doses and only partial regions are exposed, such as in cardiac and cranial CT examinations.

5.5 Radiation Dose Descriptors in CT

Because of its unique geometry, there are some radiation dose descriptors unique to CT.

5.5.1 CT Dose Index

CT dose index (CTDI) is based on measuring the absorbed dose in cylindrical polymethyl methacrylate (PMMA) phantoms 16 (for adult head and infant) and 32 cm (for adult body) in diameter. The index is measured from one axial CT scan and is calculated by dividing the total absorbed dose by the product of slice thickness and the number of slices. CTDI is defined by the following equation:

$$\text{CTDI} = \left(\frac{1}{nT}\right)\int_{-\infty}^{\infty} D(z)\mathrm{d}z$$

where n is the number of slices, T is the slice thickness, and $D(z)$ is the dose profile along the z-axis from a single acquisition (Figure 5.2).

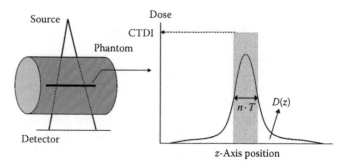

FIGURE 5.2
A conceptual diagram of the computed tomography dose index (CTDI).

1. CTDI_{100}

   CTDI_{100} is measured in units of exposure (coulomb/kg, C/kg) and is converted to absorbed dose (mGy). A pencil-type ionization chamber that has a 100 mm active length is inserted within the phantom's holes to measure the absorbed dose. Therefore, CTDI_{100} is defined and calculated using the absorbed dose within a 100 mm length along the z-axis within the chamber.

2. Weighted CTDI

   Absorbed doses between central and peripheral regions of an object are different in CT scans. To take this difference into consideration, the weighted CTDI (CTDI_w) is defined by the following equation:

   $$\text{CTDI}_\text{w} = \frac{1}{3}\text{CTDI}_{100,c} + \frac{2}{3}\text{CTDI}_{100,p}$$

   where $\text{CTDI}_{100,c}$ is CTDI_{100} at the center of the phantom and $\text{CTDI}_{100,p}$ is the averaged CTDI_{100} at four points along the periphery of the phantom. Thus, CTDI_w represents the average absorbed dose over the in-plane (x and y) direction.

3. Normalized CTDI_w

   Normalized CTDI_w ($n\text{CTDI}_\text{w}$) is CTDI_w per 100 mAs.

4. Volumetric CTDI

   To represent the dose for a consecutive CT scan, it is essential to take pitch, gaps, or overlaps into consideration. Volumetric CTDI (CTDI_{vol}) is defined by the following equations:

   $$\text{CTDI}_{\text{vol}} = \frac{nT}{I}\text{CTDI}_\text{w} \text{ (for sequential scans)}$$

   $$\text{CTDI}_{\text{vol}} = \frac{1}{p}\text{CTDI}_\text{w} \text{ (for helical scans)}$$

   where I is the table increment between each scan. From these equations, the local absorbed dose for a specific CT protocol can be obtained.

TABLE 5.2

Normalized Effective Dose Per DLP for Adults and Pediatric Patients of Various Ages for Various Body Regions

Region of Body	k (mSv·mGy^{-1}·cm^{-1})				
	<1-Year Old	1-Year Old	5-Year Old	10-Year Old	Adult
Head and neck	0.013	0.0085	0.0057	0.0042	0.0031
Head	0.011	0.0067	0.0040	0.0032	0.0021
Neck	0.017	0.012	0.011	0.0079	0.0059
Chest	0.039	0.026	0.018	0.013	0.014
Abdomen and pelvis	0.049	0.030	0.020	0.015	0.015
Trunk	0.044	0.028	0.019	0.014	0.015

Source: Data from ICRP Publication 102, *Ann ICRP*, 37(1): 1–79, 2007.

CTDI$_{vol}$ is the most familiar dose parameter because it is displayed on the console of CT scanners. One should know that although CTDI$_{vol}$ is not the absorbed dose of an actual patient, patient organ doses may be estimated from it [7,8].

5.5.2 Dose-Length Product

Dose-length product (DLP) represents the total dose over a whole scan and is defined by the following equation:

$$DLP = CTDI_{vol} \cdot \text{exposure length}$$

The unit of DLP is mGy·cm. To understand the meaning of DLP, it is important to know that DLP is not the exposed dose of an actual patient, but the patient effective dose can be estimated from DLP using the following equation:

$$E = k_E \cdot DLP$$

where k_E is the effective dose conversion factor (mSv·mGy^{-1}·cm^{-1}) that depends on patient age and scanning regions (Table 5.2) [3].

5.5.3 Multiple Scan Average Dose

Multiple scan average dose (MSAD) was also devised as a dose descriptor in CT. In this descriptor, dose profiles from consecutive multiple scans are added, and the maximum dose is treated as MSAD, which is an absorbed dose for a certain part of a patient. The dose can be measured for a scan using a specific CT protocol after placing a dosimeter at a certain position. The dosimeter that is used should be small, such as a thermoluminescent or fluoroglass type [9]. Theoretically, MSAD and CTDI are equivalent dose values because MSAD equals the dose value integrated over the dose profile for one rotation, which is equal to CTDI (Figure 5.3).

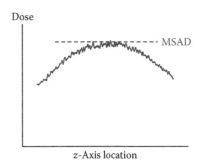

FIGURE 5.3
Dose profile when multiple scans are performed. The maximum dose is treated as the multiple scan average dose (MSAD), which is an absorbed dose for a certain part of a patient.

5.6 Methods for CTDI$_{100}$ Measurement

5.6.1 Phantoms

As described above, cylindrical PMMA phantoms that are 16 cm (for adult head and infant) and 32 cm (for adult body) in diameter (Figure 5.4) are used for CTDI$_{100}$ measurement. The phantoms are 15 cm in length, 1.19 ± 0.01 g·cm^{-3} in density, and have one hole at the center and four holes along the periphery (1 cm inside from the top, right, bottom, and left) of the phantoms for inserting a pencil-type ionization chamber. The holes not used for measurement are blocked with PMMA dummy plugs.

5.6.2 Ionization Chamber

A pencil-type ionization chamber 100 mm in active length and 3 mL in volume (Figure 5.5) is generally used. Before use, the chamber should be calibrated and the calibration factor for each energy obtained. The air temperature and pressure in the room must be measured to convert exposure doses into absorbed doses.

5.6.3 Methods

CTDI$_{100}$ is measured from one axial CT scan after inserting an ionization chamber within one of the holes of

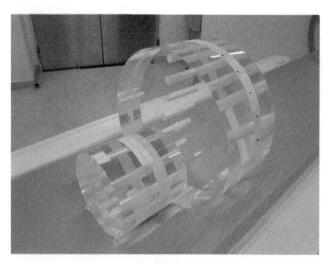

FIGURE 5.4
Photograph of polymethyl methacrylate phantoms, which correspond to an adult head and an infant (16 cm diameter) and an adult body (32 cm diameter).

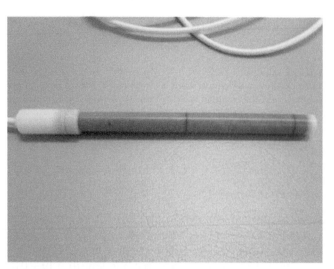

FIGURE 5.5
Photograph of an ionizing chamber specialized for CT dose measurement (10X5-3CT; Radcal, Monrovia, CA).

the phantom (Figure 5.6). Measurements at each point should be performed at least three times. The integral dose for one axial CT scan obtained from the measurement is calculated from the following equation:

$$\text{Integral dose} = \int_{-L/2}^{L/2} E(z)\,dz$$

where L is the sensitive length of the chamber and $E(z)$ is the dose profile.

Next, the integral dose is divided by the product of the slice thickness (mm) and number of slices; in MDCT, the latter product is equal to the x-ray beam width along the z-axis. The calculated value gives $CTDI_{100}$ in units of exposure.

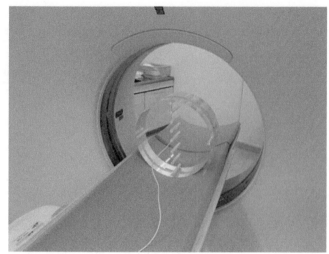

FIGURE 5.6
Setup for the measurement of $CTDI_{100}$.

The dose in units of exposure can be converted into the absorbed dose using the following equation:

$$D = XFk_{T,P}\frac{W}{e}$$

where D is the absorbed dose (Gy), X is the dose in units of exposure (C/kg), F is the calibration factor of the chamber, $k_{T,P}$ is the air density correction factor, W is the value for the average energy required for electrons to produce an ion pair in dry air (33.97 eV), and e is the elementary electric charge (1.6×10^{-19} C). W/e is equivalent to 33.97 J/C. The air density correction factor can be calculated using the following equation:

$$k_{T,P} = \left(\frac{273.2 + T}{273.2 + 22}\right)\frac{1013}{P}$$

where T is the air temperature (°C) and P is the air pressure (hPa).

5.7 Dose Measurement for Area Detector CT

Since the introduction of CTDI, CT technology has evolved and various CT scanners have been developed. A recent development is the 320-slice MDCT scanner, which uses a wide-area detector with a z-axis coverage of 160 mm. Using such a wide-area detector, the entire heart or brain may be covered in a single axial scan [10]. However, trends toward wider z-axis collimations and toward longer scanning lengths tend to limit the accuracy of $CTDI_{100}$-based parameters for estimating the CT dose because $CTDI_{100}$ excludes contributions from radiation scattered beyond the relatively short (100 mm) range of integration along the z-axis. This leads to underestimation of the CT dose, and the error increases with increasing width of the z-axis collimation [11].

In addition to the 320-slice MDCT, some MDCTs have z-axis collimations broader than 100 mm. Therefore, a 100 mm pencil-type ionizing chamber is insufficiently long to register all of the primary radiation, let alone all of the scatter radiation.

To solve this problem, the American Association of Physicists in Medicine Task Group 111 [12] reported a new measurement method based on a unified theory for axial, helical, fan-beam, and cone-beam scanning with or without z-axis translation of the patient table. In this method, a water-filled, polyethylene, or PMMA phantom that has an active length of at least 45 cm and a thimble ionizing chamber that has an active length of 20–35 mm and a volume of at least 0.6 cm³ are used. When the dose is measured, the thimble ionization chamber is placed in the phantom hole and centered at the phantom central plane, which corresponds to the midpoint of the scanning range. Next, the phantom's central axis is aligned with the scanner's axis of rotation, and the measurements are performed using axial or helical scanning. Helical scanning is relatively more convenient than axial scanning. Cumulative dose values at the phantom central plane can be easily measured by this method.

5.8 Diagnostic Reference Levels

Diagnostic reference levels (DRLs) are dose levels or levels of activity in medical radiodiagnostic or radiopharmaceutical procedures for groups of standard-sized patients. The key issue that governs medical radiodiagnostic or radiopharmaceutical examinations is the establishment and use of DRLs.

DRLs are taken from easily measured quantities, usually the absorbed dose in air or in a tissue-equivalent material at the surface of a standardized phantom or representative patient. $CTDI_{vol}$ and DLP are generally used for DRLs in CT. DRLs are intended for use as a simple test for identifying situations where the patient dose level is unusually high or low.

If the doses exceed relevant DRLs, there should be a local review of the procedures and the equipment to determine whether the protection has been optimized. If not optimized, measures aimed at reduction of the doses should be taken. It is important to know that DRLs do not provide a line separating good and bad levels and that they contribute to good medical radiodiagnostic or radiopharmaceutical procedures [13].

DRLs do not apply to radiation therapy and have no direct linkage to the numerical values of the dose limits

TABLE 5.3

DRLs for Pediatric Patients

Examination	$CTDI_w$ (mGy)[a]	$CTDI_{vol}$ (mGy)[a]	DLP (mGy·cm)
Chest: ≤1-year old	23	12	204
Chest: 5-year old	20	13	228
Chest: 10-year old	26	17	368
Head: ≤1-year old	28	28	270
Head: 5-year old	43	43	465
Head: 10-year old	52	51	619

Data are given as third quartile (75%) values [3].

[a] Calculated values of $CTDI_w$ and $CTDI_{vol}$ relate to the 16 cm diameter dosimetry phantom.

or dose constraints. In practice, these values are chosen as percentile points on the observed distribution of doses to patients. The values should be selected by professional medical bodies in conjunction with national health and radiological protection authorities and reviewed at intervals that represent a compromise between the necessary stability and long-term changes in the observed dose distributions. The selected values could be specific to a country or region. One of the examples of DRLs for CT examinations is shown in Table 5.3 [3].

The main purposes of using DRLs are as follows:

- To improve a regional, national, or local distribution of observed results for a general medical imaging task by reducing the frequency of unjustified high or low values.

- To promote attainment of a narrower range of values that represent good practice for a more specific medical imaging task.

- To promote attainment of an optimum range of values for a specified medical imaging protocol.

5.9 Patient Dose Measurement/ Simulation in CT

5.9.1 Actual Measurement Method

In this method, an anthropomorphic phantom, small dosimeters, and an actual CT scanner are used.

5.9.1.1 Anthropomorphic Phantom

Anthropomorphic phantoms are designed to investigate organ doses (Figure 5.7). For a specific manufacturer, these phantoms range in sizes appropriate for newborns to adults. Each phantom is cut into thin transverse sections having grids of holes for placement of small

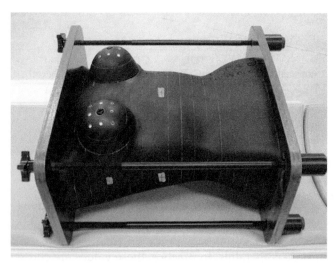

FIGURE 5.7
An anthropomorphic phantom (RAN110; The Phantom Laboratory, Salem, NY) used for the measurement of the patient dose in a CT procedure.

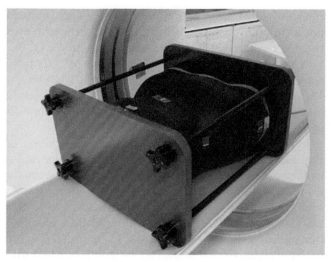

FIGURE 5.8
Setup for the measurement of the patient dose in CT by using an anthropomorphic phantom.

dosimeters, and soft tissue-, bone-, and lung-equivalent materials are used in all aspects of the phantom.

5.9.1.2 Small Dosimeter

Sectioned and drilled phantoms accept small dosimeters such as thermoluminescent dosimeters (TLDs) or radiophotoluminescent glass dosimeters (RPLDs).

In previous reports, TLDs were used most frequently. In general, LiF and BeO, which have low effective atomic numbers, have low energy dependencies within the energy range generally used in CT, but they also have low sensitivities. Mg_2SiO_4 and $CaSO_4$, which have high effective atomic numbers, have high energy dependencies and high sensitivities. There are some limitations of using TLDs. For example, the thermoluminescent signal disappears during reading, and reading cannot be performed repeatedly. Moreover, the differences in dose values among dosimeters are relatively high.

Recently, RPLDs also have been used frequently. Compared with TLDs, the advantages of RPLDs include good reproducibility of readout values, little fading effect, low energy dependence, and better dose linearity [14]. The radiophotoluminescent signal does not disappear during reading. The energy dependency within the energy range generally used in CT is relatively high, and TLDs or RPLDs must be calibrated with the effective energy used. One of the methods for calibration is to compare dose values with those of an ionizing chamber using a diagnostic x-ray system. The chamber and TLDs or RPLDs are placed adjacent to each other at the same distance from the x-ray focus in an irradiated field.

If an anthropomorphic phantom is drilled to accommodate various dosimeters, other types of small dosimeters such as small ion chambers or optically stimulated luminescent dosimeters can also be used. Radiographic or radiochromic film may also be used instead of small dosimeters. The film is placed between any two contiguous sections, and the sections are then sealed with black tape to prevent any exposure of the film to light.

5.9.1.3 Methods

When TLDs or RPLDs are used as small dosimeters, they should be annealed beforehand. To exclude the dose of localizer radiographs from the results, localizer radiographs should be obtained first after placing the phantom on the CT table. After obtaining localizer radiographs, the relative positions of the four corners of the phantom are marked on the CT table using certain markers (e.g., tape and a felt-tip pen) to maintain the phantom in the same position for subsequent CT acquisitions, and the phantom is removed from the table. Then, multiple small dosimeters are placed at the drilled holes that are located corresponding to targeted tissues and organs. The maximum number of small dosimeters possible should be used. Thereafter, the phantom is replaced on the CT table using the previous made reference marks. The measurement should be performed at least three times using separate sets of small dosimeters to reduce uncertainty and random error. The setup for measurement is shown in Figure 5.8. Small dosimeters that are used to measure background radiation should not be placed at the phantom.

After scanning, the small dosimeters are removed from the phantom, and the dose values are read after adequate time has passed (for TLDs) or preheating has been performed (for RPLDs) to stabilize the obtained values. Examples of adequate times are 1 hour for BeO and from 12 to 24 hours for $CaSO_4$ (see operation manuals).

As shown in the following equation, the absorbed dose for each organ is obtained by multiplying the averaged value of the organ or tissue, calibration factor, and the ratio of mass energy-absorption coefficients for each organ or tissue to air:

$$D_T = (M_T - M_B)k_C \frac{(\mu_{en}/\rho)_T}{(\mu_{en}/\rho)_A}$$

where M_T is the averaged value from the small dosimeters placed at locations corresponding to each organ or tissue, M_B is the background value, k_C is the calibration factor, $(\mu_{en}/\rho)_T$ is the mass energy-absorption coefficient for each organ or tissue, and $(\mu_{en}/\rho)_A$ is the mass energy-absorption coefficient for air [15].

If the mass energy-absorption coefficient cannot be obtained for a specific organ or tissue, the value for soft tissue should be used. In addition, the absorbed dose for bone surface can be calculated from the following equation:

$$D_{bone\_surface} = (M_{bone\_surface} - M_B)k_C B_i \frac{(\mu_{en}/\rho)_{cortical\_bone}}{(\mu_{en}/\rho)_A}$$

where $D_{bone\_surface}$ is the absorbed dose for bone surface, $M_{bone\_surface}$ is the averaged value from the small dosimeters placed at locations corresponding to the bone surface, B_i is the weight ratio of the bone where the small dosimeters are placed [16], and $(\mu_{en}/\rho)_{cortical\_bone}$ is the mass energy-absorption coefficient for the cortical bone. The absorbed dose for bone marrow can be calculated from the following equation:

$$D_{bone\_marrow} = (M_{bone\_marrow} - M_B)k_C M_i \frac{(\mu_{en}/\rho)_{bone\_marrow}}{(\mu_{en}/\rho)_A}$$

where D_{bone_marrow} is the absorbed dose for bone marrow, M_{bone_marrow} is the averaged value from the dosimeters placed at locations corresponding to the bone marrow, M_i is the weight ratio of the bone marrow where the small dosimeters are placed [16], and $(\mu_{en}/\rho)_{bone\_marrow}$ is the mass energy-absorption coefficient for the bone marrow. The absorbed dose for the skin can be calculated from the following equation:

$$D_{skin} = (M_{skin} - M_B)k_C \frac{A_{exposed}}{A_{total}} \frac{(\mu_{en}/\rho)_{skin}}{(\mu_{en}/\rho)_A}$$

where D_{skin} is the absorbed dose for the skin, M_{skin} is the averaged value from the small dosimeters placed at locations corresponding to the skin, $A_{exposed}$ is the exposed skin area of a patient (phantom), A_{total} is the total skin area of a patient (phantom), and $(\mu_{en}/\rho)_{skin}$ is the mass energy-absorption coefficient for the skin. The total skin area can be estimated using the following equation:

$$A_{total} = 0.63(\text{height})^2$$

where the unit of height is meter.

5.9.2 Simulation Method

Without using anthropomorphic phantoms and small dosimeters, the absorbed dose for each organ or tissue can be calculated using dose simulation software. One example is ImPACT CT Patient Dosimetry Calculator software (St George's Hospital, London, UK) (Figure 5.9) [17]. This software uses the National Radiological Protection Board Monte Carlo dose datasets produced in Report SR250 (Health Protection Agency Centre for Radiation, Chemical and Environmental Hazards, Didcot, UK). It provides normalized organ dose data for irradiation of a mathematical (medical internal radiation dose [MIRD]) phantom. By entering acquisition parameters on the spreadsheet, organ doses and $CTDI_{vol}$ can be calculated. The effective dose can also be calculated, but strictly, it is different from the true effective dose because it is defined not in the MIRD phantom but in the reference person in ICRP Publication 103. However, the calculated effective dose may be useful for comparing doses from different diagnostic procedures, scanners, or hospitals. One of the limitations of this method is that the use of automatic tube current modulation (ATCM) cannot be reflected in organ dose calculation.

5.10 Effective Doses for Various CT Procedures

Table 5.4 shows a list of effective doses found in previous reports of CT procedures [18]. Coronary angiogram shows the highest effective dose for various CT procedures.

5.11 Techniques and Technologies to Optimize Patient Dose in CT Procedures

There are some useful techniques and technologies for the optimization of the patient dose in CT procedures.

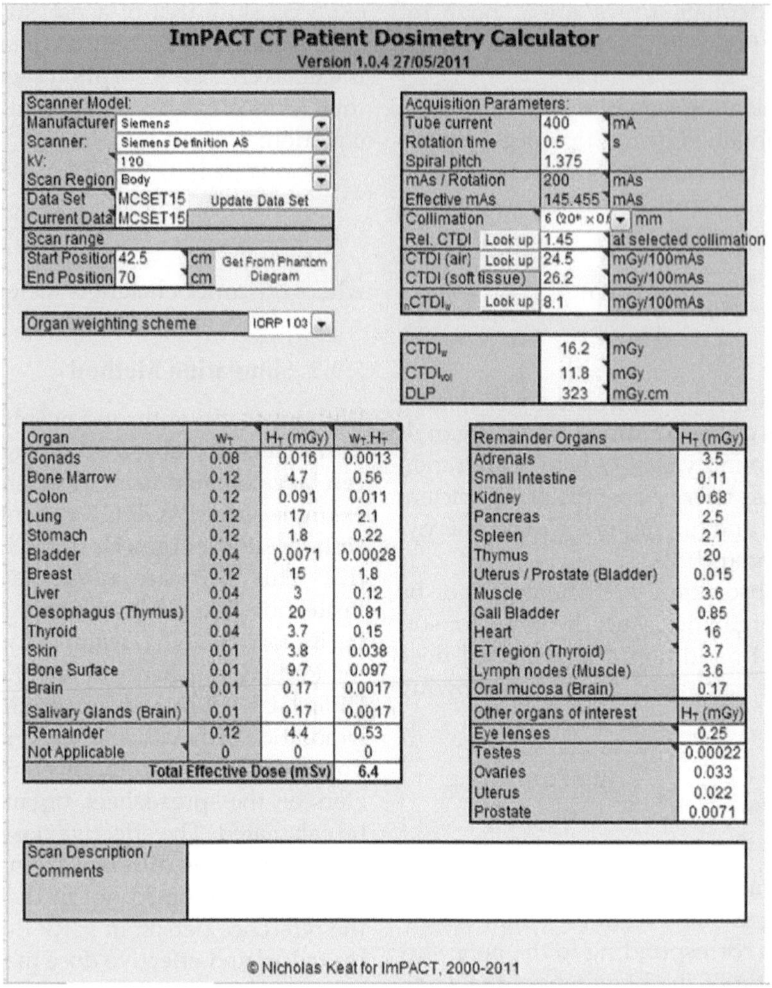

ImPACT CT Patient Dosimetry Calculator
Version 1.0.4 27/05/2011

Scanner Model:
Manufacturer: Siemens
Scanner: Siemens Definition AS
KV: 120
Scan Region: Body
Data Set: MCSET15   Update Data Set
Current Data: MCSET15
Scan range
Start Position: 42.5 cm   Get From Phantom Diagram
End Position: 70 cm

Organ weighting scheme: ICRP 103

Acquisition Parameters:
Tube current: 400 mA
Rotation time: 0.5 s
Spiral pitch: 1.375
mAs / Rotation: 200 mAs
Effective mAs: 145.455 mAs
Collimation: 6 (20* × 0.f) mm
Rel. CTDI Look up 1.45 at selected collimation
CTDI (air) Look up 24.5 mGy/100mAs
CTDI (soft tissue) 26.2 mGy/100mAs
$_n$CTDI$_w$ Look up 8.1 mGy/100mAs

CTDI$_w$ 16.2 mGy
CTDI$_{vol}$ 11.8 mGy
DLP 323 mGy.cm

Organ	w_T	H_T (mGy)	$w_T.H_T$
Gonads	0.08	0.016	0.0013
Bone Marrow	0.12	4.7	0.56
Colon	0.12	0.091	0.011
Lung	0.12	17	2.1
Stomach	0.12	1.8	0.22
Bladder	0.04	0.0071	0.00028
Breast	0.12	15	1.8
Liver	0.04	3	0.12
Oesophagus (Thymus)	0.04	20	0.81
Thyroid	0.04	3.7	0.15
Skin	0.01	3.8	0.038
Bone Surface	0.01	9.7	0.097
Brain	0.01	0.17	0.0017
Salivary Glands (Brain)	0.01	0.17	0.0017
Remainder	0.12	4.4	0.53
Not Applicable	0	0	0
Total Effective Dose (mSv)			6.4

Remainder Organs	H_T (mGy)
Adrenals	3.5
Small Intestine	0.11
Kidney	0.68
Pancreas	2.5
Spleen	2.1
Thymus	20
Uterus / Prostate (Bladder)	0.015
Muscle	3.6
Gall Bladder	0.85
Heart	16
ET region (Thyroid)	3.7
Lymph nodes (Muscle)	3.6
Oral mucosa (Brain)	0.17

Other organs of interest	H_T (mGy)
Eye lenses	0.25
Testes	0.00022
Ovaries	0.033
Uterus	0.022
Prostate	0.0071

Scan Description / Comments

© Nicholas Keat for ImPACT, 2000-2011

FIGURE 5.9
An example of dose simulation software (ImPACT CT Patient Dosimetry Calculator). (Data from Impact, St. George's Healthcare NHS Trust, London, http://www.impactscan.org/ctdosimetry.htm [accessed Feb 26, 2013].)

TABLE 5.4

List of Effective Doses Found in Previous Study Reports for CT Procedures

Examination	Average Effective Dose (mSv)	Values Reported in Literature (mSv)
Head	2	0.9–4.0
Neck	3	
Chest	7	4.0–18.0
Chest for pulmonary embolism	15	13–40
Abdomen	8	3.5–25
Pelvis	6	3.3–10
Three-phase liver study	15	
Spine	6	1.5–10
Coronary angiography	16	5.0–32
Calcium scoring	3	1.0–12
Virtual colonoscopy	10	4.0–13.2

Source: Data from Mettler FA Jr, Huda W, Yoshizumi TT, Mahesh M, Radiology, 248(1): 254–263, 2008.

5.11.1 mA (mAs) Adjustment

Dose and mA (mAs) are proportionally related. The amount of image noise is inversely proportional to the square root of mA (mAs). An excessive increase in mA (mAs) causes an increase in the patient dose, but excessive mA (mAs) reduction can adversely affect image quality and decrease lesion detectability. Therefore, the operator should use mA (mAs) that provides the optimal patient dose.

ATCM is often used to optimize the patient dose in CT procedures. There are four types of ATCM: angular (xy-axis) modulation, z-axis modulation, organ-based modulation, and electrocardiogram (ECG)-gated modulation.

5.11.1.1 xy-Axis Modulation

X-rays are significantly less attenuated in the antero-posterior direction and more attenuated in the lateral

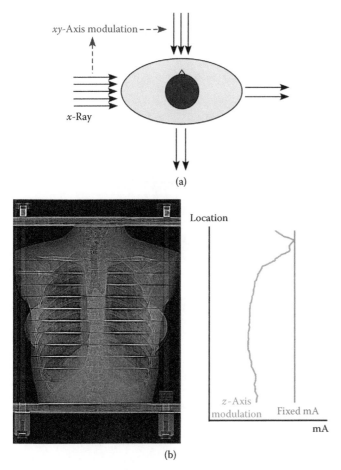

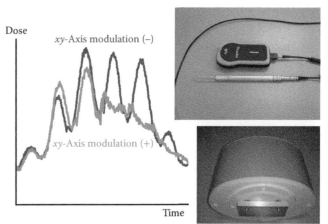

FIGURE 5.11
An example of dose profiles with and without *xy*-axis modulation. These profiles were acquired using the CT Dose Profiler and an elliptical cylindrical phantom.

FIGURE 5.10
Conceptual diagrams of (a) *xy*-axis modulation and (b) *z*-axis modulation.

direction (Figure 5.10). Therefore, the tube current should also be adjusted within one gantry rotation by modulating it in a sinusoidal manner on the basis of the assumption. The tube current varies according to the attenuation information on the CT projection radiograph or in near real-time according to the measured attenuation from the previous 180° projection.

In some implementations of angular dose modulation, an increase in tube current may be allowed in the shoulder region, whereas in other implementations, the tube current is not allowed to exceed the initial value prescribed by the operator [19].

An example of dose modulation along the *xy*-axis is shown in Figure 5.11. These profiles were acquired using the CT Dose Profiler (RTI Electronics, Mölndal, Sweden) and an elliptical cylindrical phantom (Kyoto Kagaku, Kyoto, Japan) when helical CT scans were performed with and without *xy*-axis modulation, which varies the tube current in near real-time according to the measured attenuation from the previous 180° projection. The dose profiles gradually stabilized because the tube current could be adjusted properly.

5.11.1.2 z-Axis Modulation

Tube current is adjusted according to the anatomical regions of the patients. Unlike *xy*-axis modulation, *z*-axis modulation is performed to produce relatively uniform noise levels across the various regions of the anatomy (Figure 5.10). The tube current is modulated to provide the desired level of image quality at the chosen attenuation. *z*-Axis modulation can adjust the tube current to maintain a user-chosen noise level or image quality and uses at least a single localizer radiograph to calculate the attenuation profile of the patients. The tube current is dynamically modulated in the *z*-direction based on the basis of the prior calculations from the localizer radiograph.

The results specified per anatomical region as mAs reduction in percent are shown in Table 5.5 [20].

The simultaneous combination of *xy*- and *z*-axis modulations involves variation of the tube current both during gantry rotation and along the *z*-axis of the patient. This is the most comprehensive approach to CT dose reduction because the dose is adjusted according to the patient-specific attenuation in all three planes.

5.11.1.3 Organ-Based Modulation

To reduce the dose to radiosensitive organs, such as the breast, thyroid, and eye lens, an organ-based modulation technique (X-CARE; Siemens Healthcare, Erlangen, Germany) was developed (Figure 5.12). In this technique, the tube current is decreased by 75% from the reference scan's tube current for an angular range of approximately 120° over the anterior surface of the head, symmetric to the median plane of the patient. During

TABLE 5.5

Results Specified Per Anatomical Region as mAs Reduction in Percent

	mAs Reduction (%)	
Region	Patients	Cadavers
Head	18	11
Shoulder	53	40
Thorax	22	27
Abdomen	15	23
Pelvis	25	34
Extremity	39	27

Source: Data from Greess H, Wolf H, Baum U et al., *Eur Radiol*, 10(2): 391–394, 2000.

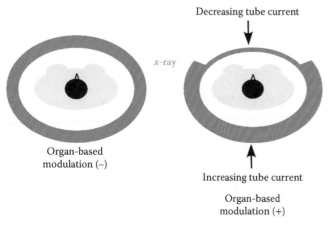

FIGURE 5.12
A conceptual diagram of organ-based modulation.

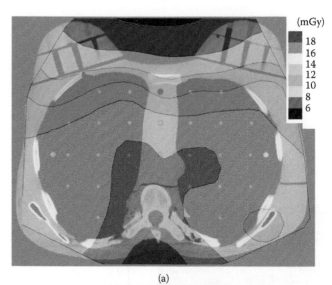

(a)

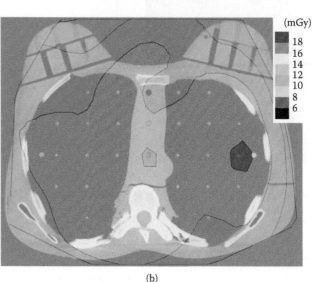

(b)

FIGURE 5.13
Absorbed dose distributions within a single section (a) with and (b) without organ-based modulation.

the remaining 240° of the scanning range, the tube current is increased by 25% so that the noise levels remain low [21]. However, a limitation is that the technique cannot be applied with high helical pitch.

In thoracic CT procedures, organ-based modulation can reduce the absorbed dose for the breast about 22% without changing the CT values and noise levels compared with those of the reference [22]. The absorbed dose distributions within a single section with and without organ-based modulation are shown in Figure 5.13. Exposure to multiple diagnostic radiographic examinations during childhood and adolescence increases the risk of breast cancer among women with scoliosis [23]. Therefore, organ-based modulation is preferable for specific groups of patients, such as children and young women, in whom the risk of breast cancer might be increased by thoracic CT.

5.11.1.4 ECG-Gated Modulation

This method applies high tube current over a limited range of heart phases (e.g., diastole phase) to ensure low noise during the phase while reducing the tube current during the remaining heart phases to reduce the patient dose (Figure 5.14).

FIGURE 5.14
Different types of electrocardiogram (ECG)-gated modulation.

Another ECG-gated modulation is to employ prospectively gated axial scans in which x-rays are turned on only during the required heart phase and turned off completely at other heart phases. However, this method can only be used for patients whose heart rate is low and stable.

One study demonstrated that ECG-gated modulation can reduce 3.4%–9.2% of the doses absorbed by thoracic organs compared with the reference dose in retrospectively ECG-gated helical scans, and prospectively gated axial scans can reduce 66.1%–71.0% of the doses absorbed by thoracic organs compared with the reference dose in retrospectively ECG-gated helical scans with ECG-gated modulation [24].

5.11.2 kVp Adjustment

Dose is approximately proportional to the square of kVp. Both mA (mAs) and kVp should be adjusted according to patient size to optimize the patient dose. In children and small adults, reduction of kVp is effective for reducing the patient dose while maintaining a desired contrast-to-noise ratio (CNR) [25].

To achieve this, a new tool (CARE kV; Siemens Healthcare) that automatically adjusts the optimal kVp setting for each individual patient for each specific CT procedure was developed recently. Information from localizer radiographs is used to optimize kVp (and mAs) so that a user-chosen CNR is maintained with the lowest dose. At present, kVp cannot be modulated during the scan.

However, changes in kVp result in a change in x-ray photon energy and changes in x-ray photon energy also result in a change in the tissue CT value. Therefore, variation in kVp also causes a substantial change in image contrast.

5.11.3 Selection of the Optimal Reconstruction Kernel

Reconstruction kernels themselves are not directly related to patient dose, but the patient dose may be reduced by selecting an optimal reconstruction kernel.

Iterative reconstruction is one of the algorithms for generating cross-sectional images from measured projections of an object. The algorithm has been applied to single-photon emission CT or positron emission tomography. In CT, however, this method has not been used because of its significantly slower calculation speed compared with that of filtered back projection, which is the standard CT image reconstruction algorithm.

In CT, various new image reconstruction systems that use iterative reconstruction algorithms have been developed recently. Using these systems, patient dose reduction can be achieved while maintaining image quality.

For example, Adaptive Statistical Iterative Reconstruction (GE Healthcare, Milwaukee, WI) focuses only on modeling of the statistical properties of the imaging chain instead of modeling the entire CT system. In addition, the new Model-Based Iterative Reconstruction system (GE Healthcare), whose brand name is Veo, uses a model of the scanning system itself to improve image quality. It tries to model the optics of the CT system by taking into consideration the noise properties, actual size and shape of the focal spot, detector cells, and image voxels. Iterative Reconstruction in Image Space (Siemens Healthcare) reduces image noise in the iterative loop process, but raw data are utilized in the image improvement process. However, the new Sinogram Affirmed Iterative Reconstruction system (Siemens Healthcare) uses raw data for the iterative loop process (Figure 5.15). Other manufacturers have also developed original reconstruction systems that use iterative reconstruction algorithms.

5.11.4 Selection of Optimal Pitch

In SDCT, increasing pitch decreases the dose without affecting image noise. In MDCT, increasing pitch not only decreases the dose but also increases image noise. If the other parameters are constant, the patient dose within the acquisition range and acquisition time can be reduced when the pitch is increased.

However, in MDCT, additional scans at the start and end of a helical scan are needed for image interpolation in the helical scans because data interpolation between two points must be performed for all projection angles. This is called an over-ranging scan and contributes an additional dose to the patient. Commonly, an additional half rotation is needed at the start and end of a helical scan. Therefore, the region of over-ranging scans decrease when pitch decreases.

A technology to reduce the additional dose to the patient is active collimation. An active collimator can block x-rays that are not required for image interpolation at the start and end of a helical scan.

5.11.5 Selection of Optimal Image Thickness and Image Noise

Thinner image thicknesses can be easily obtained using MDCT systems. When thinner image thicknesses are used, the partial volume effect decreases but image noise increases. To obtain thinner image thicknesses with lower image noise, an increased radiation dose is needed. However, the CNR and visibility of small

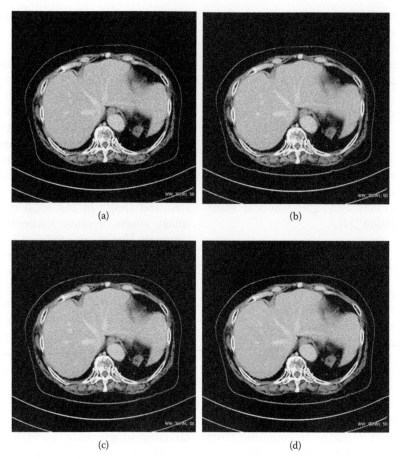

FIGURE 5.15

Differences of images reconstructed with Sinogram Affirmed Iterative Reconstruction (SAFIRE). Images reconstructed (a) without SAFIRE, (b) with SAFIRE using strength 1, (c) with SAFIRE using strength 3, and (d) with SAFIRE using strength 5.

lesions can improve despite increased noise when thinner image thicknesses are used [26].

Doses need not be necessarily increased to obtain the same image noise as achieved with greater image thicknesses even if lesser image thicknesses are required for multiplanar or 3D reformations.

5.11.6 Selection of an Optimal Bowtie Filter (or Scan Field of View)

Different types of filters are available for insertion in front of the x-ray tube. An inherent flat-shaped filter, which comprises aluminum or copper, absorbs most of the low-energy x-ray photons (Figure 5.16). In addition, bowtie filters, which barely absorb x-ray photons at the center but absorb off-axis x-ray photons, reduce the surface dose to the patient without substantially increasing image noise. In general, the optimal bowtie filter is selected when the optimal scan field of view is chosen. Therefore, one should choose the optimal scan field of view according to the anatomical size and scan region of the patient.

5.11.7 Application of Selective Organ Shielding

If an organ-based modulation technique (Section 5.11.1.3) cannot be applied, selective organ shielding may be effective for reducing the radiation dose to radiosensitive organs such as the breast, thyroid, and eye lens.

For example, breast shielding is achieved by applying a commercially available latex sheet over the breasts (Figure 5.17). The sheet contains bismuth and can attenuate many x-ray photons that would be absorbed by the breasts [27]. Some study reports have recommended the use of selective organ shielding because diagnostic image quality is not seriously affected by the shielding [28,29]; however, some studies have not recommended the use of selective organ shielding because of their impact on CT numbers, artifacts, and image noise [30,31]. Therefore, it is difficult to judge whether shielding should be used.

5.11.8 Optimization of the Number of Scans

When multiple CT scans are performed, the patient dose increases. For example, one study reported

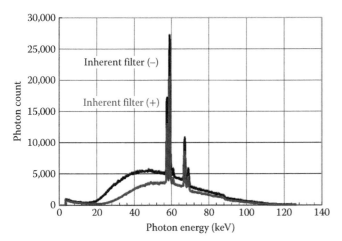

FIGURE 5.16
An x-ray spectrum for a peak tube voltage of 120 kVp with and without an inherent flat-shaped filter.

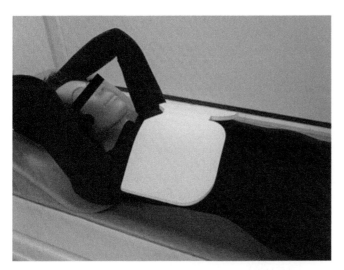

FIGURE 5.17
Photograph of a commercially available latex sheet comprising bismuth (AttenuRad; F & L Medical Products, Vandergrift, PA).

FOCUS POINT: USE OF SELECTIVE ORGAN SHIELDING IN COMBINATION WITH ATCM

There is some debate on whether selective organ shielding should be used, but there is no doubt that it can reduce the radiation dose absorbed by a radiosensitive organ. Moreover, there is no doubt that ATCM is effective for optimizing the patient dose in CT procedures.

At present, it is worthwhile to ask whether selective organ shielding in combination with ATCM is an outstanding approach. It can be argued that it is not. When ATCM is applied, it uses at least a single localizer radiograph to calculate the attenuation profile of the patient and dynamically modulates the tube current on the basis of the prior calculations from the localizer radiograph in many ATCM systems. Therefore, ATCM cannot calculate the attenuation profile of the patient correctly if a shield is placed over a radiosensitive organ. Although the issue can be avoided by placing a shield after obtaining the localizer radiograph, the shield may prevent patient dose optimization achieved by ATCM and images with the quality needed for diagnosis may not be obtained. Moreover, one specific ATCM system modulates the tube current according to the near real-time attenuation information from the previous 180° projection during the scan. Therefore, this type of ATCM cannot correctly calculate attenuation information even if the shield is placed over a radiosensitive organ after obtaining the localizer radiograph.

that detectability of hepatocellular carcinoma was improved with four-phase CT scans [32], but another study reported that four-phase CT scans did not improve the detection of hepatocellular carcinoma compared with three-phase CT scans [33]. Optimization of the number of scans is difficult, but each CT scan may increase the probability of cancer incidence, and therefore, the number of repetitions should be kept as low as possible.

5.11.9 Application of Dual-Source CT

Dual-source CT systems are equipped with two x-ray tubes and two corresponding detectors mounted onto the rotating gantry with an angular offset of 90°. By using two x-ray tubes and two corresponding detectors simultaneously to acquire complementary data, the minimum exposure time is reduced by a factor of 2 compared with that of a single-source CT system. Moreover, the maximum table feed per rotation in a helical scan can be increased by a factor of 2 compared with that in a single-source CT.

This acquisition method using a 128-slice dual-source CT system (Flash Spiral; Siemens Healthcare) is especially useful for pediatric and ECG-triggered cardiac CT procedures. In ECG-triggered cardiac CT, the entire cardiac volume can be scanned within a fraction of one cardiac RR cycle. At a rotation time of 0.28 seconds, the scan time of the entire heart is less than 0.3 seconds at a temporal resolution of 75 ms. Using this acquisition method, the effective dose can be reduced to less than 2 mSv [34].

5.11.10 Application of Area Detector CT

In the 320-slice MDCT scanner, which is generally termed area-detector CT, the maximum coverage is 16 cm at the scanner isocenter. Using the scanner, the entire heart can be acquired in a single gantry rotation. In the ECG-triggered cardiac CT procedure, the entire cardiac volume can be scanned within a fraction of one cardiac RR cycle. The 320-slice MDCT scanner has a standard temporal resolution of approximately 175 ms, which is half of the gantry rotation time. Because the temporal resolution in 320-slice MDCT is longer than that of dual-source CT (75 ms), heart rate control may be necessary to achieve good image quality. Using this acquisition method, the effective dose can be reduced to less than 5 mSv [35].

5.11.11 Application of Newly Developed Detectors

CT scanners basically turn x-rays into light using a scintillator, which is composed of materials such as cadmium tungstate. The generated light is converted into electrical signals by a photo diode.

One manufacturer has used a new scintillator that comprises a new garnet gemstone material (Gemstone Detector; GE Healthcare). It provides increased x-ray reaction speed, great light output, high transparency, low afterglow, low radiation dose, and environmental and temperature stability. Another manufacturer has also used a new scintillator that comprises praseodymium-doped gadolinium oxysulfide (Quantum Detector; Toshiba Medical Systems, Tochigi, Japan). This scintillator also provides high absorption efficiency, high transparency, fast decay time, low afterglow, and low radiation dose.

On the other hand, one manufacturer has developed a new detector system (Stellar Detector; Siemens Healthcare) with an analog-to-digital converter that is integrated with the photodiode, which significantly reduces the electronic noise. It can provide high-signal output with a low radiation dose. The new detector system may be loaded into existing CT systems.

5.12 Conclusion

In this chapter, the radiation-induced risks, dose levels, CT dose descriptors, methods for dose measurement and simulation, DRLs, effective doses for various CT procedures, and techniques and technologies for optimization of the patient dose in CT procedures were described. Understanding CT dose descriptors is necessary for the evaluation of CT doses, and familiarity with the techniques and technologies available for optimization of the patient dose in CT procedures is useful for optimization of CT scanning protocols.

Justification of CT use is a responsibility of both clinicians and radiologists, and optimization of CT protocols is a responsibility of both radiologists and radiographers. Although risks from CT procedures are probably small, all clinicians, radiologists, and radiographers must recognize that each CT scan may increase the probability of cancer incidence.

References

1. Mettler FA Jr, Thomadsen BR, Bhargavan M et al. Medical radiation exposure in the U.S. in 2006: Preliminary results. *Health Phys* 2008; 95(5): 502–507.
2. Valentin J (Editor). The 2007 Recommendations of the International Commission on Radiological Protection, ICRP Publication 103. *Ann ICRP* 2007; 37(2–4): 1–332.
3. Managing patient dose in multi-detector computed tomography (MDCT), ICRP Publication 102. *Ann ICRP* 2007; 37(1): 1–79.
4. 1990 Recommendations of the International Commission on Radiological Protection, ICRP Publication 60. *Ann ICRP* 1991; 21(1–3): 1–201.
5. Committee to Assess Health Risks From Exposure to Low Levels of Ionizing Radiation, Board on Radiation Effects Research, Division of Earth and Life Studies, National Research Council of the National Academies. *Health risks from exposure to low levels of ionizing radiation: BEIR VII phase 2.* Washington, DC: National Academies Press, 2006.
6. Pregnancy and medical radiation, ICRP Publication 84. *Ann ICRP* 2000; 30(1): 1–44.
7. Huda W, Sterzik A, Tipnis S, Schoepf UJ. Organ doses to adult patients for chest CT. *Med Phys* 2010; 37(2): 842–847.
8. Matsubara K, Koshida K, Noto K, Shimono T, Yamamoto T, Matsui O. Relationship between specific organ doses and volumetric CT dose indices in multidetector CT studies. *J Med Imaging Radiat Oncol* 2011; 55(5): 493–497.
9. Shope TB, Gagne RM, Johnson GC. A method for describing the doses delivered by transmission x-ray computed tomography. *Med Phys* 1981; 8(4): 488–495.
10. Shinno T. [Element technology for area detector CT–Aquilion ONE™]. *Jpn J Radiol Technol* 2008; 64(6): 734–743.
11. Boone JM. The trouble with CTDI100. *Med Phys* 2007; 34(4): 1364–1371.
12. Comprehensive methodology for the evaluation of radiation dose in X-ray computed tomography, AAPM Task Group Report 111. College Park, MD: American Association of Physicists in Medicine, 2010.

13. Radiological protection in medicine, ICRP Publication 105. *Ann ICRP* 2007; 37(6): 1–64.

14. Hsu SM, Yeh SH, Lin MS, Chen WL. Comparison on characteristics of radiophotoluminescent glass dosemeters and thermoluminescent dosemeters. *Radiat Prot Dosimetry* 2006; 119(1–4): 327–331.

15. Tissue substitutes in radiation dosimetry and measurement, ICRU Report 44. Bethesda, MD: International Commission on Radiation Units and Measurements, 1989.

16. Basic anatomical & physiological data for use in radiological protection: The skeleton, ICRP Publication 70. *Ann ICRP* 1995; 25(2): 1–80.

17. ImPACT Group: CT dosimetry tool. Impact, St. George's Healthcare NHS Trust, London. http://www.impactscan.org/ctdosimetry.htm (accessed Feb 26, 2013).

18. Mettler FA Jr, Huda W, Yoshizumi TT, Mahesh M. Effective doses in radiology and diagnostic nuclear medicine: A catalog. *Radiology* 2008; 248(1): 254–263.

19. McCollough CH, Bruesewitz MR, Kofler JM Jr et al. CT dose reduction and dose management tools: Overview of available options. *Radiographics* 2006; 26(2): 503–512.

20. Greess H, Wolf H, Baum U et al. Dose reduction in computed tomography by attenuation-based on-line modulation of tube current: Evaluation of six anatomical regions. *Eur Radiol* 2000; 10(2): 391–394.

21. Wang J, Duan X, Christner JA, Leng S, Grant KL, McCollough CH. Bismuth shielding, organ-based tube current modulation, and global reduction of tube current for dose reduction to the eye at head CT. *Radiology* 2012; 262(1): 191–198.

22. Matsubara K, Sugai M, Toyoda A et al. Assessment of an organ-based tube current modulation in thoracic computed tomography. *J Appl Clin Med Phys* 2012; 13(2): 3731.

23. Doody MM, Lonstein JE, Stovall M, Hacker DG, Luckyanov N, Land CE. Breast cancer mortality after diagnostic radiography: Findings from the U.S. Scoliosis Cohort Study. *Spine* 2000; 25(16): 2052–2063.

24. Matsubara K, Koshida K, Noto K et al. Estimation of organ-absorbed radiation doses during 64-detector CT coronary angiography using different acquisition techniques and heart rates: A phantom study. *Acta Radiol* 2011; 52(6): 632–637.

25. Huda W, Scalzetti EM, Levin G. Technique factors and image quality as functions of patient weight at abdominal CT. *Radiology* 2000; 217(2): 430–435.

26. Wedegärtner U, Yamamura J, Nagel HD et al. [Image quality of thickened slabs in multislice CT chest examinations: Postprocessing vs. direct reconstruction]. *Rofo* 2007; 179(4): 373–379.

27. Hopper KD, King SH, Lobell ME, TenHave TR, Weaver JS. The breast: In-plane x-ray protection during diagnostic thoracic CT—Shielding with bismuth radioprotective garments. *Radiology* 1997; 205(3): 853–858.

28. Fricke BL, Donnelly LF, Frush DP et al. In-plane bismuth breast shields for pediatric CT: Effects on radiation dose and image quality using experimental and clinical data. *AJR Am J Roentgenol* 2003; 180(2): 407–411.

29. Yilmaz MH, Yaşar D, Albayram S et al. Coronary calcium scoring with MDCT: The radiation dose to the breast and the effectiveness of bismuth breast shield. *Eur J Radiol* 2007; 61(1): 139–143.

30. Vollmar SV, Kalender WA. Reduction of dose to the female breast in thoracic CT: A comparison of standard-protocol, bismuth-shielded, partial and tube-current-modulated CT examinations. *Eur Radiol* 2008; 18(8): 1674–1682.

31. Kalra MK, Dang P, Singh S, Saini S, Shepard JA. In-plane shielding for CT: Effect of off-centering, automatic exposure control and shield-to-surface distance. *Korean J Radiol* 2009; 10(2): 156–163.

32. Murakami T, Kim T, Takamura M et al. Hypervascular hepatocellular carcinoma: Detection with double arterial phase multi-detector row helical CT. *Radiology* 2001; 218(3): 763–767.

33. Kim SK, Lim JH, Lee WJ et al. Detection of hepatocellular carcinoma: Comparison of dynamic three-phase computed tomography images and four-phase computed tomography images using multidetector row helical computed tomography. *J Comput Assist Tomogr* 2002; 26(5): 691–698.

34. Matsubara K, Koshida H, Sakuta K et al. [Evaluation of an exposed-radiation dose on a dual-source cardiac computed tomography examination with a prospective electrocardiogram-gated fast dual spiral scan]. *Jpn J Radiol Technol* 2012; 68(1): 59–64.

35. Seguchi S, Aoyama T, Koyama S, Fujii K, Yamauchi-Kawaura C. Patient radiation dose in prospectively gated axial CT coronary angiography and retrospectively gated helical technique with a 320-detector row CT scanner. *Med Phys* 2010; 37(11): 5579–5585.

Section II

Neck–Brain

6

Imaging of the Paranasal Sinuses and Ear

Thomas J. Vogl and Ahmed M. Tawfik

CONTENTS

6.1 Pathology of the Paranasal Sinuses

6.1.1 Anatomy of the Nose and Paranasal Sinuses

The lateral nasal wall shows three projections: the superior, middle, and inferior turbinate bones (or conchae). Beneath each turbinate bone lies a respectively named meatus [1]. The paranasal sinuses are four pairs, named for the bones of the skull they pneumatize. The nasal cavity and sinuses are lined by ciliated mucus-secreting epithelium. The cilia act to propel the mucus toward the sinus ostium, which drains into the nose [2].

The maxillary antrum consists of a roof (orbital floor), floor, anterior wall, medial wall (lateral wall of the nose), and posterolateral wall [3]. The maxillary antrum secretions drain into the superomedial sinus ostium, then through the infundibulum, which is the space located lateral to the uncinate process and medial to the inferomedial border of the orbit. The uncinate process is the superior extension of the lateral nasal wall. The infundibulum communicates with the middle meatus through the hiatus semilunaris, which is the gap between the free superior edge of uncinate process and the largest ethmoid air cell, the ethmoidal bulla [2,3].

The entire complex of the maxillary ostium, infundibulum, uncinate process, hiatus semilunaris, ethmoid bulla, and middle meatus makes up the ostiomeatal complex or ostiomeatal unit (Figure 6.1) [4], which acts as the common drainage pathway of the frontal, maxillary, and anterior ethmoid air cells [3].

The frontal sinuses show great variations in aeration and septations [5]. The floor of the frontal sinuses slope medially and secretions drain inferomedially through the frontal recess, which is an hourglass narrow space between the frontal sinus and the middle meatus [3].

The ethmoid sinuses are divided into groups of cells (up to 18) by bony basal lamellae that extend laterally to the lamina papyracea and superiorly to the fovea ethmoidalis [3]. The lamellae also serve as attachments for the turbinates. The basal lamella of the middle turbinate

is the most important, as it divides the ethmoid into anterior and posterior groups of cells that drain into the middle and superior meati, respectively [1] (Figure 6.2). The sphenoid sinuses drain into the sphenoethmoidal recess, which lies above the superior nasal concha [3].

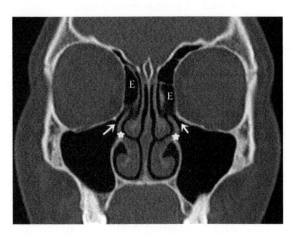

FIGURE 6.1
Normal anatomy of the ostiomeatal unit. The maxillary ostium (arrows) enters the infundibulum, which is the space between uncinate process (asterisks) and the largest ethmoid air cell or ethmoid bulla (E).

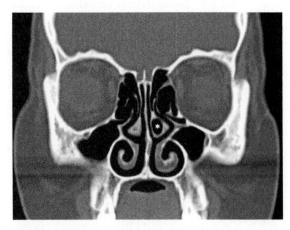

FIGURE 6.2
Left middle turbinate concha bullosa (asterisk).

BOX 6.1 ANATOMIC VARIANTS OF THE SINONASAL REGION

Location	Description	Clinical relevance
Middle turbinate	Concha bullosa (pneumatized middle turbinate)[a] Paradoxic middle turbinate (middle turbinate convex toward lateral instead of the normal medial direction)	Encroachment on the middle meatus and infundibulum
Uncinate process	Lateral deviation of the free edge of uncinate process Pneumatized uncinate process	Narrowing of the hiatus semilunaris and infundibulum
Nasal septum	Deviated nasal septum with or without septal spur	Narrowing of middle meatus
Ethmoid cells	Agger nasi cells (inferior and anterolateral to the frontal recess)	Narrowing of the frontal recess
	Haller cells (infraorbital ethmoid cells)	Narrowing of the infundibulum
	Onodi cells (pneumatized posterior ethmoid cells above sphenoid sinus)	Increase surgical risk to optic nerves
	Large ethmoid bulla	Obstruct the ostiomeatal complex
Lamina papyracea	Medial deviation or dehiscence	Increased surgical risk of orbital injury
Cribriform plate	Asymmetric height or deep olfactory fossa	Increased surgical risk of intracranial penetration
Sphenoid sinus	Extensive pneumatization	Cavernous sinus, carotid artery, optic nerve complications Increased surgical risk

Sources: Data from Laine, F.J., and Smoker, W.R., *AJR Am. J. Roentgenol.*, 159, 849–857, 1992 [1]; Earwaker, J., *Radiographics*, 13, 381–415, 1993 [6]; Polavaram, R. et al., *Otolaryngol. Clin. North Am.*, 37, 221–242, 2004 [7]; Beale, T.J. et al., *Semin. Ultrasound CT MR.*, 30: 2–16, 2009 [5].

[a] See Figure 6.2.

The anatomy of the paranasal sinuses is subject to many variations, some of them are clinically relevant and should be identified and reported by the radiologist interpreting a computed tomography (CT) scan of the sinuses (Box 6.1).

6.1.2 Congenital Anomalies of the Face and the Nose

Congenital anomalies of the face and sinonasal region may occur as isolated malformation or as a part of more complex syndrome. Cleft lip and cleft palate are the most common anomalies [8]. Anomalies causing nasal obstruction are usually detected in the neonatal period. Other anomalies may present later on.

Choanal atresia may be unilateral or bilateral and the obstruction is mostly bony or bony and membranous [9]. Bilateral complete atresia result in early neonatal severe respiratory distress and is diagnosed by failure of catheter to pass through the nose [10]. CT is indicated to delineate the obstructing bony or cartilaginous plate and the associated structural deformities, usually thickened vomer and medial pterygoid plate [9].

Congenital dacryocystocele is collection of fluid in the lacrimal sac due to failure of canalization of the lacrimal

drainage system both above and below the lacrimal sac [9]. It presents as a mass in the medial canthus of an infant or a child [8].

An encephalocele is the protrusion of intracranial contents through a defect in the cranium or skull base [8]. They are classified according to the defect site as anterior (sincipital), occipital, and basal (Figure 6.3). Anterior encephaloceles are further classified as frontonasal, nasoethmoidal, and nasoorbital [11].

Nasal gliomas are uncommon, congenital heterotopic masses of glial tissue in or around the nose. In contrast to encephaloceles, they are not connected to the cerebrospinal fluid (CSF) spaces. They typically present in infancy, are very slowly growing, and have no malignant potential [8].

6.1.3 Facial Trauma

CT is the modality of choice for evaluation of facial trauma. Axial and coronal images provide most of the information. In complex and displaced fractures, 3D reconstructions allow better communication with the surgeons and are helpful in preoperative planning [12]. Facial fractures are usually multiple, complex, and asymmetric but tend to fall into various categories and classifications.

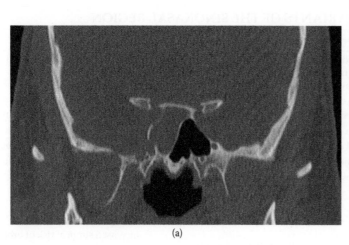

(a)

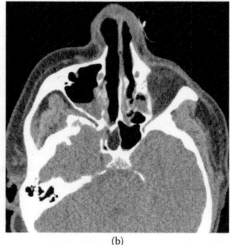

(b)

FIGURE 6.3
Encephalocele. (a) Coronal bone algorithm CT shows a defect in the wall of the right sphenoid sinus. (b) Axial soft-tissue algorithm CT shows herniated cerebral content in the right sphenoid sinus.

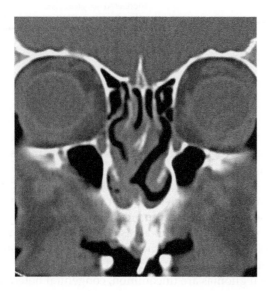

FIGURE 6.4
Nasal trauma. Coronal CT image shows traumatic septal deviation convexity to the left.

Nasal fractures are common and usually involve the thinner, distal third of the nasal bones. More severe fractures are associated with fractures of the anterior bony nasal septum (Figure 6.4), the ethmoid, and the frontal process of the maxilla [8,12].

Orbital blowout fractures usually involve the orbital floor due to a blunt trauma to the orbit. The force of the blow is absorbed by the anterior rim of the orbit and increased pressure is transmitted to the weaker orbital floor, which fractures with or without herniation of orbital fat and inferior rectus muscle. A medial blowout fracture involving the lamina papyracea is less common.

Orbital blow-in fractures are least common and occur when the orbital floor fracture segments are displaced upward into the orbit, impinging on the inferior orbital muscles or the globe [8,12].

Le Fort fractures result from direct anterior facial injuries. Le Fort I is a horizontal fracture extending across the floor of the maxillary sinuses above the dentition line of the superior alveolar ridge resulting in a "floating palate." Le Fort II fracture (pyramidal fracture) occurs vertically through the maxilla and across the upper nasal-ethmoid bone complex and back to the pterygoid plates. The zygoma is left intact with a "floating maxilla." Le Fort III is the most severe fracture type, resulting in separation of the entire facial skeleton from the skull base, or "floating face." The fracture line runs across the root of the nose, then bilaterally through the orbital walls to involve the frontozygomatic sutures, and from the orbital floor down across the back of each maxilla to the lower portion of the pterygoid plates. The zygomatic arches also are fractured [8,12].

A tripod zygomatic fracture is the result of a lateral facial trauma with three main fracture sites: through the lateral orbital wall, separating the zygoma and maxilla, and through the zygomatic arch [8].

CT findings after trauma other than fractures include intrasinus hemorrhage, subcutaneous edema, subcutaneous hematomas, and foreign bodies. Complications of facial trauma include vascular injuries of the ethmoidal and internal maxillary arteries, optic nerve injury from fractures through the orbital apex, or CSF leak due to associated dural tear. Patients with CSF leak are at increased risk of meningitis. CT after intrathecal contrast administration is the modality of choice for evaluation of suspected CSF leak [8].

6.1.4 Inflammatory Diseases of the Paranasal Sinuses

CT is the modality of choice for imaging of sinusitis and had a great impact on the advances in its management. Multi-detector CT isotropic imaging with axial and coronal (and may be sagittal) thin section reformats has replaced conventional direct coronal CT imaging for the evaluation of sinusitis. A low-dose technique is used and contrast material is not routinely given unless complications are suspected.

6.1.4.1 Acute Sinusitis

Acute sinusitis (viral or secondary bacterial infection) is a very common disease that is generally not an indication for CT imaging unless orbital or intracranial spread is suspected.

Orbital complications are secondary to direct or venous spread through the valveless venous connections with the ethmoid sinuses. Children are at higher risk for orbital complications including orbital edema or cellulitis, subperiosteal phlegmon or abscess, and intraorbital abscess. Intracranial complications are less common and usually complicate frontal sinusitis. They include sinus thrombosis, meningitis, epidural, subdural, and brain abscess [13].

6.1.4.2 Chronic Sinusitis

Chronic sinusitis results from persistent or repeated episodes of acute inflammation. CT is the imaging study of choice in adult and pediatric chronic sinusitis patients. Findings of sinus disease include opacification of the normally aerated sinus lumen and mucosal thickening. An air–fluid level denotes acute inflammation while thickening and sclerosis of the bony walls of the sinus is indicative of chronic disease [3]. Contrast material, although not routinely given, may enable differentiation of the components of an opacified maxillary sinus into three concentric rings: low-attenuation submucosal edema, enhancing mucosa, and low-attenuation secretions.

The extent of inflammatory sinus disease as seen on CT could be assigned into one of five patterns (Box 6.2) [14]. The infundibular pattern refers to focal obstruction of the maxillary sinus ostium and ethmoid infundibulum, associated with maxillary sinusitis. The Ostomeatal unit pattern refers to ipsilateral maxillary, frontal, and anterior ethmoid sinus disease due to obstruction of the middle meatus. The sphenoethmoidal recess pattern refers to sphenoid and posterior ethmoid sinus inflammation caused by sphenoethmoidal recess obstruction. The sinonasal polyposis pattern refers to diffuse nasal and paranasal sinus polyps associated with infundibular enlargement, convexity of the ethmoid sinus walls, and thinning of ethmoid trabecula and bony nasal septum. The sporadic (unclassifiable) pattern does not appear to be related to the known mucous drainage patterns [4,14].

6.1.4.3 Retention Cysts and Polyps

Retention cysts are common incidental findings caused by obstruction of a submucosal gland [4]. Polyps on the other hand may be caused by inflammation or more commonly by allergy where they are often multiple and involve the nose as well (Figure 6.5). Maxillary and other sinus retention cysts and polyps usually cannot be differentiated on imaging. They both appear as homogeneous soft-tissue density masses with smooth, convex borders (Figure 6.6) [4]. Multiple or single lesions may be present; most are small and clearly do not fill the entire sinus cavity.

On occasion, a maxillary sinus polyp may expand and prolapse through the sinus ostium, presenting as a nasal polyp. These are referred to as antrochoanal polyps, which represent 4%–6% of all nasal polyps. Most are unilateral solitary lesions (Figure 6.7).

6.1.4.4 Mucocele

Mucoceles result from obstruction of a sinus ostium and accumulation of secretions [13]. On CT, the sinus becomes completely filled and airless, and the sinus

---

BOX 6.2 CT PATTERNS OF SINUSITIS

Infundibular pattern	Disease limited to infundibulum and adjacent maxillary sinus. Frontal and ethmoid sinuses are preserved
Ostiomeatal unit pattern	Disease involves middle meatus, adjacent anterior and middle ethmoidal, and maxillary and frontal sinuses
Sphenoethmoidal recess pattern	Disease involves sphenoid sinus and ipsilateral posterior ethmoid cells
Sinonasal polyposis	Polypoid lesions fill the nasal cavity and the sinuses bilaterally
Unclassifiable	Apparently not related to known mucous drainage patterns

Source: Data from Babbel, R. et al., *Am. J. Neuroradiol.*, 13, 903–912, 1992 [14].

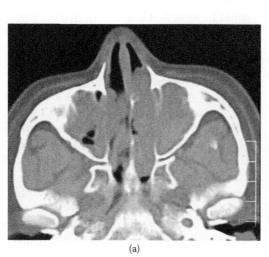

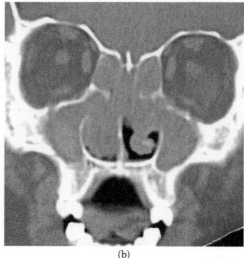

(a)   (b)

FIGURE 6.5
Sinonasal polyposis. Axial (a) and coronal (b) CT images show soft-tissue opacification of both maxillary sinuses extending into the nasal cavities with obliteration of both ostiomeatal units (OMUs).

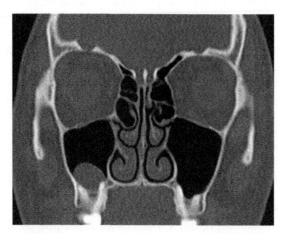

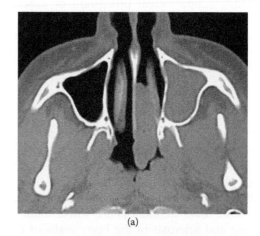

(a)

FIGURE 6.6
Polyp or retention cyst. Coronal CT image shows a polyp or a retention cyst in the right maxillary sinus. Note the patent OMU.

cavity is expanded as the bony walls are remodeled outward. Sinus expansion differentiates a mucocele from an obstructed sinus. Frontal mucoceles are most common (60%–65%) (Figure 6.8), followed by ethmoid sinuses (20%–25%), and then maxillary and sphenoid sinuses [1]. Mucoceles become symptomatic when they are large enough to cause mass effects such as proptosis or palpable swelling.

6.1.4.5 *Fungal Sinusitis*

Allergic fungal sinusitis is a benign disease caused by a hypersensitivity reaction to fungi in the sinuses. Most patients have a history of atopy or asthma. A predisposing factor is sinus obstruction due to local lesions such as nasal polyps, a deviated septum, or inflamed mucosa

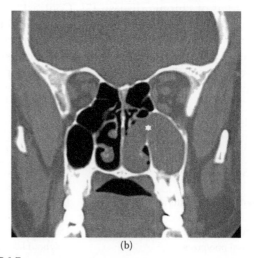

(b)

FIGURE 6.7
Antrochoanal polyp. Axial (a) and coronal (b) CT images show a solitary polyp filling the left maxillary antrum and extending through widened ostium (asterisk) into the nasal cavity.

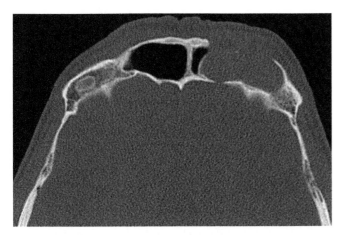

FIGURE 6.8
Sinus mucocele. Axial CT image shows mucocele of the left frontal sinus.

from chronic sinusitis [3]. Invasive fungal sinusitis primarily occurs in association with immunosuppression especially with leukemia, organ transplantation, or diabetes mellitus.

The most commonly affected sinuses are the maxillary or ethmoid. Air–fluid levels in the sinuses are very unlikely and suggest bacterial infection. CT findings that suggest fungal sinusitis include punctuate central calcifications; a combination of bone thickening, erosion, and remodeling; as well as disease extension to the cheek. High-density material within the maxillary sinus is seen with mycetomas. Invasive fungal infections have a propensity for orbital, cavernous sinus, and neurovascular structure invasion [2,3,4].

6.1.4.6 Functional Endoscopic Sinus Surgery

Since the early 1990s, functional endoscopic sinus surgery (FESS) has become the most accepted surgical treatment for sinonasal inflammatory disease. The main aim of FESS is to restore the normal function of mucociliary drainage system of the sinuses. Preoperative imaging, and in particular CT, plays a major role in patient selection, surgical planning, minimizing surgical risk, and optimizing the patient benefits from FESS. The radiologic report should cover all relevant points that are of special interest to the surgeon (Box 6.3).

6.1.5 Tumors of the Nose and Paranasal Sinuses

Sinonasal tumors are generally uncommon, comprising only 3% of head and neck malignancies [15]. Despite their low incidence, a very wide variety of tumors can arise in the sinonasal region, broadly classified into epithelial or mesenchymal (Boxes 6.4 and 6.5). The most common sinonasal malignancy is squamous cell carcinoma (SCC). Because bone destruction is a hallmark of

---

BOX 6.3 KEY POINTS OF CT OF THE SINUSES BEFORE FESS

Sinus diseases	Extent, location, bony walls, mimics of inflammatory diseases, mucocele, and fungal sinusitis
Ostiomeatal unit and other drainage pathways	Patency of ostiomeatal unit, sphenoethmoidal recess, and frontal recess
Anatomic variants	Nasal septum deviation, concha bullosa, deviated uncinate process, and large ethmoid bulla
Critical variants	Dehiscence of lamina papyracea, asymmetry of cribriform plate, and cephalocele
Complications	Brain, orbit, or soft-tissue spread

Source: Data from Hoang, J.K. et al., *AJR Am. J. Roentgenol.* 194, 527–536 [16].

BOX 6.4 PATHOLOGIC TYPES OF SINONASAL TUMORS

Epithelial tumors
Salivary tumors
Neuroectodermal and neural tumors
Lymphoproliferative tumors
Vascular tumors
Muscle tumors
Fibrous tumors
Bony and cartilaginous tumors

Sources: Data from Som, P.M., and Brandwein, M.S., *Head and Neck Imaging*, Mosby, St. Louis, 2003 [17]; Mafee, M.F. Imaging of the nasal cavity and paranasal sinuses. In: Mafee M.F., Valvassori, G.E., Becker, M., eds. *Imaging of the Head and Neck.* 2nd ed. Stuttgart; New York: Thieme; 2005: 353–474 [8].

---

sinonasal tumors, CT is invaluable in their diagnostic workup. The radiologist may be the first to suspect a tumor during CT imaging of inflammatory sinus disease. Magnetic resonance imaging (MRI) has an important complementary role in differentiation of tumors from inflammations and secretions as well as defining extensions, including perineural and perivascular spread [18].

6.1.5.1 Benign Sinonasal Tumors

6.1.5.1.1 Osteoma

Osteomas arising in paranasal sinuses are common incidental findings on plain radiographs. They may remain asymptomatic or cause headache or sinus symptoms. Uncommonly, they obstruct the frontal sinus and

BOX 6.5 OVERVIEW OF SINONASAL TUMORS AND TUMORLIKE LESIONS

Benign	Malignant
Common	*Common*
Osteoma	Squamous cell carcinoma
Papilloma	Lymphoma
Juvenile nasopharyngeal angiofibroma	Adenoid cystic carcinoma
Polyp	Melanoma
Retention cyst	Metastases
Uncommon	*Uncommon*
Choanal polyp	Olfactory neuroblastoma
Pleomorphic adenoma	Extramedullary plasmacytoma
Hamartoma	Osteosarcoma
Hemangioma	Chondrosarcoma
Granuloma	Fibrous histiocytoma
Inverted granuloma	Malignant melanoma
Histiocytosis X	
Lipoma	
Chondroma	
Fibroma	

Source: Modified from Vogl, T.J., *Diagnostische und Interventionelle Radiologie*, Springer, Berlin; Heidelberg, 2011 [19].

require urgent surgery [17]. On CT (Figure 6.9), they are seen as very dense sclerotic (ivory osteomas) to less dense (cancellous osteomas) homogeneous masses mostly arising in the frontal sinus. Pneumocephalus may be present. Multiple sinus osteomas can be a manifestation of Gardner's syndrome, one of the intestinal polyposis syndromes [20].

6.1.5.1.2 Papilloma

Inverted papillomas are benign tumors that most commonly occur in males in their fifth decade or older. The classic site of origin is in the lateral nasal wall near the middle turbinate. On CT (Figure 6.10), they appear as unilateral polypoid nasal masses with calcifications and bone remodeling [20]. Fungiform papillomas commonly affect males but in a younger age group and characteristically arise on the nasal septum [8].

6.1.5.1.3 Juvenile Nasopharyngeal Angiofibroma

Juvenile nasopharyngeal angiofibroma is a benign but locally invasive tumor almost exclusive to male

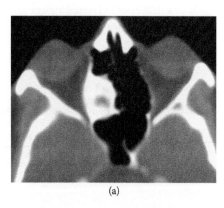
(a)

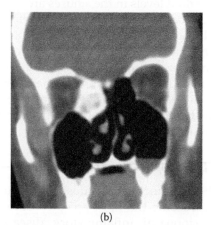
(b)

FIGURE 6.9
Osteoma. Axial (a) and coronal (b) CT images show an osteoma in the right ethmoid.

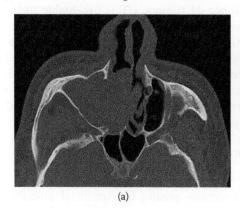
(a)

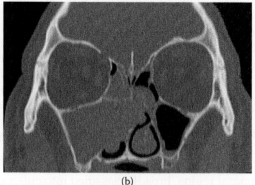
(b)

FIGURE 6.10
Inverted papilloma. Axial (a) and coronal (b) CT images show soft-tissue mass in the right maxillary sinus and nasal cavity with bone remodeling.

adolescents [21]. Earliest symptoms include nasal obstruction and epistaxis [22]. Angiofibromas arise in the posterior nasal cavity and the pterygopalatine fossa. They fill the nasopharynx asymmetrically and one side could always be assigned as the primary origin. Widening of the pterygopalatine fossa and bowing of posterior antral wall by an intensely enhancing mass are the hallmarks of angiofibroma on CT. Intracranial and intraorbital extensions should be carefully sought for and may require complementary MRI [22].

6.1.5.2 Malignant Sinonasal Tumors

6.1.5.2.1 Squamous Cell Carcinoma

SCC is the commonest sinonasal malignancy [15]. Nearly half SCCs of the sinonasal region arise in the maxillary antrum and one-fourth in the nasal cavity, followed by ethmoid sinuses and lastly sphenoid and frontal sinuses [23]. On CT, sinonasal carcinomas usually show some heterogeneity and slight to moderate enhancement. The key finding is the associated bone destruction, which is commonly aggressive, while bone remodeling is uncommon (Figure 6.11) [4]. It is very important to document the tumor extensions for accurate staging (Box 6.6).

6.1.5.2.2 Adenoid Cystic Carcinoma

Adenoid cystic carcinomas are salivary tumors that arise in the sinonasal minor salivary glands, most commonly in the maxillary antrum followed by the nasal cavity [17]. A characteristic feature of this tumor is perineural invasion [23].

6.1.5.2.3 Olfactory Neuroblastoma

Olfactory neuroblastomas are tumors of the neural crest arising in olfactory mucosa of the superior nasal fossa. The tumor has bimodal age distribution peaking in the second and sixth decades [13]. According to Kadish staging system, olfactory neuroblastomas confined to the nasal cavity are classified as stage A, those with disease in the nasal cavity and one or more paranasal sinuses are stage B, and those with disease extending beyond the nasal cavity and paranasal sinuses are stage C [24].

On CT, olfactory neuroblastomas appear as homogeneous, enhancing masses with or without calcification and with associated bone remodeling. They commonly extend into the ipsilateral ethmoid and maxillary sinuses and rarely involve the sphenoid

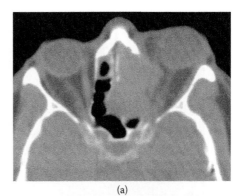

(a)

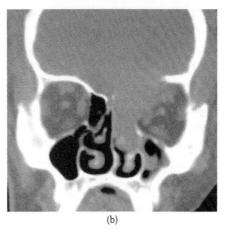

(b)

FIGURE 6.11
Sinonasal carcinoma. Axial (a) and coronal (b) CT images show a large mass in the left nasal cavity and ethmoid with extensive bone destruction and intracranial and intraorbital extension.

BOX 6.6   T-STAGING OF MAXILLARY ANTRUM CARCINOMA

T1: Tumor confined to antral mucosa with no bone erosion or destruction

T2: Tumor with erosion or destruction infrastructure, hard palate, and/or middle nasal meatus

T3: Tumor invasion into skin of cheek, posterior maxillary sinus wall, floor of medial orbital wall, and anterior ethmoid sinus

T4: Massive tumor with invasion of cribriform plate, posterior ethmoids, sphenoid, nasopharynx, ptyergoid plates, base of skull, or orbit

Source: Data from Fleming, I. et al., *American Joint Committee on Cancer Staging Manual*, Lippincott Raven, Philadelphia, 1997 [25].

---

sinuses. Large tumors can extend to involve both sides of the nasal cavity and the paranasal sinuses [17]. Documentation of intracranial extension is crucial for surgical planning.

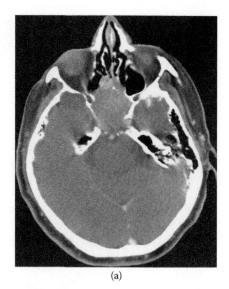
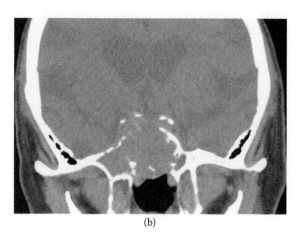

(a)   (b)

FIGURE 6.12
Sinonasal lymphoma. Enhanced axial (a) and coronal (b) CT images show a large homogeneous soft-tissue mass filling the sphenoid sinuses with bone thinning and destruction and extra-sinus extension.

6.1.5.2.4 Lymphoma

Sinonasal lymphoma is a type of extranodal lymphoma more common in Asians [17]. They commonly arise from the nasal cavity or maxillary sinuses and appear on CT as bulky homogeneous soft-tissue masses that enhance moderately (Figure 6.12) [21,26]. Bone remodeling is more common than aggressive bone invasion. The treatment is by combined local irradiation and chemotherapy [26].

6.1.5.2.5 Rhabdomyosarcoma

Rhabdomyosarcoma is the commonest soft-tissue sarcoma in children. In the head and neck, they tend to arise in the orbit, followed by the middle ear, the nasopharynx and sinonasal region, as well as other sites. On CT, the tumor masses enhance moderately and there is usually combined bone remodeling and destruction [17].

6.2 Pathology of the Ear

6.2.1 Anatomy of the Ear and Temporal Bone

The temporal bone consists of five parts: the squamous, mastoid, petrous, tympanic, and styloid. The anatomy is complex with many important structures in close relation to each other. Radiologically important anatomic regions include external auditory canal (EAC), middle ear, mastoid, inner ear, and internal auditory canal (IAC) (Figures 6.13 and 6.14).

6.2.1.1 External Auditory Canal

The EAC is lined by dermis. The wall of the lateral third is fibrocartilaginous and the wall of the medial two-thirds is bony. The floor, anterior, and most of posterior walls of the EAC are formed by the tympanic portion, and the roof is formed by the squamous portion of the temporal bone [27].

6.2.1.2 Middle Ear Cavity

The middle ear, or tympanic cavity, is a cleft-like space within the temporal bone. It could be divided into three parts: the mesotympanum (tympanic cavity proper), opposite the tympanic membrane; the epitympanum (attic), above the level of the tympanic membrane; and the hypotympanum, inferior to the level of the tympanic membrane [28].

The medial wall of the tympanic cavity is formed by the bony capsule of the inner ear and presents an important landmark, the promontory, which is a smooth bony prominence produced by the bulging basal turn of the cochlea. Above the promontory there is a horizontal ridge overlying the facial nerve canal, and immediately above this is the bulge due to the lateral semicircular canal (SCC). Above and behind the promontory lies the oval window, closed by the footplate of the stapes. Below and behind the promontory is the round window [27,28]. The lateral wall of the tympanic cavity is formed by the tympanic membrane and the squamous

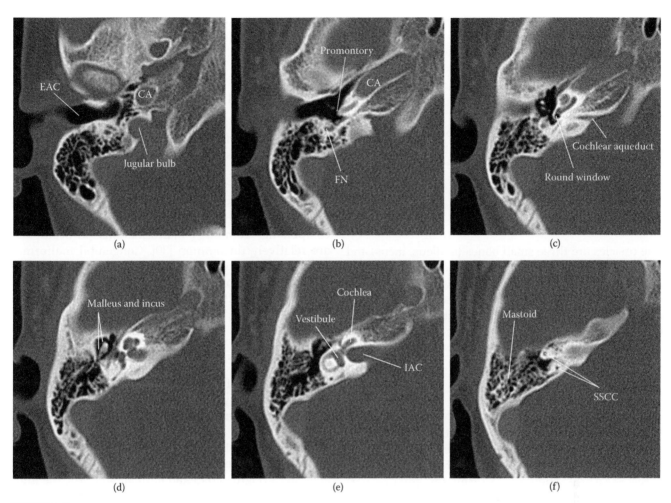

FIGURE 6.13
(a–f) Normal axial CT anatomy of the temporal bone. CA, carotid artery; EAC, external auditory canal; FN, facial nerve; IAC, internal auditory canal; and SSCC, superior semicircular canal.

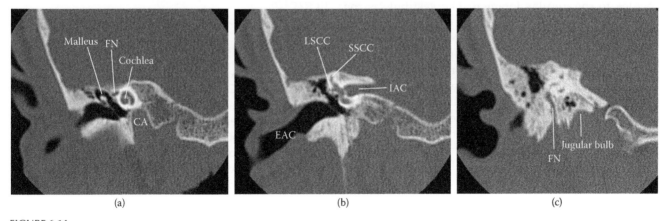

FIGURE 6.14
(a–c) Normal coronal CT anatomy of the temporal bone. CA, carotid artery; EAC, external auditory canal; FN, facial nerve; IAC, internal auditory canal; LSCC, lateral semicircular canal; and SSCC: superior semicircular canal.

bone above it. The inferior margin of the squamous bone is a pointed bony spicule called the scutum [29]. The anterior wall of the tympanic cavity is wider above than below and corresponds to the thin bony covering of the carotid canal. At the upper part of the anterior wall is the tympanic orifice of the Eustachian tube (ET) [27]. The upper part of the posterior wall of the tympanic cavity communicates with the mastoid through the aditus ad antrum. Below the aditus and behind the oval window is a hollow projection called the pyramidal eminence. There are two recesses in the posterior wall: the sinus tympani, which is the space medial to the pyramidal eminence, and the facial recess, which lies lateral to the pyramidal eminence [28]. The roof of the tympanic cavity is formed by a thin plate of bone, the tegmen tympani, which separates the cranial and tympanic cavities. The floor is a thin plate of bone that separates the tympanic cavity from the internal jugular vein [27].

6.2.1.3 Ossicular Chain

The ossicles are three small bones (malleus, incus, and stapes) extending across the tympanic cavity. The malleus is the outermost bone, attached to the tympanic membrane by its manubrium. The head of the malleus, located in the epitympanum, articulates with the body of the incus. The long process of the incus articulates with the head of the stapes. The footplate of the stapes is attached to the oval window [29].

6.2.1.4 Inner Ear

The inner ear consists of a bony labyrinth in which the membranous labyrinth is embedded. The bony labyrinth consists of the cochlea, the vestibule, and three SCCs [28]. The cochlea forms the anterior part of the labyrinth, it is a conical snail-shaped structure that winds two- and three-quarter turns around a central axis (the modiolus). The cochlear aqueduct is a small channel that extends from the basal turn of the cochlea to the jugular foramen. The vestibule is the central part of the bony labyrinth, continuous anteriorly with the cochlea, and posteriorly with the SCCs. In its lateral wall is the oval window. At the posterior part of the medial wall is the opening of the vestibular aqueduct. The bony SCCs are three in number, superior, posterior, and lateral, and are situated above and behind the vestibule. The superior and posterior SCCs are both arranged in a vertical orientation at right angles to one another. The lateral SCC makes an angle about 30° with the horizontal plane [27].

6.2.1.5 Internal Auditory Canal

The IAC transmits the 7th and 8th cranial nerves. Its lateral opening is the porus acusticus and its medial opening is the fundus. The facial nerve travels in the anterosuperior aspect of the canal, the cochlear branch of the vestibulocochlear nerve travels in the

anteroinferior aspect of the canal, and the superior and inferior vestibular branches travel in the posterior half of the canal [29].

6.2.2 Congenital Anomalies of the Ear

Both the external and middle ears develop from closely linked mesodermal and endodermal precursors while the inner ear is ectodermal in origin. Significant anomalies of the external ear are therefore usually accompanied by middle ear anomalies while inner ear anomalies usually occur independently. Because mesenchyme is involved in the development of all ear components, combined malformations do occur, but are relatively uncommon [30]. Congenital malformations of the temporal bone could be genetic (isolated or syndromal) or nongenetic. High-resolution thin section CT is well suited for imaging of most of these anomalies.

6.2.2.1 External Ear

Malformations of the external ear are termed "congenital aural dysplasias." Malformation of the auricle is referred to as microtia [28]. According to severity of the dysplasia, the EAC could be totally absent, atretic or stenotic, and the stenosis may be fibrous or bony plate or both [31]. CT is the method of choice for imaging of EAC anomalies (Figures 6.15 and 6.16). In all cases, the middle ear should be simultaneously evaluated for associated malformations especially of the malleus and incus, the facial nerve canal, as well as the degree of pneumatization of the middle ear, which is commonly reduced in size [28].

6.2.2.2 Middle Ear

Anomalies of the middle ear are either associated with those of the EAC or less commonly isolated. The ossicles may be dysplastic in shape, hypoplastic in size, malrotated, adherent to each other or to other tympanic structures, or totally absent. The incudostapedial and incudomalleal joints may be absent or fused [31,32]. Anomalies of the tympanic facial nerve include caudal displacement and bony dehiscence [27].

6.2.2.3 Inner Ear

The majority of patients with congenital sensorineural hearing loss (SNHL) have anomalies of the hearing mechanism that are beyond the resolution of imaging [30]. For those with gross anatomic or structural

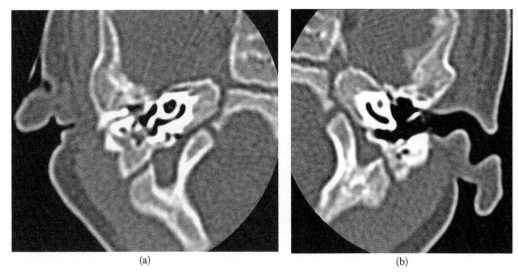

(a)   (b)

FIGURE 6.15
External auditory canal (EAC) atresia. (a) The right auricle is hypoplastic and the right EAC is completely atretic with associated middle ear malformation. (b) Normal left side for comparison.

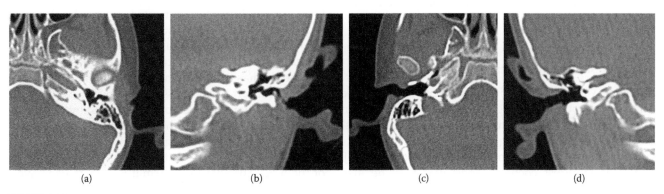

(a)   (b)   (c)   (d)

FIGURE 6.16
External auditory canal (EAC) stenoses. Axial (a) and coronal (b) CT images show stenoses of the left EAC, with normal size and aeration of the left tympanic cavity and ossicular deformity. (c, d) Normal right side for comparison.

malformations, high-resolution thin section CT provides excellent evaluation of the bony labyrinth (Box 6.7). MRI has an important complementary role because it is able to show the membranous labyrinth and the contents of the IAC [33].

6.2.2.4 Cochlea

Anomalies of the cochlea could be classified into complete aplasia or nondevelopment of the inner ear (Michel aplasia), a common cochlear and vestibular cavity with no internal structures, cochlear aplasia with formation of the vestibule and SCCs, cochlear hypoplasia, and incomplete partition of the cochlea [31]. The Mondini malformation is one of the best-known cochlear anomalies and describes incomplete partition of the cochlea

---

BOX 6.7   INNER EAR ANOMALIES

Cochlear anomaly
Labyrinthine (Michel's) aplasia
Common cavity
Cochlear aplasia, vestibule and semicircular canals present
Cochlear hypoplasia
Incomplete partition of the cochlea (Mondini)

Normal cochlea
Dysplasia of the vestibule and lateral semicircular canal
Large vestibular aqueduct
Aplasia and hypoplasia of the vestibulocochlear nerve
Semicircular canal dehiscence

Source: Data from Krombach, G.A. et al., *Eur. Radiol.* 18, 319–330, 2008 [30].

with fused middle and apical cochlear turns while the basal turn is present [30].

6.2.2.5 Semicircular Canals

The lateral SCC is the last to form and is the most commonly affected SCC. CT can show widening and shortening of the malformed SCC. Dysplasia of the vestibule is commonly associated [31]. SCC dehiscence is another anomaly defined as a defect of the bony covering, usually the roof of the superior SCC, which is best depicted on coronal CT images. This anomaly could result in sound-induced vertigo and nystagmus because changes in pressure with sound are transmitted through the defect into the vestibular apparatus [30].

6.2.2.6 Vestibule

Isolated vestibular anomalies are rare and the most common anomaly is a combined widened lateral SCC and widened vestibule [31].

6.2.2.7 Vestibular Aqueduct

The large vestibular aqueduct syndrome is one of the commonest causes of progressive SNHL in children that could be accurately diagnosed by CT [31]. The vestibular aqueduct is enlarged if its diameter exceeds 1.5 mm, measured in the middle of the aqueduct [33]. Subtle or manifest cochlear anomalies may be also present [32].

6.2.2.8 Internal Auditory Canal and the Vestibulocochlear Nerve

The normal width of the IAC is between 2 and 8 mm. An IAC less than 2 mm in width is stenotic and an MRI should be acquired to rule out aplasia of the vestibulocochlear nerve, which is a cause of SNHL from birth [31].

6.2.2.9 Facial Nerve

The facial nerve may be aplastic or hypoplastic or have an abnormal course either in isolation or in association with other anomalies of the temporal bone. Aplasia and hypoplasia result in congenital facial palsy [28]. Documentation of the course of facial nerve canal is crucial in preoperative imaging of the temporal bone in general.

6.2.2.10 Congenital Vascular Anomalies

6.2.2.10.1 Aberrant Internal Carotid Artery

Aberrant Internal Carotid Artery is a rare anomaly due to absence of the vertical petrous segment of ICA, which is replaced by the more lateral inferior tympanic and caroticotympanic arteries. This anomaly could result in vascular tinnitus and conductive hearing loss (HL) with a pulsatile mass seen behind the tympanic membrane. CT shows a soft-tissue mass in the middle ear contiguous with the horizontal carotid artery and indenting the promontory. The mass enhances avidly with contrast. Magnetic resonance angiography or computed tomography angiography shows the far lateral displacement of the ICA. An otherwise normal ICA may also have a laterally displaced course (Figure 6.17) [34].

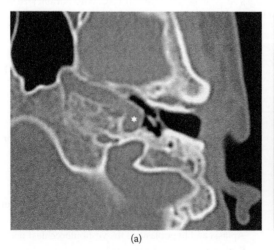
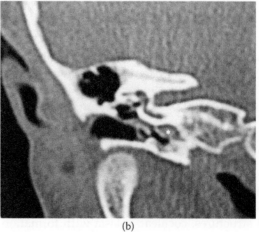

(a)   (b)

FIGURE 6.17
Lateralized course of the internal carotid artery (ICA). Axial (a) and coronal (b) CT images show a laterally displaced left ICA (asterisk) but with intact bony canal.

6.2.2.10.2 *Persistent Stapedial Artery*

Another uncommon arterial anomaly that may result in pulsatile tinnitus is a persistent stapedial artery. CT can show this small vascular structure along the promontory and in between the stapes crura. It continues superiorly to supply the middle meningeal artery and CT can show absence of the foramen spinosum, which normally transmits the middle meningeal artery when it originates from the internal maxillary artery [32,33].

6.2.2.10.3 *High Jugular Bulb*

The jugular bulb dome is normally beneath the floor of the tympanic cavity. A higher location of the jugular bulb is commonly an incidental finding on CT, but may cause vascular tinnitus or conductive HL (Figure 6.18). Moreover, the bony covering of the jugular bulb or the jugular plate may be thin or dehiscent resulting in increased risk of injury during middle ear surgical procedures [34].

6.2.3 Temporal Bone Trauma

The classic classification of temporal bone fractures according to their orientation relative to the petrous bone axis into longitudinal and transverse fractures is still widely used, although many fractures were recently found to have an oblique course or mixed components [35]. CT is the modality of choice for imaging of temporal bone fractures and the diagnosis should include the identification of injury to critical structures and complications (Box 6.8), which are more clinically relevant than simple classification of fractures [36].

6.2.3.1 **Longitudinal Fractures**

Longitudinal fractures are more common and usually result from a blunt temporal or parietal trauma (Figure 6.19) [37]. Hemotympanum is common and bleeding through the ear occurs when the tympanic membrane is breached. The fracture line usually involves the EAC and crosses the middle ear cavity so that ossicular dislocation is frequently associated, most commonly involving the incus due its relatively weak support. Traumatic subluxation of the incudo-stapedial joint is more common than that of incudo-malleal joint [36,37]. Longitudinal fractures follow the paths of least resistance and usually deflect anterior to the otic capsule [35].

6.2.3.2 **Transverse Fractures**

Transverse fractures are perpendicular to the long axis of the petrous pyramid and typically result from a blunt occipital trauma [35]. A transverse fracture could result in SNHL when it involves either the bony labyrinth or the fundus (lateral most aspect) of the IAC causing cochlear nerve transection (Box 6.9) [36]. CSF leak could occur with disruption of the middle ear roof. A perilymphatic fistula occurs due to the communication between the middle and inner ears and results in SNHL, vertigo, and nystagmus [37]. Air can follow a fracture line from the middle ear into the labyrinth, causing a pneumolabyrinth. Facial nerve injury is twice as common with transverse as with longitudinal fractures [35].

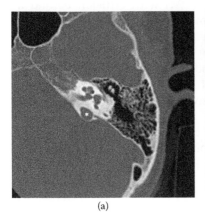 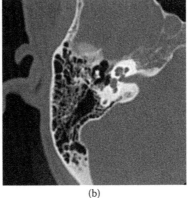 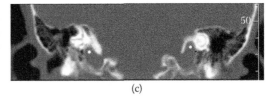

| (a) | (b) | (c) |

FIGURE 6.18

High jugular bulb. (a) Axial CT image shows the high left jugular bulb (asterisk) reaching the level of the epitympanum and internal auditory canal. (b) Axial CT image of the right side at the same level for comparison. (c) Coronal CT image shows the higher level of the left jugular bulb (asterisk) compared to the right side.

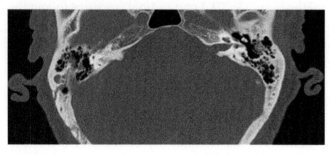

FIGURE 6.19
Temporal bone fracture. Axial CT image shows longitudinal fracture of the right temporal bone.

6.2.4 Inflammatory Diseases of the Ear and Temporal Bone

Temporal bone inflammations could be classified according to their location: [1] external ear, [2] middle ear and mastoid, [3] inner ear, and [4] petrous apex.

6.2.4.1 External Ear

6.2.4.1.1 External Otitis

External otitis is a common condition caused by many pathogens. It is usually clinically assessed and is not an indication for imaging.

6.2.4.1.2 Necrotizing External Otitis

An aggressive destructive osteomyelitis of the temporal bone was once termed "malignant otitis externa" due to the associated high mortality rate in the past. It is generally a disease of elderly diabetics and most commonly caused by the gram negative bacilli, *Pseudomonas aeruginosa* [38].

Typically, the disease starts at the osseous–cartilaginous junction of the EAC as focal osteitis and extends into the soft tissue beneath the EAC. Otalgia is usually present at this stage. As the disease progresses, there is extension into the infratemporal fossa and may also extend into the parotid or temporo-mandibular joint (TMJ) or soft tissues of the neck. CT is the method of choice for evaluation of bone destruction and extensions. The integrity of facial nerve canal should be evaluated because facial palsy is a known complication. Further extension into the skull base could cause other cranial nerve palsies and inadequately treated cases may present also with intracranial complications such as meningitis, abscess, or sinus thrombosis [38,39].

6.2.4.2 Middle Ear

6.2.4.2.1 Otitis Media and Mastoiditis

Because the pneumatized regions of the temporal bone are contiguous, inflammation of the middle ear may involve the other pneumatized spaces (mastoid, petrous apex, and perilabyrinthine air cells). Repeated middle ear infections in infancy and inflammatory changes of the air cell mucosa cause the subepithelial connective tissue to fibrose, and hence, growth and pneumatization of air spaces are impaired, resulting in a small mastoid cavity with sclerotic bony walls [39].

Acute otitis media (OM) with effusion behind an intact tympanic membrane is common in children, often following a respiratory tract infection. Uncomplicated acute OM is readily treated medically and is not an indication for imaging. Acute OM, however, may persist into a more chronic stage or be complicated by erosive mastoiditis, facial palsy, or labyrinthitis.

OM is considered chronic if the effusion persists more than three months and is usually associated with ET obstruction [39]. CT shows effusion as air–fluid levels in the tympanic or mastoid cavities. In adults with spontaneous effusion, the nasopharynx should be also evaluated for the presence of neoplastic obstruction of ET. Chronic suppurative otitis media indicates the presence of otorrhea, or ear discharge, for more than 6 weeks. Otorrhea occurs through a tympanic membrane perforation or a tympanostomy tube. CT shows the presence of inflammatory granulation tissue as soft-tissue density in the middle ear cavity with no ossicular displacement or bone erosions (Figure 6.20) [39].

Mastoiditis could be associated with infection spread from the mucosa to the bone and CT is the best modality to show erosions of the mastoid septa. Extension through mastoid cortical defects may cause a subperiosteal abscess in the postauricular region. If the infection spreads inferiorly into the neck deep to the sternocleidomastoid fascia, a Bezold abscess results. Other severe complications could occur due to intracranial spread such as dural sinus thrombosis, meningitis, or intracranial abscess [38].

6.2.4.2.2 Cholesteatoma

A cholesteatoma is a sac lined with stratified squamous epithelium and filled with keratin debris and could be congenital or acquired. Most middle ear cholesteatomas are acquired and occur as sequelae of chronic OM and perforated tympanic membrane [29]. A small proportion of acquired cholesteatomas occur in retraction pockets of the pars flaccida of the tympanic

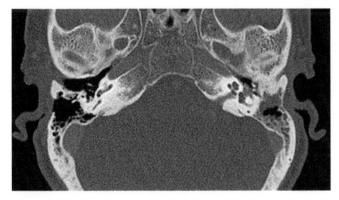

FIGURE 6.20
Otitis and mastoiditis. Axial CT image shows partial opacification of the mastoid and tympanic cavity.

membrane without infection [39]. Congenital cholesteatomas are epidermoid cysts occurring anywhere in the temporal bone, more commonly in the anterior tympanic cavity [29].

Acquired cholesteatomas arising in the pars flaccida extend into Prussak's space, which is limited laterally by the pars flaccida, medially by the neck of the malleus, and inferiorly by the short process of the malleus. On CT, Prussak's space cholesteatomas displace the malleus head medially and erode the adjacent bony scutum. Prussak's space opens posteriorly into the epitympanum, and from there, the mass easily extends posteriorly in the superior incudal space to the posterolateral attic and then through the aditus ad antrum to the antrum and mastoid air cells. Widening of the aditus is often an important imaging diagnostic finding [29,39].

Cholesteatomas arising from the pars tensa are much less common and often involve the facial recess laterally and then the more medial sinus tympani. Superior extension into the attic will displace the ossicles laterally. Pars tensa cholesteatomas tend to extend initially toward the medial wall of the middle ear and come into contact early with the otic capsule. Fistulous formation to the lateral SCC is, therefore, more commonly seen than in the pars flaccida cholesteatoma [29,39].

The key finding of cholesteatoma on CT is an expansile soft-tissue mass associated with bone erosion (Figure 6.21) (see Box 6.10 for differential diagnosis) [29]. Cholesteatomas may erode the scutum, ossicles, tegmen tympani, and bony labyrinth. The long process of the incus (best seen on coronal CT) is the most commonly eroded ossicle followed by the lenticular process and the stapes crura [38]. The lateral SCC region should be carefully assessed to rule out a labyrinthine fistula. Just _inferior to this is the tympanic facial canal, which may or may not be covered by bone as normal variants. Imaging of the brain is required when CT shows

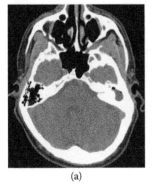
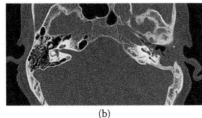
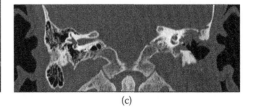

(a) (b) (c)

FIGURE 6.21
Cholesteatoma. Axial soft-tissue algorithm (a) and axial and coronal bone algorithm (b, c) CT images show partial left mastoidectomy and soft-tissue density filling the tympanomastoid cavity.

erosion of the tegmen tympani to rule out intracranial spread of infection (see Box 6.11 for complications of cholestaeatoma) [39].

6.2.4.3 Inner Ear

6.2.4.3.1 Labyrinthitis

Inflammation of the membranous labyrinth could be viral, bacterial, autoimmune, or systemic. Viral labyrinthitis is a cause of congenital SNHL due to cytomegalo virus or rubella infection. In adults, viral labyrinthitis could be caused by mumps, varicella-zoster, or measles. Bacterial labyrinthitis might be caused by extension from meningitis or from middle ear infections through the round window or development of a labyrinthine

fistula. MRI rather than CT is the method of choice for evaluation of labyrinthitis [29,30].

6.2.4.3.2 Labyrinthitis Ossificans

Pathologic ossification can occur as a sequel of labyrinthitis as well as other conditions such as otosclerosis, labyrinthine artery occlusion, leukemia, and temporal bone tumors. The process usually starts by fibrosis in the basal turn of cochlea and progresses to new bone formation extending from basal to apical turns [39]. MRI is more sensitive at the early fibrosis stage but the ossification stage is very clearly shown by CT [30]. The diagnosis of labyrinthitis ossificans is very important if cochlear implantation is planned [32].

6.2.4.3.3 Otosyphilis

Labyrinthine involvement can occur in congenital syphilis or less commonly in the secondary or tertiary stages of acquired infection and results in permeative, or "moth-eaten," demineralization of the cochlea and otic capsule best seen on CT. The differential diagnosis includes otosclerosis, Paget's disease, and osteogenesis imperfecta [33,39].

6.2.4.4 Petrous Apex

6.2.4.4.1 Aeration of the Petrous Apex

The petrous apex is filled with marrow in two-thirds and pneumatized in about one-third of the normal subjects so that it is liable for inflammatory conditions extending from middle ear infections (Figure 6.22) [41].

6.2.4.4.2 Petrous Apex Effusion

Simple effusion may be due to obstruction of pneumatized air cells and usually has no clinical significance [29].

BOX 6.10   THE DIFFERENTIAL DIAGNOSIS OF A DESTRUCTIVE MIDDLE EAR AND TEMPORAL BONE LESION

Inflammatory (common)
Cholesteatoma
Mastoiditis, chronic otitis
Mastoidectomy
Petrous apicitis
Necrotizing external otitis (malignant otitis externa)
Cholesterol granuloma
Inflammatory granulomas (TB)
Tumors (uncommon)
Benign schwannomas
  Langerhans cell histiocytosis
  Dermoid cyst
Malignant squamous cell carcinoma
  Metastases
  Rhabdomyosarcoma

Source: Modified from Vogl, T.J., *Diagnostische und Interventionelle Radiologie*, Springer, Berlin; Heidelberg, 2011 [40].

BOX 6.11   COMPLICATIONS OF CHOLESTEATOMA

Ossicular erosion
Labyrinthine fistula
Facial nerve canal invasion
Tegmen tympani erosion
Intracranial infection (meningitis, abscess, and sinus thrombosis)

Source: Data from Nemzek, W.R., and Swartz, J.D, *Head and Neck Imaging*, Mosby, St. Louis, 2003 [39].

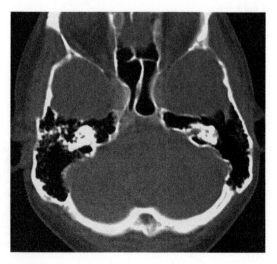

FIGURE 6.22
Bilateral extensive aeration of the petrous apex.

6.2.4.4.3 Mucocele

This is an uncommon lesion in the petrous apex caused by obstruction of the air cells and excessive mucus production causing expansion and remodeling [41].

6.2.4.4.4 Acute Petrositis

Acute petrositis is caused by spread from middle ear infection into the petrous apex and adjacent intracranial structures and can result in Gradenigo's syndrome. This syndrome includes a triad of middle ear infection with otorrhea, pain behind the eye due to trigeminal ganglionitis, and lateral rectus palsy secondary to involvement of the 6th nerve at the tip of the petrous apex. Other cranial nerve palsies are also commonly affected [39]. CT shows debris and fluid within petrous apex air cells. Lysis of bony septa and disruption of the adjacent bony cortex enable differentiation of this condition from simple petrous apex effusion (Figure 6.23) [29]. When evaluating this condition, it is also important to exclude any intracranial complications such as meningitis, abscess, or sinus thrombosis [39,42].

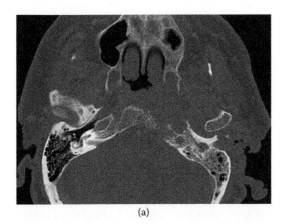

(a)

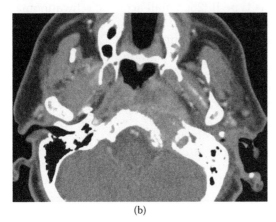

(b)

FIGURE 6.23
Petrositis. Axial bone algorithm (a) and contrast-enhanced CT (b) images show a destructive lesion in the left petrous apex.

6.2.4.4.5 Cholesterol Granuloma

This is an expansile, erosive lesion that occurs in the middle ear, mastoid, or petrous apex. It is thought to arise as a result of obstruction with repeated microhemorrhages, which in turn cause a giant cell reaction to cholesterol deposits. On CT, the differential diagnosis of an expansile petrous apex lesion besides CG is the less common cholesteatoma and mucocele (Box 6.12) [42]. The MRI appearance is classically that of high signal intensity on all sequences, secondary to the presence of extracellular methemoglobin [41]. However, a potential pitfall in MRI diagnosis of CG is petrous apex effusion with high protein content and high T1 signal intensity. Both conditions are easily differentiated by CT findings of nonexpansile air cell opacification with intact bone septation [39].

6.2.4.4.6 Cholesteatoma

Most cholesteatoma of the petrous apex are primary, arising from epithelial rests [41]. Acquired lesions are usually an extension from an aggressive middle ear cholesteatoma. On CT, a cholesteatoma is a smooth-walled, expansile lesion. MRI could distinguish a cholesteatoma (low signal intensity on T1-weighted images and higher signal intensity on T2-weighted images) from CG (bright on all pulse sequences) [39].

6.2.5 Otosclerosis and Other Temporal Bone Dysplasias

The temporal bone is affected by several types of diseases and dysplasias, most of them involve other bones as well. Otosclerosis is a type of dysplasia confined to the temporal bone. Temporal bone dysplasias may result

---

BOX 6.12   DIFFERENTIAL DIAGNOSES OF DESTRUCTIVE LESION OF THE PETROUS APEX

Petrositis

Cholesterol granuloma

Cholesteatoma

Metastases

Mucocele

Sarcoidosis

Epidermoid

Plasmacytoma

Chordoma

Chondrosarcoma

Source: Modified from Vogl, T.J., *Diagnostische und Interventionelle Radiologie*, Springer, Berlin; Heidelberg, 2011 [40].

in HL or cranial nerve compression. High-resolution CT is very sensitive to subtle changes of bone thickness and architecture and is the gold standard imaging modality for such conditions.

6.2.5.1 Otosclerosis

It is a slowly progressive disorder that is twice as common in females, mostly in their second and third decades. The disease is unique to the temporal bone manifesting as focal replacement of regular endochondral bone by immature highly vascularized spongy bone that eventually calcifies [30]. Two types occur: fenestral and cochlear (retrofenestral).

6.2.5.2 Fenestral Otosclerosis

In fenestral ostosclerosis, the fissula ante fenestram (region anterior to the oval window) is the most common site of otosclerosis and can be affected first. Conductive HL occurs secondary to fixation of the stapes footplate by the abnormal bone. CT shows focal lucent areas or less commonly sclerotic foci around the oval window region [30,33].

6.2.5.3 Cochlear (Retrofenestral) Otosclerosis

Cochlear or retrofenestral otosclerosis is less common than the fenestral type and patients present with sensorineural in addition to conductive HL. Demineralization occurs in the otic capsule surrounding the cochlea, sometimes giving the CT appearance of a "fourth turn" of the cochlea [30,33]. Later on, those focal areas remineralize and become harder to detect on CT.

6.2.5.4 Fibrous Dysplasia

Fibrous dysplasia is a disease of unknown etiology characterized by slowly progressive replacement of normal bone by dysplastic fibro-osseous tissue. It may be monostotic or polyostotic [29]. Temporal bone affection often leads to HL [33]. The most common CT findings include bone expansion, increase in bone thickness, and loss of trabecular pattern with mixed lytic and sclerotic areas or ground glass densities. EAC stenosis is common and there may be impingement on the IAC as well [28].

6.2.5.5 Paget's Disease (Osteitis Deformans)

Paget's disease is a chronic progressive disease usually affecting several bones including the pelvis, femur, skull, tibia, and spine. The disease usually passes through serial phases of osteolytic, mixed, osteoblastic, and remodeling bone changes. Temporal bone affection

leads to HL, which may be sensorineural, conductive, or mixed [28]. On CT, there is demineralization and increase in size of bone with focal areas of increased bone thickness in a mosaic pattern (cotton wool appearance). The central skull base is also commonly affected [29].

6.2.6 Temporal Bone Tumors

The clinical presentation of temporal bone tumors and cerebellopontine angle (CPA) tumors usually overlap because both regions are traversed by the 5th through 12th cranial nerves.

The commonest presentation that requires imaging evaluation to rule out the possibility of tumor is that of SNHL, tinnitus, and disequilibrium, and the commonest cause is acoustic schwannoma. MRI is the preferred modality for this indication, and CT is considered complementary. CT is, however, commonly requested for patients presenting with pulsatile tinnitus or jugular foramen syndrome to rule out paraganglioma or other jugular foramen tumors. Other indications for CT imaging include conductive HL, retrotympanic mass, or a clinically identified tumor of the external ear.

6.2.6.1 Acoustic Schwannoma and Other Cerebellopontine Angle Lesions

Acoustic schwannomas are the most common tumors of the CPA region (60%–90%). Despite the term "acoustic," most schwannomas arise from the vestibular, rather than the acoustic, division of the 8th cranial nerve [43]. They commonly present by progressive unilateral SNHL, often associated with tinnitus or disequilibrium due to pressure on the 8th cranial nerve. Bilateral schwannomas are the hallmark of neurofibromatosis type II [28]. Small acoustic schwannomas may be confined within the IAC. More commonly, they have a rounded component in the CPA and a small stem extending into the IAC resulting in the characteristic ice-cream cone appearance [29]. On noncontrast CT of the temporal bones, acoustic schwannomas tend to enlarge the IAC compared to healthy side (Figure 6.24). A large CPA tumor usually shows dense homogeneous contrast enhancement [43].

Meningiomas are the second most common CPA tumors, but they account for only 5%–10% of CPA tumors. Unlike acoustic schwannomas, meningiomas present with symptoms of pressure on the cranial nerves or cerebellum more commonly than HL. They usually have a broad base against the posterior petrous wall presenting an obtuse bone tumor angle. On noncontrast CT, meningiomas are usually hyperdense and calcifications are common. Meningiomas of the CPA are eccentric to the IAC, which is rarely enlarged. The commonest bony change associated with meningioma is bony hyperostosis [29,43].

Other CPA tumors include epidermoid cysts, arachnoid cysts, schwannomas of other cranial nerves, and other less common tumors (Box 6.13). Some vascular lesions may also cause compression symptoms on the cranial nerves simulating CPA tumors, the commonest is vertebrobasilar dolichoectasia. On CT, a basilar artery of diameter more than 4.5 mm is considered ecstatic, and elongation may be considered when the basilar artery extends lateral to the clivus margin [43].

6.2.6.2 Internal Auditory Canal Tumors

Most of the IAC tumors are schwannomas of the 8th cranial nerve (acoustic schwannomas). Facial nerve schwannomas arising in the IAC are usually indistinguishable from acoustic schwannomas, unless extension into the labyrinthine segment of facial nerve canal is recognized [44]. Other uncommon tumors of the IAC include meningiomas, hemangiomas, metastases, and others (Box 6.14).

6.2.6.3 Paragangliomas and Other Jugular Foramen Tumors

Jugular foramen tumors often present with combinations of 9th, 10th, and 11th cranial nerve palsies, HL, and tinnitus. The most common jugular foramen tumors are paragangliomas (glomus tumors). Paragangliomas occur more commonly in middle-aged women. They are slowly growing, locally

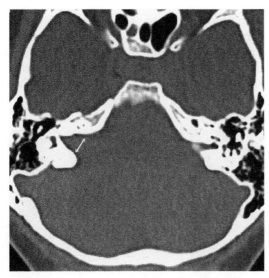

FIGURE 6.24
Acoustic schwannoma. Bone algorithm axial CT shows smooth widening of the right internal auditory canal by an intracanalicular schwannoma.

BOX 6.13 DIFFERENTIAL DIAGNOSIS OF CEREBELLOPONTINE ANGLE (CPA) LESIONS

Primary tumors of the CPA
Acoustic schwannoma
Meningioma
Epidermoid
Arachnoid cyst
Schwannoma of the 5th, 7th, 9th, 10th, and 11th nerves
Primary melanoma
Hemangioma
Lipoma, dermoid, and teratoma
Secondary tumors of the CPA
Paraganglioma
Chondrosarcoma
Chordoma
Extension of cerebellar tumors
Metastases
Vascular lesions
Aneurysm
Arteriovenous malformation
Vertebrobasilar dolichoectasia

Source: Data from Maya, M.M. et al., *Head and Neck Imaging*, Mosby, St. Louis, 2003 [43].

BOX 6.14 DIFFERENTIAL DIAGNOSIS OF INTERNAL AUDITORY CANAL MASS LESIONS

Inflammatory
Arachnoiditis
Sarcoidosis
Meningitis
Neuritis
Vascular
Anterior inferior cerebellar artery loop or aneurysm
Arteriovenous malformation
Neoplastic
Acoustic schwannoma[a]
Facial schwannoma
Hemangioma
Meningioma
Metastasis
Glioma
Lipoma
Osteoma
Lymphoma
Arachnoid cyst

Sources: Data from Maya, M.M. et al., *Head and Neck Imaging*, Mosby, St. Louis, 2003 [43]; Vogl, T.J., *Diagnostische und Interventionelle Radiologie*, Springer, Berlin; Heidelberg, 2011 [40].
[a] Most common.

invasive tumors that rarely metastasize. Only large paragangliomas can present with signs of catecholamine release [43]. Paragangliomas of the jugular foramen, or glomus jugulare tumors, arise in the jugular foramen from the paraganglionic tissue in the adventitia of the jugular bulb or along the tympanic and auricular branches of glossopharyngeal and vagus nerves, respectively [45]. On CT, early signs are enlargement of the jugular foramen with small erosions and irregularities of its smooth bony margins (Figure 6.25). The tumor tends to extend along paths of least resistance, but larger tumors may result in extensive bone destruction. Erosion of the jugular plate with extension into the middle ear is common [43,46]. Paragangliomas are vascular tumors and always enhance avidly with contrast.

Schwannomas of the 9th, or less commonly 10th and 11th, cranial nerves may arise in the jugular foramen. Unlike paragangliomas, they usually result in symmetrical smooth expansion of the jugular foramen with sharp thin sclerotic rims [47]. Other lesions of the jugular foramen include meningiomas, carcinomas, and metastases (Figures 6.26 and 6.27) (Box 6.15).

6.2.6.4 Middle Ear Tumors

Most intratympanic masses are nonneoplastic. The most common tumor is paraganglioma or glomus tympanicum originating from paraganglionic tissue in the middle ear [43,46]. Glomus tympanicum tumors often present early with pulsatile tinnitus and conductive HL. Otoscopy may reveal a pulsatile retrotympanic mass.

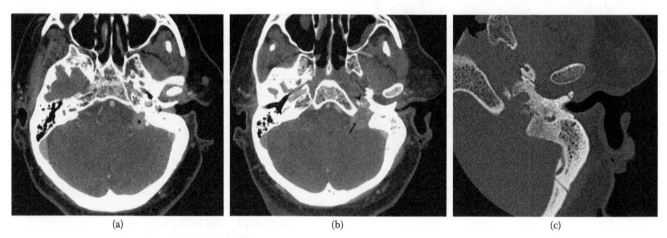

(a)   (b)   (c)

FIGURE 6.25
Paraganglioma (a) axial contrast-enhanced CT shows an enhancing mass (asterisks) in the left jugular fossa and left tympanic cavity. (b) Axial contrast-enhanced CT image at another level shows the enhancing mass (arrow) eroding the anterior part of the left carotid canal (arrowhead). (c) Bone algorithm CT image shows asymmetric widening of the left jugular fossa.

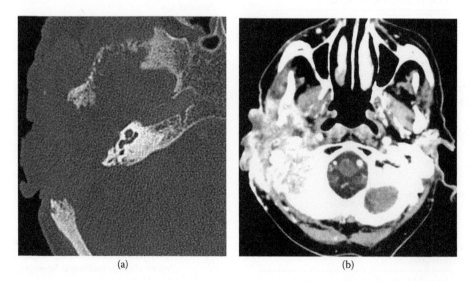

(a)   (b)

FIGURE 6.26
Squamous cell carcinoma of the temporal bone. Axial bone algorithm (a) and contrast-enhanced CT (b) images show a large mass infiltrating the skin, soft tissue, and the right temporal bone.

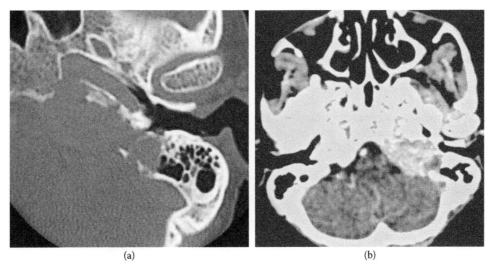

(a)   (b)

FIGURE 6.27
Temporal bone metastases. Axial bone algorithm (a) and contrast-enhanced CT (b) images show aggressive destruction of the left petrous temporal bone by a large enhancing mass.

BOX 6.15   DIFFERENTIAL DIAGNOSIS OF JUGULAR FORAMEN MASS LESIONS

Nonneoplastic
Asymmetric jugular foramen
Cholesteatoma (congenital or acquired)
High jugular bulb
Neoplastic
Paraganglioma
Schwannoma of the 9th, 10th, 11th cranial nerves
Meningioma
Metastasis
Squamous cell carcinoma
Plasmacytoma or multiple myeloma
Chondrosarcoma
Chordoma
Fibrosarcoma
Hemangiopericytoma

Source: Modified from Vogl, T.J., *Diagnostische und Interventionelle Radiologie*, Springer, Berlin; Heidelberg, 2011 [40].

BOX 6.16   DIFFERENTIAL DIAGNOSIS OF MIDDLE EAR MASS LESIONS

Nonneoplastic
Congenital/acquired cholesteatoma
Cholesterol granuloma (cyst)
Dehiscent jugular bulb
Aberrant/laterally placed carotid
Persistent stapedial artery
Histiocytosis
Neoplastic
Paraganglioma
Facial/chorda tympani schwannoma
Hemangioma
Squamous/adenocarcinoma
Rhabdomyosarcoma
Metastases

Source: Data from De Foer, B. et al., *Neuroimaging Clin. N. Am.,* 19, 339–366, 2009 [46].

Small glomus tympanicum tumors are usually confined to the middle ear at the promontory. Large lesions may completely fill the middle ear and extend into the mastoid or the EAC but the ossicles are typically spared [46]. Other middle ear tumors include cholesterol granuloma (CG), hemangioma, facial nerve, or chorda tympani schwannomas (Box 6.16). Malignant tumors are rare and include SCC and rhabdomyosarcoma.

6.2.6.5 External Auditory Canal Tumors

The most common benign tumors of the EAC are exostoses and osteomas. Exostoses are sessile, broad-based bony masses arising deep in the EAC. They usually occur bilaterally, secondary to prolonged exposure to cold seawater or other chronic irritation. Exostoses typically cause stenosis but not occlusion of the EAC. Osteomas are much less common, solitary, pedunculated bony growths of mature bone, often arising in the outer portion of the bony EAC [28,43].

SCCs are the commonest malignancy of the ear. They may be preceded by long history of chronic ear infection. They can extend into the middle ear and often result in destruction of the bony EAC and extend into the surrounding soft tissue [46]. Other malignant EAC tumors are rare.

References

1. Laine FJ, Smoker WR. The ostiomeatal unit and endoscopic surgery: Anatomy, variations, and imaging findings in inflammatory diseases. *Am J Roentgenol* 1992; 159: 849–857.

2. Zinreich SJ, Albayram S, Benson ML, Oliverio PJ. Sinonasal cavities: The ostiomeatal complex and functional endoscopic surgery. In: Som PM, Curtin HD, eds. *Head and Neck Imaging.* St. Louis: Mosby; 2003: 149–173.

3. Momeni AK, Roberts CC, Chew FS. Imaging of chronic and exotic sinonasal disease: Review. *Am J Roentgenol* 2007; 189: 35–45.

4. Dym RJ, Masri D, Shifteh K. Imaging of the paranasal sinuses. *Oral Maxillofac Surg Clin North Am.* 2012; 24:175–189.

5. Beale TJ, Madani G, Morley, SJ. Imaging of the paranasal sinuses and nasal cavity: Normal anatomy and clinically relevant anatomical variants. *Semin Ultrasound CT MR* 2009; 30: 2–16.

6. Earwaker J. Anatomic variants in sinonasal CT. *Radiographics* 1993; 13: 381–415.

7. Polavaram R, Devaiah AK, Sakai O, Shapshay SM. Anatomic variants and pearls—Functional endoscopic sinus surgery. *Otolaryngol Clin North Am* 2004; 37: 221–242.

8. Mafee, MF. Imaging of the nasal cavity and paranasal sinuses. In: Mafee MF, Valvassori, GE, Becker, M, eds. *Imaging of the Head and Neck.* 2nd ed. Stuttgart; New York: Thieme; 2005: 353–474.

9. Ramsden JD, Campisi PFV. Choanal atresia and choanal stenosis. *Otolaryngol Clin North Am* 2009; 42: 339–352.

10. Baxter DJG, Shroff M. Congenital midface abnormalities. *Neuroimaging Clin N Am* 2011; 21: 563–584.

11. Parmar H, Gujar S, Shah G, Mukherji SK. Imaging of the anterior skull base. *Neuroimaging Clin N Am* 2009; 19: 427–439.

12. Mehta N, Butala P, Bernstein, MP. The imaging of maxillofacial trauma and its pertinence to surgical intervention. *Radiol Clin North Am* 2012; 50: 43–57.

13. Rao VM, El-Noueam KI. Sinonasal imaging. Anatomy and pathology. *Radiol Clin North Am* 1998; 36: 921–939.

14. Babbel R, Harnsberger H, Sonkens J, Hunt S. Recurring patterns of inflammatory sinonasal disease demonstrated on screening sinus CT. *AJNR Am J Neuroradiol* 1992; 13: 903–912.

15. Resto VA, Deschler DG. Sinonasal malignancies. *Otolaryngol Clin North Am* 2004; 37: 473–487.

16. Hoang JK, Eastwood JD, Tebbit CL, Glastonbury CM. Multiplanar sinus CT: A systematic approach to imaging before functional endoscopic sinus surgery. *AJR Am J Roentgenol* 2010; 194: 527–536.

17. Som PM, Brandwein MS. Sinonasal cavities: Tumors and tumor-like conditions. In: Som PM, Curtin HD, eds. *Head and Neck Imaging.* St. Louis: Mosby; 2003: 261–373.

18. Branstetter BF IV, Weissman JL. Role of MR and CT in the paranasal sinuses. *Otolaryngol Clin North Am* 2005; 38: 1279–1299.

19. Vogl TJ. Gesichtsschaedel, nasennebenholen und orbita. In: Vogl TJ, Reith W, Rummeny EJ, eds. *Diagnostische und Interventionelle Radiologie.* Berlin; Heidelberg: Springer; 2011b: 397–413.

20. Melroy CT, Senior BA. Benign sinonasal neoplasms: A focus on inverting papilloma. *Otolaryngol Clin North Am* 2006; 39: 601–617.

21. Das S, Kirsch, CFE. Imaging of lumps and bumps in the nose: A review of sinonasal tumours. *Cancer Imaging* 2005; 5: 167–177.

22. Blount A, Riley, KO, Woodworth, BA. Juvenile nasopharyngeal angiofibroma. *Otolaryngol Clin North Am* 2011; 44: 989–1004.

23. Loevner LA, Sonners AI. Imaging of neoplasms of the paranasal sinuses. *Neuroimaging Clin N Am* 2004; 14: 625–646.

24. Kadish S, Goodman M, Wine C. Olfactory neuroblastoma: A clinical analysis of 17 cases. *Cancer* 1976; 37: 1571–1576.

25. Fleming I, Cooper J, Henson D, Hutter RVP, Kennedy BJ, Murphy GP, O'Sullivan B, Sobin LH, Yarbro JW. *American Joint Committee on Cancer Staging Manual.* 5th ed. Philadelphia: Lippincott Raven; 1997.

26. Aiken AH, Glastonbury C. Imaging Hodgkin and non-Hodgkin lymphoma in the head and neck. *Radiol Clin North Am* 2008; 46: 363–378.

27. Curtin HD, Sanelli PC, Som, PM. Temporal bone: Embryology and anatomy. In: Som PM, Curtin HD, eds. 4th ed. St. Louis: Mosby; 2003: 1057–1091.

28. Valvassori GE 2005. Imaging of the temporal bone. In: Mafee MF, Valvassori, GE, Becker, M, eds. *Imaging of the Head and Neck.* Stuttgart; New York: Thieme; 2005: 3–133.

29. Davidson, HC. Imaging of the temporal bone. *Magn Reson Imaging Clin N Am* 2002; 10: 573–613.

30. Krombach GA, Honnef D, Westhofen M, Di Martino E, Günther RW. Imaging of congenital anomalies and acquired lesions of the inner ear. *Eur Radiol* 2008; 18: 319–330.

31. Mukerji SS, Parmar HA, Ibrahim M, Mukherji SK. Congenital malformations of the temporal bone. *Neuroimaging Clin N Am* 2011; 21: 603–619.

32. Rodriguez K, Shah RK, Kenna M. Anomalies of the middle and inner ear. *Otolaryngol Clin North Am* 2007; 40: 81–96.

33. Shah LM, Wiggins RH. Imaging of hearing loss. *Neuroimaging Clin N Am* 2009; 19: 287–306.

34. Romo LV, Casselman JW, Robson CD. Temporal bone: Congenital anomalies. In: Som PM, Curtin HD, eds. *Head and Neck Imaging.* St. Louis: Mosby; 2003: 1109–1171.

35. Swartz JD, Curtin HD. Temporal bone: Trauma. In: Som PM, Curtin HD, eds. *Head and Neck Imaging.* St. Louis: Mosby; 2003: 1230–1244.

36. Zayas JO, Feliciano YZ, Hadley CR, Gomez AA, Vidal JA. Temporal bone trauma and the role of multidetector CT in the emergency department. *Radiographics* 2011; 31: 1741–1755.

37. Swartz JD. Temporal bone trauma. *Semin Ultrasound CT MR* 2001; 22: 219–228.

38. Lemmerling MM, De Foer B, Verbist, BM, VandeVyver V. Imaging of inflammatory and infectious diseases in the temporal bone. *Neuroimaging Clin N Am* 2009; 19: 321–337.

39. Nemzek WR, Swartz JD. Temporal bone: Inflammatory disease. In: Som PM, Curtin HD, eds. *Head and Neck Imaging*. St. Louis: Mosby; 2003: 1173–1229.

40. Vogl TJ. Felsenbein und mittlere schaedelbasis. In: Vogl TJ, Reith W, Rummeny E, eds. *Diagnostische und Interventionelle Radiologie*. Berlin; Heidelberg: Springer; 2011: 362–383.

41. Schmalfuss IM. Petrous apex. *Neuroimaging Clin N Am* 2009; 19: 367–391.

42. Isaacson B, Kutz JW, Roland PS. Lesions of the petrous apex: Diagnosis and management. *Otolaryngol Clin North Am* 2007; 40: 479–519.

43. Maya MM, Lo, WWM, Kovanlikaya, I. Temporal bone tumors and cerebellopontine angle lesions. In: Som PM, Curtin HD, eds. *Head and Neck Imaging*. St. Louis: Mosby; 2003: 1057–1091.

44. Wiggins RH III, Harnsberger HR, Salzman KL, Shelton C, Kertesz TR, Glastonbury CM. The many faces of facial nerve schwannoma. *Am J Neuroradiol* 2006; 27: 694–699.

45. Caldemeyer KS, Mathews VP, Azzareli B. The jugular foramen: A review of anatomy, masses, and imaging characteristics. *Radiographics* 1997; 17: 1123–1139.

46. De Foer B, Kenis C, Vercruysse, JP, Somers T, Pouillon M, Offeciers E, Casselman JW. Imaging of temporal bone tumors. *Neuroimaging Clin N Am* 2009; 19: 339–366.

47. Eldevik OP, Gabrielsen TO, Jacobsen EA. Imaging findings in schwannomas of the jugular foramen. *Am J Neuroradiol* 2000; 21: 1139–1144.

7

Head and Neck

Irfan Celebi

CONTENTS

7.1 Introduction

Despite growing technology, the radiological assessment of head and neck lesions has still some difficulties in certain cases because of the complex anatomy of this region, the small and mobile structures it harbors, and the apposition of the mucosal surfaces in the neutral position. Computed tomography (CT) is the standard modality for head and neck imaging and is more commonly used compared to magnetic resonance imaging (MRI). The introduction of multi-detector row CT has contributed to these properties [1–3]. Using multi-detector CT (MDCT), the entire neck can be imaged in 2–4 seconds. The short acquisition time increases patient cooperation, improves the diagnostic value of the scans, and makes it more convenient for patients who have difficulty tolerating MRI, and it also eliminates motion artifact. Advances in MDCT technology have also resulted in scans with lower radiation doses. Improvements in the spatial and temporal resolution enable better imaging of small, moveable anatomical structures, such as the larynx. Conversely, for evaluating regions involving predominantly soft-tissue structures (e.g., the nasopharynx and the parapharyngeal space [PPS]), MRI is superior to CT.

7.2 Sinonasal Imaging

High-resolution CT has become more valuable for imaging the sinonasal cavity, especially given the importance of the anatomy of the ostiomeatal complex in inflammatory diseases and endoscopic surgery. For evaluating both disease extent and bone structures, MDCT devices make excellent contributions. On the other hand, MRI is better for assessing intracranial and intraorbital complications.

Both CT and MRI can be used to evaluate sinonasal cavity tumors before treatment, but MRI is clearly superior for tumor mapping. MRI has superior soft-tissue contrast for distinguishing the tumor from the surrounding inflammation (Figure 7.1). CT enables a detailed examination of bone structure, investigation of calcifications, which is important for differentiating some tumors, and identification of anatomical landmarks in the skull base. It is the imaging study of

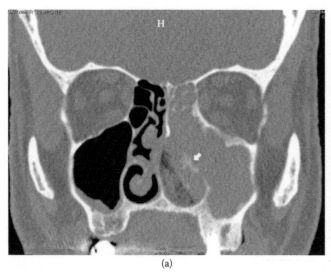

(a)

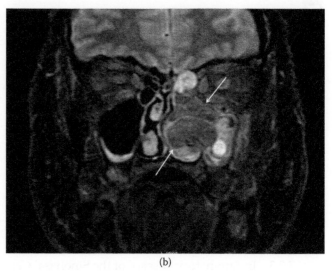

(b)

FIGURE 7.1
Coronal bone computed tomography (CT) scan (a) and T2-weighted magnetic resonance imaging (T2W MRI) (b) of the sinonasal cavity. In this case, no obvious, demarcated mass is seen on CT; however, there is an osseous destruction in the medial antral wall (arrow). It is difficult to determine the boundaries of the tumor because of accompanying inflammation. However, coronal T2W MRI, fat-suppressed (b), clearly reveals the boundaries of the tumor (arrows). This patient had an inverted papilloma. T2W MRI reveals the border of the mass and differentiated the tumor from the secretion.

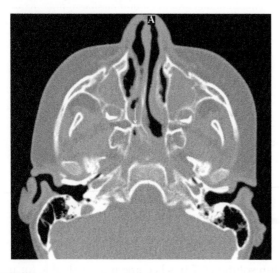

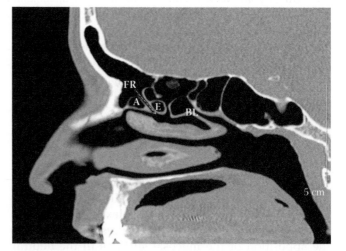

FIGURE 7.2
Axial bone CT scan. Unilateral bony atresia is evident on the right side (arrow). Note the hypoplasia of the posterior nasal cavity on the side of choanal atresia.

FIGURE 7.3
Normal sagittal reformatted CT scan. FSDP, frontal sinus drainage pathway (dashed line); A, Agger nasi cell; E, ethmoid cell; BL, basal or ground lamella that demarcates the anterior ethmoid air cells from the posterior ethmoid cells.

choice to evaluate patients suggestive of choanal atresia (Figure 7.2). Choanal atresia is the most common congenital abnormality of the nasal cavity. It can be unilateral or bilateral and atresia can be caused by a bony, membranous, or mixed type obstruction.

7.2.1 Normal Anatomy

The terminology used for describing the paranasal cavity and the sinonasal drainage pathways may be subjective because of the multiple anatomic variations. For

example, the best way to describe the frontal sinus passageway (known as frontoethmoid recess), which has the most complex and variable drainage, is frontal sinus drainage pathway (FSDP). FSDP is a surgically difficult to reach region because of its relation to both the orbita and the anterior skull base, and it is difficult to assess by standard axial and coronal CT images. The advent of multiplanar CT imaging with the addition of sagittal reconstructions greatly improves the understanding of FSDP [4] (Figure 7.3).

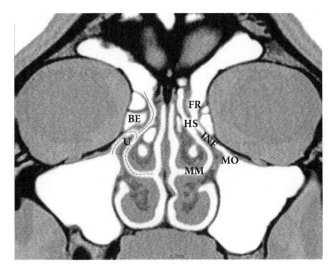

FIGURE 7.4
Normal coronal CT scan (negative contrast view) at the level of the ostiomeatal complex. FR, frontal recess (long thin line on the opposite side); HS, hiatus semilunaris (small dashed line on the opposite side); INF, infundibulum (small thin line on the opposite side); MO, primary maxillary ostium; MM, middle meatus (long dashed line on the opposite side); U, uncinate process; BE, ethmoid bulla.

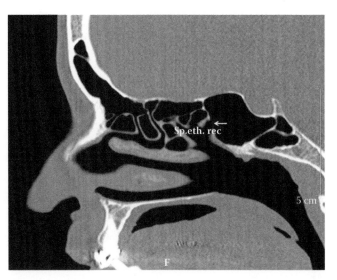

FIGURE 7.5
Normal sagittal reformatted CT scan at the level of the sphenoid ostium (arrow). Sp.eth.rec. = sphenoethmoid recess.

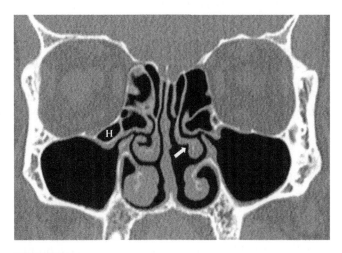

FIGURE 7.6
Normal coronal CT scan shows Haller cell (H) on the right side and paradoxic left middle turbinate (arrow).

The nasal septum, which consists of cartilaginous and osseous components, divides the nasal respiratory passageway shaped as a pyramid from the middle into two fossae. Each nasal fossa has three projections along the lateral wall, which are formed by the superior, middle, and inferior turbinates or concha. The turbinates divide the nasal cavity into three distinct air passages: the superior, middle, and inferior meati. Each respective meatus is lateral to its corresponding turbinate.

The maxillary, frontal, and anterior ethmoid sinuses drain into the middle meatus, which lies inferolateral to the middle turbinate. This region is called the anterior ostiomeatal complex or unit and incorporates the maxillary sinus ostium, infundibulum, uncinate process, hiatus semilunaris, ethmoid bulla, middle turbinate, and middle meatus (Figure 7.4).

The superior meatus drains the posterior ethmoid air cells and, more posteriorly, the sphenoid sinus (via the sphenoethmoidal recess) (Figure 7.5). The inferior meatus receives drainage from the nasolacrimal duct.

7.2.2 Anatomic Variations

Although sinonasal anatomy varies significantly from patient to patient, there are some specific variations that occur repeatedly within the population.

Paradoxic curvature and concha bullosa of the middle turbinate are probably the most common form among all of the variations. Normally, the convexity of the middle turbinate bone is directed medially toward the nasal septum. When paradoxically curved, the convexity of the bone is directed laterally toward the lateral

sinus wall (Figure 7.6). A concha bullosa is an aerated turbinate, most often the middle turbinate (Figure 7.7). Middle turbinates, which are highly aerated, are related to a higher prevalance of ipsilateral sinus disease [5,6].

The other variations are the following: infraorbital ethmoid cells, also known as Haller cells (Figure 7.6), which are the extension of the ethmoid air cells inferiorly and laterally forming the roof of the maxillary ostium; sphenoethmoid cells, known as Onodi cells, which are posterior ethmoid cells extending into the sphenoid bone, situated either adjacent to or impinging upon the optic nerve [7]; and Agger nasi cells, which are the most anterior cells of the ethmoid labyrinth that have extended anterior and into the lacrimal bone. In the sagittal plane, Agger nasi cells are located anterior and below the frontal recess (Figure 7.3).

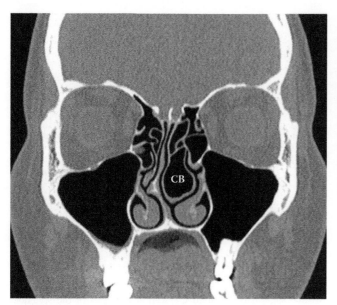

FIGURE 7.7
Concha bullosa. Coronal plane sinus CT shows large, pneumatized left middle turbinates (CB).

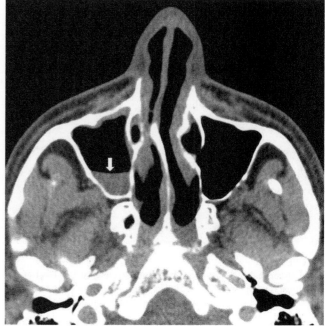

FIGURE 7.8
Axial CT scan shows a right maxillary sinus mucoid attenuation air–fluid level (arrow). Clinically, this patient had acute bacterial sinusitis.

Ethmoid bulla, which is the largest air cell in the anterior ethmoid complex (Figure 7.4), may vary in size and may prolapse into the middle nasal meatus or ethmoid infundibulum. It can narrow these structures when it is enlarged.

7.2.3 Inflammatory Disease of the Sinonasal Cavities

Inflammatory disease is the most common pathology involving the paranasal sinuses and nasal cavity. It primarily results from interference of mucociliary clearance because of the compromise of the drainage portals (ostiomeatal channels) of the individual sinus cavities or ventilation disturbance. Mild mucoperiosteal thickening (<3 mm) is primarily found in the maxillary and ethmoid sinuses. It is not uncommon and may be seen in asymptomatic individuals. There is a ciliated cuboidal epithelium in the sinonasal cavity mucosa that secretes mucus. This is called a mucous blanket. The movement of this mucous blanket is called mucociliary clearance. Functional endoscopic sinus surgery, which is widely accepted, aims to restore sinus drainage via the normal anatomic drainage pathways, thus allowing normal mucociliary clearance.

Acute sinusitis is characterized by the presence of air–fluid levels (Figure 7.8) and is typically caused by a viral upper respiratory tract infection. Changes in chronic sinusitis include mucoperiosteal thickening and osseous thickening of the sinus wall. The imaging findings are nonspecific and should be correlated with the clinical history and physical examination. Chronic sinusitis is usually a result of repeated episodes of acute or subacute sinusitis. Changes including hypertrophy, polypoid thickening, areas of some atrophy, and fibrosis occur as a result of repeated inflammation in the mucosa.

Retention cysts are mucous retention cysts, which occur because of inflammatory obstruction of seromucinous glands, or serous retention cysts, which occur because of accumulation of serous fluid. Retention cysts have a rounded appearance with a typical smooth and convex outer surface. They are mostly found on the basis of the maxillary sinuses. They are incidentally detected in most examinations and cannot be distinguished from solitary polyps with imaging. Mucocele is similar to retention cysts, but different than a single mucous gland becoming obstructed, the entire sinus is obstructed. An expanded, airless sinus cavity filled with fairly homogeneous mucoid attenuation (10–18 HU) secretions on CT is diagnostic of a mucocele [8]. Infected mucocele, mucopyocele, is easily diagnosed if the inflamed sinus mucosa shows a thin line inside the sinus bone wall and if the sinus is completely full.

Chronic inflammation results in mucosal hypertrophy, which causes mucosal redundancy and polyp formation. Nasal polyps have been associated with intolerance to aspirin. Allergy, inflammations, infections, vasomotor rhinitis, and cystic fibrosis are also

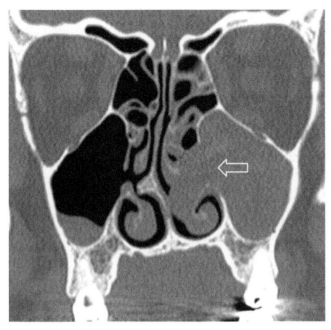

FIGURE 7.9
Coronal computed tomography scan shows a polypoid mass opacifying completely the left maxillary sinus with extension into the nasal cavity (open arrow) consistent with antrochoanal polyp.

associated with polyp formation. On CT scan, a typical antrochoanal polyp appears as a soft-tissue polyp completely filling a maxillary sinus. The infundibular region is usually widened, and the antral mass is extruded into the nasal cavity via the middle meatus (Figure 7.9).

Fungal sinusitis, which was once considered a rare disorder, is now reported with increasing frequency throughout the world. Fungal sinus infections can have a variety of forms depending on the host's immune system and other factors. They are divided into noninvasive and invasive subgroups. The invasive group consists of acute invasive fungal sinusitis, chronic invasive fungal sinusitis, and chronic granulomatous invasive fungal sinusitis, whereas noninvasive fungal sinusitis is composed of allergic fungal sinusitis and fungus ball (fungal mycetoma). These five subtypes have different clinical and radiological features. Acute invasive fungal sinusitis is rarely seen in healthy individuals. It is a rapidly progressing infection seen predominantly in immunocompromised patients and patients with poorly controlled diabetes. It is the most lethal form of fungal sinusitis. The reported mortality is 50%–80% [9].

As inflammation is spread intraorbitally and intracranially, the sinus wall shows rapid aggressive bone destruction. The intracranial extension of the disease from the sphenoid sinus causes cavernous sinus thrombosis and even carotid artery invasion, occlusion, or pseudoaneurysm. This results with fatal cerebral infarct and hemorrhage. All patients at risk for

acute invasive fungal sinusitis should be investigated for obliteration of the periantral fat that is a sign of such extension [10].

In chronic invasive fungal sinusitis, symptoms directly related to the invasive disease take months or years to develop. The disease is usually persistent and recurrent. Noncontrast CT shows a hyperattenuating soft-tissue collection in one or more of the paranasal sinuses. Mottled lucencies or irregular bone destruction may be seen in the paranasal sinuses. Chronic invasive fungal sinusitis and malignant neoplasm may not be differentiated based on imaging findings [11,12]. CT findings of allergic fungal sinusitis show opacified ethmoid and maxillary sinuses with high-density material without osseous destruction, often in conjunction with allergic rhinitis and asthma. The high density is not pathognomonic for fungal infection.

Wegener's granulomatosis shows nonspecific inflammatory changes in the sinonasal cavities. Often aggressive findings such as nasal septal perforation and orbital involvement are seen. Intracranial extension of the disease occurs occasionally.

7.2.4 Neoplastic Disease of the Paranasal Cavities

Nasal and paranasal tumors can be benign or malignant that can be broadly classified as either epithelial or mesenchymal. The mucosal lining of the nose, the schneiderian membrane, is derived from ectoderm, which is different from the rest of the upper respiratory tract mucosa being derived from the endoderm.

Different types of schneiderian papilloma, that is fungiform, inverted, and cylindrical, can occur within the nasal cavity. CT shows a soft-tissue mass within the nasal cavity, arising from the lateral nasal wall and extending into the maxillary sinus for inverted papilloma (Figure 7.1a). The mass is usually heterogeneous and often has radiodensities confusing calcification. These radiodensities within the lesion are actually foci of residual bone. The nasal septum usually remains intact, but the mass can cause a bowing to the opposite side.

Juvenile nasopharyngeal angiofibroma: These tumors occur typical in adolescent males. The patient presents with epistaxis. This is a benign tumor that can be very locally aggressive. The pterygopalatine fossa is often already involved at the time of diagnosis. The tumor originates from fibrovascular stroma of the nasal wall adjacent to the sphenopalatine foramen. CT scan shows an enhancing nasal cavity/nasopharyngeal mass that extends to the pterygopalatine fossa (Figure 7.10).

Olfactory neuroblastoma (ONB): This tumor is also known as esthesioneuroblastoma. It originates from the neurosensory body cells in the olfactory epithelium in

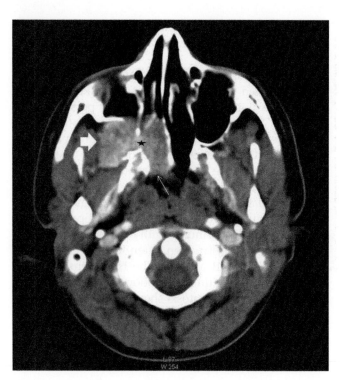

FIGURE 7.10
Axial CT scan reveals juvenile nasopharyngeal angiofibroma centered at sphenopalatine foramen (star). Mass is diffusely enhanced with contrast medium and extends pterygopalatine/infratemporal fossa (thick arrow) and the nasal cavity/nasopharynx (thin arrow).

the superior nasal fossa. On biopsy, it is usually seen as a solitary soft-tissue nasal polyp that may bleed profusely. CT scan shows an avidly enhancing lesion in the upper nasal cavity invading the skull base. When there are peripheral cysts along the tumor–brain interface, an esthesioneuroblastoma with intracranial extension should be considered.

There are many diagnostic possibilities of a unilateral polypoid nasal mass with calcifications, but it is most likely to be either an ONB or an inverted papilloma. A nasal septal mass with calcification is either a chondroid tumor or the result of fungal disease [13].

The tissues from where malignancies can originate within the paranasal sinuses and nasal cavity include the squamous epithelium, lymphoid tissue, and minor salivary gland. Therefore, the corresponding malignancies are squamous cell carcinoma (SCCA), lymphoma, and minor salivary gland tumors. SCCA is the most common malignant tumor in the sinonasal cavities. It is often seen in the maxillary sinus; 20%–30% are in the nasal cavity and 10%–15% are in the ethmoid sinuses. Cancer in the sphenoid or frontal sinuses is extremely rare, accounting for only 5% of such cancers. CT shows opacified maxillary sinus with bone destruction. These nonspecific findings do not allow differentiation from non-Hodgkin's lymphoma

or a minor salivary gland malignancy. Previously, the maxillary antrum was divided into an infrastructure and a suprastructure. However, this classification was soon modified into an infrastructure, a mesostructure, and a suprastructure, with the lines of division being drawn on a coronal view of the sinuses through the antral floor and the antral roof. According to this system, tumors limited to the mesostructure and infrastructure require a partial or total maxillectomy, whereas tumors that involve the suprastructure require a total maxillectomy and possible orbital exenteration [13].

The radiologist must be aware of the critical areas of tumor extension that will alter a surgical or irradiation treatment plan to achieve the best tumor mapping and staging. This accurate information is now available through the improved imaging technology. These critical areas include tumor extension into the floor of the anterior and middle cranial fossae, the pterygopalatine fossa, the orbits, and the palate [13]; and the radiologist should always evaluate fat planes in the pterygopalatine fossa, inferior orbital fissure, foramen rotundum, and Vidian (pterygoid) canal for possible perineural tumor spread.

7.3 Skull Base

The skull base is simply the bottom of the skull. It extends from the nose anteriorly to the occipital protuberance posteriorly. It is composed of the ethmoid, sphenoid, occipital, temporal, and frontal bones [14]. Both vascular and neural structures pass through several foramina of the skull base.

Any lesion from the paranasal sinuses and nasal cavity may extend to involve the skull base. Although various primary malignant neoplasms of the skull base are described, most malignant lesions of the skull base are metastatic in origin. There is a large number of possible lesions that occur in the skull base. Determination of the position of apparent origin of a mass or pathology narrows the list to a few possibilities.

In the petrous apex of the temporal bone (T-bone), the first task is to locate the lesion and exclude lesions arising in the jugular foramen, in the internal auditory canal, or in the petro-occipital fissure. A lesion centered in the jugular fossa is almost always a paraganglioma or schwannoma. Rarely a meningioma or metastasis can occur in this area.

A mass that causes permeative and infiltrative changes in the adjacent osseous structures, rather than erosion and remodeling, thus resulting with an expansion of the jugular fossa, is compatible with glomus jugulare tumor. On the other hand, schwannoma causes remodeling and expansion of the jugular foramen rather than destructive changes. Dynamic contrast examinations via multislice CT, which enables a rapid scan, are very valuable in distinguishing these two lesions and showing the hypervascularity of globus tumors.

Cholesterol cyst, cholesteatoma (epidermoid), petrous carotid aneurysm, arachnoid cyst, and mucocele are the cystic or expansile lesions of the petrous bone. These lesions cannot be differentiated by CT alone. Usually, MRI is necessary and contributes to the diagnosis.

Meningioma is the most common lesion in this area that shows internal enhancement. This tumor originates from the dura. It usually follows the dura along the outside of the petrous bone rather than appearing to originate from within the apex. Meningiomas that originate from within the apex are extremely rare.

CT shows an expansile ground-glass density osseous lesion in fibrous dysplasia, which is a common benign fibro-osseous lesion. It is usually unilateral and involves contiguous bones in the head and neck. On the other hand, Paget's disease is a common disease, and the etiology is unknown. It is seen in elderly people but usually before the age of 40. Any bone can be affected. However, the skull and the skull base involvements are common, whereas isolated involvement of the petrous apex is extremely rare.

Two types of infection can involve the petrous apex: petrous apicitis and malignant (or necrotizing) otitis externa. Infection can reach the petrous apex via the middle ear. Osteomyelitis is developed as a result. As the apex infection continues, a classic pattern may evolve. Gradenigo's syndrome is characterized by a draining ear, deep head pain, and the sixth nerve palsy. The sixth nerve passes through the Dorello's canal, which is a small channel along the apex.

Infection of the center skull base can give the appearance of tumor. Pseudotumor or nonspecific orbital inflammatory disease can enhance in the anterior cavernous sinus (Tolosa–Hunt syndrome) with obliteration of the fat in the superior orbital fissure and orbital apex. This appearance can mimic lymphoma and other infiltrative diseases.

Chordoma is a tumor arising from the notochord remnant. It is rare and often occurs in the clivus (Figure 7.11). This tumor is usually placed in the midline, in contrast with chondrosarcoma that arises from the cartilage of the petroclival synchondrosis. Therefore, chondrosarcoma locates off-midline. Both tumors have similar density on CT and signal pattern on MRI.

Cephalocele is defined as a herniation of cranial contents through a bone defect in the skull (meningocele, meninges + cerebrospinal fluid (CSF);

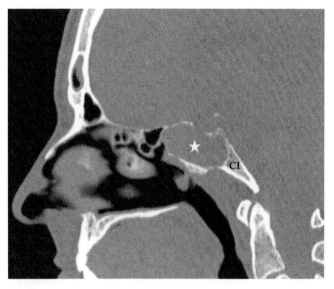

FIGURE 7.11
Sagittal reformatted CT scan shows a soft-tissue mass in the upper clivus (Cl) opacifying completely sphenoid sinus (star). This patient had a chordoma. In this case, the mass mimicking sphenoid sinus mucocele.

meningoencephalocele, meninges + CSF + brain tissue). Transethmoid and sphenoid cephaloceles can be present as a nasal mass later in life, whereas occipital cephaloceles are typically diagnosed at birth. Cephalocele should always be included in the differential diagnosis of nasal masses particularly in young patients and whenever suspected, MRI should be done.

7.4 Orbit

The orbits are bordered by periosteum, known as the periorbita. They are separated from the optic bulbus by Tenon's capsule. There are two recesses that contain the globes (optic bulbus); extraocular muscles; blood vessels; lymphatics; 2nd, 3rd, 4th, 5th, and 6th nerves; adipose and connective tissues; and most of the lacrimal apparatus. The orbital septum and the lids are located anteriorly. The apex of the orbit is directed posteriorly and medially. It is formed by the optic canal and the superior orbital fissure. The optic canal, and the superior and the inferior orbital fissures allow various structures to enter and leave the orbits. The optic canal has up to 9 mm length. It contains the optic nerve and ophthalmic artery in adults. Just lateral and inferolateral to the optic canal is the superior orbital fissure, which communicates with the middle cranial fossa and transmits the oculomotor, trochlear and abducens

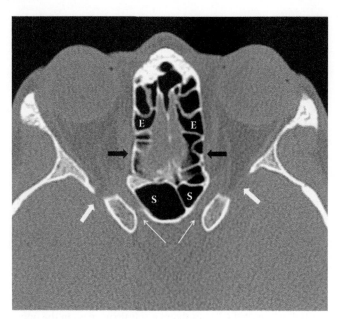

FIGURE 7.12
Normal axial CT scan through the optic canal (arrows); superior orbital fissure (thick white arrows); lamina papricea (thick black arrows); S, sphenoid sinus; E, ethmoid sinuses.

nerves, and the terminal branches of the ophthalmic nerve and ophthalmic veins (Figure 7.12). The inferior orbital fissure that separates the inferior and lateral walls of the orbit at the posterior aspect is bounded above by the greater wing of the sphenoid, below by the maxilla and the orbital process of the palatine bone, and laterally by the zygomatic bone or the zygomatico-maxillary suture.

Both CT and MRI are valuable for the imaging of the orbit, and each has different benefits. MRI has superior soft-tissue contrast resolution especially for intraocular, intramuscular lesions, and optic nerve pathology. On the other hand, CT is the modality of choice for the evaluation of calcification, such as in retinoblastoma, in a child with leukocoria, or for bony fracture following trauma.

Muscle cone is formed by the extraocular muscles (superior, inferior, medial, and lateral rectus; superior oblique; and levator palpebrae superior). A fibrous septum separates the retrobulbar space into intra- and extraconal spaces. When identifying an intraconal lesion, an essential issue is whether the lesion arises from the optic nerve sheath complex or is extrinsic to it. The optic nerve sheath complex is composed of the optic nerve and the surrounding perioptic nerve sheath. The optic nerve sheath contains three layers; the pia mater, the arachnoid, and the dura. The pia mater is highly vascular and attached tightly to the optic nerve. The subarachnoid space is filled with CSF in continuity with the intracranial subarachnoid space. The subdural space

surrounding the optic nerve, however, has no direct connection to the intracranial subdural space. The most common lesion arising from the optic nerve sheath complex is either an optic nerve glioma or an optic sheath meningioma.

Optic gliomas often occur between the ages of two and eight years, extend anteriorly and posteriorly along the optic nerve, and often involve the optic chiasm. In adults this tumor occurs rarely but is highly malignant. Bilateral optic gliomas are pathognomonic for neurofibromatosis type 1.

Meningioma is a benign tumor arising from arachnoid cells within the optic nerve sheath. They are typically solid, tubular, highly enhancing, well-defined masses, which classically show "tram-track" appearance caused by tumor enhancement or calcification on either side of the optic nerve.

Schwannomas of the optic nerve sheath commonly occur in the superior portion of the orbit because there are more sensory nerves in that location. The optic nerve is an extension of the brain and does not have schwann cells. Therefore, schwannoma does not arise from the optic nerve.

A variety of vascular lesions may develop in the orbit. The four lesions we will consider include capillary hemangioma, lymphangioma, cavernous hemangioma, and varix.

Capillary hemangioma is the most common orbital tumor of infancy. CT shows a lobulated, avidly enhancing mass without calcification usually in the superior aspect of the orbit.

Lymphangioma is one of the most common orbital tumors of childhood, and occur in an older group of children (3–15 years) [15]. On CT scan, lymphangioma appears as poorly circumscribed, often heterogeneous masses of increased density in the extraconal or intraconal space. Bony expansion may be present, calcification is rare, and minimal or marked contrast enhancement may be present.

Cavernous hemangioma is the most common benign orbital tumor in adults. It is often seen in middle-aged women. It is most commonly located in the intraconal space, although can occur anywhere in the orbit. Well-demarcated margin, ovoid shape, and homogeneous delayed or prolonged enhancement are characteristic findings for cavernous hemangioma.

Wright et al. have emphasized that it is artificial and unnecessary to separate orbital venous malformations (OVMs) as lymphangioma and orbital varices, and that both should be considered as OVM according to their origin, clinical symptoms, and treatment [16,17]. Orbital varix is the pathological enlargement of the venous channels in the orbita, both of its afferent and efferent vessels are in venous nature. The

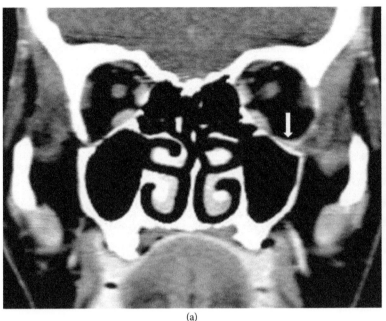
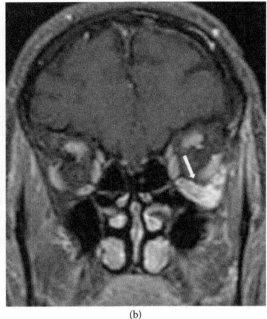

(a)   (b)

FIGURE 7.13
Contrast-enhanced coronal plane reformatted image (a) obtained in the supine position. Careful examination revealed an indistinct, dense soft-tissue lesion in the inferior aspect of the left orbit (arrow). A coronal plane contrast-enhanced T2-weighted MRI (b) of the same patient, obtained in the prone position during a Valsalva maneuver, clearly shows the orbital varix (arrow).

distensibility of OVM affects the clinical and radiological behavior. The histopathological structures of distensible and nondispensible lesions do not differ. However, nondistensibles show more thrombosis and hemorrhage [18].

Contrast-enhanced orbital CT scan is reported to be reliable in imaging OVM [19]. However, varices may not be shown via standard CT, even with contrast material, or may only be shown as minimal dilation of involved veins. OVM tends to collapse and may not be shown via routine CT scan or MRI. In this case Valsalva's maneuver may help expose the varices (Figure 7.13).

Idiopathic inflammatory syndromes of orbit are also known as orbital pseudotumors. These are nongranulomatous orbital inflammatory disorders and their etiology is unknown. Among orbital disorders, after Graves' disease, pseudotumor is the next most common ophthalmologic disease and the second most common cause of exophthalmos. There is a group of diverse disease entities that can mimic pseudotumors. Diagnosis of this disease is usually made by exclusion of other disease based on the history, the clinical course of the disease, the response to steroid therapy, and the laboratory tests and biopsy in a limited number of cases [20]. Imaging findings of orbital pseudotumor are nonspecific and variable. The disease is often rapidly developing, and in the acute phase presents with painful proptosis, restricted eye movement, chemosis, and ophthalmoplegia. Orbital pseudotumor occurs anywhere in the orbit and often involves the lacrimal gland, extraocular muscles, intraorbital fat, optic nerve sheath complex, eyelid, and sclera. Extraocular muscle involvement is often seen in the superior and lateral rectus muscles.

Thyroid ophthalmopathy (Graves' disease) occurs most commonly in middle-aged women. This condition is the result of an inflammatory infiltration of the orbital muscles and orbital connective tissue. CT findings are enlargement of the extraocular muscles and lacrimal glands, and increase in volume and edema of the intraorbital fat. The inferior and medial rectus muscles are more commonly affected; however, their tendinous insertions tend to be spared.

CT findings of lymphoma and other lymphoid tumors are similar to those of idiopathic orbital inflammation (pseudotumor) and sarcoidosis. The lacrimal gland is most commonly affected in sarcoidosis.

Choroidal osteoma is a benign tumor that is typically found in young white girls. On a CT scan, it appears as a platelike calcified thickening of the posterior ocular wall, typically in the juxtapapillary region; unlike drusen, calcification typically does not involve the center of the optic disc (Figure 7.14) (The list of the differential diagnosis of some orbital lesions is in Tables 7.1 through 7.3.) [13].

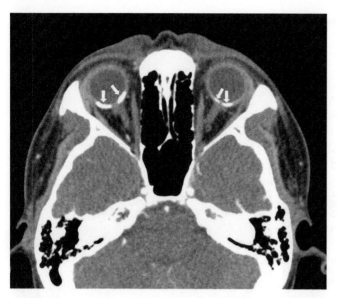

FIGURE 7.14
Choroidal osteoma. Axial CT scan shows a peripapillary plaque-like calcification (arrows), compatible with choroidal osteoma. Typically, the center of the optic disc is not involved.

TABLE 7.1

Intraconal (Central Orbital) Lesions

More Common	Less Common
Cavernous hemangioma	Capillary hemangioma
Optic nerve meningioma	Peripheral nerve tumors
	Neurofibroma
	Schwannoma
Optic nerve glioma	Leukemia
Optic nerve granulomatous disease (sarcoid)	Hematocele
Optic neuritis (multiple sclerosis)	Optic nerve sheath cyst
Lymphoma	Colobomatous cyst
Pseudotumor	Hemangioblastoma (optic nerve)
Lymphangioma	Chemodectoma (ciliary ganglion)
Venous angioma	Necrobiotic xanthogranuloma
Varix	Lipoma
Arteriovenous malformation	Amyloidosis
Carotid cavernous fistula	
Hemangiopericytoma	
Rhabdomyosarcoma	
Metastasis	
Orbital cellulitis and abscess	

TABLE 7.2

Extraconal (Peripheral Orbital) Lesions

More Common	Less Common
Capillary hemangiomas	Amyloidosis
Cholesterol granulomas	Fibrous histiocytoma
Dermoids and epidermoids	Hemangiosarcoma
Lacrimal gland lesions	Hemangiopericytoma
Inflammation	
Lymphoma	
Pseudotumor	
Sarcoidosis	
Epithelial tumors	Hematic cyst
Lymphangiomas	Lipoma
Peripheral nerve tumors	Orbital encephalocele
Plasmacytomas	Wegener's granulomatosis
Rhabdomyosarcomas	
Sarcoidosis	

TABLE 7.3

Differential Diagnosis of Metastatic Orbital Calcification

Congenital
  Fanconi's syndrome (proximal renal tubular dysfunction)
  Milk–alkali syndrome
  Renal tubular acidosis
Endocrine
  Hyperparathyroidism, primary or secondary
  Hypoparathyroidism
  Pseudohypoparathyroidism
Idiopathic-sarcoidosis
  Infectious
    Cytomegalovirus
    Leprosy
    Osteomyelitis
    Syphilis
    Toxoplasmosis
    Tuberculosis
Toxic
  Excessive ingestion of calcium phosphate or alkali
  Vitamin D intoxication
Traumatic immobilization
  Neoplastic
    Bronchogenic carcinoma
    Metastatic involvement of bone
    Multiple myeloma
    Parathyroid adenoma
    Parathyroid carcinoma

Source: Modified from Froula PD et al., *Mayo Clin Proc*, 1993, 68, 256–257.

7.5 Temporal Bone

Recent developments in the multi-detector row CT provide better anatomic resolution for imaging thin anatomical structures such as skull base and T-bone within a shorter acquisition time. However, this technique is unreliable in differentiating fluids and soft tissue filling the mastoid air cells and middle ear because of partial volume averaging effects. Therefore, CT scan mainly provides information in the extension of disease, and about the destruction in the bone structure, especially ossicular structures.

The most common diseases involving the T-bone are inflammatory in nature and include cholesteatomas.

Serous otitis media is the most common cause of hearing loss in children. Sterile serous fluid fills the middle ear and sometimes the entire mastoid air cell system. CT shows opacification of the tympanic cavity and pneumatized mastoid air cells without bone sclerosis or bone destruction. Rhabdomyosarcoma or Langerhans cell histiocytosis should be considered if aggressive bone destruction or cranial nerve impairment is noted. Acute coalescent mastoiditis also causes a breakdown of the trabecular pattern of the mastoid. Acute otomastoiditis is the result of bacterial infection. Complications include coalescent mastoiditis, subperiosteal abscess, dural sinus thrombosis, meningitis, brain abscess, labyrinthitis, and petrous apicitis. Chronic otomastoiditis is the result of eustachian tube disfunction. Complications include tympanic membrane retraction, acquired cholesteatoma, granulation tissue, cholesterol granuloma, postinflammatory ossicular fixation, and noncholesteatomatous ossicular erosions [21].

CT findings of chronic mastoiditis are a nonhomogeneous clouding of the mastoid antrum and air cells with sclerotic changes of the mastoid air cells. Granulation tissue is probably the most common cause of middle ear debris, and is diagnosed by CT with its lack of bony erosion or ossicular displacement [22].

Suppurative mastoiditis is generally a bacterial infection. Pus is present in the middle ear. Coalescent mastoiditis and extraosseous abscess formation are possible. Bezold's abscess can occur along the sternocleidomastoid muscle. Infection may extend to the petrous apex and may cause Gradenigo syndrome with abducens nerve palsy and trigeminal neuralgia. In chronic suppurative otitis media and mastoiditis, the residual portion of the tympanic membrane is usually thickened and visible. In chronic adhesive otitis media, CT shows thickened portions of the tympanic membrane retracted to the promontory and a contracted middle ear space. Erosion of the long process of the incus commonly occurs in chronic otitis media, and the malleus handle is often foreshortened.

The presence of bone erosion of the scutum, ossicles, lateral semicircular canal (labyrinthine fistula), and tegmen tympani suggests secondary acquired cholesteatoma. A cholesteatoma is an epidermoid cyst that histologically consists of desquamating stratified squamous epithelium. These cysts are middle ear masses resulting from accumulation of keratin debris because of the migration of the squamous epithelium. They may be either congenital (2%) or acquired (98%). Congenital form originates from epithelial rests within or adjacent to the T-bone. Acquired form originates from the stratified squamous epithelium of the tympanic membrane. These begin as localized tympanic membrane retraction pockets. A soft tissue arising within Prussac

space, which is located medial to the pars flaccida (superior recess of the tympanic membrane) between scutum and the neck of the malleus, with subtle erosion of the scutum and medial displacement of the ossicules is a characteristic of cholesteatoma (Figure 7.15). Automastoidectomy refers to spontaneous evacuation of cholesteatoma after extensive bone destruction, mimicking surgery. Cholesterol granuloma is a specific subtype of granulation tissue. It is histopathologically different from cholesteatoma because it is lined by fibrous connective tissue rather than keratinized stratified squamous epithelium. Cholesterol granulomas cannot be distinguished on CT from congenital cholesteatoma and mucoceles of the petrous apex. However, it is easy to diagnose the cholesterol granuloma on MRI, by defining a bright lesion characterized by a short T1 and long T2 relaxation time.

Congenital abnormalities of the ear are variable and most of them are mentioned together with the syndromes. Atresia of the external auditory canal (EAC) is commonly seen in boys and degree of atresia can be variable (Figure 7.16). Awareness of congenital vascular variants involving the T-bones is important as they may mimic glomus tumors or complicate middle ear surgery. An aberrant or ectopic carotid artery is formed by collateral blood flow, substituting the cervical and vertical petrous portions of the internal carotid artery (ICA), through branches of the external carotid artery [23]. The aberrant artery enters the T-bone through an enlarged inferior tympanic canaliculus and then undulates through the tympanic cavity to enter the horizontal portion of the carotid canal through a dehiscence in the carotid plate (Figure 7.17).

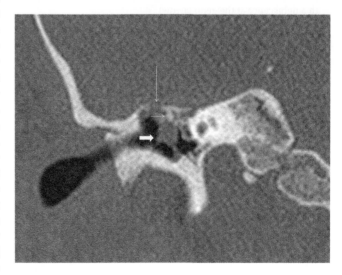

FIGURE 7.15
Prussac cholesteatoma. Coronal temporal-bone CT scan shows a soft-tissue mass (thick arrow) abuts the tympanic membrane. Ossicules (thin arrow) are medially displaced and eroded. There is also an erosion in the tegmen tympani (long thin arrow).

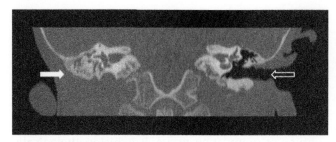

FIGURE 7.16
Coronal CT shows very thick right atretic bony plate with no aeration of the tympanic cavity (thick arrow). Ossicules are not identified. On the opposite side, normal external auditory canal is seen (open arrow).

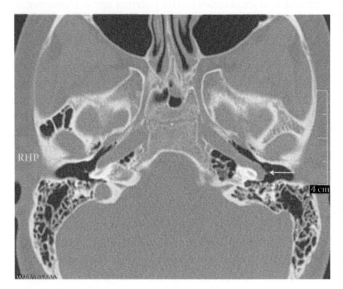

FIGURE 7.17
Axial high-resolution CT images through both temporal bones. The left aberrant carotid artery is reaching over the cochlear promontory with a dehiscence at the genu (arrow).

The stapedial artery is normally a transient embryonic vessel that is regressed by the third fetal month [23]. Persistence of the stapedial artery is rare too. It may or may not be associated with an aberrant carotid artery [24]. Although congenital vascular variants involving the middle ear are rare, awareness of these variants is important. Patients may present with pulsatile tinnitus or conductive hearing loss but many remain asymptomatic and are identified incidentally. They may mimic a glomus tumor or other vascular neoplasms and complicate middle ear surgery if not recognized in advance. Puncture of the aberrant carotid artery may result in serious complications such as hemorrhage and stroke [25].

Glomus jugulare and glomus tympanicum (Figure 7.18) are the paragangliomas arising at the level of the jugular foramen and tympanic cavity (especially around the cochlear promontory) respectively. These tumors are highly vascular and may show permeative or infiltrative changes in the adjacent osseous structures.

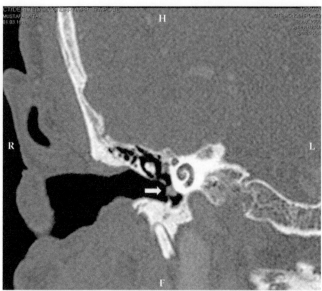

FIGURE 7.18
Glomus tympanicum. Coronal temporal-bone CT shows a small tympanicum paraganglioma in the lower-middle ear cavity (arrow). Tumor slightly bulging against tympanic membrane and abutting cochlear promontory.

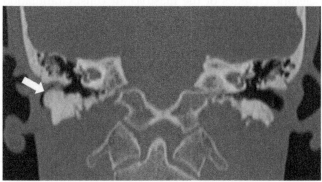

FIGURE 7.19
Coronal temporal-bone computed tomography scan shows a local osseous density mass lesion (arrow) within the external auditory canal, consistent with a benign osteoma.

Osteoma is a benign slow-growing pedunculated bony lesion within the EAC (Figure 7.19). Differential considerations for EAC osteomas include exostosis. Differentiation between EAC osteomas and exostosis may not be crucial as treatment is essentially the same. Several studies have found a high prevalence of EAC exostosis in cold-water sports enthusiasts, leading to name "surfer's ear."

7.6 Suprahyoid Neck

The aerodigestive tractus over the hyoid bone level is divided into compartments that include the nasopharynx, oropharynx, and nasal/oral cavity. The nasopharynx lies above the oropharynx, separated by a horizontal line drawn along the hard and soft palates. Both nasopharynx and oropharynx are collectively known as the visceral space, using the space's nomenclature. A visceral fascia surrounds the visceral space. Most pathologies of the visceral space are processes involving the epithelial lining of the pharynx. The most common malignancy in this space is the SCCA. The imaging methods are usually unable to differentiate between SCCA and other malignancies; therefore, the primary role of imaging is accurate tumor mapping. A noninfiltrating, homogeneously enhancing mass located on the posterior mucosal surface of the nasopharynx may be either a low-grade tumor or a prominent adenoidal tissue, and clinical correlation should be requested.

The PPS, which extends from the skull base to the level of the greater cornu of the hyoid bone, is next to the pharynx. Actually this space is divided by the tensor-styloid-vascular fascia into prestyloid and poststyloid compartments. This fascia extending from the styloid process to the tensor veli palatini muscle and crosses posteriorly in the PPS fat. Prestyloid PPS may also be referred to as the PPS in practice (true PPS). The space posterior to this fascia should be referred to as the carotid sheath (carotid space). The displacement pattern of the PPS fat indicates the possible space of origin of a lesion and helps limit the differential diagnosis based on the contents of that space. Adipose tissue is the primary content of the PPS. Other contents are arteries, veins, and minor salivary gland rests. Primary lesions of the PPS are rare, although lipoma or minor salivary gland

tumors can occur. PPS tumors generally present as asymptomatic masses [26]. Eighty percent of PPS tumors are benign, and 20% are malignant [26]. Paragangliomas that involve the PPS originate from either the vagal (glomus vagale tumor) or the carotid bodies (glomus caroticum or carotid body tumor). They are characteristically hypervascular in nature and show early enhancement in the arterial phase, and early washout in dynamic examination (hypervascular mass) (Figure 7.20). Schwannoma also occurs in similar locations; however, enhancement may result from the progressive extravascular accumulation of contrast material (hypovascular mass). Dynamic scans must be obtained during the vascular filling phase for differentiation of a hypervascular and a hypovascular mass. This occurs within 10–20 seconds after contrast administration. After this time, the contrast is in an equilibration phase in both vascular and hypovascular lesions, and any distinction between the modes of contrast accumulation is impossible. Hypovascular lesions have a slow contrast filling, and a prolonged washout phase because of a paucity of veins. For this reason dynamic CT evaluation should be used instead of routine contrast-enhanced CT scans to critically assess lesion vascularity. Pleomorphic adenomas of the PPS generally originate from the deep lobe of the parotid gland, but can also occur from the extraparotid minor salivary gland or ectopic salivary tissue (Figure 7.21). This tumor is differentiated from the neurogenic tumors by displacement of the PPS fat and the confirmation of its prestyloid compartment in location.

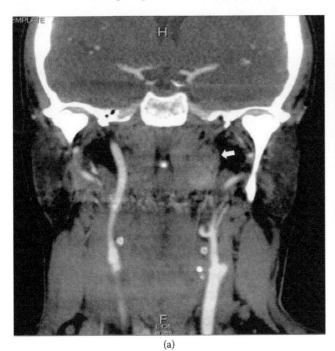
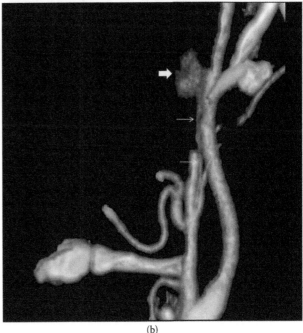

(a) (b)

FIGURE 7.20
Coronal CT angiogram and volume-rendered image. Maximum intensity projection CT scan (a) from a dynamic series shows the tumor vascularity in the early phase, and volume-rendered images (b) (thick arrow). Note the feeding artery (thin arrows).

Masticator space (MS) is enclosed by the split layers of the superficial layer of the deep cervical fascia (SLDCF). It extends from the skull base to the inferior border of the mandible. Infections and inflammatory lesions are the most common lesions arising in this location. Since inflammation and abscess originating from dental infection and osteomyelitis are more easily identified on CT compared to MRI, CT should be the initial modality of choice for the evaluation of infections or inflammatory lesions of the MS. In a case of tumor invasion of the MS places, the branches of V3 are at risk for perineural spread, which is a particular feature with some tumors, such as adenoid cystic carcinoma. Tumor invading the muscles of the MS may cause trismus. Lymphoma is an exception to this rule [27].

Parotid space (PS) contains the parotid gland, and the facial nerve that divides the parotid into a superficial and deep lobe. The SLDCF splits to enclose the PS. The parotid gland and lymph nodes are the structures that may give rise to pathology within the PS. The parotid gland is the only salivary gland that has lymph nodes within its capsule. Neither CT nor MRI can differentiate benign from malignant disease with certainty. Most parotid masses are benign (80%) and most of these are pleomorphic adenomas (benign mixed cell tumors). The space, in which the submandibular gland is located, is limited above by the mucosa in the floor of the mouth and caudally by the SLDCF as it extends from the hyoid

bone to the mandible. Submandibular gland stones constitute between 80% and 90% of all salivary gland stones and are easily diagnosed by CT. Noncontrast CT is required for the detection of parotid and submandibular gland stones (Figure 7.22).

Retropharyngeal space is also known as retrovisceral space. This is a potential space that lies posterior to the pharyngeal constrictor muscles and upper esophagus. More specifically, in its upper regions, this space lies between the buccopharyngeal fascia anteriorly, and the alar fascia posteriorly. On either side, the cloison sagittale separates the retropharyngeal space from the more laterally positioned PPS. It extends from the skull base below between the sixth cervical and fourth thoracic vertebrae, where the alar fascia fuses with the visceral fascia. This space serves as a potential conduit for the spread of tumor or infection from the pharynx to the mediastinum. Most of the pathologies, which arise from this space, are metastatic adenopathy, lymphoma, or abscess/cellulitis.

Prevertebral space is a potential space that exists between the prevertebral fascia and the vertebrae, extending from skull base to the coccyx.

Grodinsky and Holyoke [28] described the danger space as lying between the alar fascia ventrally and the prevertebral fascia dorsally. This space extends from the skull base to the posterior mediastinum to the level just

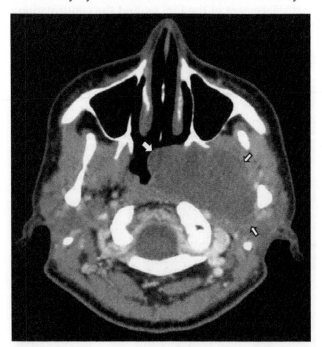

FIGURE 7.21
Axial contrast-enhanced CT scan shows a huge pleomorphic adenoma into the prestyloid compartment of the left parapharyngeal space (open arrows). The mass has displayed the pharyngeal wall medially (thick arrow). This was an extraparotid pleomorphic adenoma arising from minor salivary gland rest cells.

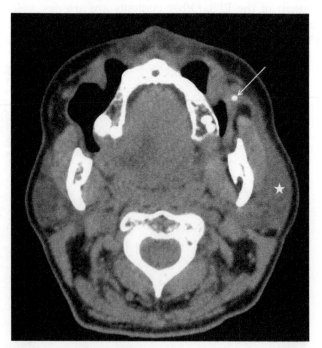

FIGURE 7.22
Non-enhanced puffed-cheeks axial CT scan. To eliminate artifacts related to the dental restoration material, scan is obtained with the head in hyperflexion. A small sialolith (arrow) can be visualized in the left distal Stensen's duct. In this technique, the distance to the ductal orifice can be measured easily. Note the increased density in the left parotid consistent with sialadenitis (star).

above the diaphragm, where the fused alar and visceral fascia, in turn, fuse with the prevertebral fascia.

Below the hard palate lie the oral cavity and oropharynx. These two areas are divided by a ring of structures. These include the circumvallate papillae (located along the posterior aspect of the tongue), tonsillar pillars, and the soft palate. Traditional compartments of oral cavity are important for describing the spread of superficial mucosal-based lesions. When evaluating a patient with pathology in the mucosal superficial space, it is important to determine within which space the pathology lies (e.g., buccal, gingival, palatal, retromolar, lingual, and sublingual). Lesions originating from the superficial mucosal space may invade deep to the mucosal space. These lesions may show transspatial extention resulting in poor prognosis. The oral cavity tumors can easily be assessed by inspection and palpation; however, these malignancies can be overlooked until they grow large. Puffed-cheek technique is radiologically very useful in demonstrating the presence of gingivobuccal/gingivolabial lesions and its extensions.

Oral cavity contains the anterior two-thirds of the tongue, the mouth floor, mandibular and maxillary alveolus, hard palate, lips, and cheeks [29]. It is located in the anterior of the soft palate, anterior tonsillar pillars, and the circumvallate papilla of the tongue [29]. CT has important limitations in patients with oral cavity tumors. Oral vestibula separates teeth and gingival mucosa from the cheek in the posterior and from the lip mucosa in the anterior. In neutral position, the buccal and gingival mucosa are in contact and difficult to differentiate with conventional CT scan. Small mucosa tumors can be overlooked. Evaluation of which mucosa surface the tumor originates from and whether the opposite side mucosa was invaded can be difficult because of the contact of these mucosa. Amalgam artifacts due to dental occlusal restorations in most adult patients make it more difficult for the radiologist. Visual inspection and bimanual palpation are the main issues in the diagnosis of these lesions [30]. CT and MRI are used as complementary to clinical examination for the assessment of deep tissue invasion and the demonstration of metastatic lymph nodes [31–35]. Puffed-cheek CT is a new imaging technique for evaluation of oral vestibular pathologies. The problem gingivobuccal tumors create for the radiologist can be overcome with the puffed-cheek maneuver (Figure 7.23). Puffed-cheek CT allows a better and more detailed assessment compared to the conventional (nonpuffed) examination in mucosal disease of the oral cavity.

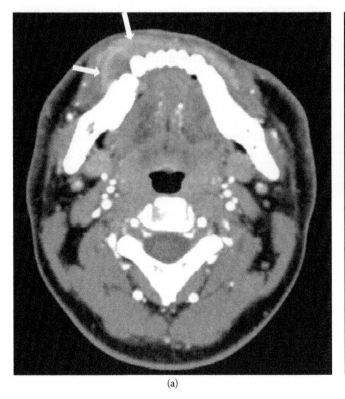

(a)

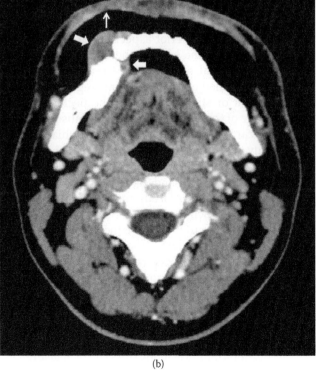

(b)

FIGURE 7.23
Contrast-enhanced axial CT images. Gingivobuccal mass (double arrows) originating from the mandibular gingiva. Although the mass can be identified on the images obtained during a routine scan (a), it is not possible to determine that labial mucosa is attached or not. On images obtained with the puffed-cheek technique (b), the tumor is seen to originate from the right gingival mucosa with invasion both labial and lingual sides (thick arrows). Labial mucosa is intact (small arrow).

The term ranula refers to an epithelial-lined retention cyst that occurs primarily within the sublingual space above the mylohyoid muscle (simple form). It is usually a consequence of prior trauma or inflammation. Diving or plunging ranula is a mucocele that develops from the rupture of the wall of a simple ranula. Therefore, the simple ranula is a true cyst that has an epithelial lining; however, the diving ranula is a pseudocyst. Its wall has both epithelium and inflammatory elements and it usually extends below the mylohyoid muscle. On CT, ranula is shown as simple fluid containing lesions centered in the sublingual space, with or without extension to the submandibular space, and without associated enhancing component. If the cyst has become infected, the cyst wall enhances and becomes thicker.

Embryologic anomalies of the branchial (pharyngeal) arches manifest as cysts, fistulae, and sinuses, either external or internal. Most authors think that branchial cleft cysts result from incomplete obliteration of the epithelial-lined cervical sinus. The branchial anomalies are classified as first, second, third, and fourth, according to their proposed pouch, or cleft of origin. The first branchial cleft anomalies are periauricular or periparotid thin-wall cystic lesion. Patients typically present in young ages, with parotid swelling and fewer. The second branchial cleft anomalies account more than 95% of all branchial disorders [36,37] and cysts are far more common than sinuses or fistulas. The typical presentation is a thin-walled, low attenuation cystic mass that is located along the anterior aspect of the sternocleidomastoid muscle, at the level of the carotid bifurcation. The third branchial anomalies are rare. On imaging, the cyst is identified either in the same region as second branchial cyst or slightly lower in the neck along the anterior edge of the sternocleidomastoid muscle and lateral to the carotid sheath. The fourth branchial anomalies are only a few documented anomalies. On imaging, they usually appear as solitary, often infected cysts, just anterior to the thyroid gland, usually on the left side. A fourth branchial pouch cyst adjacent to the larynx, like a third branchial pouch cyst, must be differentiated from a laryngocele or saccular cyst (see the larynx).

Lymphatic malformations, also known as lymphangiomas or cystic hygromas, are very important for the differential diagnosis of congenital or developmental cystic masses in the neck, usually in the posterior cervical space. They can be unilocular or multilocular. Presence of fat density within the cyst suggests dermoid, which is also in the differential diagnosis.

Arteriovenous malformations (AVMs) are developmental malformations of the vascular system that result in the abnormal communication between arteries and veins. They are characterized by a tangle of enhancing serpiginous vessels that are not associated with a surrounding soft-tissue mass. They are believed to be of congenital origin and are usually discovered in childhood. Diagnosis is made clinically by noting a soft fullness in the lower neck. That is most prominent when the patient is supine, or phonates in the erect position, and then disappears when the patient is erect and breathes normally.

7.7 Infrahyoid Neck

Imaging plays an important role in the management of neck disease and CT is the method of reference. As a rule, the examination should completely cover the entire head and neck region because diseases located in the neck can extend or disseminate from the suprahyoid neck, or be caused by a process in this region. Therefore, the scanning area should extend from the skull base (EAC) to the thoracic inlet (superior aspect of the manubrium).

Thyroglossal duct cysts are common congenital abnormalities or developmental cystic lesions. They are usually located in the midline anterior neck. They can occur anywhere along the course of the thyroglossal duct, between the foramen cecum and thyroid, and are often seen around the level of the hyoid. The CT findings show a unilocular or multilocular cystic mass with peripheral enhancement. Recurrent infection or hemorrhage may increase the attenuation of the cystic component, and cause thickening of the enhancing rim. Normally, there should be no solid enhancing component of a thyroglossal duct cyst. The presence of an intracystic solid enhancing mass may represent residual thyroid tissue. A coexisting papillary carcinoma should be suspected with this finding and it should be conveyed to the referring physician. The typical cyst is deep into or embedded in the infrahyoid strap muscles.

Dermoid or epidermoid cysts are located superficial to the strap muscle. Differentiation of a dermoid and epidermoid is often difficult by imaging; however, the presence of fat strongly suggests a dermoid.

Involvement of the Delpian node (prelaryngeal lymph node) can be as a result of diffuse nodal involvement in SCC, or in isolation from direct lymphatic spread of laryngeal cancer through the anterior commissure. Thyroid carcinomas may also involve this node.

7.7.1 Larynx and Hypopharynx

The diagnostic evaluation of the larynx and hypopharynx is primarily done with endoscopy. However, cross-sectional imaging also plays an inevitable complementary role, because it enables one to evaluate the deep structures of the larynx. The laryngoscopic visualization of the laryngeal ventricle, the subglottic region, and the hypopharynx is restricted. Clinical suspicion of submucosal spread or lesion extension into deeper tissues requires radiological imaging.

The region of the true cords, false cords, and intervening ventricle is particularly important in organizing the anatomy of the larynx (Figure 7.24). A small recess at the level of the false cord, projects superiorly from the anterior laryngeal ventricle into the paraglottic fat. This recess is called the laryngeal saccule or appendix. It lies between the quadrangular membrane and the thyroid cartilage. Dilatation of the saccule causes a supraglottic cyst called a laryngocele.

Radiological methods have difficulties in detailed identification of normal laryngeal anatomic structures because of the small size and mobility of this organ. In this regard, certain respiratory maneuvers have been used extensively during laryngeal MDCT to enable much better visualization of the larynx [38]. MDCT scanners have enabled us to capture the dynamic changes in the vocal cords during phonation, inspiration, or expiration.

Use of the Valsalva and modified Valsalva maneuvers, phonation, and inspiration has been described for radiographic studies and has been adopted in sectional imaging with advances in technology [39–41].

The larynx is the second most common site of head and neck cancer, and laryngeal tumors are the eleventh most common form of cancer among men worldwide [42].

Nearly, all laryngeal malignancies (>90%) are SCCAs [43]. Carcinoma of the larynx arises in the supraglottic region (30%), glottis (65%), or subglottic region (5%) [43]. Tumors of the true cords usually present at a fairly early stage unlike the supraglottic region, because they interfere with normal vocalization [44].

When performing cross-sectional imaging for a laryngeal or hypopharyngeal tumor, these questions should be answered: Does the tumor invade the supraglottis, glottis, subglottis, pyriform sinus, retrocricoarytenoid region, or posterior pharyngeal wall? Is there invasion of the paraglottic space or preepiglottic space? Is there cartilage invasion or invasion of the soft tissue of the neck? The term transglottic carcinoma generally refers to tumors that involve both the glottis and supraglottis at the time of diagnosis.

A variety of benign and malignant tumors of nonsquamous cell origin may occur in the larynx and hypopharynx [45,46]. These tumors are rare as they are less than 5% of all tumors of this region. The majority of non-neoplastic diseases do not require imaging. However, CT is useful in some situations, such as the delineation of abscess formation in inflammatory conditions and the evaluation of the extent of laryngeal fractures caused by severe blunt trauma.

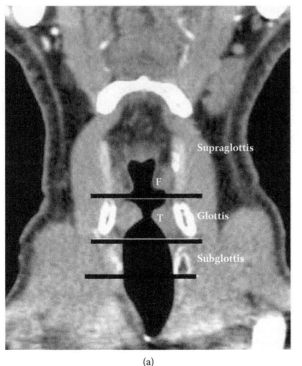

(a)

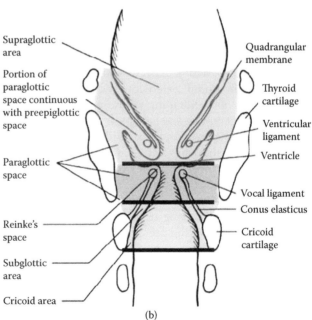

(b)

FIGURE 7.24

Normal laryngeal anatomy. Coronal contrast-enhanced CT scan (a) and schematic representation (b). Black lines determine the laryngeal regions. Supraglottis, green area; glottis, pink area; subglottis, blue area. F, false cords; T, true cords.

7.8 Lymph Nodes

The lymphatic system consists of a number of nodes, mucosa-associated lymphoid tissue (Waldeyer's ring in the head and neck), the spleen, and the thymus. Waldeyer's ring connects the nasopharyngeal adenoids, the palatine tonsils, and the lingual tonsils. Efferent lymphatic vessels carry lymph from peripheral lymph nodes and eventually, via the thoracic duct on the left side and the right lymphatic duct, to the blood through the great veins in the root of the neck.

Even if a hyperplastic or reactive cervical node has a normal imaging appearance, a variety of diseases may still have affected it. In most of these cases, the precise pathology may not be predicted on imaging. It is the pathologist who determines the diagnosis in the final analysis. On imaging, the assessment of size criteria and nodal architecture are used to evaluate SCCA metastasis. Metastases should be considered in a patient with primary malignancy, if the lymph node exceeds 1.5 cm in level II, or 1 cm in anywhere else in the neck. If the lymph node has a low density in its center, this is considered as abnormal, regardless of the size of the node. Such a metastatic node will classically be enlarged, have central tumor necrosis, and have extracapsular tumor spread. However, even when all of these imaging criteria are present, the histology may still reveal some form of lymphoma or infectious process [47]. It must always be remembered that in patient with a head and neck tumor, hyperplastic-appearing lymph nodes may still contain microscopic metastases. This highlights a persistent limitation of clinical and radiographic evaluation.

When a primary neoplasm of the head and neck is detected, it is vital to assess the lymph nodes for tumor staging. The presence of a single ipsilateral malignant node reduces the patient's expected survival by 50%. An extracapsular nodal extension reduces survival by an additional 50%. Mapping of the primary upper aerodigestive tract tumor site is critical to the imaging study, in the evaluation of a patient with cervical nodal metastasis. The relationship between various primary sites and the location and frequency of cervical metastasis has been well studied [48,49] (Table 7.4).

Nasopharyngeal carcinoma is one of the few head and neck primary tumors having no relationship between primary tumor size and the presence of nodal disease. In other words, a large tumor may have no nodal metastasis, whereas small tumors may present with diffuse, bilateral cervical metastases.

Nasopharyngeal carcinoma and thyroid carcinoma are two primary head and neck tumors that their distribution of nodal metastases and the prognosis associated with such regional metastases are sufficiently different from those of the other.

TABLE 7.4

Head and Neck Primary Tumor Sites and Their Correlation with Cervical Nodal Metastasis

Primary Site	Common Nodal Levels	Nodes (%)	Bilateral Nodes (%)
Oral tongue	I, II, III	34–65	11.8
Floor of the mouth	I, II	30–59	7.8
Retromolar trigone			
Anterior tonsillar pillar	I, II, III	39–56	8.8
Soft palate	II	37–56	25.0
Nasopharynx	II, III, IV, V (22.3%)	86–90	32.8
Oropharynx	II, III, V (10.9%)	50–71	20.2
Tonsillar fossa	I, II, III, IV, V (9%)	58–76	13.0
Hypopharynx	II, III, IV, V (8.4%)	52–72	9.0
Base of the tongue	II, III, IV, V (6.7%)	50–83	21.3
Supraglottic larynx	II, III, IV	31–54	22.5

The number and the specific chains of lymph nodes involved may also suggest a diagnosis. Diffuse nodal disease suggests a systemic process such as infectious mononucleosis, acquired immune deficiency syndrome, sarcoidosis, or lymphoma, especially if suboccipital nodes are involved. Unilateral involvement of lymph nodes is less specific. They can be found in many diseases including metastatic carcinoma, lymphoma, tuberculosis, and a variety of local infections. Nodes found in the infraomohyoid neck, without supraomohyoid nodes, suggest that the source of the nodes lies in the thyroid, in the cervical esophagus, or in a primary tumor caudal to the clavicles, most often in the lung or breast.

Lymph nodes with tuberculous involvement show multiple rim-enhancing cystic masses in the neck (Figure 7.25), particularly in the posterior triangle. Necrotic metastases (most often from SCCA or papillary thyroid carcinoma) and intranodal necrosis or abscess from bacterial infection always should be considered as a differential diagnosis.

In 1999, addressing specific issues raised in both the American Joint Committee on Cancer and the American Academy of Autolaryngology-Head and Neck Surgery classifications, and bringing the anatomic detail and reproducibility of imaging to nodal classification were suggested [50]. The classification can be applied to either the clinical examination or the imaging studies using landmarks readily identified with either. This is not meant to replace the clinical assessment. It is recommended rather to allow clinicians and radiologists to use the same system.

A consistent scanning technique must be used to provide reproducible nodal levels, when the imaging-based classification is used. Such consistency includes patient positioning and gantry angulation for CT scan.

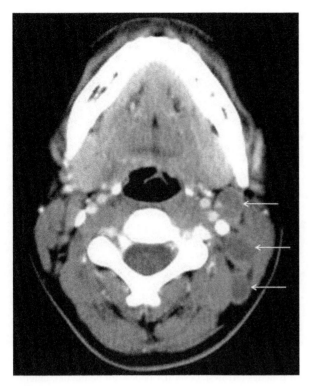

FIGURE 7.25
Axial contrast-enhanced CT shows multiple rim-enhancing cervical lymph nodes with central necrosis on the left side (arrows) in a patient with tuberculosis.

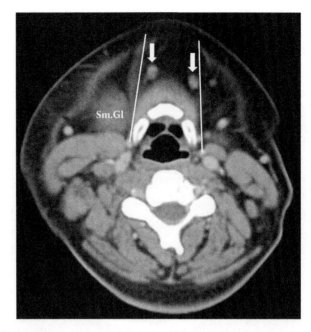

FIGURE 7.26
Level IA lymph nodes (arrows). The medial edge of the anterior belly of the digastrics muscle (dm) separates levels IA and IB. The line represents the border. Sm.Gl = Submandibular gland.

There is no single method of performing CT of the neck. However, the following technique is used by many head and neck radiologists and slight variations from this approach do not change the nodal levels. The axial plane referred to in this classification is obtained with the patient's head in a comfortable neutral position with the hard palate perpendicular to the tabletop and the shoulders down as far as possible. The scanner gantry is aligned along the inferior orbitomeatal plane and, if possible, the examination is performed with the administration of intravenous contrast material to allow the best possible differentiation of nodes from vessels. The recommended field of view is 16 × 18 cm. The CT examination is performed as contiguous 3 mm scans from the skull base to the manubrium or as a helical study reconstructed as contiguous 2 or 3 mm slices. The helical technique uses 3 mm thick scans with a 3 mm gap and a pitch of 1:1.

7.8.1 The Imaging-Based Classification

This classification was designed to be easily and readily usable. Each side of the neck should be evaluated separately.

Level I includes all nodes above the hyoid bone, below the mylohyoid muscle, and anterior to a transverse line drawn on each axial image through the posterior edge of the submandibular gland. Thus, level I nodes include the previously classified submental and submandibular nodes. They can be subclassified into levels IA and IB.

Level IA includes the nodes that lie between the medial margins of the anterior bellies of the digastric muscles, above the hyoid bone, and below the mylohyoid muscle (previously classified as submental nodes) (Figure 7.26).

Level IB includes the nodes that lie below the mylohyoid muscle, above the hyoid bone, posterior and lateral to the medial edge of the anterior belly of the digastric muscle, and anterior to a transverse line drawn on each axial image tangent to the posterior surface of the submandibular gland on each side of the neck (previously classified as submandibular nodes) (Figure 7.27).

Level II extends from the skull base, at the lower level of the bony margin of the jugular fossa, to the level of the lower body of the hyoid bone. Level II nodes are present anterior to a transverse line drawn on each axial image through the posterior edge of the sternocleidomastoid muscle and lie posterior to a transverse line drawn on each axial scan through the posterior edge of the submandibular gland. A node present within 2 cm of the skull base located anterior, lateral, or posterior to the carotid sheath, is classified as a level II node. If the node is located medial to the ICA, it is classified as a retropharyngeal node. Caudal to 2 cm below

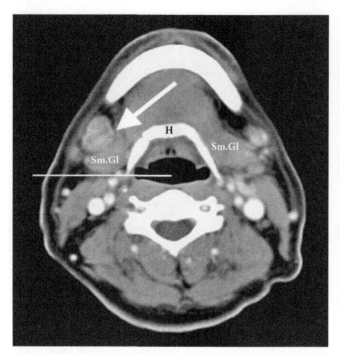

FIGURE 7.27
Level IB lymph nodes (arrow). The dorsal edge of the submandibular gland (Sm.Gl) separates levels I and II.

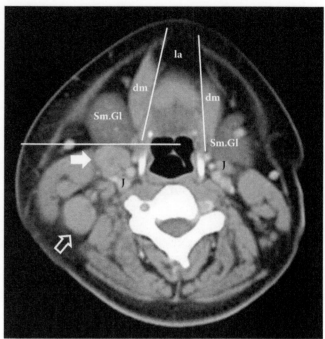

FIGURE 7.28
Level II nodes (arrows). Level IIA nodes can be medial, anterior, or lateral to the vein (thick arrow). Level IIB nodes are posterior to the jugular vein and are not touching the vein (open arrow). Sm.Gl, submandibular gland; dm, digastrics muscle.

the skull base, level II nodes can be located anterior, lateral, medial, and posterior to the internal jugular vein. Level II nodes can be subclassified into levels IIA and IIB (Figure 7.28).

Level IIA nodes are level II nodes those are located posterior to the internal jugular vein and are inseparable from the vein or that are located anterior, lateral, or medial to the vein (previously classified as upper internal jugular nodes).

Level IIB nodes are level II nodes (previously classified as upper spinal accessory nodes) those are located posterior to the internal jugular vein and have a fat plane separating the nodes and the vein.

Level III nodes are located between the level of the lower body of the hyoid bone and the level of the lower margin of the cricoid cartilage arch. These nodes are located anterior to a transverse line drawn on each axial image through the posterior edge of the sterno-cleidomastoid muscle. Level III nodes are also found lateral to the medial margin of either the common carotid artery or the ICA. On each side of the neck, the medial margins of these arteries separate level III (lateral) nodes from level VI (medial) nodes. Level III nodes were previously known as the mid jugular nodes (Figure 7.29).

Level IV nodes are located between the level of the lower margin of the cricoid cartilage arch and the level of the clavicle on each side as seen on each axial scan. These nodes lie anterior and medial to an oblique line

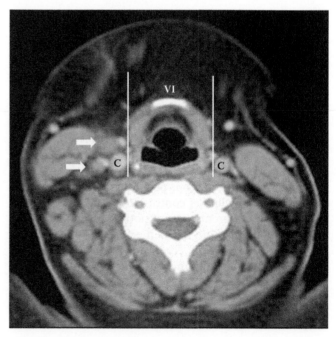

FIGURE 7.29
Level III nodes are also known as middle jugular nodes (arrows).

drawn through the posterior edge of the sternocleidomastoid muscle and the posterolateral edge of the anterior scalene muscle on each axial image. The medial aspect of the common carotid artery is the landmark

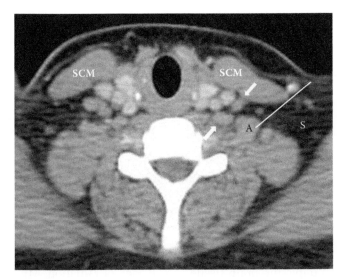

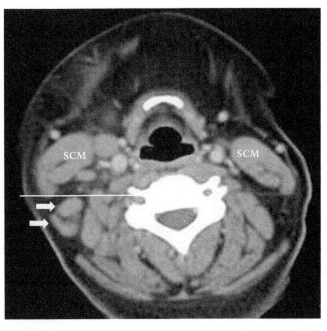

FIGURE 7.30
Level IV nodes are also known as inferior jugular nodes (arrows). A, anterior scalene muscle; S, supraclavicular fossa; SCM, sterno-cleidomastoid muscle. Below the bottom of the hyoid, the line passing through the medial border of the carotid arteries separates level IV nodes from VI. (Courtesy of Dr. Nezahat Erdoğan and Dr. Eşref Kızılkaya.)

FIGURE 7.31
Level V nodes (arrows). The back edge of the sternocleidomastoid muscle separates levels II, III, and IV from level V. (Courtesy of Dr. Nezahat Erdoğan and Dr. Eşref Kızılkaya.)

that separates level IV nodes (lateral to this artery) from level VI nodes (medial to this artery). Level IV nodes were previously known as the low jugular nodes (Figure 7.30).

Level V nodes extend from the skull base, at the posterior border of the attachment of the sternocleidomastoid muscle, to the level of the clavicle as seen on each axial scan. Level V nodes are all located anterior to a transverse line drawn on each axial scan, through the anterior edge of the trapezius muscle. Between the levels of the skull base and the bottom of the cricoid arch, these nodes are situated posterior to a transverse line drawn on each axial scan through the posterior edge of the sternocleidomastoid muscle (Figure 7.31). Between the axial level of the bottom of the cricoid arch and the level of the clavicle, level V nodes lie posterior and lateral to an oblique line through the posterior edge of the sternocleidomastoid muscle and the posterolateral edge of the anterior scalene muscle. Level V nodes can be subdivided into VA and VB nodes.

Level VA (upper level V) nodes are located between the skull base and the level of the lower margin of the cricoid cartilage arch, behind the posterior edge of the sternocleidomastoid muscle.

Level VB (lower level V) nodes are located on each side between the level of the lower margin of the cricoid cartilage arch and the level of the clavicle as seen on each axial scan. They are behind an oblique line through the posterior edge of the sternocleidomastoid muscle and the posterolateral edge of the anterior scalene muscle.

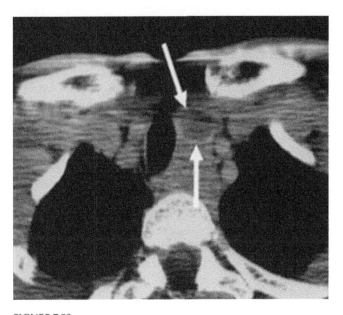

FIGURE 7.32
Level VI nodes (arrows). The upper border of the manubrium separates levels VI and VII. (Courtesy of Dr. Nezahat Erdoğan and Dr. Eşref Kızılkaya.)

Level VI nodes are located inferior to the lower body of the hyoid bone, superior to the top of the manubrium, and between the medial margins of the left and right common carotid arteries or the ICAs. They are the visceral nodes (Figure 7.32).

Level VII nodes are located caudal to the top of the manubrium in the superior mediastinum, between the medial margins of the left and right common carotid arteries. These superior mediastinal nodes extend caudally to the level of the innominate vein.

Supraclavicular nodes are located at or caudal to the level of the clavicle and lateral to the carotid artery on each side of the neck, as seen on each axial scan.

Retropharyngeal nodes are the nodes within 2 cm caudal to the skull base. They are located medial to the ICAs.

7.9 Dynamic Maneuvers in Head and Neck

Despite advances in technology, there may still be difficulties in the radiological assessment of certain head and neck lesions. These difficulties arise because of the complex anatomy of this region, the small and mobile structures it contains, and the apposition of mucosal surfaces in the neutral position. Certain maneuvers have been described in literature to overcome these difficulties [41,51]. We review the use of the puffed-cheek technique, phonation and inspiration, the Valsalva, and the modified Valsalva maneuver, with possible applications in head and neck imaging.

Puffed-cheek CT is a new imaging technique for evaluating oral vestibular pathologies. The patient is asked to close the mouth and fully puff the cheeks. The entire oral cavity, from the hard palate to the mandible, is scanned with a continuous spiral scan, following contrast material administration. By puffing the cheeks, the oral vestibule is filled with air, which by creating a negative contrast separates the buccal and labial mucosas from the gingival mucosa. This allows both mucosal surfaces to be assessed separately. The buccinator muscle, the pterygomandibular raphe, and the retromolar trigone can be better delineated. Assessment of loss of mucosal pliability because of the accompanying submucosal fibrosis, which is commonly observed in oral cavity cancers, is also facilitated. Puffed-cheek CT allows a better and more detailed assessment of the gingivobuccal tumors compared to the conventional (nonpuffed) CT examination.

Patients with laryngeal neoplasm usually have difficulty during the time required for MR scanning because of breathing problems. However, with today's faster imaging, examination in different respiratory phases is now possible. If the precise tumor localization and borders are vague, and the true and false cords cannot be accurately distinguished in a laryngeal CT scan done during superficial respiration or apnea, the examination is indicated to be repeated during inspiration and by applying phonation maneuver to the patient. Problems in precise documentation of the tumor borders of vocal cord tumors can be overcome via multiphase larynx

examination done by applying inspiration, "i" phonation, and Valsalva's maneuvers [41].

Because the varix may be completely collapsed or barely visible when the patient is lying supine, any time an orbital varix is suspected, obtaining additional CT sections during Valsalva's maneuver is recommended.

CSF leakage occurs as a result of communication of the subarachnoid space with the extracranial regions, in the presence of an osseous and dural defect in the skull base. Most cases are posttraumatic, with iatrogenic cases due to previous otorhinolaryngological or neurosurgical procedures being common [52]. Plain, thin-section coronal CT scans are generally used to show bony defects. The site of CSF leakage can be identified via MRI or CT cisternography; however, because of the superior geometrical resolution of MR imaging in depicting brain tissue and its lack of radiation, MRI cisternography is usually the method of choice. For CT cisternography, approximately 3–10 mL of nonionic low-osmolar contrast material and, for MRI cisternography, 0.5–1 mL of gadopentate-based contrast material diluted with 4 mL saline are administered intrathecally by lumbar puncture. The patient is kept in the Trendelenburg position until the contrast material reaches the basal cisterns. In cases of slow flow rhinorrhea, cisternography is carried out after provocative maneuvers, such as sneezing or the Valsalva maneuver. These maneuvers should not be used in conditions with increased intracranial pressure, such as trauma or an intracranial mass. The demonstration of contrast material in the sinonasal cavities or the middle ear, together with the presence of a skull base defect, is diagnostic.

Modified Valsalva's maneuver is different from Valsalva's maneuver. It was first described by Jonsson as "a method of examination of the hypopharynx and the upper passage way" in 1934 [53]. Expiration is forced not against the closed glottis but against the resistance of the closed nose and mouth cavities. The major effects of the modified Valsalva maneuver are to open the rosenmuller fossa and to distend the laryngeal ventricule and priform sinuses [51].

References

1. Baum U, Greess H, Lell M, Nömayr A, Lenz M. Imaging of head and neck tumors—methods: CT, spiral-CT, multislice-spiral-CT. *Eur J Radiol* 2000; 33(3): 153–160.
2. Rydberg J, Buckwalter KA, Caldemeyer KS et al. Multisection CT: Scanning techniques and clinical applications. *Radiographics* 2000; 20: 1787–1806.
3. Blum A, Walter F, Ludig T, Zhu X, Roland J. Multislice CT: Principles and new CT-scan applications. *J Radiol* 2000; 81: 1597–1614.

4. DelGaudio JM, Hudgins PA, Venkatraman G, Beningfield A. Multiplanar computed tomographic analysis of frontal recess cells: Effect on frontal isthmus size and frontal sinusitis. *Arch Otolaryngol Head Neck Surg* 2005; 131(3): 230–235.

5. Bolger WE, Butzin CA, Parsons DS. Paranasal sinus bony anatomic variations and mucosal abnormalities: CT analysis for endoscopic sinus surgery. *Laryngoscope* 1991; 101(1 Pt 1): 56–64.

6. Zinreich SJ, Mattox DE, Kennedy DW, Chisholm HL, Diffley DM, Rosenbaum AE. Concha bullosa: CT evaluation. *J Comput Assist Tomogr* 1988; 12(5): 778–784.

7. Stammberger HR, Kennedy DW. Paranasal sinuses: Anatomic terminology and nomenclature. The anatomic terminology group. *Ann Otol Rhinol Laryngol Suppl* 1995; 167: 7–16.

8. Perugini S, Pasquini U, Menichelli F et al. Mucoceles in the paranasal sinuses involving the orbit: CT signs in 43 cases. *Neuroradiology* 1982; 23(3): 133–139.

9. Waitzman AA, Birt BD. Fungal sinusitis. *J Otolaryngol* 1994; 23(4): 244–249.

10. Silverman CS, Mancuso AA. Periantral soft-tissue infiltration and its relevance to the early detection of invasive fungal sinusitis: CT and MR findings. *Am J Neuroradiol* 1998; 19(2): 321–325.

11. Stringer SP, Ryan MW. Chronic invasive fungal rinosinusitis. *Otolaryngol Clin Nort Am* 2000; 33(2): 375–387.

12. Sarti EJ, Blaugrund SM, Lin PT, Camins MB. Paranasal sinus disease with intracranial extension: Aspergillosis versus malignancy. *Laryngoscope* 1988; 98(6 Pt 1): 632–635.

13. Som PM, Brandwein MS. Tumors and tumor-like conditions. In: Som PM, Curtin HD, eds. *Head and Neck Imaging*. 4th ed. St. Louis, MO: Mosby; 2003:261–373.

14. Lustrin ES, Robertson RL, Tilak S. Normal anatomy of the skull base. *Neuroimaging Clin N Am* 1994; 4(3): 465–478.

15. Caro PA, Mahboubi S, Faerber EN. Computed tomography in the diagnosis of lymphangiomas in infants and children. *Clin Imaging* 1991; 15(1): 41–46.

16. Wright JE, Sullivan TJ, Garner A, Wulc AE, Moseley IF. Orbital venous anomalies. *Ophthalmology* 1997; 104: 905–913.

17. Wright JE. Orbital vascular anomalies. *Trans Am Acad Ophthalmol Otolaryngol* 1974; 78: OP606–OP616.

18. Lacey B, Rootman J, Marotta TR. Distensible venous malformations of the orbit: Clinical and hemodynamic features and a new technique of management. *Ophthalmology* 1999; 106: 1197–1209.

19. Shields JA. *Diagnosis and Management of Orbital Tumors*. Philadelphia, PA: WB Saunders; 1989:140–143.

20. Weber AL, Vitale RL, Sabates NR. Pseudotumor of the orbit. Clinical, pathologic and radiologic evaluation. *Radiol Clin North Am* 1999; 37: 151–168.

21. Swartz JD, Harnsberger HR, Mukherji SK. The temporal bone. Contemporary diagnostic dilemmas. *Radiol Clin North Am* 1998; 36(5): 819–853.

22. Swartz JD, Harnsberger HR (eds). *Imaging of the Temporal Bone*. 3rd ed. New York, NY: Thieme Medical Publishers; 1998.

23. Lasjaunias P, Moret J, Manelfe C, Théron J, Hasso T, Seeger J. Arterial anomalies at the base of the skull. *Neuroradiology* 1977; 13: 267–272.

24. Moreano EH, Paparella MM, Zelterman D, Goycoolea MV. Prevalence of facial canal dehiscence and of persistent stapedial artery in the human middle ear: A report of 1000 temporal bones. *Laryngoscope* 1994; 104: 309–320.

25. Celebi I, Oz A, Yildirim H. A case of an aberrant internal carotid artery with a persistent stapedial artery: Association of hypoplasia of the A1 segment of the anterior cerebral artery. *Surg Radiol Anat* 2011; 34(7): 665–670.

26. Olsen KD. Tumors and surgery of the parapharyngeal space. *Laryngoscope* 1994; 104(5 Pt 2 Suppl 63): 1–28.

27. Stambuk HE, Patel SG. Imaging of the parapharyngeal space. *Otolaryngol Clin N Am* 2008; 41: 77–101.

28. Grodinsky M, Holyoke E. The fasciae and fascial spaces of the head, neck and adjacent regions. *Am J Anat* 1938; 63: 367–408.

29. American Joint Committee on Cancer. Lip and oral cavity. In: Greene FL, ed. *AJCC Cancer Staging Manual*. 7th ed. New York, NY: Springer; 2010:29–35.

30. Sharma PK, Schüller DE, Baker SR. Malignant neoplasms of the oral cavity. In: Cummings CW, Fredrickson MJ, Harker LA, Krause CJ, Richardson MA, Schuller DE, eds. *Otolaryngology: Head and Neck Surgery*. 3rd ed. St Louis, MO: Mosby CD online (CD-ROM); 1999.

31. Alvi A, Myers EN, Johnson JT. Cancer of the oral cavity. In: Myers EN, Suen JY, eds. *Cancer of the Head and Neck*. 2nd ed. Philadelphia, PA: Saunders; 1996:321–361.

32. Thabet HM, Sessions DG, Gado MH, Gnepp DA, Harvey JE, Talaat M. Comparison of clinical evaluation and computed tomographic diagnostic accuracy for tumors of the larynx and hypopharynx. *Laryngoscope* 1996; 106: 589–594.

33. Zbaren P, Becker M, Lang H. Pretherapeutic staging of laryngeal carcinoma: Clinical findings, computed tomography and magnetic resonance imaging compared with histopathology. *Cancer* 1996; 77: 1263–1273.

34. Zbaren P, Becker M, Lang H. Pretherapeutic staging of hypopharyngeal carcinoma: Clinical finding, computed tomography, and magnetic resonance imaging compared with histopathologic evaluation. *Arch Otolaryngol head Neck Surg* 1997; 123: 908–913.

35. Ferri T, De Thomasis G, Quaranta N, Bacchi G, Bottazzi D. The value of CT scans in improving laryngoscopy in patients with laryngeal cancer. *Eur Arch Otorhinolaryngol* 1999; 256: 395–399.

36. Benson MT, Dalen K, Mancuso AA, Kerr HH, Cacciarelli AA, Mafee MF. Congenital anomalies of the branchial apparatus: Embryology and pathologic anatomy. *Radiographics* 1992; 12: 943–960.

37. Liston SL, Siegel LG. Branchial cysts, sinuses, and fistulas. *Ear Nose Throat J* 1979; 58: 9–17.

38. Connor S. Laryngeal Cancer: How does the radiologist help? *Cancer Imaging* 2007; 7: 93–103.

39. Rubesin SE, Jones B, Donner MW. Contrast pharyngography: The importance of phonation. *Am J Roentgenol* 1987; 148: 269–272.

40. Kim BS, Ahn KJ, Park YH. Usefulness of laryngeal phonation CT in the diagnosis of vocal cord paralysis. *Am J Roentgenol* 2008; 190: 1376–1379.

41. Celebi I, Basak M, Ucgul A, Yildirim H, Oz A, Vural C. Functional imaging of larynx via 256-slice multi-detector computed tomography in patients with laryngeal tumors: A faster, better and more reliable pre-therapeutic evaluation. *Eur J Radiol* 2011; 81(4): e541–547.

42. Chu EA, Kim YJ. Laryngeal cancer: Diagnosis and pre-operative work-up. *Otolaryngol Clin North Am* 2008; 41: 673–695.

43. Becker M, Burkhardt K, Dulguerov P, Allal A. Imaging of the larynx and hypopharynx. *Eur J Radiol* 2008; 66: 460–479.

44. Murakami R, Furusawa M, Baba Y et al. Dynamic helical CT of T1 and T2 glottic carcinomas: Predictive value for local control with radiation therapy. *Am J Neuroradiol* 2000; 21: 1320–1326.

45. Becker M. Larynx and hypopharyx. *Radiol Clin N Am* 1998; 36(5): 891–9205.

46. Becker M. Larynx and hypopharyx. In: Valvassori G, Mafee M, eds. *Imaging of the Head and Neck*. New York, Stuttgart: Thieme; 2004:731–777.

47. Som PM, Brandwein MS. Lymph Nodes. In: Som PM, Curtin HD, eds. *Head and Neck Imaging*. 4th ed. St. Louis, MO: Mosby; 2003:1865–1934.

48. Van den Brekel MW, Stel HV, Castelijns JA et al. Cervical lymph node metastasis: Assessment of radiologic criteria. *Radiology* 1990; 177(2): 379–384.

49. Cummings B. Radiation therapy and the treatment of the cervical lymphs nodes. In: Cummings C, Fredrickson J, Harker L et al, eds. *Otolaryngology Head and Neck Surgery*. Vol 2. 2nd ed. St Louis, MO: Mosby Year Book; 1993;1626–1648.

50. Som P, Curtin H, Mancuso A. An imaging-based classification for the cervical nodes designed as an adjunct to recent clinically based nodal classifications. *Arch Otolaryngol Head and Neck Surg* 1999; 125: 388–396.

51. Henrot P, Blum A, Thoussaint B, Troufleau P, Stines J, Roland J. Dynamic maneuvers in local staging of head and neck malignancies with current imaging techniques: Principles and clinical applications. *Radiographics* 2003; 23: 1201–1213.

52. Aarabi B, Leibrock LG. Neurosurgical approaches to cerebrospinal fluid rhinorrhea. *Ear Nose Throat J* 1992; 71: 300–305.

53. Jonsson G. A method for examination of the hypopharynx and upper way passages. *Acta Radiol* 1934; 15: 125.

8

Computed Tomography Imaging of Brain Tumors

Jonathan K. Park and Whitney Pope

CONTENTS

8.1 Epidemiology

Primary central nervous system tumors comprise a group of mostly fatal conditions in the United States as well as worldwide, with expected 5- and 10-year survival rates of 29.1% and 25.3%, nationally [1]. In the United States, the incidence rate of all primary brain and central nervous system tumors is 19.9 cases per 100,000 person-years [2] or 14 in every 100,000 people [3–7]. The annual global incidence of brain tumors is slightly higher in men (3.7 per 100,000) than in women (2.6 per 100,000) [1,8]. However, in the United States, this rate is higher in women (21.3 per 100,000 person-years) than in men (18.3 per 100,000 person-years) [2]. Men also have higher rates of primary malignant brain tumors, whereas in comparison, women have higher rates of nonmalignant tumors, primarily meningiomas [1].

Compared to primary brain tumors, metastatic brain tumors arising from other primary cancer types are substantially more common and affect over 150,000 patients each year in the United States alone [9–11]. Of the new primary brain tumors that are diagnosed, approximately 60% are malignant and 45% are gliomas [2]. Malignant gliomas are the second leading cause of cancer mortality in people under the age of 35, the fourth leading cause in those under the age of 54, and result in approximately 13,000 mortalities yearly [2]. Epidemiological data suggests that children under the age of 14 and patients over the age of 70 have a higher incidence of primary brain tumors compared to other age groups [12]. The median age at diagnosis for primary brain tumors is between 54 and 58 years [3–7].

8.2 Classification

In 1926, Harvey Cushing and Percival Bailey published one of the first classification systems for gliomas with 14 different glial tumor subtypes [13]. Since this initial classification, significant advances in classifying brain tumors histologically have been made. In particular, the World Health Organization (WHO) has embarked on creating a standard classification system for brain tumors in an effort to correlate histology with prognosis [14–17]. The WHO approach incorporates multiple characteristics to construct a malignancy scale based on histologic tumor features. There are a large number of histologically different tumors arising within the brain (Table 8.1) and several factors that assist in making an appropriate differential diagnosis.

Although advances in imaging have allowed for increasing sophistication in the characterization of brain tumors, the neuroradiologist still relies greatly upon traditional criteria, such as neuraxis location and patient age, to suggest the possibility of specific histologic diagnoses. For instance, the majority of intracranial brain tumors occur in adults and are mostly located supratentorially; glioblastoma is the most common intra-axial supratentorial adult neoplasm [2]. In contrast, the posterior fossa is a rare site for primary brain tumor in adults and an infratentorial, intra-axial mass in an adult is more likely to be secondary to infarct, hemorrhage, or metastasis [18]. In comparison, brain tumors much more commonly develop infratentorially in children older than one year than in adults [19], whereas secondary metastatic lesions in children are less common. Supratentorial tumors in children are more likely to involve midline structures than peripheral cerebral hemispheres. Thus, in summary, the age of the patient and tumor site provide crucial information in constructing a differential diagnosis.

TABLE 8.1

Classification of Primary Intracranial Central Nervous System Tumors

1. Glial Cell Tumors (Gliomas)
   a. Low-grade gliomas (WHO I–II)
      i. Pilocytic astrocytoma (WHO I)
      ii. Maxopapillary ependymoma (WHO I)
      iii. Subependymal giant cell astrocytoma (WHO I)
      iv. Subependymoma (WHO I)
      v. Ependymoma (WHO II)
      vi. Astrocytoma (WHO II)
      vii. Oligodendroglioma (WHO II)
      viii. Mixed oligoastrocytoma (WHO II)
   b. Anaplastic gliomas (WHO III)
      i. Anaplastic astrocytoma (WHO III)
      ii. Anaplastic oligodendroglioma (WHO III)
      iii. Anaplastix mixed oligodendroglioma (WHO III)
   c. Glioblastoma (WHO IV)
   d. Special subtypes
      i. Pleomorphic xanthoastrocytoma
      ii. Desmoplastic infantile astrocytoma
      iii. Gliofibroma
      iv. Choroid plexus papilloma
      v. Choroid plexus carcinoma
2. Neuronal and Mixed Neuronal-Glial Tumors
   a. Neuronal tumors
      i. Gangliocytoma
      ii. Neurocytoma
   b. Mixed neuronal-glial tumors
      i. Ganglioglioma and anaplastic ganglioglioma
      ii. Desmoplastic infantile ganglioglioma
      iii. Dysembryoplastic neuroepithelial tumors
3. Medulloblastoma
   a. Medulloblastoma
   b. Nodular medulloblastoma
   c. Medullomyoblastoma
   d. Melanotic medulloblastoma
4. Meningeal Tumors
   a. Meningioma
   b. Atypical meningioma
   c. Anaplastic meningioma
   d. Meningioma variants (Meningiothelial, fibrous, transitional, psammamatous, angiomatous, microcystic, secretory, metaplastic, etc.)

8.3 Computed Tomography

Since its introduction into clinical practice in 1974, computed tomography (CT) is a well-accepted and widely available imaging modality. Following its subsequent introduction, magnetic resonance imaging (MRI) gradually became the primary modality of choice for brain tumor imaging, particularly because of its increased sensitivity for the detection of most brain tumors and depth of anatomic detail provided [20–28]. CT nevertheless can provide valuable supplementary information and, in situations where MRI is not available or contraindicated (e.g., patients with pacemakers or other implanted metallic devices), serves as the primary imaging modality for brain tumors. Furthermore, patients presenting initially with symptoms related to brain tumors are likely to be imaged first with CT, necessitating a thorough understanding of the CT appearance of tumors for the neuroradiologist.

The density scale for CT generally ranges from −1000 to +1000 Hounsfield unit (HU), with 0 corresponding with water and −1000 with air. Fat is usually in the −40 to −100 HU range. White matter and gray matter are in the 30–50 HU range; increased cell density results in greater Hounsfield units on CT. Hematomas range from approximately 50–80 HU, and calcifications generally 150 HU or greater. Dense bone and metal are at the highest Hounsfield unit range. High protein concentrations result in greater Hounsfield unit values (such as clotted blood and sinus secretions) (Figure 8.1a–e).

The particular strengths of CT in brain tumor assessment include its ability to detect calcification, particularly

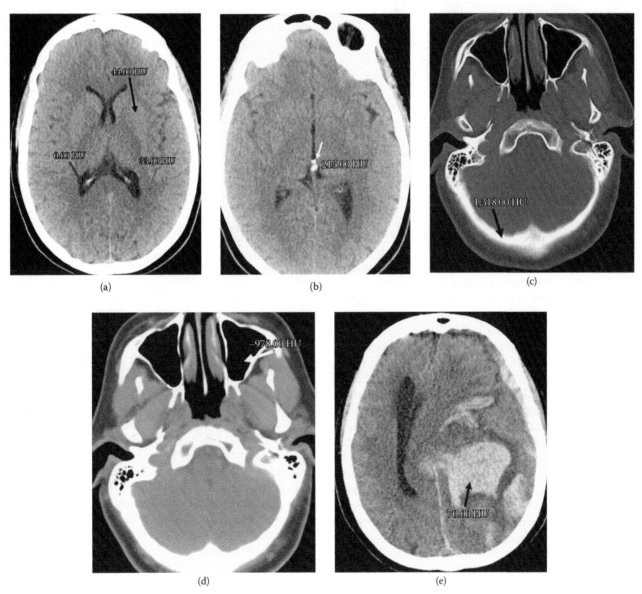

(a)   (b)   (c)

(d)   (e)

FIGURE 8.1
Computed tomography (CT) brain density values. (a) Noncontrast axial CT through the level of the basal ganglia. Gray matter (black arrow pointing to left basal ganglia) has slightly higher density than white matter (blue arrow pointing to left periventricular white matter). Water measure approximately 0 HU on CT (red arrow pointing to cerebrospinal fluid in the atrium of the right lateral ventricle). (b) Calcified pineal gland (white arrow). Calcifications measure 150 HU or greater. (c) Right occipital bone measuring over 1000 HU (black arrow). Dense bone and metal are at the highest spectrum of CT density. (d) Air in left maxillary sinus (white arrow). Air measures approximately −1000 HU. (e) 93-Year-old female on warfarin with supratherapeutic international normalized ratio with large left hemispheric hematoma (black arrow). Acute blood on CT ranges from 50 to 80 HU.

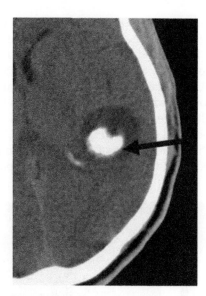

FIGURE 8.2
Calcification in an oligoastrocytoma. CT remains superior to magnetic resonance imaging (MRI) in identifying calcifications and is often seen in multiple types of tumors, including oligodendroglioma and astrocytoma.

MRI has largely become the primary imaging modality for the evaluation and assessment of brain tumors, multiple contrast administration strategies have been previously developed and described for optimal CT evaluation of tumors. For instance, delayed scanning following contrast administration is useful in honing the differential diagnosis of brain tumors; delay times ranging from 15 minutes to 3 hours have been reported to be beneficial in diagnosis [29–32]. The dynamics of contrast enhancement may also reflect the vascular function of tumors [33]; for instance, contrast shows a tendency to remain in malignant gliomas, while washing out rapidly from nonglial tumors such as meningiomas [29,34–37]. An additional strategy to improve lesion detection is utilizing a higher dose of contrast as this show not only better lesions, but also as many as 50% more metastatic lesions not visible with lower doses [4,29–31,38,39]. Thus, both noncontrast and contrast-enhanced series with axial, coronal, and sagittal reconstructions are recommended for brain tumor detection with CT, and double-dose delayed scanning may be used as well to improve lesion detection [32,38,40].

if MRI is confined to conventional sequences. For example, oligodendrogliomas and oligoastrocytomas frequently show particularly dense peripheral calcification (Figure 8.2). Although gradient-echo, T_2-weighted MRI sequences are more sensitive to calcifications than standard sequences and may be used as supplementary aids, CT remains superior in its ability to identify calcifications with great accuracy. Because different tumor types often have overlapping imaging findings, the identification of calcifications is useful in limiting the differential diagnosis. Other than oligodendrogliomas, other commonly calcified tumors include craniopharyngiomas, gangliogliomas, meningiomas, pineal gland tumors, low-grade astrocytomas, and ependymomas.

In spite of this strength, a potential pitfall must be noted in regard to CT detection of calcifications; calcified lesions can at times present a diagnostic dilemma on CT because the density of calcium may mask subtle density increase from CT contrast agents, whereas on T_1-weighted MRI sequences, calcium shows low signal intensity, thus more easily identifying enhancement of neoplastic matrix within even densely calcified tumors.

Certain primary tumors, such as high-grade gliomas, and some types of metastases have a tendency to exhibit both acute and chronic hemorrhage. Although acute hemorrhage is visible on both types of modalities, CT is useful for showing that the early stages of hemorrhage are higher density than surrounding brain.

When obtaining CT for the evaluation of brain tumors, examinations should include both noncontrast and iodinated contrast-enhanced series. Although again

8.4 Strategies for Tumor Diagnosis

Although imaging does not replace the neuropathologist, it does provide useful information to predict the histopathology. The structural abnormalities suggesting the presence of brain tumors include morphological changes of the brain parenchyma and cerebrospinal fluid (CSF) spaces. These findings may be subdivided into direct and indirect signs.

- *Direct signs*: Brain tumors will often exhibit abnormal density on CT images in comparison to normal brain on noncontrast scans. Gliomas, in particular, tend to show low density. The appearance may vary further following iodinated contrast administration. Enhancement patterns should be observed for homogeneity or nonhomogeneity, rapidity of enhancement, and ring enhancement with regular versus irregular wall thickness.

- *Indirect signs*: Changes include alteration of normal anatomic structures secondary to tumor infiltration, displacement of adjacent structures, mass effect on the ventricular system with possible obstructive hydrocephalus, sulcal effacement, and cisternal distortion.

Certain tumor characteristics should always be assessed for, regardless of modality. These include lesion border definition, presence of associated hemorrhage, cystic components, intratumoral necrosis, calcifications, peritumoral edema, and extension across the midline. Careful assessment for these features is critical in predicting tumor type, as well as in directing therapy. Other disease-specific findings are also notable on CT and will be discussed later under specific diseases. Precise tumor localization is also necessary, and differentiation should always be made between intra-axial and extra-axial lesions as this typically leads to substantially different possible diagnoses. Although the limits of tumor infiltration should be assessed, it should be noted that this is not always accurately feasible. Infiltrating tumors may exhibit clear-cut borders on MRI that do not correlate with histopathologic findings, whereas on CT, these same lesions can exhibit ill-defined borders [41].

Neuroimaging also plays a critical role for therapy monitoring. Images should be evaluated carefully for mass effect, hydrocephalus, hemorrhage, infarct, midline shift, as well as positioning of ventricular catheters. Whenever tumor resection is incomplete, an immediate post-therapy, contrast-enhanced study should be obtained, with a subsequent follow-up study at a later time. Examples of typical postoperative changes are provided in Figure 8.3. The definite diagnosis of tumor progression or recurrence may only be made on the basis of imaging findings that show convincing enlargement of tumor on follow-up examinations. With regard to radiation therapy, both CT and MRI are ineffective in differentiating between radiation necrosis and tumor recurrence, and positron emission tomography (PET) may be superior because of its depiction of metabolic activity [42].

Hemorrhage into a pre-existing tumor also presents a potentially complex problem in differential diagnosis as its high density on CT can obscure underlying tumor [43]. Furthermore, peripheral ring enhancement can be seen as part of the normal evolution of hematomas [44]. When confronted with a hemorrhagic lesion, the following five diagnostic factors can be carefully evaluated for clues to confirming or excluding an underlying tumor [43].

1. *Location*: Aneurysms and hypertensive hemorrhages have preferred locations (such as the basal cisterns); thus, an atypical location should always evoke the diagnosis of underlying tumor.

2. *Edema*: Although edema may occur in the setting of an acute hematoma, the presence of persistent or exuberant edema indicates an underlying lesion.

3. *Heterogeneity*: Depending on hematoma age, uncomplicated hematomas tend toward homogeneity; while a tumor nodule is sometimes identifiable within a heterogeneous hematoma on imaging, contrast enhancement may be beneficial in these cases.

4. *Hemosiderin*: The presence of hemosiderin is more readily assessable on MRI. Absent, decreased, or irregular hemosiderin deposits within a hematoma have been associated with brain tumors.

5. *Evolution*: A delay in the normal timing of hematoma evolution is strongly indicative of an underlying tumor.

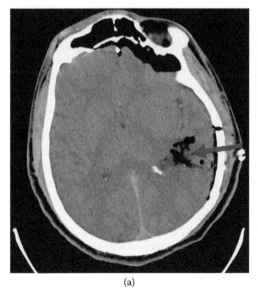 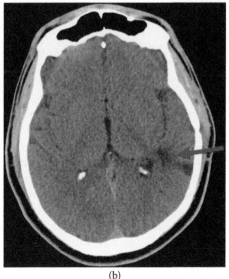

(a) (b)

FIGURE 8.3

(a) Immediate postoperative change following tumor resection shows intracranial air (arrow). CT density for air is approximately −1000. (b) Scan obtained 9 months later shows resolution of immediate postsurgical changes. A resection cavity at the original tumor site remains.

8.5 Specific Tumor Types

In the following sections, individual brain tumor types will be reviewed. First off, gliomas will be reviewed, with a focus on astrocytomas. Subsequently, a variety of other tumors where CT has particular utility in predicting the diagnosis will be discussed. These include calcified tumors and skull base tumors, in addition to several other types. Potential false positives that may be encountered will be reviewed as well.

8.5.1 Glial Cell Tumors

Gliomas are tumors arising from astrocytes, oligodendrocytes, or ependymal cells. According to the WHO classification [14–16], gliomas are subdivided into either diffuse or localized subtypes, which are graded from I to IV in order of increasing malignancy and worse prognosis. Diffuse gliomas can then be further subdivided into astrocytomas, oligodendrogliomas, and mixed oligoastrocytomas, depending on the particular histological features of the tumor. Glioblastoma, or grade IV astrocytomas, can be subdivided into primary and secondary glioblastomas. Secondary glioblastomas arise from malignant transformation of grade II/III gliomas, as opposed to primary glioblastomas, which arise de novo. Ependymomas and choroid plexus tumors, which are also considered of glial origin, constitute most of the remaining proportion of primary brain tumors in adults. The relatively benign group of localized gliomas includes pilocytic astrocytomas, giant cell astrocytomas affiliated with tuberous sclerosis, and pleomorphic xanthoastrocytomas.

8.5.1.1 Low-Grade Astrocytomas (WHO Grade II)

8.5.1.1.1 General

Low-grade astrocytomas are diffusely infiltrative gliomas comprising neoplastic astrocytes and typically have ill-defined boundaries, low cellularity, and few nuclear atypia [16,17]. Lacking malignant features such as endothelial microvascular proliferation, high mitotic activity and proliferation rate, and microscopic necrosis, low-grade astrocytomas are typically of low aggressivity compared to high-grade tumors. They are relatively slow growing and invade rather than destroy adjacent parenchyma. Grade II astrocytomas are most commonly found in the cerebral hemispheres of young adults, with a peak incidence in the third and fourth decades. Their route of spread is via the white matter tracts, and neurological deficits tend to be minor in relation to lesion size at time of presentation [45].

It was recently shown that low-grade astrocytomas and oligodendrogliomas contain an activating mutation of the isocitrate dehydrogenase I gene (IDH1) and to a lesser extent IDH2 [46,47]. These conserved mutations are associated with prolonged survival, O(6)-methylguanine-DNA methyltransferase (MGMT) methylation, and an associated hypermethylation phenotype [48]. Approximately 70%–80% of grade II/III gliomas are positive for the IDH1 mutation [49]. Many secondary glioblastomas harbor the mutation, whereas only about 5%–10% of all primary glioblastomas are positive [50]. IDH1 mutation is thought to be an early event in gliomagenesis [51]. It is associated with *TP53* mutation and not other classical hallmarks of glioblastoma, such as epidermal growth factor amplification or mutation, or Phosphatase and tensin homolog (PTEN) deletion [52]. This suggests an alternate oncogenic pathway in secondary glioblastomas [53,54].

8.5.1.1.2 CT Appearance

Grade II astrocytomas show low CT density and are not expected to enhance following contrast administration because of their intact blood–brain barrier [45]. Most low-grade gliomas are diffusely infiltrating but some appear well circumscribed, and in this group may show mild to moderate inhomogeneous enhancement [55]. In theory, relatively little enhancement should be expected with low-grade astrocytomas, with high-grade tumors showing more extensive enhancement; however, CT has not proved reliable in differentiating between tumor grades [45]. In addition, since this group of tumors infiltrates diffusely, they may produce only minor expansion of involved structures and thus may be missed on nonenhanced CT; however, calcifications may be seen in 10%–20% of low-grade astrocytomas, which is a useful diagnostic feature [56] (Figure 8.4). Calcification is infrequent in high-grade tumors unless the lesion has progressed from a low-grade malignancy [45].

8.5.1.2 Anaplastic Astrocytomas (WHO Grade III)

8.5.1.2.1 General

Anaplastic astrocytomas are malignant astrocytomas with many of the histological features of grade II astrocytomas, but lacking the endothelial microvascular proliferation and necrosis found in glioblastomas. The peak age of incidence is in the fifth decade [45]. Anaplastic astrocytomas are typically more highly cellular compared to low-grade astrocytomas and exhibit mitotic activity (Ki-67), typically around 12%–14% [57,58]. However, they do not show necrosis, which is a diagnostic criteria for glioblastoma. The presence of gemistocytes is usually a poor prognostic indicator; the presence of at least 20% gemistocytes usually warrants classification as an anaplastic astrocytoma [59].

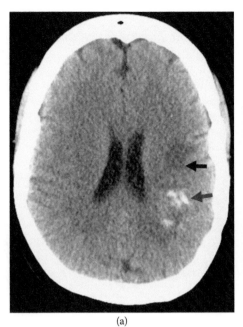
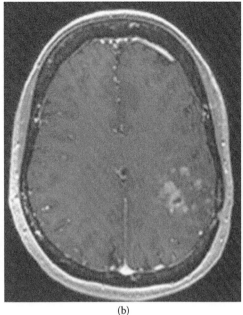

(a)   (b)

FIGURE 8.4
Grade II astrocytoma. (a) Noncontrast axial CT shows an ill-defined mass in the left posterior cerebrum with moderate perilesional edema (black arrow) and foci of internal calcifications (red arrow). Calcifications are seen in 10%–20% of low-grade astrocytomas. Although this tumor had features of oligodendroglioma, it was pathologically proven to be an astrocytoma. (b) Axial postcontrast axial T_1 image in same patient shows mild enhancement. While this lesion demonstrates enhancement expected of a higher grade tumor, it was biopsy-proven to be a grade II astrocytoma.

8.5.1.2.2 CT Appearance

Anaplastic astrocytomas represent the histological progression point between Grade II and Grade IV astrocytomas; there may be overlap with imaging findings as well. Grade III astrocytomas are primarily of low density with areas of irregular or ring enhancement, following contrast administration. Compared to grade II astrocytomas, they tend to show more mass effect but rarely calcify or show cyst formation [45].

8.5.1.3 Glioblastoma: WHO Grade IV

8.5.1.3.1 General

Glioblastoma, previously referred to as glioblastoma multiforme, is the most malignant and common primary brain tumor, comprising nearly 54% of all primary gliomas [2]. Glioblastomas occur with a peak in the sixth decade, and patterns in glioblastoma location suggest that the most frequent area of tumor occurrence migrates from posteriorly with increasing age. Glioblastomas are highly infiltrative, proliferative, and aggressive brain tumors with a very poor patient prognosis, despite advances in therapy. Median survival for patients with glioblastoma is around 14.6 months (radiotherapy and temozolomide) and 12.1 months for radiotherapy alone [60].

Microscopically, glioblastomas exhibit markedly elevated cellularity and anaplasia with giant cells and mitotic figures. There is increased vascularity with endothelial proliferation and necrosis. Hemorrhage is common and tends to occur in high-grade gliomas [61]; the presence of necrosis is a major histological criteria for Grade IV [62]. Stereotactic biopsy is generally directed toward areas of enhancement seen on MRI or CT and may indicate foci of high-grade tumors.

As with all astrocytomas, glioblastomas infiltrate diffusely, but on neuroimaging and even sometimes histopathology, may give the false impression of having well-circumscribed margins. In reality, tumor cells are present throughout adjacent areas of apparent edema and even in areas of brain that appear normal on imaging [55,62,63]. Tumor spread occurs not only along white matter tracts, but also leptomeningeally and subependymally around ventricular walls into CSF [56]. Secondary to the ill-defined and infiltrating nature of these tumors, it is not possible to achieve total surgical resection.

8.5.1.3.2 CT Appearance

The heterogeneous histological appearance of glioblastoma is also reflected in the CT appearance. Typically noted is a mass with a thick ring of contrast enhancement with central low density indicating necrosis, which is seen in approximately 95% of these tumors (Figure 8.5). A surrounding low-density change usually indicates edema, although nonenhancing tumor also is typically having low density. Peritumoral edema is much more

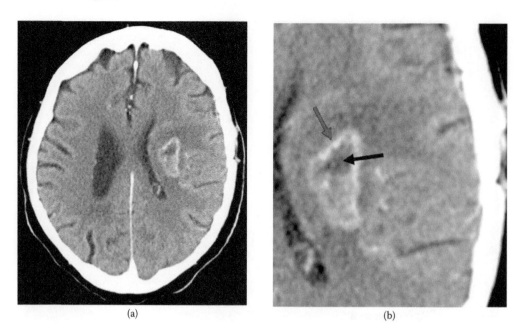

(a)   (b)

FIGURE 8.5
(a) Contrast-enhanced axial CT showing glioblastoma with ring enhancement, internal hypodensity, as well as peritumoral edema and mass effect on the lateral ventricle. (b) Close-up view of imaging findings. Red arrow indicates coarse and irregular ring enhancement, whereas black arrow indicates internal hypodensity likely representing necrosis.

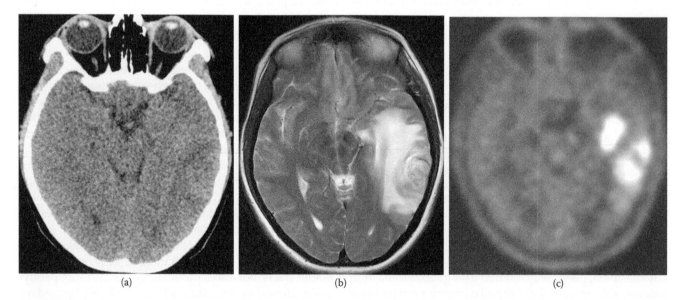

(a)   (b)   (c)

FIGURE 8.6
Glioblastoma. (a) Noncontrast axial CT shows faint density irregularities involving the left temporal lobe. (b) Tumoral changes are much more obvious on axial T_2 image. There is significant vasogenic edema on this view that was not readily seen on noncontrast CT. (c) Axial fluorine-18-L-dihydroxyphenylalanine positron emission tomography scan shows multifocal avid radiotracer uptake involving the left temporal lobe, corresponding with tumor.

obviously seen on MRI (Figure 8.6). Inhomogeneous patchy enhancement may be noted throughout the mass as well. Areas of new enhancement on subsequent scans can indicate disease progression, or recurrence, or treatment change (so-called pseudoprogression). Pseudoprogression typically occurs within 3 months of the end of chemoradiation therapy and then slowly resolves without change in treatment. This phenomenon is more common with the current treatment paradigm of radiation with temozolomide than previously. Following treatment, edema surrounding the resection cavity is common; postoperative, follow-up scans should

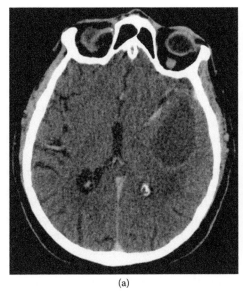 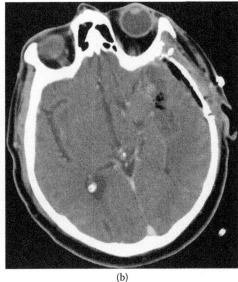

(a)   (b)

FIGURE 8.7
Glioblastoma. (a) Postcontrast axial CT shows a hypodense left hemispheric mass with mass effect, which was ultimately diagnosed as glioblastoma. (b) Immediate postresection scan shows air within the intracranial cavity and interval removal of hypodense tumor. An initial scan should be performed during the first few days after surgery; contrast enhancement frequently develops at the resection margins after 3–4 days and can persist up to 6 months following procedure.

show diminished edema and mass effect, although this is often better depicted by MRI.

To document postsurgical change, an initial scan should be performed during the first few days following surgery, when contrast enhancement is not yet seen secondary to the procedure (Figure 8.7). Contrast enhancement frequently develops at the resection margin after 3–4 days [64] and typically lasts for 3–4 weeks, but may be visible up to 6 months postprocedure [65]. Hemorrhagic fluid is often present at the operative site, which with CT is not easily distinguishable from areas of enhancement. This factor, along with the fact that enhancement may be secondary to nonspecific reaction in adjacent tissues (such as subacute to chronic peri-resectional ischemia) versus residual disease, renders interpretation of postoperative CT unreliable at times [45]. Thus, serial scanning is needed to distinguish these postsurgical changes from true recurrent disease [63,66].

Dural enhancement is not usually detected with CT, unless there has been a craniectomy. The dural enhancement may be relatively thick, precluding definitive differentiation between true recurrence versus other etiologies such as infection [45].

Both chemotherapy and radiation therapy can produce changes within the brain that must be differentiated from malignancy. White matter changes, vascular occlusion, cranial nerve damage, and possible secondary malignancies may occur. The risk of radiation damage is dependent on total dose administered, as well as the method of radiation delivery [67].

With improvement in the survival duration of patients with glioblastomas, the time available for development of delayed radiation effects is also increasing [67]. Following radiation, there is usually a time delay before imaging changes and symptoms manifest themselves. These changes are generally characterized at the time in which they appear as acute (first months); early delayed (3 weeks–3 months); and delayed (6 months–years) [45]. Chemotherapy can potentiate the development of these findings as well, and radiation and chemotherapy induced damage can resemble each other [45].

Acute changes are usually not visible with imaging, but are nonspecific when seen, and are likely secondary to damage to capillary endothelium with resultant vasogenic edema [68]. Although reactions are generally not severe, diffuse cerebral edema can occur, resulting in brain (tonsillar) herniation and death [45].

With early delayed damage, symptoms of somnolence or focal deficits are thought to be secondary to demyelination [45,67,68]. Low-density change in the deep white matter, basal ganglia, and cerebral peduncles may be seen on CT [67,69,70]. Changes in the primary tumor secondary to necrosis may occur and should not be confused with disease progression [70].

Late radiation damage to the white matter may be focal or diffuse, but both appear to be related to endothelial damage, preferably involving small arteries and arterioles [45]. Seventy percent of changes are seen between six months and two years of treatment [45].

Initial imaging changes are generally seen in the subependymal white matter but later extend peripherally to the gray-white junction; the corpus callosum, internal capsule, posterior fossa, and basal ganglia are usually spared [45]. Changes are accompanied by sulcal and ventricular enlargement secondary to atrophy, without significant mass effect [71,72].

Mineralizing microangiopathy is sometimes seen in children; 25%–30% of children treated with intrathecal methotrexate and cranial irradiation will show calcifications months following therapy [45,73] and are readily shown on CT secondary to basal ganglia (particularly putaminal) and basal ganglia calcifications [45]. Calcifications are secondary to necrosis and do not generally cause symptoms [67].

Focal radiation necrosis is another late radiation change that is identifiable with CT and is indistinguishable from recurrence. Contrast-enhanced CT will depict an irregular or ring-enhancing mass lesion centered in the white matter [67,71,72], with central nonenhancing necrosis and low-density edema. To further complicate the diagnosis, radiation necrosis can result in increasing mass effect and also can occur in tandem with recurrence. For this reason, metabolic imaging using PET may be helpful for differentiation of these etiologies [42], although PET also is not 100% accurate.

8.5.2 Miscellaneous Calcifications

As discussed earlier, CT is particularly useful for the detection and characterization of calcified tumors. Other than astrocytomas, tumors commonly presenting with calcifications include oligodendrogliomas, craniopharyngiomas, and meningiomas.

8.5.2.1 Oligodendroglioma (WHO Grade II)

8.5.2.1.1 General

Oligodendroglioma is the third most common glioma overall, accounting for 2%–5% of primary brain tumors and 5%–18% of all glial neoplasms, overall [74,75]. Other oligodendrogliomal origin tumors include anaplastic oligodendrogliomas and mixed oligoastrocytomas. Almost two-thirds of patients with oligodendrogliomas present with seizures [76]. Most oligodendrogliomas occur in adults with a peak incidence in the fourth and fifth decades [75,77,78]. Patients with anaplastic tumors are usually slightly older, with a peak in the sixth and seventh decades. Only a small proportion (approximately 6%) of tumors arise in children [75,79].

The vast majority of oligodendroglial tumors occur in the supratentorial brain with the frontal lobe being the most common site (50%–65%) [80]. The temporal lobe (47%) is the next most common location, and the parietal (7%–20%) and occipital lobes (1%–4%) are the less common sites of lobar involvement [80]. The cerebellum (3%), brain stem, spinal cord (1%), leptomeninges (also called "oligodendrogliomatosis"), cerebellopontine angle, ventricles, retina, and optic nerve are even less common sites [80].

Histopathological analysis reveals moderately cellular tumor with typically monotonous pattern of uniformly rounded hyperchromatic nuclei surrounded by clear cytoplasm, resulting in a classic "fried-egg" appearance [80]. A branching network of capillaries is also common, producing a "honeycomb" or "chicken-wire" pattern [80]. Microcalcifications are seen in 90% of tumors [80], and mucoid or cyst degeneration is also frequently noted [80]. Cortical gray matter involvement is a highly distinctive feature [80]. There is a propensity for loss of heterozygosity on chromosome 19q in 50%–80% of these tumors and on chromosome 1p in 40%–92% [80]. These findings are strongly affiliated with classic histopathologic findings seen in well-differentiated oligodendrogliomas [80].

8.5.2.1.2 CT Appearance

Oligodendrogliomas typically manifest as round or oblong, sharply marginated masses involving the cortex or subcortical white matter [80]. Approximately 60% of lesions are hypodense while 23% are isodense, and 6% hyperdense [81]. Calcifications, generally coarse in nature, are noted between 20% and 91% of tumors [80,81] and are an imaging hallmark; because of the superiority of CT in depicting calcifications, CT serves a particularly useful role in diagnosing oligodendrogliomas (Figure 8.8). Cystic degeneration and hemorrhage are also occasionally seen and if the mass is sufficiently exophytic, calvarial erosion may also be noted [81].

Subtle ill-defined enhancement is noted in 15%–20% of tumors and is associated with high-grade tumors [81]. This may be better appreciated on MRI (Figure 8.6). Calcification, vasogenic edema, and enhancement are also less commonly noted in children than in adults [80]. The contrast enhancement pattern is commonly in a "dot-like" lacy pattern, but many tumors do not enhance at all [82].

Intraventricular oligodendrogliomas are rare, and some literature reports noted that many of these tumors had different imaging traits compared to those arising in the parenchyma [80]. These lesions were usually hyperdense on CT compared to normal parenchyma, and almost all had contrast enhancement [80].

Diffuse involvement of cisternal and subarachnoid spaces characterizes diffuse leptomeningeal

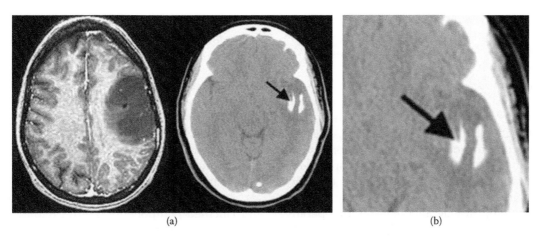

FIGURE 8.8
Oligodendroglioma. (a) Juxtaposed postcontrast axial T_1 (left) and noncontrast axial CT (right). Note the dense calcification in this peripherally located tumor (arrow) that is much more appreciable on CT scan, hence CT retains an integral role in diagnosing and characterizing these tumors. Contrast enhancement may be subtle or sometimes not seen at all. (b) Close-up view of axial CT shows dense and bulky calcifications characteristic of oligodendroglioma.

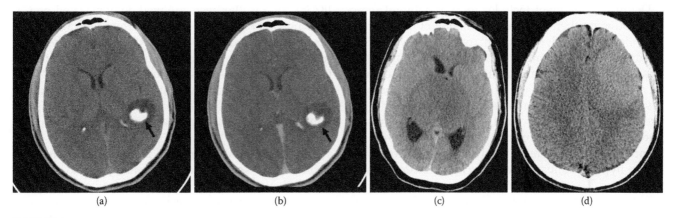

FIGURE 8.9
Oligoastrocytoma. (a, b) Pre- and postcontrast images show a hypodense mass with large internal calcification. Final pathology showed oligoastrocytoma. Differentiation with oligodendroglioma may be difficult at times using imaging as the tumors can present with similar findings. (c) Axial noncontrast CT image shows a large bithalamic heterogeneous mass that was shown to be an oligoastrocytoma upon histological analysis. No definite calcifications are seen, and calcifications are less common in mixed histology tumors. (d) Axial noncontrast CT image shows a large, nearly isodense left frontal lobe mass. Although this lesion has a nonspecific appearance, it was also confirmed to histologically to be an oligoastrocytoma.

oligodendroglioma [80]. Meningeal calcification has also been noted on CT in primary leptomeningeal oligodendroglioma [80].

The usual imaging appearance of an oligodendroglioma is more variable compared to an oligodendroglioma [83], reflecting the presence of necrosis, cystic degeneration, and hemorrhage. Occasionally, a ringlike enhancement pattern may be seen and the appearance may mimic a glioblastoma [83].

No unique features on imaging allow differentiation between mixed oligoastrocytoma and oligodendroglioma (Figure 8.9) [82]. Calcifications are less common with mixed forms (14%), but enhancement is more common (50%) [77,81].

8.5.2.2 Craniopharyngioma

8.5.2.2.1 General

Craniopharyngiomas occur at a rate of 0.5–2.0 cases per million per year worldwide, with 30%–50% of cases occurring during childhood and adolescence [84]. There is a bimodal distribution as tumors typically affect patients in the 5–14 and 50–74 years age ranges [85]. Craniopharyngiomas account for 1.2%–4% of pediatric intracranial tumors and 3% of adult intracranial tumors [85].

Histologically, craniopharyngiomas arise from the squamous epithelial rests of Rathke's cleft in the sellar and suprasellar region of the central nervous system.

The histopathological subtypes include the adamaninomatous and squamous-papillary variants; the adaminomatous type in particular is over-represented in pediatric patients [85].

Presenting symptoms are often related to increased intracranial pressure and include headache and nausea. Accompanying symptoms often include signs of visual impairment such as bitemporal hemianopsia, caused by optic chiasm compression by tumor. Additional visual findings include central visual defects, papilledema, and optic atrophy. Systemic manifestations of tumor-induced hypopituitarism such as growth delay, vigilance deficit, and polydipsia may also develop. Preoperative endocrinopathies may also be seen and include diabetes insipidus, as well as deficiencies of growth hormone, gonadotropins, adrenocorticotropic hormone, and thyrotropin stimulating hormone. Hypothalamic disturbance resulting in weight gain from loss of appetite control is a late but notable symptom.

Definitive treatment includes total or subtotal resection, radiation therapy, or a combination of these strategies. Before definitive treatment, patients may undergo a temporizing intervention to treat hydrocephalus, such as a shunt or surgical implantation of an intracystic catheter to allow CSF drainage around the tumor. Complete resection is the historical first-line treatment, aiming to preserve postoperative visual, hypothalamic, pituitary, and neuropsychiatric function. It is favored when the tumor does not intimately involve vital structures such as the hypothalamus, optic nerve and chiasm, or pituitary gland. Gross total removal can be achieved from 45% to 90% of patients and yields a reported 5-year control rate in the range of 70%–90% [86]. Because of tumor proximity to the optic nerve, optic chiasm, oculomotor nerve, and carotid arteries, radical resection is unfortunately offered in a fraction of cases only. Complete removal of the cystic and solid components of tumor is not always achieved despite best efforts, and recurrence may develop at the resection margin.

8.5.2.2.2 CT Appearance

Although the initial diagnosis of craniopharyngioma may be made with MRI, CT can be used to confirm the diagnosis. MRI shows a heterogenous mass with variable signal densities reflecting its solid, cystic, and calcified components (Figure 8.10). Once craniopharyngioma is diagnosed with MRI, CT facilitates detection of the classic intracystic calcifications that are seen in >90% of cases [87]. The lesion localizes to the suprasellar region exclusively in up to a third of cases, with a rare proportion that are exclusively intrasellar, and the rest are both intrasellar and suprasellar [87,88]. Suprasellar cysts are well demonstrated on CT; although there may be a simple, rounded cyst, many are lobulated and can be quite extensive [45]. Cyst contents are usually of slightly higher CT density than CSF and occasionally show hemorrhage as well [45]. The cyst wall may show contrast enhancement on CT, but more commonly, the nodule in the cyst wall is the enhancing component and also often shows calcifications (Figure 8.10) [45].

The differential diagnosis for craniopharyngioma includes Rathke's cleft cysts, pituitary adenomas, epidermoid tumors, germinomas, Langerhans cell histiocytosis, aneurysms, arachnoid cysts, inflammatory variations, hypothalamic and optic tract gliomas, and

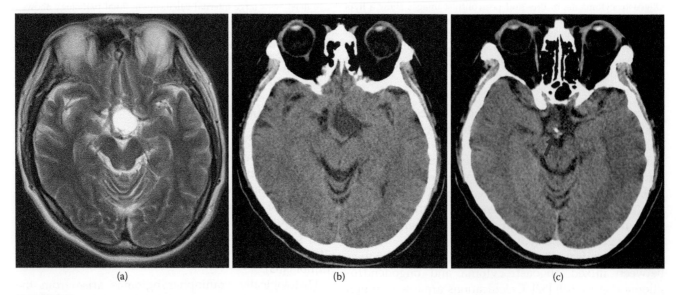

(a)	(b)	(c)

FIGURE 8.10
Craniopharyngioma. (a) Axial T_2 image confirms cystic mass in the suprasellar cistern that is consistent in appearance with craniopharyngioma. (b) Axial noncontrast CT shows a cystic lesion centered in the suprasellar cistern. (c) Axial noncontrast CT depicts punctate calcifications in the lesion's right posterolateral margin (arrow), which is seen in over 90% of craniopharyngiomas.

colloid cysts of the third ventricle [89]. In particular, craniopharyngiomas bear the most imaging resemblance to Rathke's cleft cysts. In comparison to craniopharyngiomas, Rathke's cleft cysts are more commonly intrasellar, homogeneous, typically located between the anterior and posterior pituitary, and lacking in calcifications.

With regard to therapy monitoring, radiation treatment can lead to a transient enlargement of the solid component during radiation and the tumor shrinkage itself may be prolonged over months (mean of 29 months; range of 6–68 months) [90]. Cystic change is less predictable, with enlargement occasionally seen after radiation within the first 3–6 months [91,92], and cyst shrinkage occurring with conservative treatment or no intervention at all. Thus, to differentiate treatment effect from recurrence, longer follow-up is necessary.

Recurrence most often occurs 2–5 years following treatment but can occur within the first 12 months or as remotely as over 30 years later [93]. Recurrence after surgery is best seen on MRI and appears as enlarging cysts or refractory solid enhancing tumor seeded along the surgical route [94]. With respect to surveillance, serial follow-up must be performed within 3 months of the attempted resection therapy because of the high propensity for recurrence in this time period [95]; surveillance then may be spaced out regularly in 6–12 month intervals.

8.5.3 Skull Base Tumors

Tumors arising from the skull base by nature intimately involve the bones of the skull base. Although current characterization always involves MRI, CT retains a particularly crucial role in helping to define extent of bony involvement and relationship with adjacent osseous structures. Common differential considerations in skull base lesions will be addressed here.

8.5.3.1 Chordoma

8.5.3.1.1 General

Chordomas are slow-growing but locally aggressive tumors representing up to 1% of intracranial tumors and 4% of primary bone tumors [96]. Intracranial chordomas represent one-third of all chordomas [96]. There are two histologic subtypes, typical chordomas and chondroid chordomas, the latter resembling low-grade chondrosarcomas. Because these tumors are derived from embryonic remnants of the notochord, they may be found intracranially and extracranially anywhere along the course of the notochord from its cranial to sacral extent. These tumors typically arise in the clival region, but may also arise elsewhere including the nasopharynx, maxilla, paranasal sinuses, or intradural region [97].

Symptoms vary with lesion location and proximity to critical neurovascular structures, reflecting specific sites of extension from the clivus (mainly sellar, parasellar, and retroclival areas and, occasionally, the sphenoid sinus) [96]. The most common initial complaints are diplopia related to cranial nerve palsy and headache (usually occipital or retro-orbital); the abducens nerve is the most commonly affected cranial nerve [96].

Although intracranial chordomas are generally slow growing and rarely metastasize, their close relation to critical structures and extremely high rate of local recurrence have often resulted in high mortality in the past [96]. Complete surgical removal is the preferred treatment for locally aggressive chordomas, but its application is limited by tumor encasement of critical neurovascular structures and brain stem adherence. When possible, gross total resection is preferred because it correlates with superior long-term survival and lower recurrence than subtotal resection [98]. Most cases require combined subtotal surgery, followed by radiation to halt the growth of residual tumor. Although advances in skull base surgery and radiation therapy offer the potential for cure, prognosis remains suboptimal, with 5-year survival rates in the range of 54%–79% [97,99,100].

8.5.3.1.2 CT Appearance

The imaging capabilities provided by MRI and CT allow precise characterization of tumors, leading to superior treatment and cure rates [96]. In particular, tumor extension to the skull base and relationship to adjacent neural structures are shown in detail. Both CT and MRI are usually required for pre-therapy evaluation by neurosurgeons and radiation oncologists to plan treatment [96]. Thus, familiarity with the imaging features of chordoma is essential in facilitating optimal management.

High-resolution CT with bone and soft-tissue algorithms is sensitive for detecting skull base lesions [96]. Thin axial and coronal slices with and without iodinated contrast are recommended. Although CT is accurate for depicting bone abnormalities, the ability to show posterior fossa soft-tissue structures is limited by beam-hardening artifact [101]. MRI, in this regard, offers the advantage of providing excellent tissue contrast and anatomic detail [96].

The classic appearance of intracranial chordomas with high-resolution CT is a well-circumscribed, expansile soft-tissue mass centered on the clivus, with extensive lytic bony destruction of adjacent bone (Figure 8.11) [45,96]. The main clue to diagnosis is the location of the mass in the midline with epicenter in the posterior aspect of the clivus [45]. The bulk of the tumor is usually

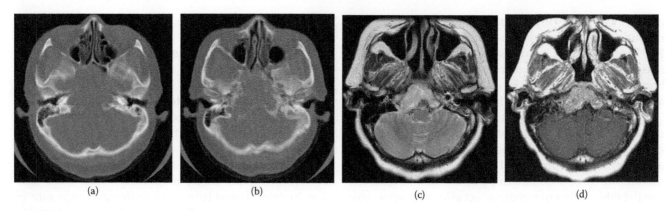

(a)   (b)   (c)   (d)

FIGURE 8.11
Chordoma. (a, b) Axial noncontrast CT images show an expansile, lytic lesion centered in the clivus. The lesion arises from the midline and lacks ground-glass density. There is extensive bony remodeling, with probable compromise of the hypoglossal canals and some effacement of the left jugular foramen. (c) Axial T_2 image in the same patient shows a T_2-hyperintense mass arising from the chordoma with mild extension into the premedullary space without significant compression on the medulla. (d) Axial postcontrast T_1 image shows homogeneous enhancement of clival mass; final diagnosis was a clival chordoma.

hyperattenuating relative to the adjacent neural axis. Intratumoral calcifications appear irregular and are usually thought to represent sequestra from bony destruction rather than dystrophic calcifications of the tumor itself [96]. The chondroid variant, in particular, is more likely to show real intratumoral calcifications. Following contrast administration, there is moderate to marked tumor enhancement (Figure 8.11); solitary or multiple low-attenuation areas are sometimes seen best within the soft-tissue mass and likely represent myxoid and gelatinous material seen on gross pathology [101,102].

The classic midline clival chordoma can spread anteriorly, laterally, posteriorly, inferiorly, and superiorly, thus affecting the sellar area, petrous apex-middle cranial fossa, prepontine cistern, foramen magnum-nasopharynx, and optic chiasm-third ventricle, respectively [96]. Usually, more than one of these regions are involved. Anterior tumor extension can involve the sphenoid sinus, and less likely the posterior ethmoid sinus. Anteroinferior extension can affect the nasopharynx and parapharyngeal space. Posteroinferior extension leads to involvement of the jugular fossa and foramen magnum, with erosion of the atlas and other cervical vertebrae [96]. Intracranial chordomas may arise in the sellar and parasellar areas; lateral extension of these tumors can invade the middle cranial fossa, whereas posterior extension can affect the petrous apex. Intracranial chordomas can grow into basal cisterns with brain stem compression. Furthermore, intracranial chordomas commonly encroach onto the anterior visual pathway and cranial nerves in the prepontine cistern and cavernous sinus, resulting in visual and cranial nerve abnormalities [96].

The lesion most commonly confused with chordomas are chondrosarcomas [96]. Other differential diagnoses include clival meningioma, nasopharyngeal malignancies, plasmacytoma, lymphoma, and craniopharyngiomas. Rhabdomyosarcoma should also be considered in pediatric patients. Less common differential diagnoses include metastases, aggressive pituitary adenomas, histiocytosis X, dermoid and epidermoid cysts, trigeminal neuroma, and fibrous dysplasia [96].

8.5.3.2 Chondrosarcoma

8.5.3.2.1 General

Chondrosarcomas are a rare group of tumors arising from cartilage, enchondral bone, or primitive mesenchymal cells in the brain or meninges [103]. Head and neck chondrosarcomas account for 6.7% of all reported sites of occurrence [104]. Intracranially, they arise most commonly adjacent to the sella, in the cerebellopontine angle, and near the convexity [105]. Parasellar lesions occasionally extend through the skull base and typically spread by local invasion. Even when removed surgically, chondrosarcomas may recur, but systemic metastases are infrequent and usually occur only with aggresssssive variants [106].

8.5.3.2.2 CT Appearance

As with chordomas, MRI is best suited to show disease extent when assessing chondrosarcomas (Figure 8.12). CT, however, still retains an important complementary role for the evaluation of calcifications, which are helpful in differential diagnosis [106]. CT also is helpful in the evaluation of subtle bone erosions. The most common bone changes are a combination of erosion and destruction, usually with a narrow zone of transition (Figure 8.12). Matrix calcification is a hallmark of these lesions, similar to that seen when these lesions are seen elsewhere in the body [107]. There is typically minimal to moderate contrast enhancement seen with CT [103].

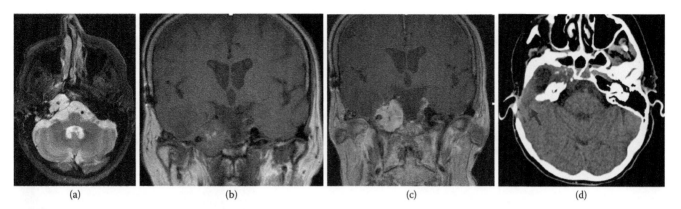

(a)	(b)	(c)	(d)

FIGURE 8.12
Chondrosarcoma. (a) Axial T_2-weighted magnetic resonance (MR) shows T_2 hyperintensity in the right petrous apex near the petro-clival synchondrosis, with internal signal voids corresponding to calcifications. MRI also plays an important role in characterization of chondrosarcomas. (b) T_1-weighted, coronal, noncontrast MRI shows an isointense mass containing scattered calcifications abutting the right internal carotid artery. There is right temporal encephalomalcia and evidence of right craniotomy related to prior treatment. (c) Post-contrast T1-weighted coronal MRI demonstrates enhancement of the right sided mass abutting the internal carotid artery. (d) Axial CT without contrast through the skull base shows erosion of the right petrous temporal apex by an isodense mass (arrow) that contains stippled calcifications (not well seen on this image). A clue to differentiating this tumor from chordoma is that chordomas tend to be in the midline.

Chondrosarcomas may be commonly confused with chordomas [96]. Unlike intracranial chordomas, which are located in the midline skull base, most chondrosarcomas arise along the petro-occipital fissure. When chondrosarcomas are in the midline, differentiation is difficult. Since the tumors can have similar MRI signal intensities, linear, globular, or arclike calcifications seen on CT with chondrosarcomas can help to differentiate them from intracranial chordomas [96]. Meningiomas may also be difficult to differentiate; however, contrast enhancement with CT tends to be more confluent with meningioma. Furthermore, although meningioma can show hyperostosis, chondrosarcoma and chordoma are essentially lytic lesions [103].

8.5.3.3 Fibrous Dysplasia

8.5.3.3.1 General

Fibrous dysplasia is a developmental anomaly of the mesenchymal precursor of bone, manifesting as a defect in osteoblastic differentiation and maturation [106]. About 70%–80% of cases are monostotic. Although calvarial involvement is usually monostotic, the skull base and facial bones are commonly affected in polyostotic forms. Up to half of patients with polyostotic fibrous dysplasia have skull and facial involvement, whereas 10%–25% of patients with the monostotic form exhibit involvement of these areas [108]. The sphenoid, frontal, maxillary, and ethmoid bones are most commonly involved, followed by occipital and temporal bones [108].

Common presenting symptoms include cranial asymmetry and facial deformity. Involvement of the optic canal and sphenoid wing may encroach on the optic

nerve and result in blindness. Symptoms referable to the orbit include exophthalmos and visual impairment.

8.5.3.3.2 CT Appearance

Three radiologic appearances of fibrous dysplasia of the skull have been described: pagetoid, sclerotic, and cystic. The sclerotic type most commonly involves the skull base and sphenoid bone [108]. Widened diploic spaces and osseous expansion, along with hazy sclerotic lesions, are commonly seen. Foraminal encroachment on the skull base is readily seen on CT. Expansile lesions with abrupt transitions zones between the lesion and normal bone are common. The imaging appearance will vary based on the underlying histological composition (Figure 8.13).

8.5.3.4 Pilocytic Astrocytoma (WHO Grade I)

8.5.3.4.1 General

A tumor of childhood with a peak incidence between 5 and 15 years, pilocytic astrocytoma accounts for 30%–40% of intracranial pediatric tumors [109]. These most commonly occur in the cerebellar hemispheres but are also found in the floor of the third ventricle, thalamus, and basal ganglia [45]. Those associated with neurofibromatosis generally occur in the optic chiasm and nerves [110]. Histologically, pilocytic astrocytomas show characteristic alternating patterns of compact bipolar pilocytic (hairlike) astrocytes and loosely aggregated astrocytes, the latter of which often undergo microcystic degeneration [111,112]. These tumors are generally low-grade and almost never recur following complete surgical excision; even those that are incompletely resected are slow growing and do not undergo malignant transformation [110].

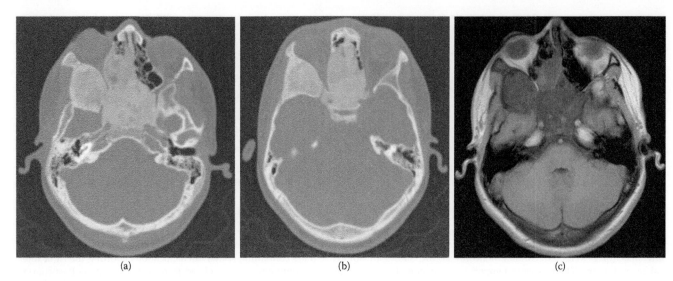

(a)   (b)   (c)

FIGURE 8.13
Fibrous dysplasia. (a, b) Noncontrast axial CT images show ground-glass opacity and bony expansion of the sphenoid bone and greater wing of the right sphenoid bone, and posterior ethmoid air cells on the right. The right superior orbital fissure is also deformed. Findings are compatible with fibrous dysplasia. (c) Noncontrast axial T_1 images in the same patient show bony expansion of the sphenoid bone, greater wing of the sphenoid on the right, and right posterior ethmoid air cells. T_1 hypointensity is noted.

8.5.3.4.2 *CT Appearance*

Pilocytic astrocytomas have a characteristic appearance of a grossly cystic nature, with a richly vascular mural tumor nodule in the cyst wall (Figure 8.14). These tumors tend to be found around the third ventricle supratentorially and the fourth ventricle infratentorially. Lesions are sharply demarcated with smooth margins except when located in the optic chiasm or nerves, where they tend to grow along the optic pathway and give a multilobulated or dumbbell appearance. With CT, the tumor matrix appears hypodense or isodense (Figure 8.14) with strong contrast enhancement. The pattern of strong contrast enhancement helps differentiate these tumors from low-grade fibrillary astrocytomas, which usually present as hypodense, nonenhancing masses [110]. This finding is likely secondary to tumor vascularity or lack thereof. Surrounding edema is frequently absent, also likely related to the low malignancy potential.

Tumor calcification is rare and tends to be fleck-like when seen. Formation of micro- or macrocysts is also common, and macrocysts are rare in lesions along the optic pathways or in the third ventricle. The differential diagnosis includes craniopharyngioma, germinoma, metastases, and invasive pituitary adenoma in the region of the optic chiasm; medulloblastoma and ependymoma in the posterior fossa; and intraventricular or subependymal oligodendroglioma and ependymoma in the paraventricular cerebral hemisphere [110].

8.5.3.5 *Meningioma*

8.5.3.5.1 *General*

Meningiomas are typically benign, slow-growing tumors arising from arachnoidal cells of the meninges. They account for approximately 15% of all primary brain tumors and are the second most common primary intracranial tumor after glioblastomas [45]. The peak age of prevalence is between 40 and 60, and there is an increased incidence in women, 3:2, compared to men [45]. Multiple meningiomas are found with neurofibromatosis 2 and are also the most common intracranial malignancy induced by prior radiation therapy [45].

Meningiomas are most commonly found adjacent to the falx, with the next being the meninges adjacent to suture lines [45]. Skull base meningiomas are also not uncommon [106]. Morphologically, two common types are seen: the flat, "en plaque" variety and the lobulated or spherical mass which indents adjacent parenchyma [45].

Resectability is the single greatest factor predicting patient prognosis. The overall recurrence rate of meningiomas is 21%. If a tumor is excised entirely with its dural attachment, the recurrence rate diminishes to 5%–9%, as compared with 39% for tumors where there is only partial excision. The relationship of the tumor to adjacent intracranial structures ultimately determines respectability, and thus prognosis. Thus, it is important to precisely localize the tumor and to give an accurate assessment of adjacent structures [45].

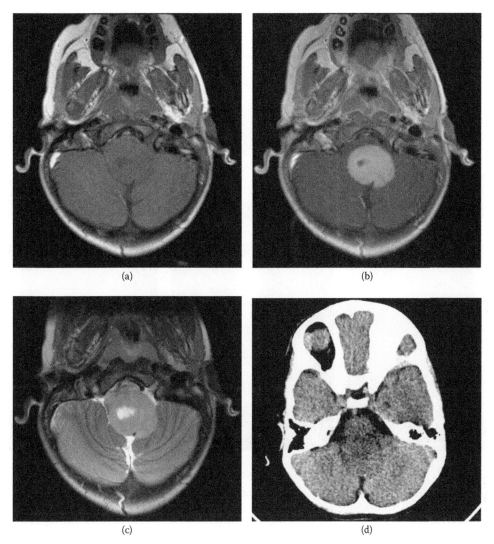

(a)

(b)

(c)

(d)

FIGURE 8.14
Pilocytic astrocytoma. (a, b) Sharply demarcated mass arising from the region of the fourth ventricle with cystic and solid components. Pre- and postcontrast axial T_1 images show marked homogeneous contrast enhancement, which is characteristic of pilocytic astrocytomas. (c) Axial T_2 image clearly shows cystic component within the mass. Note the lack of significant edema around the tumor, which is characteristic. (d) Axial nonenhanced CT scan shows regional hypodensity in the region of the tumor. Hypodensity or isodensity to surrounding brain matter is an expected finding. Although an abnormality is visible, the mixed cystic and solid components are better depicted on MRI.

8.5.3.5.2 CT Appearance

The typical imaging appearance is a well-defined hyperdense mass arising from dura and displacing adjacent brain (Figure 8.15) [45]; however, 25%–33% may be isodense and rarely may also be hypodense [113]. Calcifications are seen in 20%–25%, which are well demonstrated on CT scan [45]. Hyperostosis, or less commonly, bone destruction may occur in 15%–20% of cases (Figure 8.15) [45]. Following contrast injection, nearly all meningiomas will show intense enhancement [113]. Edema can be seen in adjacent white matter parenchyma in up to 60% of cases as well [113] and can be extensive.

Smaller meningiomas are usually best seen with CT as they have relaxation times similar to brain parenchyma on MRI [106]. Focal areas of hyperostosis are best seen with bone windows and may be the only abnormality seen with smaller lesions; the soft-tissue component, when present, usually enhances intensely after contrast administration [106].

Precise lesion localization and definition of the relationship to adjacent structures are critical roles of the neuroradiologist in tumor assessment as these factors dictate the extent of respectability. The most common tumor locations are in Sections 8.5.3.6 through 8.5.3.11.

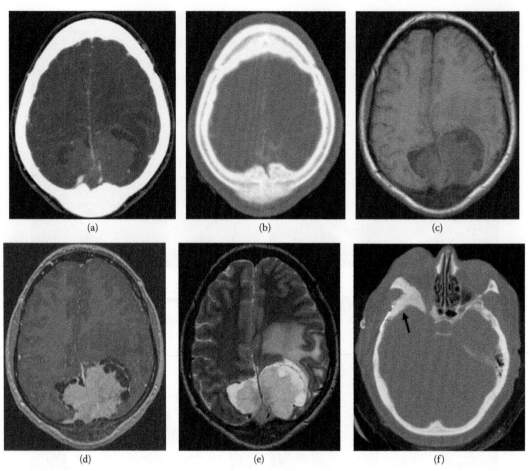

FIGURE 8.15

Meningioma. (a, b) Axial postcontrast CT images on soft tissue and bone windows. Large posterior parietal dural-based mass with significant enhancement and hyperostosis. (c, d) Axial pre- and postcontrast T_1 images showing an avidly enhancing mass with significant mass effect. It is not as well circumscribed as a typical meningioma and findings were overall consistent with anaplastic meningioma. (e) Axial T_2 image in the same patient shows significant vasogenic edema, and again is suggestive of a more aggressive process than a classic benign meningioma. (f) Axial noncontrast CT image in a different patient. Postoperative film following meningioma resection; there is marked hyperostosis of the right greater sphenoid wing (arrow), secondary to a sphenoid wing meningioma. Hyperostosis may be seen in approximately 15%–20% of meningiomas. There has been a right anterior craniotomy with resection of part of the right orbital roof.

8.5.3.6 Parasagittal and Convexity Meningiomas

The majority of meningiomas (45%) are found in these sites. The most important feature in preoperative assessment is involvement of the superior sagittal sinus; 25% of intracranial meningiomas are in the parasagittal group and of these, half will either partially or completely obliterate the superior sagittal sinus on presentation [45]. If the sinus is completely obliterated before surgery, the tumor may be safely removed. However, if the middle third of the sinus is only partially obliterated, total meningioma excision cannot be achieved as attempts at abrupt obliteration of the sinus are likely fatal; unfortunately, 60% of parasagittal meningiomas involve this middle third of the sinus, whereas only 13% involve the anterior third which may be safely surgically obliterated [45].

Convexity meningiomas arising adjacent and growing into the sylvian fissure must be assessed with regard to their proximity to the middle cerebral artery branches.

8.5.3.7 Sphenoid Wing Meningiomas

These lesions account for 15%–20% of all meningiomas total and are commonly of the "en plaque" variety and involve adjacent bone, leading to hyperostosis. The tumor traverses bone to involve adjacent structures such as the orbit, optic canal, temporal fossa, and possibly the temporalis muscle. The en plaque variety is usually accompanied by slowly progressive, unilateral, and painless exophthalmos; headache and numbness in the distribution of cranial nerves V1 and V2, and seizures may also be seen [106]. Resection needs to be extensive and can lead to neurological deficits in its own right; thus, radical surgery is often delayed in efforts to preserve remaining function for as long as possible [45].

8.5.3.8 Olfactory Groove Meningiomas

These tumors account for 5%–10% of all meningiomas, and aside from personality changes, often produce few symptoms; thus, they tend to attain larger sizes by the time of presentation. Given their location, they indent the inferior portions of the frontal lobe and may extend superiorly into the inferior aspect of the interhemispheric fissure. They occasionally may extend through the floor of the anterior cranial fossa, resulting in CSF leaks. With regard to surgical planning, the relationship to the anterior cerebral artery must be assessed [45].

8.5.3.9 Parasellar Meningiomas

Approximately 5%–10% of meningiomas arise from the tuberculum sellae, and they grow up and over the planum sphenoidale to displace the optic chiasm and pituitary stalk posteriorly. Tumors may also arise from the adjacent sellar diaphragm and impact structures abutting the suprasellar cistern. Tumor relationship to adjacent major vessels must also be assessed before surgery [45].

8.5.3.10 Cavernous Sinus Meningiomas

Meningiomas of the cavernous sinus invade the sinus itself and encase the internal carotid artery. They may extend posteriorly to involve the tentorium cerebelli and invade down the posterior aspect of the clivus; total resection of these meningiomas is not feasible [45].

8.5.3.11 Posterior Fossa Meningiomas

Meningiomas of the posterior fossa may arise from either the clivus or the petrous bone. If arising from the petrous bone, they often have broad bases laterally and medially and indent adjacent brain stem structures. They may extend into the internal auditory canal, with enhancement being shown within the canal. CSF may even become trapped laterally, leading to a cystic appearance in relation to the tumor. These lesions are the second most common tumors of the cerebellopontine angle [45].

8.5.3.12 Others

Finally, approximately 5% of meningiomas do not have dural attachments and may be found in the ventricles or arise from the diploic space [45]. Because arachnoid cells can be found accompanying cranial nerves, it is not surprising that meningiomas can also be found adjacent to and traversing various skull base foramina [106]. Although these meningiomas can cause foraminal erosion and simulate schwannomas, grossly destructive changes in the skull base may also be seen; in these cases, it may be difficult to distinguish these tumors from malignant processes [106].

8.5.4 False Positives

Although tumors on CT often show cysts or calcifications, benign pathologies may also be present with these findings. Cystic lesions arising in the area of the pituitary gland may represent Rathke's cleft cysts (Figure 8.16). Large aneurysms often present with calcifications and could mimic a calcified tumor (Figure 8.17). Although enhancement is frequently seen

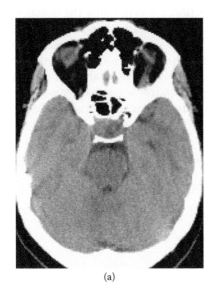
(a)

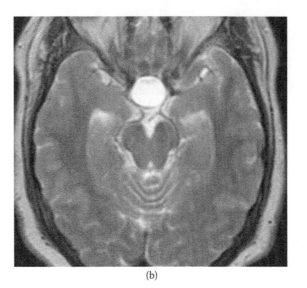
(b)

FIGURE 8.16
Rathke's cleft cyst showed on (a) noncontrast axial CT and (b) axial T_2 images.

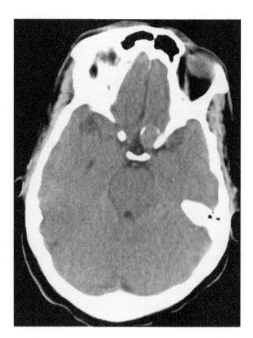

FIGURE 8.17
Calcified structure anterior and to the left of the dorsum sellae represents a large aneurysm.

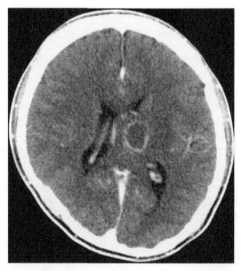

FIGURE 8.18
Just to the left of the midline there is a structure with smooth ring enhancement. Although ring enhancement may be seen with glioblastoma, this lesion represents an abscess. Compare with ring-enhancing glioblastoma in Figure 8.5.

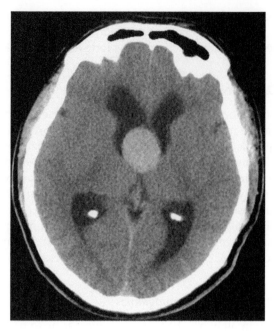

FIGURE 8.19
Colloid cyst. Large homogeneous hyperdense cystic lesion arising from the anterior portion of the third ventricle represents a colloid cyst.

lesions represent just a small subset of non-neoplastic pathologies mimicking tumors, but serve as a reminder to consider alternative etiologies when assessing lesions on CT.

8.6 Conclusion

Despite advances in MRI for the imaging of brain tumor, CT retains an important role in tumor characterization and detection. CT is not only the initial imaging modality for patients initially presenting with unknown brain tumors, but is also particularly useful for showing certain tumor characteristics such as calcifications, osseous involvement, and cystic change. Thus, a familiarity with the imaging characteristics of various brain tumors on CT is essential for the neuroradiologist.

with tumors, non-neoplastic lesions can also calcify; as an example, abscesses characteristically present with ring enhancement (Figure 8.18). Finally, colloid cysts may also mimic tumors; on CT, they are with high density secondary to proteinaceous contents, and arise from the anterior aspect of the third ventricle just posterior to the foramen of Monro (Figure 8.19). The aforementioned

References

1. Bondy ML, Scheurer ME, Malmer B, Barnholtz-Sloan JS, Davis FG, Il'yasova D, Kruchko C, McCarthy BJ, Rajaraman P, Schwartzbaum JA et al. Brain tumor epidemiology: Consensus from the Brain Tumor Epidemiology Consortium. *Cancer* 2008; 113(7 Suppl): 1953–1968.
2. CBTRUS. *Primary Brain Tumors in the United States 2004-2008.* Chicago, IL: Central Brain Tumor Registry of the United States, 2012.

3. Preston-Martin S. Epidemiology of primary CNS neoplasms. *Neurol Clin* 1996; 14(2): 273–290.

4. Davis FG, McCarthy BJ. Current epidemiological trends and surveillance issues in brain tumors. *Expert Rev Anticancer Ther* 2001; 1(3): 395–401.

5. Osborne RH, Houben MP, Tijssen CC, Coebergh JW, van Duijn CM. The genetic epidemiology of glioma. *Neurology* 2001; 57(10): 1751–1755.

6. Wrensch M, Minn Y, Chew T, Bondy M, Berger MS. Epidemiology of primary brain tumors: Current concepts and review of the literature. *Neuro-oncology* 2002; 4(4): 278–299.

7. Hess KR, Broglio KR, Bondy ML. Adult glioma incidence trends in the United States, 1977-2000. *Cancer* 2004; 101(10): 2293–2299.

8. Parkin DM, Whelan SL, Ferlay J, Teppo L, Thomas DB *Cancer Incidence in Five Continents*. Lyon, France: IARC Press, 2002.

9. Soffietti R, Ruda R, Mutani R. Management of brain metastases. *J Neurol* 2002; 249(10): 1357–1369.

10. Langer CJ, Mehta MP. Current management of brain metastases, with a focus on systemic options. *J Clin Oncol* 2005; 23(25): 6207–6219.

11. Bajaj GK, Kleinberg L, Terezakis S. Current concepts and controversies in the treatment of parenchymal brain metastases: Improved outcomes with aggressive management. *Cancer Invest* 2005; 23(4): 363–376.

12. Legler JM, Ries LA, Smith MA, Warren JL, Heineman EF, Kaplan RS, Linet MS. Cancer surveillance series [corrected]: Brain and other central nervous system cancers: Recent trends in incidence and mortality. *J Natl Cancer Inst* 1999; 91(16): 1382–1390.

13. Bailey P, Cushing H. *A Classification of the Tumors of the Glioma Group on a Histogenetic Basis with a Correlated Study of Prognosis*. Philadelphia, PA: JB Lippincott, 1926: 95.

14. Kleihues P, Burger P, Scheithauer B. Histological classification of CNS tumours. In: Sobin L, ed. *Histological Typing of Tumours of the Central Nervous System*. Berlin, Germany: Springer-Verlag, 1993: 1–105.

15. Kleihues P, Cavenee W. *Pathology and Genetics of Tumours of the Nervous System*. Lyon, France: IARC Press, 2000.

16. Kleihues P, Louis DN, Scheithauer BW, Rorke LB, Reifenberger G, Burger PC, Cavenee WK. The WHO classification of tumors of the nervous system. *J Neuropathol Exp Neurol* 2002; 61(3): 215–225; discussion 226–229.

17. Louis DN, Ohgaki H, Wiestler OD, Cavenee WK, Burger PC, Jouvet A, Scheithauer BW, Kleihues P. The 2007 WHO classification of tumours of the central nervous system. *Acta Neuropathol* 2007; 114(2): 97–109.

18. Bilaniuk LT. Adult infratentorial tumors. *Semin Roentgenol* 1990; 25(2): 155–173.

19. Pollack IF. Brain tumors in children. *N Engl J Med* 1994; 331(22): 1500–1507.

20. Brant-Zawadzki M, Badami JP, Mills CM, Norman D, Newton TH. Primary intracranial tumor imaging: A comparison of magnetic resonance and CT. *Radiology* 1984; 150(2): 435–440.

21. Brant-Zawadzki M, Davis PL, Crooks LE, Mills CM, Norman D, Newton TH, Sheldon P, Kaufman L. NMR demonstration of cerebral abnormalities: Comparison with CT. *AJR Am J Roentgenol* 1983; 140(5): 847–854.

22. Lee BC, Kneeland JB, Cahill PT, Deck MD. MR recognition of supratentorial tumors. *AJNR Am J Neuroradiol* 1985; 6(6): 871–878.

23. Healy ME, Hesselink JR, Press GA, Middleton MS. Increased detection of intracranial metastases with intravenous Gd-DTPA. *Radiology* 1987; 165(3): 619–624.

24. Russell EJ, Geremia GK, Johnson CE, Huckman MS, Ramsey RG, Washburn-Bleck J, Turner DA, Norusis M. Multiple cerebral metastases: Detectability with Gd-DTPA-enhanced MR imaging. *Radiology* 1987; 165(3): 609–617.

25. Bydder GM, Steiner RE, Young IR, Hall AS, Thomas DJ, Marshall J, Pallis CA, Legg NJ. Clinical NMR imaging of the brain: 140 Cases. *AJR Am J Roentgenol* 1982; 139(2): 215–236.

26. Alfidi RJ, Haaga JR, El-Yousef SJ, Bryan PJ, Fletcher BD, LiPuma JP, Morrison SC, Kaufman B, Richey JB, Hinshaw WS et al. Preliminary experimental results in humans and animals with a superconducting, whole-body, nuclear magnetic resonance scanner. *Radiology* 1982; 143(1): 175–181.

27. Young IR, Burl M, Clarke GJ, Hall AS, Pasmore T, Collins AG, Smith DT, Orr JS, Bydder GM, Doyle FH et al. Magnetic resonance properties of hydrogen: Imaging the posterior fossa. *AJR Am J Roentgenol* 1981; 137(5): 895–901.

28. Young IR, Randell CP, Kaplan PW, James A, Bydder GM, Steiner RE. Nuclear magnetic resonance (NMR) imaging in white matter disease of the brain using spin-echo sequences. *J Comput Assist Tomogr* 1983; 7(2): 290–294.

29. Hatam A, Bergvall U, Lewander R, Larsson S, Lind M. Contrast medium enhancement with time in computer tomography. Differential diagnosis of intracranial lesions. *Acta Radiol Suppl* 1975; 346: 63–81.

30. Norman D, Enzmann DR, Newton TH. Optimal contrast dosage in cranial computed tomography. *AJR Am J Roentgenol* 1978; 131(4): 687–689.

31. Norman D, Stevens EA, Wing SD, Levin V, Newton TH. Quantitative aspects of contrast enhancement in cranial computed tomography. *Radiology* 1978; 129(3): 683–688.

32. Hayman LA, Evans RA, Hinck VC. Delayed high iodine dose contrast computed tomography: Cranial neoplasms. *Radiology* 1980; 136(3): 677–684.

33. Gado MH, Phelps ME, Coleman RE. An extravascular component of contrast enhancement in cranial computed tomography. Part I. The tissue-blood ratio of contrast enhancement. *Radiology* 1975; 117(3 Pt 1): 589–593.

34. Bergvall B. Temporal course of contrast medium enhancement in differential diagnosis of intracranial lesions with computed tomography. In: Salamon G, ed. *Advance in Cerebral Angiography*. Berlin, Germany: Springer-Verlag, 1975: 346–348.

35. Komatsu K, Tsuyumu M, Tsuruoka S, Fukumoto T, Takei H, Ohie K, Yamaguchi T, Okada K, Hiratsuka H, Inaba Y. [CT diagnosis of brain tumors—Sequential study of delayed enhanced CT and radioisotope delayed scan (author's transl)]. *Neurol Med Chir* (Tokyo) 1978; 18(4): 287–293.

36. Sato O, Kanazawa I, Kokunai T, Yamashita M. [A study of the delayed scan in the enhanced computed tomography for intracranial tumors (author's transl)]. *Neurol Med Chir* (Tokyo) 1977; 17(2 Pt 2): 123–128.

37. Steinhoff H, Aviles C. Contrast enhancement response of intracranial neoplasms: Its validity for the differential diagnosis of tumors in CT. In: Lanksch W, Kazner E, eds. *Cranial Computed Tomography*. New York, NY: Springer-Verlag, 1976: 151–163.

38. Davis JM, Davis KR, Newhouse J, Pfister RC. Expanded high iodine dose in computed cranial tomography: A preliminary report. *Radiology* 1979; 131(2): 373–380.

39. Davis PC, Hudgins PA, Peterman SB, Hoffman JC Jr. Diagnosis of cerebral metastases: Double-dose delayed CT vs contrast-enhanced MR imaging. *AJNR Am J Neuroradiol* 1991; 12(2): 293–300.

40. Shalen PR, Hayman LA, Wallace S, Handel SF. Protocol for delayed contrast enhancement in computed tomography of cerebral neoplasia. *Radiology* 1981; 139(2): 397–402.

41. Balériaux D, Bank W, Matos C. The brain. In: Vanel D, Stark D, eds. *Imaging Strategies in Oncology*. New York, NY: John Wiley & Sons, 1993: 1–36.

42. Di Chiro G. Positron emission tomography using [18F] fluorodeoxyglucose in brain tumors. A powerful diagnostic and prognostic tool. *Invest Radiol* 1987; 22(5): 360–371.

43. Atlas SW, Grossman RI, Gomori JM, Hackney DB, Goldberg HI, Zimmerman RA, Bilaniuk LT. Hemorrhagic intracranial malignant neoplasms: Spin-echo MR imaging. *Radiology* 1987; 164(1): 71–77.

44. Zimmerman RD, Leeds NE, Naidich TP. Ring blush associated with intracerebral hematoma. *Radiology* 1977; 122(3): 707–711.

45. Britton J. Primary tumours of the central nervous system. In: Husband J, Reznek R, eds. *Imaging in Oncology*. London, UK: Taylor & Francis Group, 2004: 711–787.

46. Parsons DW, Jones S, Zhang X, Lin JC, Leary RJ, Angenendt P, Mankoo P, Carter H, Siu IM, Gallia GL et al. An integrated genomic analysis of human glioblastoma multiforme. *Science* 2008; 321(5897): 1807–1812.

47. Yan H, Parsons DW, Jin G, McLendon R, Rasheed BA, Yuan W, Kos I, Batinic-Haberle I, Jones S, Riggins GJ et al. IDH1 and IDH2 mutations in gliomas. *N Engl J Med* 2009; 360(8): 765–773.

48. Noushmehr H, Weisenberger DJ, Diefes K, Phillips HS, Pujara K, Berman BP, Pan F, Pelloski CE, Sulman EP, Bhat KP et al. Identification of a CpG island methylator phenotype that defines a distinct subgroup of glioma. *Cancer Cell* 2010; 17(5): 510–522.

49. Weller M, Wick W, von Deimling A. Isocitrate dehydrogenase mutations: A challenge to traditional views on the genesis and malignant progression of gliomas. *Glia* 2011; 59(8): 1200–1204.

50. Ichimura K, Pearson DM, Kocialkowski S, Bäcklund LM, Chan R, Jones DT, Collins VP. IDH1 mutations are present in the majority of common adult gliomas but rare in primary glioblastomas. *Neuro-oncology* 2009; 11(4): 341–347.

51. Watanabe T, Nobusawa S, Kleihues P, Ohgaki H. IDH1 mutations are early events in the development of astrocytomas and oligodendrogliomas. *Am J Pathol* 2009; 174(4): 1149–1153.

52. van den Bent MJ, Dubbink HJ, Marie Y, Brandes AA, Taphoorn MJ, Wesseling P, Frenay M, Tijssen CC, Lacombe D, Idbaih A et al. IDH1 and IDH2 mutations are prognostic but not predictive for outcome in anaplastic oligodendroglial tumors: A report of the European Organization for Research and Treatment of Cancer Brain Tumor Group. *Clin Cancer Res* 2010; 16(5): 1597–1604.

53. Huse JT, Holland EC. Targeting brain cancer: Advances in the molecular pathology of malignant glioma and medulloblastoma. *Nat Rev Cancer* 2010; 10(5): 319–331.

54. Huse JT, Phillips HS, Brennan CW. Molecular subclassification of diffuse gliomas: Seeing order in the chaos. *Glia* 2011; 59(8): 1190–1199.

55. Castillo M, Scatliff JH, Bouldin TW, Suzuki K. Radiologic-pathologic correlation: Intracranial astrocytoma. *AJNR Am J Neuroradiol* 1992; 13(6): 1609–1616.

56. Osborn A. *Neuroradiology*, Chapter 13. Saint Louis, MO: Mosby, 1994: 529–578.

57. Montine TJ, Vandersteenhoven JJ, Aguzzi A, Boyko OB, Dodge RK, Kerns BJ, Burger PC. Prognostic significance of Ki-67 proliferation index in supratentorial fibrillary astrocytic neoplasms. *Neurosurgery* 1994; 34(4): 674–678; discussion 678–679.

58. Raghavan R, Steart PV, Weller RO. Cell proliferation patterns in the diagnosis of astrocytomas, anaplastic astrocytomas and glioblastoma multiforme: A Ki-67 study. *Neuropathol Appl Neurobiol* 1990; 16(2): 123–133.

59. Krouwer HG, Davis RL, Silver P, Prados M. Gemistocytic astrocytomas: A reappraisal. *J Neurosurg* 1991; 74(3): 399–406.

60. Stupp R, Mason WP, van den Bent MJ, Weller M, Fisher B, Taphoorn MJ, Belanger K, Brandes AA, Marosi C, Bogdahn U et al. Radiotherapy plus concomitant and adjuvant temozolomide for glioblastoma. *N Engl J Med* 2005; 352(10): 987–996.

61. Tervonen O, Forbes G, Scheithauer BW, Dietz MJ. Diffuse "fibrillary" astrocytomas: Correlation of MRI features with histopathologic parameters and tumor grade. *Neuroradiology* 1992; 34(3): 173–178.

62. Watanabe M, Tanaka R, Takeda N. Magnetic resonance imaging and histopathology of cerebral gliomas. *Neuroradiology* 1992; 34(6): 463–469.

63. Tovi M. MR imaging in cerebral gliomas analysis of tumour tissue components. *Acta Radiol Suppl* 1993; 384: 1–24.

64. Rao CV, Kishore PR, Bartlett J, Brennan TG. Computed tomography in the postoperative patient. *Neuroradiology* 1980; 19(5): 257–263.

65. Elster AD, DiPersio DA. Cranial postoperative site: Assessment with contrast-enhanced MR imaging. *Radiology* 1990; 174(1): 93–98.

66. Lanzieri CF, Som PM, Sacher M, Solodnik P, Moore F. The postcraniectomy site: CT appearance. *Radiology* 1986; 159(1): 165–170.

67. Valk PE, Dillon WP. Radiation injury of the brain. *AJNR Am J Neuroradiol* 1991; 12(1): 45–62.

68. Hecht-Leavitt C, Grossman RI, Curran WJ Jr, McGrath JT, Biery DN, Joseph PM, Nelson DF. MR of brain radiation injury: Experimental studies in cats. *AJNR Am J Neuroradiol* 1987; 8(3): 427–430.

69. Graeb DA, Steinbok P, Robertson WD. Transient early computed tomographic changes mimicking tumor progression after brain tumor irradiation. *Radiology* 1982; 144(4): 813–817.

70. Yamashita J, Handa H, Yumitori K, Abe M. Reversible delayed radiation effect on the brain after radiotherapy of malignant astrocytoma. *Surg Neurol* 1980; 13(6): 413–417.

71. Curnes JT, Laster DW, Ball MR, Moody DM, Witcofski RL. MRI of radiation injury to the brain. *AJR Am J Roentgenol* 1986; 147(1): 119–124.

72. Tsuruda JS, Kortman KE, Bradley WG, Wheeler DC, Van Dalsem W, Bradley TP. Radiation effects on cerebral white matter: MR evaluation. *AJR Am J Roentgenol* 1987; 149(1): 165–171.

73. Dean BL, Drayer BP, Bird CR, Flom RA, Hodak JA, Coons SW, Carey RG. Gliomas: Classification with MR imaging. *Radiology* 1990; 174(2): 411–415.

74. Engelhard HH, Stelea A, Mundt A. Oligodendroglioma and anaplastic oligodendroglioma: Clinical features, treatment, and prognosis. *Surg Neurol* 2003; 60(5): 443–456.

75. Mørk SJ, Lindegaard KF, Halvorsen TB, Lehmann EH, Solgaard T, Hatlevoll R, Harvei S, Ganz J. Oligodendroglioma: Incidence and biological behavior in a defined population. *J Neurosurg* 1985; 63(6): 881–889.

76. Nijjar TS, Simpson WJ, Gadalla T, McCartney M. Oligodendroglioma. The Princess Margaret Hospital experience (1958-1984). *Cancer* 1993; 71(12): 4002–4006.

77. Shaw EG, Scheithauer BW, O'Fallon JR, Tazelaar HD, Davis DH. Oligodendrogliomas: The Mayo Clinic experience. *J Neurosurg* 1992; 76(3): 428–434.

78. Dehghani F, Schachenmayr W, Laun A, Korf HW. Prognostic implication of histopathological, immunohistochemical and clinical features of oligodendrogliomas: A study of 89 cases. *Acta Neuropathol* 1998; 95(5): 493–504.

79. Tice H, Barnes PD, Goumnerova L, Scott RM, Tarbell NJ. Pediatric and adolescent oligodendrogliomas. *AJNR Am J Neuroradiol* 1993; 14(6): 1293–1300.

80. Koeller KK, Rushing EJ. From the archives of the AFIP: Oligodendroglioma and its variants: Radiologic-pathologic correlation. *Radiographics* 2005; 25(6): 1669–1688.

81. Lee YY, Van Tassel P. Intracranial oligodendrogliomas: Imaging findings in 35 untreated cases. *AJR Am J Roentgenol* 1989; 152(2): 361–369.

82. Lee C, Duncan VW, Young AB. Magnetic resonance features of the enigmatic oligodendroglioma. *Invest Radiol* 1998; 33(4): 222–231.

83. Cairncross JG, Ueki K, Zlatescu MC, Lisle DK, Finkelstein DM, Hammond RR, Silver JS, Stark PC, Macdonald DR, Ino Y et al. Specific genetic predictors of chemotherapeutic response and survival in patients with anaplastic oligodendrogliomas. *J Natl Cancer Inst* 1998; 90(19): 1473–1479.

84. Bunin GR, Surawicz TS, Witman PA, Preston-Martin S, Davis F, Bruner JM. The descriptive epidemiology of craniopharyngioma. *Neurosurg Focus* 1997; 3(6): e1.

85. Muller HL. Childhood craniopharyngioma—Current concepts in diagnosis, therapy and follow-up. *Nat Rev Endocrinol* 2010; 6(11): 609–618.

86. Minniti G, Esposito V, Amichetti M, Enrici RM. The role of fractionated radiotherapy and radiosurgery in the management of patients with craniopharyngioma. *Neurosurg Rev* 2009; 32(2): 125–132; discussion 132.

87. Rennert J, Doerfler A. Imaging of sellar and parasellar lesions. *Clin Neurol Neurosurg* 2007; 109(2): 111–124.

88. Warmuth-Metz M, Gnekow AK, Müller H, Solymosi L. Differential diagnosis of suprasellar tumors in children. *Klin Padiatr* 2004; 216(6): 323–330.

89. Zada G, Lin N, Ojerholm E, Ramkissoon S, Laws ER. Craniopharyngioma and other cystic epithelial lesions of the sellar region: A review of clinical, imaging, and histopathological relationships. *Neurosurg Focus* 2010; 28(4): E4.

90. Hamamoto Y, Niino K, Adachi M, Hosoya T. MR and CT findings of craniopharyngioma during and after radiation therapy. *Neuroradiology* 2002; 44(2): 118–122.

91. Hasegawa T, Kobayashi T, Kida Y. Tolerance of the optic apparatus in single-fraction irradiation using stereotactic radiosurgery: Evaluation in 100 patients with craniopharyngioma. *Neurosurgery* 2010; 66(4): 688–694; discussion 694–695.

92. Chung WY, Pan HC, Guo WY, Shiau CY, Wang LW, Wu HM, Lee LS. Protection of visual pathway in gamma knife radiosurgery for craniopharyngiomas. *Stereotact Funct Neurosurg* 1998; 70(Suppl 1): 139–151.

93. Eldevik OP, Blaivas M, Gabrielsen TO, Hald JK, Chandler WF. Craniopharyngioma: Radiologic and histologic findings and recurrence. *AJNR Am J Neuroradiol* 1996; 17(8): 1427–1439.

94. Schmalisch K, Beschorner R, Psaras T, Honegger J. Postoperative intracranial seeding of craniopharyngiomas—Report of three cases and review of the literature. *Acta Neurochir (Wien)* 2010; 152(2): 313–319; discussion 319.

95. Mortini P, Losa M, Pozzobon G, Barzaghi R, Riva M, Acerno S, Angius D, Weber G, Chiumello G, Giovanelli M. Neurosurgical treatment of craniopharyngioma in adults and children: Early and long-term results in a large case series. *J Neurosurg* 2011; 114(5): 1350–1359.

96. Erdem E, Angtuaco EC, Van Hemert R, Park JS, Al-Mefty O. Comprehensive review of intracranial chordoma. *Radiographics* 2003; 23(4): 995–1009.

97. McMaster ML, Goldstein AM, Bromley CM, Ishibe N, Parry DM. Chordoma: Incidence and survival patterns in the United States, 1973-1995. *Cancer Causes Control* 2001; 12(1): 1–11.

98. Colli B, Al-Mefty O. Chordomas of the craniocervical junction: Follow-up review and prognostic factors. *J Neurosurg* 2001; 95(6): 933–943.

99. Noël G, Feuvret L, Ferrand R, Boisserie G, Mazeron JJ, Habrand JL. Radiotherapeutic factors in the management of cervical-basal chordomas and chondrosarcomas. *Neurosurgery* 2004; 55(6): 1252–1260; discussion 1260–1262.

100. Hug EB, Loredo LN, Slater JD, DeVries A, Grove RI, Schaefer RA, Rosenberg AE, Slater JM. Proton radiation therapy for chordomas and chondrosarcomas of the skull base. *J Neurosurg* 1999; 91(3): 432–439.
101. Meyer JE, Oot RF, Lindfors KK. CT appearance of clival chordomas. *J Comput Assist Tomogr* 1986; 10(1): 34–38.
102. Whelan MA, Reede DL, Meisler W, Bergeron RT. CT of the base of the skull. *Radiol Clin North Am* 1984; 22(1): 177–217.
103. Morimoto T, Sasaki T, Takakura K, Ishida T. Chondrosarcoma of the skull base: Report of six cases. *Skull Base Surg* 1992; 2(4): 177–185.
104. Pritchard DJ, Lunke RJ, Taylor WF, Dahlin DC, Medley BE. Chondrosarcoma: A clinicopathologic and statistical analysis. *Cancer* 1980; 45(1): 149–157.
105. Braun IF. MRI of the nasopharynx. *Radiol Clin North Am* 1989; 27(2): 315–330.
106. Laine FJ, Nadel L, Braun IF. CT and MR imaging of the central skull base. Part 2. Pathologic spectrum. *Radiographics* 1990; 10(5): 797–821.
107. Lee YY, Van Tassel P. Craniofacial chondrosarcomas: Imaging findings in 15 untreated cases. *AJNR Am J Neuroradiol* 1989; 10(1): 165–170.
108. Daffner RH, Kirks DR, Gehweiler JA Jr, Heaston DK. Computed tomography of fibrous dysplasia. *AJR Am J Roentgenol* 1982; 139(5): 943–948.
109. Giannini C, Scheithauer BW. Classification and grading of low-grade astrocytic tumors in children. *Brain Pathol* 1997; 7(2): 785–798.
110. Lee YY, Van Tassel P, Bruner JM, Moser RP, Share JC. Juvenile pilocytic astrocytomas: CT and MR characteristics. *AJR Am J Roentgenol* 1989; 152(6): 1263–1270.
111. Steinhoff H, Lanksch W, Kazner E, Grumme T, Meese W, Lange S, Aulich A, Schindler E, Wende S. Computed tomography in the diagnosis and differential diagnosis of glioblastomas. A qualitative study of 295 cases. *Neuroradiology* 1977; 14(4): 193–200.
112. Marks JE, Gado M. Serial computed tomography of primary brain tumors following surgery, irradiation, and chemotherapy. *Radiology* 1977; 125(1): 119–125.
113. Sheporaitis LA, Osborn AG, Smirniotopoulos JG, Clunie DA, Howieson J, D'Agostino AN. Intracranial meningioma. *AJNR Am J Neuroradiol* 1992; 13(1): 29–37.

9

Computed Tomography Imaging of Stroke

Angelika Hoffmann and Max Wintermark

CONTENTS

9.1 Introduction

Acute stroke is a leading cause of mortality and morbidity worldwide. According to the World Health Organization, 15 million people worldwide suffer a stroke annually. In the United States, approximately 800,000 people experience a new or recurrent stroke each year and more than 140,000 die from stroke [1].

Imaging plays a central role in the evaluation of patients with acute stroke symptoms. It is key to distinguish ischemic from hemorrhagic stroke, which can be difficult clinically. The main goal in acute ischemic stroke treatment in the early phase is to rescue potentially salvageable ischemic brain tissue as fast as possible. Ischemic stroke is a highly treatable neuroemergency; early intravenous (IV) administration of recombinant tissue plasminogen activator (rtPA) remains the most beneficial, proven intervention for emergency treatment of stroke. Several interventions, including intra-arterial administration of thrombolytic agents and mechanical interventions, show great promise. Computed tomography (CT) or magnetic resonance imaging (MRI) offers important information to guide therapy, including the elimination of hemorrhage as a cause, the characterization of stroke location and subtype, as well as the assessment of tissue viability, with the exact role of these additional pieces of information remaining to be determined.

In this chapter, we will give an overview about the diagnostic information provided by the different components of the CT workup of the patients with stroke, especially those with ischemic stroke, including information about brain tissue viability status and blood–brain barrier (BBB) permeability. A multimodal acute stroke protocol contains a noncontrast CT (NCT), perfusion CT (PCT), and CT angiography (CTA), which can be performed within 10 minutes, giving treatment guidance, without substantially delaying definitive treatment.

We will structure this chapter around an adapted concept of the "four P's" of stroke (parenchyma, pipes, penumbra, and permeability) proposed by Dr. Howard Rowley and use this concept as a practical guide to explain the purpose of the components of a multimodal acute stroke CT protocol.

9.2 Parenchyma

In about 15% of cases, stroke is caused by intracerebral hemorrhage (ICH), whereas in about 85% of cases, stroke is ischemic in nature and results from decreased blood supply to the brain. Different etiologies cause ischemic stroke, such as large-artery atherosclerosis, cardioembolism, and lacunar stroke [2]. In the imaging workup of a patient with stroke, it is important to first determine whether the stroke is ischemic or hemorrhagic in nature. NCT is the main diagnostic test used for this purpose, to triage patients presenting with acute stroke symptoms.

9.2.1 Noncontrast Computed Tomography

Since the invention of the CT scanner in the 1970s, when the original systems were dedicated to head imaging [3], CT has evolved as an important and widely used imaging tool for stroke.

9.2.1.1 Is the Stroke Caused by Hemorrhage?

A fast NCT can detect ICH with high accuracy and is considered to be the gold standard for excluding ICH in the acute setting. Also, stroke mimics, such as tumor or infections, can be excluded, although these lesions are often poorly characterized.

9.2.1.2 Are Ischemic Changes Present?

In ischemic stroke, early ischemic changes may be present on the NCT scan. The hyperdense artery sign, focal tissue swelling, or hypoattenuation can be detected on narrowly windowed and leveled NCT in the first hours of a stroke by the experienced observer. Ischemia causes cerebral capillary dysfunction, resulting in cytotoxic edema, which leads to water influx into the brain [4]. This increase in water content is seen as a hypodensity on CT.

9.2.1.3 How Can Early Ischemic Changes Be Quantified?

Early ischemic changes, such as hypoattenuation or focal swelling, in the anterior circulation can be quantified topographically with the Alberta Stroke Program Early CT Score (ASPECTS), a simple and reliable score, which divides the middle cerebral artery (MCA) territory into 10 regions of interest. By weighing the 10 regions of interest based on functional importance, the ASPECTS identifies those stroke patients who are unlikely to make an independent recovery despite thrombolytic treatment [5]. To compute the ASPECTS, axial cuts of the brain CT are assessed in two standardized levels of the MCA territory, the ganglionic ASPECT region (M1–M3, insula, caudate nucleus, lentiform nucleus, and internal capsule) and the supraganglionic ASPECT region (M4–M6). The caudate nucleus is analyzed in both levels—the head of the caudate in the ganglionic level and the body and tail of the caudate in the supraganglionic level (Figure 9.1). If early ischemic changes are present in a region of interest, a single point is subtracted from 10. Thus, a score of 10 reflects a normal scan and a score of 0 reflects diffuse ischemic involvement throughout the MCA territory. Scores of 7 or less are associated with both poor functional outcome and symptomatic ICH [5]. To ensure that a lesion is truly abnormal and not caused by partial volume effect, early ischemic changes should be visible on at least two adjacent slices.

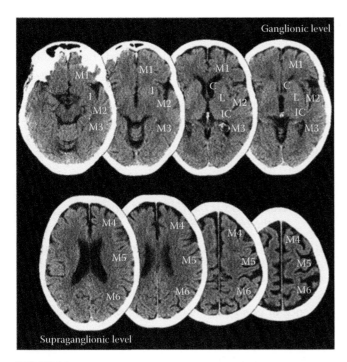

FIGURE 9.1
The two Alberta Stroke Program Early Computed Tomography levels are shown, the ganglionic level in the first row (M1–M3, insula, caudate nucleus, lentiform nucleus, and internal capsule) and the supraganglionic level in the second row (M4–M6). (Reproduced from http://www.aspectsinstroke.com.)

9.2.1.4 How Large Is the Extent of Ischemic Changes?

If infarct signs are well established in more than one-third of the hemisphere, patients are likely not to benefit from thrombolytic treatment and at risk of developing adverse outcome. This is also known as the one-third rule and is based on results of the European Cooperative Acute Stroke Study: patients with hypodensity or sulcal effacement on the initial CT covering greater than one-third of the MCA territory had an increased risk of fatal intraparenchymal hemorrhage after IV thrombolysis [6]. However, if only subtle early ischemic parenchymal changes are present, the rule might not be applicable.

9.2.1.5 Why Is It Difficult to Detect Early Ischemic Changes in the Posterior Fossa?

Early ischemic changes are more difficult to detect in patients with posterior fossa ischemia, chronic ischemia, and/or areas of leukomalacia.

Detection of early ischemic changes in the posterior fossa is mainly complicated by streak artifacts, which are primarily caused by nonlinear partial volume and beam hardening effects [7–9].

Beam hardening artifact occurs as a result of the x-ray beam attenuation passing through the dense temporal bone and is mainly independent of slice thickness [9].

Nonlinear partial volume artifact is caused by the inconstant beam attenuation in the transverse direction across the section thickness, being prominent at the level of the skull base [7]. Reducing section thickness by using thinner collimation available on multi-detector row scanners leads to decreased posterior fossa artifact and better delineation of brain parenchyma in that region, but comes at the cost of an increased radiation dose [10,11].

9.2.1.6 How High Is the Overall Sensitivity of Noncontrast Computed Tomography to Detect Acute Ischemic Stroke?

The overall sensitivity to detect early infarction signs with NCT in the 6 hour time window ranges widely between 20% and 87% with a specificity of 56%–100% reflecting only moderate interobserver agreement [12]. Compared to NCT, diffusion-weighted MRI proves to be more sensitive to detect early ischemic lesions in the setting of acute stroke [13]. Especially in detection of small infarcts or posterior fossa lesions, MR is superior to CT. Nonetheless, NCT is a very helpful tool in the emergency setting to triage stroke patients for ischemic therapy, by ruling out hemorrhage with high accuracy, in a fast and cost-effective way. In addition, CTA and PCT can be performed in the same imaging session and will be discussed in Sections 9.3.2 and 9.4.2.

9.3 Pipes

If ischemic stroke is suspected, intracranial and extracranial vessels need to be assessed for evidence of an intravascular thrombus or any other vascular pathology that might increase stroke risk.

9.3.1 Is a Thrombus Sign Visible on the Noncontrast Computed Tomography?

Some insight about vessel patency can be extracted from NCT, if the hyperdense artery sign is present (Figure 9.2). The hyperdense artery sign, which is caused by acute thromboembolism, is a very specific sign (90%–100%) and associated with poor outcome. With a CT slice thickness of 5 mm, the sign has a limited sensitivity of about 30% [14]. A higher sensitivity of 88% is reached when thin slice NCT is used [15]. Furthermore, the thrombus length adds additional important information. If the thrombus length exceeds 8 mm, the likelihood of dissolving the clot with IV rtPA is very low and is associated with poor outcome [16].

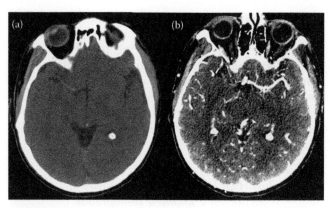

FIGURE 9.2
The hyperdense artery sign is present on noncontrast computed tomography showing an occlusion of the right middle cerebral artery. Same findings are identified on the computed tomography angiography images.

However, CTA detects arterial occlusions with a higher specificity and sensitivity than NCT, as it allows identifying primary, secondary, and increasingly tertiary branch levels of intracranial occlusion.

9.3.2 Computed Tomography Angiography

The development of spiral CT scanners in the 1990s allowed to significantly decrease the scan times per slice and consequently perform rapid acquisition of angiographic-type vascular images, overcoming the limitation of motion or breathing artifacts.

CTA is thus able to visualize the intra- and extracranial vasculature after a bolus injection of iodinated contrast material, providing truly anatomic, non-flow-dependent data.

9.3.2.1 Where Is the Occlusion Located and Why Is It Important?

CTA allows determining the presence, extent, and location of large intracranial and extracranial vessel stenosis and/or occlusion with a high overall accuracy of 95%–99% [17–19]. This information is of important prognostic value for patients with acute stroke as the presence, location, and/or level of the occlusion influence treatment decision. The initial vascular patency may be used as stroke imaging biomarker to select appropriate treatment [20].

If no occlusion is present on angiography, it is argued that those patients might not need thrombolytic therapy, in contrary to patients presenting with occlusion [20,21].

If patients present with terminal carotid T occlusions, proximal middle cerebral artery occlusion, tandem lesions, or significant thrombus burden, they tend to respond poorly to IV thrombolysis and might be better

candidates for intra-arterial thrombolysis or mechanical clot retrieval [22–24].

Furthermore, a classification called Boston Acute Stroke Imaging Scale (BASIS) has been proposed, combining the ASPECTS and CTA information [25]. This classification has been shown to improve outcome prediction in a prospectively designed study. If combined with the NIH Stroke Scale (NIHSS) score, the outcome prediction is stronger than using the BASIS or NIHSS by themselves [26].

9.3.2.2 How Good Is the Collateral Flow to the Ischemic Region?

Furthermore, CTA permits visualization of the extent of leptomeningeal collateral vessels, which provide alternative routes for blood flow in stroke and may add prognostic information in patients with acute stroke. The presence of good collateral flow is associated with less infarct growth and better outcome after ischemic stroke [27], whereas poor collateral flow is linked with hemorrhage after intra-arterial thrombolysis [28].

Collateralization on CTA has been assessed with several different grading scales; however, to implement this information into clinical decision-making, consistency in the grading of collateral flow is needed [29].

New 320-row CT scanners, which enable whole brain coverage in a single rotation allowing for time-resolved angiographic studies [30], offer further interesting applications, such as dynamic assessment of collateral flow combined with PCT (Figure 9.3).

9.3.2.3 Are Other Pathologies Present?

In addition to identifying vessel occlusion and collateral flow, CTA is becoming increasingly important as it has the ability to identify other pathologies such as arterial dissection, or intracranial aneurysms, which might prompt alternative therapeutic options.

9.3.2.4 When Is the Best Time Point in a Multimodal Stroke Protocol to Perform Computed Tomography Angiography?

CTA can be performed as second or third study of a multimodal stroke protocol either before or after PCT, which will be discussed in Section 9.4. Institutions acquiring CTA right after NCT follow the rationale that CTA provides more vital information than PCT and should be performed early to avoid patient motion, which often increases with scan time. Furthermore, venous contamination from initial PCT contrast injection can theoretically be avoided, leading to an improved arterial lesion detection and characterization. By characterizing the arterial lesion and its exact anatomical location first, the

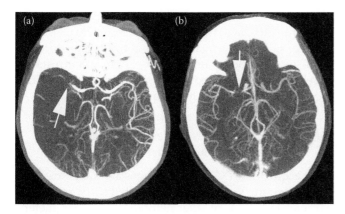

FIGURE 9.3
Computed tomography angiography maximal intensity projection images of two patients presenting with right middle cerebral artery occlusion are shown. (a) Poor collateral flow, reflected by poor filling of the arteries distal to the occlusion. (b) Good collateral flow, reflected by good filling of the arteries distal to the occlusion.

PCT slices can be placed in the area of suspicion, which was of special concern when the spatial coverage of PCT was limited.

At our institution, PCT is performed before CTA and is acquired using 40 mm slabs at two locations 7 seconds after the beginning of the IV contrast injection (40 mL of contrast material injected at 5 mL/s). The PCT source images serve as a test bolus to determine the optimal timing of CTA. The image frame where the contrast material starts appearing in the arteries is identified. The time of this image frame (e.g., image frame obtained 13 seconds after the beginning of the PCT acquisition) is added to the starting time of the so-called prep group (7 seconds), and the resulting time delay (20 seconds in this example) is used as the delay between the beginning of the IV injection of contrast material for the CTA (50–70 mL of contrast material injected at 5 mL/s) and the start of the acquisition of CTA images. Selecting the imaging frame ensures an optimal arterial phase on CTA, as very little residual venous contrast material remains from the PCT acquisition if the patient has adequate renal excretion. Some contrast material, however, will be present on CTA images. In our experience, the optimal timing of CTA imaging outweighs the disadvantage of PCT-related venous contamination. On the other hand, venous contamination on PCT images interferes with determination of accurate perfusion values on PCT maps, and thus avoiding the venous contamination on PCT images from the contrast administered for the CTA portion leads to more accurate hemodynamic parameter calculation.

If full-brain coverage CT scanners or improved large coverage toggling table acquisition techniques are used, volumetric angiographic and perfusion data can be obtained from a single contrast injection and it will render considerations about which study to perform first irrelevant [30].

9.4 Penumbra and Perfusion

In addition to determining the presence, type, and location of stroke, it is important to analyze the perfusion status, indicating the amount of cerebral blood flow (CBF) arriving at a particular brain region. Several factors, such as the occlusion site, its time course, and potential collateral pathways, influence the cerebral perfusion and the viability of cerebral tissue, and consequently treatment options. Identifying the tissue at risk, the so-called penumbra, which is the target of acute reperfusion therapies, is a main goal of modern neuroimaging in patients with stroke.

9.4.1 What Is the Penumbra?

The concept and term of ischemic penumbra arose from experimental studies and refers to hypoperfused cerebral tissue surrounding the infarct core (or irreversibly damaged tissue), in which electrical failure has occurred but oxygen and glucose supply levels are sufficient to maintain membrane homeostasis and thus cellular viability. If reperfusion occurs in a timely manner, the penumbral tissue will survive, whereas it will turn into infarction in case of persistent arterial occlusion. This evolution from ischemic penumbra to irreversible damaged tissue in absence of reperfusion is a gradual process and time dependent, as the penumbra can remain viable for hours. The temporal evolution of the penumbra or tissue at risk varies individually and depends on factors such as collateralization, severity, and duration of the ischemic event. Information about whether the tissue is still salvageable provides a physiologically relevant target for therapy and is especially important outside the conventional rtPA time window. PCT helps to characterize the ischemic penumbra, by assessing cerebral perfusion.

9.4.2 Perfusion Computed Tomography

PCT measures brain hemodynamics by tracking an intravenously injected bolus of iodinated contrast agent. After identification of the arterial input and venous outflow and application of deconvolution methods, perfusion parameters can be calculated: CBF, cerebral blood volume (CBV), and mean transit time (MTT). CBF is measured in milliliters per 100 g of brain tissue per minute and reflects the amount of blood flowing through each voxel in 1 minute. CBV is measured in milliliters per 100 g of brain tissue and refers to the blood pool content of each pixel. MTT is measured in seconds and designates the average time required by a unit of iodinated contrast to cross the capillary network in each voxel on the image. The relationship between CBV, MTT, and

CBF is described by the following equation: CBF = CBV/MTT, known as the central volume principle [31,32]. Further time parameters such as time-to-peak (TTP) or T_{max} can also be determined.

9.4.2.1 How Does Perfusion Computed Tomography Assess Tissue at Risk (Penumbra)?

In the setting of acute stroke, PCT can assess cerebral vascular autoregulation and thus provides a means to distinguish tissue that will inevitably die from tissue that may either survive or die depending on whether early reperfusion occurs [33]. In normal brain tissue, regional CBF is maintained to a constant level by cerebral vascular autoregulation despite changes in the metabolic activity of local neurons and in the local arterial perfusion pressure [33,34]. During cerebral ischemia, perfusion pressure decreases. This results in prolongation of the MTT and other time parameters such as TTP and T_{max} in both the ischemic core and the penumbra. In response, exclusively in the ischemic penumbra not in the infarct core, cerebral vascular autoregulation induces dilatation of capillaries supplying and draining the ischemic region in an attempt to maintain a constant CBF. Thus, CBV in the penumbral tissue is maintained or increased as a result of vasodilatation and recruitment of collaterals. In the infarct core, however, the autoregulation mechanisms are not functional anymore leading to a diminished CBV (Table 9.1).

9.4.2.2 Which Are the Best Parameters and Thresholds to Characterize Ischemic Core and Penumbra?

As just mentioned, the MTT in the penumbra will be prolonged, but the CBF will be normal or increased, in contrary to the infarct core where CBV will be decreased in addition to an elevated MTT. Using PCT, we have found an MTT threshold of 145% (elevated MTT of at least 145% compared with normal contralateral tissue) to best define tissue with prolonged MTT and an absolute CBV threshold value of 2.0 mL/100 g to most accurately define irreversibly infarcted tissue [35].

So far, no consensus has been reached regarding the best perfusion parameters and thresholds. The exact values, which best characterize ischemic core and penumbra, are still a topic of debate and ongoing research. They are among others complicated by the fact that different scanner manufacturers are using different algorithms to calculate perfusion parameters [36].

There is clearly a need to standardize the different perfusion methods, parameter selection, and thresholds to reliably determine core and penumbra and facilitate the clinical use of these techniques (Figure 9.4).

9.4.2.3 Which Principles Underlie the Calculation of Perfusion Parameters?

After acquisition, PCT source images are transferred to a postprocessing workstation. Dedicated software creates parametric maps of the hemodynamic parameters, which are calculated based on time–density curves of the injected contrast agent for each pixel. The time–density curves, used for CBV calculation, reflect the wash-in and wash-out of contrast material in a single pixel assuming that the contrast material is not diffusible into the brain tissue. Thus, the area under the curve of voxels located at the center of a vessel is greater than the one of those voxels containing brain parenchyma, of which the vascular volume represents only a few percent of the total volume. Based on the concept of partial volume averaging effect, the fraction of vascular volume within pixels of the brain parenchyma, or CBV, can be determined by comparison with the contrast enhancement profile in a reference pixel containing only blood, such as the center of a large vein. The CBV values can then be determined on a pixel-by-pixel basis and converted into a parametric map [31,37].

To determine MTT and CBF, commercial software suppliers use a number of different mathematic models. Two major models used are the maximum slope model and deconvolution-based mathematic methods.

The maximal slope model was initially used to determine perfusion by injecting microspheres [38,39]. It is based on the assumption that after arterial injection all particles are completely extracted (trapped in the precapillary and capillary network) at first pass through the tissue. The total number of accumulated microspheres in a specific region is thereby proportional to its perfusion and its rate of accumulation (slope of accumulation curve). When this model is applied to PCT data, the CBF in a voxel of brain tissue is considered to be the maximal slope of density increase on the time–density curve of in- and outflowing iodinated contrast agent. However, iodinated contrast agent has different flow dynamics compared to microspheres, as it is not completely extracted during the first pass. To apply the maximal slope method to PCT data, one needs to assume that, during the time of contrast injection, no contrast material has reached the venous side of the circulation. This condition could theoretically be reached with a very high injection rate of contrast agent (at least 10 mL/s). However, even with an injection rate of 20 mL/s CBF

TABLE 9.1

Change of Perfusion Parameters in Acute Ischemic Stroke

	Time Parameter	CBF	CBV
Ischemic penumbra	⇑	⇓	Normal or ⇑
Infarct core	⇑⇑	⇓⇓	⇓

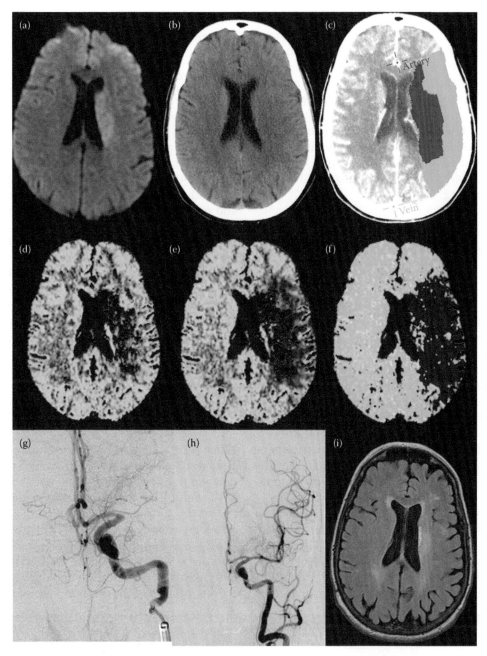

FIGURE 9.4
Sample case of a 76-year-old female presenting after wake-up stroke with a NIH Stroke Scale (NIHSS) score of 23. The diffusion-weighted image (a) shows a hyperintense left caudate nucleus. On noncontrast computed tomography (b), no hemorrhage is present; and a large penumbra can be identified with perfusion computed tomography imaging (c). The individual parametric perfusion maps are shown in the second row (cerebral blood volume [CBV], d; cerebral blood flow, e; mean transit time [MTT], f; from left to right), demonstrating decreased CBV in the area corresponding to the diffusion lesion (d) and hypoperfusion and prolonged MTT on the temporal and frontal lobe (e, f). The patient's left middle cerebral artery, initially occluded (g), was successfully recanalized with intravenous recombinant tissue plasminogen activator and mechanical embolus removal in cerebral ischemia (h). A left caudate infarct was seen on the follow-up fluid-attenuated inversion recovery images (i). The patient shows a favorable outcome at 90 days with a NIHSS score of 2.

values are underestimated as fractions of the contrast agent bolus are missed [40]. The CBF underestimation is even more pronounced at lower contrast injection rates.

The deconvolution method overcomes some limitations of the maximal slope model as it does not rely on simplified assumptions regarding the underlying vascular architecture and is reliable even for low injection rates of contrast agent [41]. MTT and CBF are determined with the time–density curves of the tracer at the arterial input and at the brain tissue of interest. The choice of the arterial input function thereby directly affects the calculation of MTT and CBF, whereas CBV is determined using a reference vein as outlined earlier [31,37]. To derive MTT and CBF parametric maps, to take the hemodynamic properties of the contrast agent in a given voxel into account, a mathematical operation known as "deconvolution" is applied. Compared to early versions of deconvolution, which were technically demanding and involved complicated time-consuming data processing, modern commercial software use modern forms of deconvolution and allow for fast and easy generation of MTT and CBF parametric maps, which makes their use suitable for the emergency setting.

9.4.2.4 Which Artery Should Be Chosen for the Arterial Input Function?

The arterial input function is estimated from a major artery assuming that it represents the exact input to the tissue. This assumption, however, is rarely true as the tissue of interest is usually located at some distance from the selected artery. Consequently, any delay of contrast agent to the tissue may cause errors in the calculation of parametric MTT and CBF maps [42].

In acute stroke patients without ipsilateral carotid artery stenosis, the selection of the arterial input function does not have a significant impact on the PCT parametric maps [43–45]. Therefore, a proximal anterior cerebral artery is usually selected as the arterial input function because it has a large caliber, is perpendicular to axial images (diminishing the risk of volume averaging with brain tissue), and can be easily and reproducibly identified [45].

In acute stroke patients with chronic vascular conditions, such as chronic internal carotid artery stenosis or giant aneurysm, delay and dispersion of the contrast agent bolus can occur. In those cases, the artery selection has significant impact on MTT and CBF calculation. Delay-corrected or delay-sensitive deconvolution

software corrects for the delay and is especially useful in those patients.

9.4.2.5 Which Vein Should Be Chosen for a Reference Venous Output Function?

The venous output function serves as a reference for CBV values, as outlined earlier. The best location for the venous output function is a voxel that has the maximal area under the time–density curve, in other words, the least amount of partial volume averaging. Usually a pixel inside the superior sagittal sinus is selected as it is large and orthogonal to axial PCT source images (Figure 9.5). Other venous structures, such as the straight sinus, are also suitable. The only requirement for CBV calculation is to have a vascular pixel without partial averaging effect and with a maximal area under the time–density curve. Thus, if no good venous structure can be identified, a large artery within the PCT slice devoid of partial volume averaging effect, such as the cavernous internal carotid artery, can also be chosen for the "venous" output function.

9.4.2.6 Why Can Abnormally Increased Mean Transit Time Values Be Seen in an Arterial Territory Even When a Patient Has No Acute Symptoms?

When using delay-sensitive deconvolution software, hemodynamically significant carotid stenosis causes a delay in transit of contrast material and thus prolonged MTT values in the supplied territory. This finding can result from the stenosis but can also be caused by collateral arteries through which the blood flows more slowly arriving at the tissue over an indirect route. It thus does not represent acute cerebral ischemia, but still has clinical relevance and should not be ignored as it reflects a decrease in cerebral vascular reserve and an

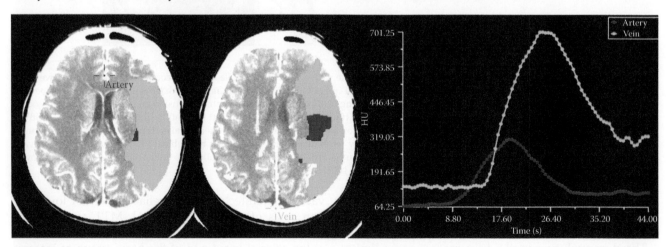

FIGURE 9.5
Perfusion computed tomography slices with selected artery and vein as well as the corresponding time curves are shown. The artery cursor is placed into the anterior cerebral artery and the vein cursor into the superior sagittal sinus.

increased likelihood of ischemia in the future. Therefore, an increased MTT derived with delay-sensitive software in patients without acute symptoms should be a reminder to review the CTA images for possible arterial stenoses or occlusions that may cause delay or dispersion of the bolus of contrast material.

When a prolonged MTT is detected using delay-insensitive or delay-corrected deconvolution PCT software or when the CTA is normal but the PCT shows an MTT abnormality in a vascular territory, a very recent transient ischemic attack might have occurred shortly beforehand.

Finally, if the PCT abnormality does not conform to a vascular territory, the possibility of a stroke mimic should be taken into consideration.

9.4.2.7 How Should Perfusion Defects Be Interpreted That Are Not Consistent with a Vascular Territory?

Many neurologic disease cause symptoms simulating cerebrovascular disease, producing an alteration of brain perfusion, which can be seen on PCT parametric maps. Findings on NCT and CTA performed along with PCT may be indicative of entities producing non-ischemic perfusion abnormalities. Examples of such entities include neoplasm, subdural hematoma, vasospasm, venous thrombosis, or even seizure-related hyper- or hypoperfusion.

The clinical presentation of seizures can sometimes be similar to ischemic stroke. Depending on the timing of the study in regard to the seizure activity, the specific pattern observed on perfusion imaging varies widely [46]. Postictal perfusion imaging shows prolonged MTT with decreased CBF and CBV, which is similar to findings in acute ischemic stroke [47]. However, perfusion alterations related to seizures do not correspond to arterial vascular territories and tend to mainly involve the cortical gray matter.

Perfusion alterations can also be detected in cerebral venous thrombosis, showing an increased MTT with preserved CBV [48]. Early diagnosis is crucial to prompt adequate treatment, which can reverse the disease. Venous thrombosis can also progress to venous infarction, which shows the same PCT findings as arterial infarction.

9.4.2.8 How Safe Is Perfusion Computed Tomography in Respect to Radiation Dose?

First of all, it should always be ensured that all CT protocols respect the as low as reasonably achievable dose principle and that CT quality is assured. Concerning a PCT study, the radiation dose for a single-slab PCT study is approximately the same as for a NCT (approximately 2–3 mSv), if performed at 80 kVp and 100 mAs, which are considered optimal acquisition parameters. Using these parameters ensures not only reduced radiation dose but also improved image quality. For instance, PCT performed with 80 kVp rather than 120–140 kVp reduces the administered radiation dose by a factor of approximately 3 and increases conspicuity of IV contrast material because of proximity to the k-edge of iodine [49].

A comprehensive stroke CT protocol including unenhanced and contrast-enhanced head CT, PCT, and CTA of the cervical and intracranial arteries can deliver a large mean effective dose (on the order of 7–8 mSv) [50]. However, not all components of such a protocol are required for each patient and dedicated stroke protocols should be tailored to specific clinical indications. This is especially important in patients with stroke who may need multiple imaging studies involving ionizing radiation during a single admission. In such patients, radiation reduction strategies should be implemented as appropriate and when feasible, MRI should be performed in the subsequent, nonemergent imaging evaluation.

The potential risks of any diagnostic test or therapeutic procedure must always be weighed against the real benefits of limiting disability and preventing death. PCT imaging is a justifiable and safe diagnostic test when appropriately and correctly performed, providing valuable information that can substantially contribute to the management of acutely ill patients with acute cerebrovascular disease.

9.5 Permeability

As explained earlier, PCT allows to determine tissue viability and thus might enable to select patients who may still profit from recanalization. A further piece of valuable information would be to identify patients at risk of complications, such as symptomatic hemorrhagic transformation. Permeability as fourth P of stroke shows promise of PCT to characterize the risk of hemorrhagic transformation, although this application is still experimental at the current stage.

By simply extending the PCT acquisitions to 210 seconds, information about the disruption of BBB can be obtained. Increased BBB permeability has been associated with an increased risk of hemorrhagic transformation [51], and imaging abnormal BBB could identify patients at risk of developing this complication. Symptomatic hemorrhagic transformation is a serious complication of acute ischemic stroke and associated with worse clinical outcome [52]. Although the definition and the magnitude of symptomatic hemorrhagic transformation are still under debate [53,54], there is consensus that minimizing its occurrence is of importance.

9.5.1 How Can Blood–Brain Barrier Measurements Be Obtained?

Quantitative measurements of BBB permeability can be obtained by applying pharmacokinetic, compartmental models to PCT data. As already mentioned, PCT relies on IV injection of an iodinated contrast agent measuring the attenuation coefficient (Hounsfield units) as a function of time on a voxel basis. The acquired source images can then be postprocessed to quantify contrast agent. The most commonly used mathematical model in ischemic stroke to calculate permeability values is the Patlak model, a one directional, two compartment method, modeling the leakage of contrast agent from the vessel lumen into the interstitial space. To generate accurate permeability values, PCT acquisitions should thereby extent at least 210 seconds [55]. Clinical studies have so far shown promising results to use BBB permeability measurements as surrogate marker for hemorrhagic transformation (Figure 9.6) [56,57].

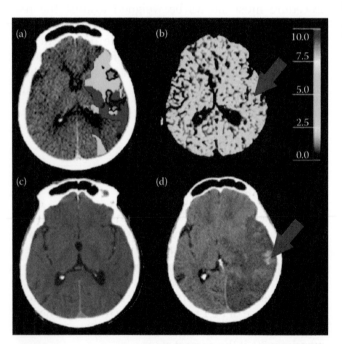

FIGURE 9.6

Blood–brain barrier permeability measurements to predict hemorrhagic transformation in a sample case: A 75-year-old woman was admitted to the emergency department with a right hemiparesis approximately 2 hours after symptom onset. Noncontrast computed tomography (NCT) (c) revealed no evidence of intracranial hemorrhage, and she was treated with intravenous recombinant tissue plasminogen activator at this time. One red arrow on the admission permeability map (b) points to a "hotspot" of sizable abnormally elevated permeability on the baseline perfusion computed tomography (a) (red, infarct core; green, penumbra; blue, increased permeability). This hotspot was situated in the same location as a focus of hemorrhage on the follow-up NCT (d) performed 23 hours later, when the patient's condition in the intensive care unit worsened. (From Hom J, Dankbaar JW, Soares BP et al., *AJNR Am J Neuroradiol*, 2011, 32, 41–48. With pemission.)

9.6 Conclusion

Neuroimaging in acute ischemic stroke is essential to determine the underlying pathology and offers important information to guide treatment decisions, including the ruling out of hemorrhage, the characterization of stroke location and subtype, as well as the assessment of tissue viability. Stroke imaging and treatment aim toward more individualized approaches. Type of stroke, location of occlusion, extent of salvageable tissue, and risk of symptomatic hemorrhagic transformation are playing an increasing role to determine the appropriate treatment strategy. Further work is necessary, however, to determine the exact role of these additional pieces of information.

References

1. Roger VL, Go AS, Lloyd-Jones DM, et al. Heart disease and stroke statistics—2011 update: a report from the American Heart Association. *Circulation* 2011; 123: e18–e209. doi:CIR.0b013e3182009701 [p.ii].
2. Adams HP, Jr, Bendixen BH, Kappelle LJ et al. Classification of subtype of acute ischemic stroke. Definitions for use in a multicenter clinical trial. TOAST. Trial of Org 10172 in Acute Stroke Treatment. *Stroke* 1993; 24: 35–41.
3. Ambrose J. Computerized transverse axial scanning (tomography). 2. Clinical application. *Br J Radiol* 1973; 46: 1023–1047.
4. Simard JM, Kent TA, Chen M et al. Brain oedema in focal ischaemia: Molecular pathophysiology and theoretical implications. *Lancet Neurol* 2007; 6: 258–268.
5. Barber PA, Demchuk AM, Zhang J et al. Validity and reliability of a quantitative computed tomography score in predicting outcome of hyperacute stroke before thrombolytic therapy. ASPECTS Study Group. Alberta Stroke Programme Early CT Score. *Lancet* 2000; 355: 1670–1674.
6. Hacke W, Kaste M, Fieschi C et al. Intravenous thrombolysis with recombinant tissue plasminogen activator for acute hemispheric stroke. The European Cooperative Acute Stroke Study (ECASS). *JAMA* 1995; 274: 1017–1025.
7. Glover GH, Pelc NJ. Nonlinear partial volume artifacts in x-ray computed tomography. *Med Phys* 1980; 7: 238–248.
8. Rozeik C, Kotterer O, Preiss J et al. Cranial CT artifacts and gantry angulation. *J Comput Assist Tomogr* 1991; 15: 381–386.
9. Mostrom U, Ytterbergh C. Artifacts in computed tomography of the posterior fossa: A comparative phantom study. *J Comput Assist Tomogr* 1986; 10: 560–566.
10. Jones TR, Kaplan RT, Lane B et al. Single- versus multi-detector row CT of the brain: Quality assessment. *Radiology* 2001; 219: 750–755.

11. Ertl-Wagner B, Eftimov L, Blume J et al. Cranial CT with 64-, 16-, 4- and single-slice CT systems-comparison of image quality and posterior fossa artifacts in routine brain imaging with standard protocols. *Eur Radiol* 2008; 18: 1720–1726.

12. Wardlaw JM, Mielke O. Early signs of brain infarction at CT: Observer reliability and outcome after thrombolytic treatment—systematic review. *Radiology* 2005; 235: 444–453.

13. Chalela JA, Kidwell CS, Nentwich LM et al. Magnetic resonance imaging and computed tomography in emergency assessment of patients with suspected acute stroke: A prospective comparison. *Lancet* 2007; 369: 293–298.

14. Leys D, Pruvo JP, Godefroy O et al. Prevalence and significance of hyperdense middle cerebral artery in acute stroke. *Stroke* 1992; 23: 317–324.

15. Kim EY, Lee SK, Kim DJ et al. Detection of thrombus in acute ischemic stroke: Value of thin-section noncontrast-computed tomography. *Stroke* 2005; 36: 2745–2747.

16. Riedel CH, Zimmermann P, Jensen-Kondering U et al. The importance of size: Successful recanalization by intravenous thrombolysis in acute anterior stroke depends on thrombus length. *Stroke* 2011; 42: 1775–1777.

17. Bash S, Villablanca JP, Jahan R et al. Intracranial vascular stenosis and occlusive disease: Evaluation with CT angiography, MR angiography, and digital subtraction angiography. *AJNR. Am J Neuroradiol* 2005; 26: 1012–1021.

18. Tan JC, Dillon WP, Liu S et al. Systematic comparison of perfusion-CT and CT-angiography in acute stroke patients. *Ann Neurol* 2007; 61: 533–543.

19. Lev MH, Farkas J, Rodriguez VR et al. CT angiography in the rapid triage of patients with hyperacute stroke to intraarterial thrombolysis: Accuracy in the detection of large vessel thrombus. *J Comput Assist Tomogr* 2001; 25: 520–528.

20. Fiebach JB, Al-Rawi Y, Wintermark M et al. Vascular occlusion enables selecting acute ischemic stroke patients for treatment with desmoteplase. *Stroke* 2012; 43: 1561–1566.

21. Ma L, Gao PY, Lin Y et al. Can baseline magnetic resonance angiography (MRA) status become a foremost factor in selecting optimal acute stroke patients for recombinant tissue plasminogen activator (rt-PA) thrombolysis beyond 3 hours? *Neurol Res* 2009; 31: 355–361.

22. Zaidat OO, Suarez JI, Santillan C et al. Response to intraarterial and combined intravenous and intra-arterial thrombolytic therapy in patients with distal internal carotid artery occlusion. *Stroke* 2002; 33: 1821–1826.

23. Rubiera M, Ribo M, Delgado-Mederos R et al. Tandem internal carotid artery/middle cerebral artery occlusion: An independent predictor of poor outcome after systemic thrombolysis. *Stroke* 2006; 37: 2301–2305.

24. Saqqur M, Uchino K, Demchuk AM et al. Site of arterial occlusion identified by transcranial Doppler predicts the response to intravenous thrombolysis for stroke. *Stroke* 2007; 38: 948–954.

25. Torres-Mozqueda F, He J, Yeh IB et al. An acute ischemic stroke classification instrument that includes CT or MR angiography: The Boston acute stroke imaging scale. *AJNR. Am J Neuroradiol* 2008; 29: 1111–1117.

26. Gonzalez RG, Lev MH, Goldmacher GV et al. Improved outcome prediction using CT angiography in addition to standard ischemic stroke assessment: Results from the STOPStroke study. *PLoS One* 2012; 7: e30352.

27. Miteff F, Levi CR, Bateman GA et al. The independent predictive utility of computed tomography angiographic collateral status in acute ischaemic stroke. *Brain* 2009; 132: 2231–2238.

28. Christoforidis GA, Karakasis C, Mohammad Y et al. Predictors of hemorrhage following intra-arterial thrombolysis for acute ischemic stroke: The role of pial collateral formation. *AJNR Am J Neuroradiol* 2009; 30: 165–170.

29. McVerry F, Liebeskind DS, Muir KW. Systematic review of methods for assessing leptomeningeal collateral flow. *AJNR Am J Neuroradiol* 2012; 33: 576–582.

30. Salomon EJ, Barfett J, Willems PW et al. Dynamic CT angiography and CT perfusion employing a 320-detector row CT: Protocol and current clinical applications. *Klin Neuroradiol* 2009; 19: 187–196.

31. Wintermark M, Maeder P, Thiran JP et al. Quantitative assessment of regional cerebral blood flows by perfusion CT studies at low injection rates: A critical review of the underlying theoretical models. *Eur Radiol* 2001; 11: 1220–1230.

32. Eastwood JD, Lev MH, Provenzale JM. Perfusion CT with iodinated contrast material. *AJR Am J Roentgenol* 2003; 180: 3–12.

33. Wintermark M, Reichhart M, Thiran JP et al. Prognostic accuracy of cerebral blood flow measurement by perfusion computed tomography, at the time of emergency room admission, in acute stroke patients. *Ann Neurol* 2002; 51: 417–432.

34. Heiss WD, Sobesky J, Hesselmann V. Identifying thresholds for penumbra and irreversible tissue damage. *Stroke* 2004; 35: 2671–2674.

35. Wintermark M, Flanders AE, Velthuis B et al. Perfusion-CT assessment of infarct core and penumbra: Receiver operating characteristic curve analysis in 130 patients suspected of acute hemispheric stroke. *Stroke* 2006; 37: 979–985.

36. Dani KA, Thomas RG, Chappell FM et al. Computed tomography and magnetic resonance perfusion imaging in ischemic stroke: Definitions and thresholds. *Ann Neurol* 2011; 70: 384–401.

37. Konstas AA, Goldmakher GV, Lee TY et al. Theoretic basis and technical implementations of CT perfusion in acute ischemic stroke, part 1: Theoretic basis. *AJNR Am J Neuroradiol* 2009; 30: 662–668.

38. Peters AM, Gunasekera RD, Henderson BL et al. Noninvasive measurement of blood flow and extraction fraction. *Nucl Med Commun* 1987; 8: 823–837.

39. Heymann MA, Payne BD, Hoffman JI et al. Blood flow measurements with radionuclide-labeled particles. *Prog Cardiovasc Dis* 1977; 20: 55–79.

40. Koenig M, Klotz E, Luka B et al. Perfusion CT of the brain: Diagnostic approach for early detection of ischemic stroke. *Radiology* 1998; 209: 85–93.

41. Eastwood JD, Provenzale JM, Hurwitz LM et al. Practical injection-rate CT perfusion imaging: Deconvolution-derived hemodynamics in a case of stroke. *Neuroradiology* 2001; 43: 223–226.

42. Calamante F, Gadian DG, Connelly A. Delay and dispersion effects in dynamic susceptibility contrast MRI: Simulations using singular value decomposition. *Magn Reson Med* 2000; 44: 466–473.

43. Sanelli PC, Lev MH, Eastwood JD et al. The effect of varying user-selected input parameters on quantitative values in CT perfusion maps. *Acad Radiol* 2004; 11: 1085–1092.

44. Bisdas S, Konstantinou GN, Gurung J et al. Effect of the arterial input function on the measured perfusion values and infarct volumetric in acute cerebral ischemia evaluated by perfusion computed tomography. *Invest Radiol* 2007; 42: 147–156.

45. Wintermark M, Lau BC, Chien J et al. The anterior cerebral artery is an appropriate arterial input function for perfusion-CT processing in patients with acute stroke. *Neuroradiology* 2008; 50: 227–236.

46. Wiest R, von Bredow F, Schindler K et al. Detection of regional blood perfusion changes in epileptic seizures with dynamic brain perfusion CT—A pilot study. *Epilepsy Res* 2006; 72: 102–110.

47. Gelfand JM, Wintermark M, Josephson SA. Cerebral perfusion-CT patterns following seizure. *Eur J Neurol* 2010; 17: 594–601.

48. Doege CA, Tavakolian R, Kerskens CM et al. Perfusion and diffusion magnetic resonance imaging in human cerebral venous thrombosis. *J Neurol* 2001; 248: 564–571.

49. Wintermark M, Maeder P, Verdun FR et al. Using 80 kVp versus 120 kVp in perfusion CT measurement of regional cerebral blood flow. *AJNR Am J Neuroradiol* 2000; 21: 1881–1884.

50. Diekmann S, Siebert E, Juran R et al. Dose exposure of patients undergoing comprehensive stroke imaging by multidetector-row CT: Comparison of 320-detector row and 64-detector row CT scanners. *AJNR Am J Neuroradiol* 2010; 31: 1003–1009.

51. Wang X, Lo EH. Triggers and mediators of hemorrhagic transformation in cerebral ischemia. *Mol Neurobiol* 2003; 28: 229–244.

52. Berger C, Fiorelli M, Steiner T et al. Hemorrhagic transformation of ischemic brain tissue: Asymptomatic or symptomatic? *Stroke* 2001; 32: 1330–1335.

53. Saver JL. Hemorrhage after thrombolytic therapy for stroke: The clinically relevant number needed to harm. *Stroke* 2007; 38: 2279–2283.

54. Gumbinger C, Gruschka P, Bottinger M et al. Improved prediction of poor outcome after thrombolysis using conservative definitions of symptomatic hemorrhage. *Stroke* 2012; 43: 240–242.

55. Hom J, Dankbaar JW, Schneider T et al. Optimal duration of acquisition for dynamic perfusion CT assessment of blood-brain barrier permeability using the Patlak model. *AJNR Am J Neuroradiol* 2009; 30: 1366–1370.

56. Aviv RI, d'Esterre CD, Murphy BD et al. Hemorrhagic transformation of ischemic stroke: Prediction with CT perfusion. *Radiology* 2009; 250: 867–877.

57. Hom J, Dankbaar JW, Soares BP et al. Blood-brain barrier permeability assessed by perfusion CT predicts symptomatic hemorrhagic transformation and malignant edema in acute ischemic stroke. *AJNR Am J Neuroradiol* 2011; 32: 41–48.

10

Neurodegenerative Diseases

Asim K. Bag, Joel K. Curé, and Philip R. Chapman

CONTENTS

10.1 Introduction

Neurodegenerative diseases (NDDs) comprise a large and complex group of neurologic disorders with variable etiologies, various affected tissues within the brain, and myriad of clinical manifestations. Most NDDs are characterized by neurologic symptoms that progress chronically and relentlessly over time. Many are age related, with peak prevalence occurring in the elderly population. With advancing life expectancies, the numbers of patients diagnosed with Alzheimer's disease (AD) and other NDDs have reached epidemic proportions.

Even though most of the NDDs have overlapping clinical and imaging manifestations, it is now possible to establish a specific diagnosis in some of the NDDs based on imaging findings in the context of clinical manifestations. Familiarity with these imaging features and clinical presentations is, thus, essential in the practice of neuroradiology. Furthermore, neuroradiologic studies may indicate the presence of disease before conclusive symptoms develop, offering the opportunity for early treatment.

10.2 General Pathological, Clinical, and Genetic Features of Neurodegenerative Disorder

NDDs encompass a large and complex group of disorders. As a group they can be difficult to diagnose, quantify, and classify. Although etiology, genetics, and histopathological findings vary and in some cases remain obscure, NDDs typically share a common end point of progressive neuronal loss and dysfunction. Przedborski et al. [1] characterized four general stages of neurodegeneration: (1) neuronal pathology including inclusion bodies, (2) neuronal cell death, (3) disappearance of cell bodies, and (4) glial proliferation.

Clinically, these diseases progress relentlessly until death and are not reversible with current therapies. Common clinical presentations include cognitive impairment, dementia, and problems with movement and balance.

Some of the NDDs have well-recognized hereditable patterns. Sporadic and familial cases are indistinguishable from each other in terms of clinical and histopathological manifestations, although familial forms of NDDs usually present earlier than the nonfamilial forms. A number of genes have been identified for specific NDD subtypes (i.e., amyloid precursor protein [APP], presenilin 1 [PSEN1], and presenilin 2 [PSEN2] for AD, and superoxide dismutase [SOD1] for amyotrophic lateral sclerosis [ALS]).

10.3 Neuroradiology of Normal Aging

Specific diagnosis of NDDs is challenging. Familiarity with the neuroimaging features of normal aging is critical in the evaluation of neuroimaging studies in patients with NDDs. Most common imaging findings associated with normal aging are diffuse volume loss, increased T2/fluid-attenuated inversion recovery (FLAIR) signal in hemispheric white matter and iron deposition in putamen and globus pallidus in a variable pattern. Unfortunately, there is significant overlap between these normal or expected age-related changes and the findings associated with NDDs, making the neuroimaging distinction difficult. Even though these findings are routinely seen in older people, they reflect the result of various insults to the brain over a lifetime. In this case, "normal" does not therefore equal "nonpathological."

10.3.1 Brain Volume Loss

Brain volume loss is documented as an expected feature of normal aging in multiple research studies, including population-based neuroimaging studies and postmortem evaluations. The rate and pattern of the volume loss is highly variable and differs between men and women. Volume loss can be diffuse and hemispheric or more focal. Although the exact mechanism is not clear, brain volume loss reflects neuronal loss from numerous insults to the brain. This results in neuroimaging findings of passive enlargement of the cerebrospinal fluid (CSF) compartments (ventricles, sulci, and basal cisterns).

Enlargement of the perivascular space (Virchow–Robin [VR] space) at the basal ganglia and pons is frequently seen in aging brain. This could be due to localized parenchymal brain tissue loss and subsequent enlargement of the CSF-like perivascular space that surround penetrating blood vessels. Differentiating VR space from a lacunar infarct is a common problem. However, Table 10.1 delineates the major differences between the two.

10.3.2 White Matter T2 Hyperintensities

Increasing prevalence of focal and confluent areas of increased T2 and FLAIR signal in the white matter is another well-recognized imaging feature of normal aging. Initially, focal punctuate T2/FLAIR hyperintensities are seen in centrum semiovale and periventricular white matter. These gradually enlarge and ultimately

TABLE 10.1

Difference between Dilated VR Space and Lacunar Infarct

	Dilated VR Space	Lacunar Infarct
Location	Inferior putamen	Superior putamen
Symmetry	Can be symmetrical	Asymmetrical
Morphology	>5 mm	<5 mm
Signal characteristics	Isointense to CSF on all sequences	Not isointense to CSF on all sequences unless there is complete cystic change

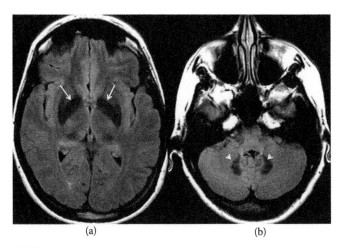

(a) (b)

FIGURE 10.1
Normal brain iron deposition. Transverse fluid-attenuated inversion recovery images (a, b) demonstrate hypointensity of the putamen (arrow) and dentate nucleus (arrowhead) in a 65-year-old man without any specific central nervous system symptom secondary to normal brain iron accumulation. Images were obtained at 3T magnet exaggerating iron-induced local magnetic inhomogeneity effect.

become more extensive and confluent. The exact pathophysiologic basis of these changes is not exactly clear. Endothelial dysfunction and atherosclerosis-induced narrowing of the microvasculature have been hypothesized for these changes.

10.3.3 Iron Deposition

Iron deposition in brain is another well-recognized age-related change. Low T2 signal as a result of iron-induced local magnetic susceptibility is initially seen in globus pallidus, red nucleus, substantia nigra, and dentate nucleus. With further aging, low T2 signal is also seen in putamen and head of the caudate nucleus. This change is more obvious in imaging with a 3T magnet compared to 1.5T magnet (Figure 10.1).

10.4 Classification of Neurodegenerative Disorders

10.4.1 Neurodegenerative Diseases with Predominant Cognitive Symptoms (Predominant Cortical Involvement)

10.4.1.1 Alzheimer's Disease

AD is a devastating NDD characterized by gradual and progressive amnestic disorder with subsequent appearance of cognitive, behavioral, and neuropsychiatric symptoms. Ultimately, deterioration of executive capacity leads to impairment of social function and activities

of daily life. Histopathologically, AD is characterized by intraneuronal neurofibrillary tangles (NFTs) and accumulation of extracellular amyloid plaques, which untimely causes neuronal dysfunction and cellular death.

AD is the most common cause of dementia, accounting for up to 60% of all cases [2]. AD is a disease of the elderly; the onset of sporadic cases is unusual before the age of 60. Age is the strongest risk factor for AD. Annual incidence of AD is as low as 0.6% for individuals of 65–69 years of age to as high as 8.4% in individuals of ≥85 years of age.

The exact etiopathologic mechanism of AD is not completely understood. The disease appears to have both environmental and genetic risk factors. Most cases of AD are considered to be nonfamilial or sporadic, without a definite distinguishing chromosomal abnormality. Familial AD comprises less than 1% of AD cases but demonstrate identical pathological features to the nonfamilial cases, with regional brain neuronal loss, NFTs, and amyloid plaques. Although sharing most features of disease phenotype, familial forms are particularly devastating because they have an earlier onset of symptoms, before the age of 65. Three genes have been identified that account for a significant number of familial cases: (1) *APP* on chromosome 21, (2) *PSEN1* on chromosome 14, and (3) *PSEN2* on chromosome 1. *APOE-ε4* allele has been linked to the development of AD. This allele increases the risk of AD by three times in heterozygotes and by 15 times in homozygotes.

Other factors are implicated to increase the epidemiological risk of AD. Vascular pathology and metabolic dysfunction appear to contribute to the final common pathway of neuronal damage and amyloid accumulation. The exact mechanisms are not known. Atherosclerosis, hypertension, and stroke may ultimately lead to brain cellular hypoperfusion and alterations in biochemical pathways that compound amyloid accumulation and neuronal toxicity. In addition, hypercholesterolemia, diabetes mellitus (insulin resistance), hypertension, smoking, metabolic syndrome, obesity, and sedentary lifestyle have recently been shown to be contributory. High physical activity, higher educational status, and higher fish consumption are likely to have protective effects on AD.

To date, the pathogenesis of AD is incompletely understood. Macroscopically there is diffuse cerebral volume loss with passive widening of the CSF compartments. Microscopically, the disease is characterized by amyloid-containing neuritic plaques and NFTs in excess of that anticipated for age-matched healthy controls. Amyloid plaques consist of a central core of β-amyloid (Aβ) protein (a 40–42 amino acid peptide derived from proteolytic cleavage of the large transmembrane APP protein) surrounded by astrocytes, microglia, and dystrophic neuritis. Neuritic plaque burden was initially

TABLE 10.2

Classification of Neurodegenerative Disorders

1. Neurodegenerative diseases with predominant cognitive symptoms (predominant cortical involvement)
   1.1 Alzheimer's disease
   1.2 Vascular dementia
       1.2.1 Dementia secondary to large vessel disease
       1.2.2 Dementia secondary to small vessel ischemic disease
       1.2.3 Cerebral amyloid angiopathy
       1.2.4 CADASIL
   1.3 Dementia with Lewy body
   1.4 Frontotemporal degeneration
       1.4.1 Behavioral-variant frontotemporal degeneration
       1.4.2 Symantic dementia
       1.4.3 Progressive nonfluent aphasia
   1.5 Dementia associated with systemic diseases

2. Neurodegenerative diseases with predominant cognitive and other neurological symptoms
   2.1 Huntington disease
   2.2 CADASIL
   2.3 Prion diseases
       2.3.1 Creutzfeldt–Jakob disease
       2.3.2 Variant Creutzfeldt–Jakob disease

3. Neurodegenerative diseases with predominant motor symptoms (Predominant Subcortical Involvement)
   3.1 Neurodegenerative diseases with abnormalities of posture and movement
       3.1.1 Parkinson disease
       3.1.2 Parkinson plus syndrome
       3.1.3 Progressive supranuclear palsy
       3.1.4 Multisystem atrophy
       3.1.5 Corticobasal-ganglionic degeneration
   3.2 Neurodegeneration with brain iron accumulation
       3.2.1 Pantothenate kinase associated neurodegeneration
       3.2.2 PLA2G6-associated neurodegenration
   3.3 Familial idiopathic basal ganglionic calcification
   3.4 Neurodegeneration with abnormal movement disorder as a part of systemic disorders
       3.4.1 Hepatolenticular degeneration (Wilson disease)

4. Neurodegenerative diseases with predominant gait disturbances
   4.1 Autosomal dominant cerebellar ataxia
   4.2 Frdriech's ataxia
   4.3 Normal pressure hydrocephalus

5. Neurodegenerative diseases with only motor symptoms
   5.1 Motor system diseases
       5.1.1 Amyotrophic lateral sclerosis
       5.1.2 Progressive muscular atrophy
       5.1.3 Primary lateral sclerosis
   5.2. Heredofamilial forms of progressive muscular atrophy

thought to correlate with disease severity, but more recently it has been hypothesized that the imbalance between the production and clearance of Aβ, particularly the more toxic Aβ1-42, plays the key role in the pathogenesis of AD. Decreased clearance of toxic Aβ isoform has been implicated as the etiopathologic basis of sporadic AD, whereas increased production of Aβ is implicated in familial AD. NFTs contain paired helical filaments of abnormally hyperphosphorylated tau proteins that occupy the cell body and extend to dendrites. The NFT-induced damage usually starts in the entorhinal cortex, spreading to the hippocampus and amygdala regions, and subsequently involving the rest of the neocortex. Unlike amyloid plaques, NFTs appear to correlate well with specific deficits, such as memory loss.

Several biomarkers of AD have been identified recently. They are grossly classified either as pathophysiologic markers that identify characteristic AD pathology or topographical markers that are less specific and used to assess downstream structural changes, particularly in the medial temporal lobes. Examples of pathophysiologic markers include CSF Aβ protein, tau and phosphorylated tau proteins, and high cerebral uptake of amyloid-specific positron emission tomography (PET) tracers (11C-labeled Pittsburg (PiB) agent, 18F-labeled PiB (Fultemetamol), 18F-Florbetapir, 18F-Florbetaben). Decreased parietotemporal fluorodeoxyglucose (FDG) uptake and medial temporal lobe atrophy identified by magnetic resonance imaging (MRI) are the topographical markers.

The typical clinical presentation of AD is an insidious progressive impairment of episodic memory with gradual emergence of aphasia, apraxia, agnosia, and executive deficits as the disease progresses. Neuropsychiatric symptoms are very common in AD patients and can occur in up to 98% of patients. Visual and auditory hallucinations are the most common perceptual abnormalities. Functional decline starts with the higher order executive functions (such as financial management) well in advance of the more basic functions relating to basic self-care.

Clinicians have been using the National Institute of Neurological and Communicative Disorders and Stroke and the Alzheimer's Disease and Related Disorders Association (NINCDS-ADRDA) clinical criteria for AD diagnosis since 1984. This classifies AD as "definite" (clinical diagnosis with histologic confirmation), "probable" (typical clinical syndrome without histologic confirmation), and "possible" (atypical clinical features or comorbid pathology but no definite identifiable explanation for dementia without histologic confirmation). Since histologic confirmation is often not possible, application of these criteria typically results in a diagnosis of "probable" or "possible" AD. With better understanding of the disease pathogenesis and availability of multiple AD biomarkers, a more recent and perhaps more practical classification system has been suggested [3]. In this new lexicon, two preclinical stages of AD ("asymptomatic at risk for AD" and "presymptomatic AD") have been described in addition to the "prodromal AD" (clinically affected patients with positive AD biomarkers). The widely accepted term mild cognitive impairment (MCI) is now included in the prodromal AD group. AD is further subclassified as AD dementia, typical AD, atypical AD, and mixed AD. Clinical diagnosis of MCI is no longer encouraged according to the newly suggested lexicon.

Imaging of AD can be grossly classified as structural/topographical imaging (computed tomography [CT] and MRI) or pathophysiologic imaging (FDG-PET, amyloid imaging).

Conventional neuroimaging with CT and/or MRI is routinely performed in the evaluation of NDD including dementia. These studies are important in offering clues suggesting AD, and also in excluding other diseases. CT scan can have a variable appearance depending on the stage of the disease. In early stage of AD, minimal brain volume loss is the usual finding, which is difficult to differentiate from normal aging pattern. With advanced disease, moderate to severe brain volume loss preferentially affecting the temporal lobes occurs.

MRI of patients with AD often demonstrates diffuse cerebral volume loss predominantly in the parietal and temporal lobes, specifically the hippocampus (Figure 10.2).

Parietal and hippocampal volume loss can support a clinical diagnosis, but cannot definitely establish the diagnosis of AD as these findings often overlap with the

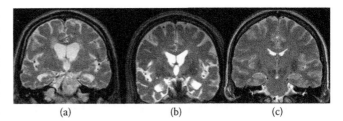

(a)   (b)   (c)

FIGURE 10.2
Variable degree of hippocampal atrophy. (a) Bilateral moderate hippocampal atrophy with prominence of temporal horns on this coronal T2-weighted sequence. The atrophy is asymmetric, more severe on the left. (b) Bilateral severe hippocampal atrophy with moderate passive enlargement of the temporal horns. (c) Normal hippocampal and temporal horn morphology.

normal aging pattern and other non-Alzheimer's dementias. Several different techniques have been described to increase the sensitivity and specificity of structural MRI such as visual, semiautomated, and automated quantification of volume loss involving entorhinal cortex, perirhinal cortex, and hippocampus. In many institutions, some form of automated or semiautomated quantification of temporal volume loss is performed. Numerous methods have been described. In our institution, we use the visual rating system of the degree of hippocampal volume loss as described by Urs et al. [4]. Medial temporal lobe atrophy score as suggested by Duara et al. [5] is also popular visual rating system used in clinical practice. Calculation of temporal horn volume and temporal horn index (ratio of temporal horn volume to lateral ventricle volume) by segmentation is another method of evaluation of AD. Both the volume and the indices are significantly larger in patients with AD than control group and correlates with the neuropsychiatric symptoms [6]. More quantitative region-of-interest-based analysis of the entorhinal cortex and hippocampus has also been described for detection of preclinical AD [7]. Voxel-based morphometry is another technique of quantification of medial temporal volume loss. Advanced MRI techniques (diffusion imaging, perfusion imaging, MR spectroscopy) have also been used in evaluation of AD with variable success.

Metabolic features of AD seen on FDG-PET vary on the stage of the disease. In early stage of the disease, there is reduced glucose metabolism in the parietotemporal association cortices as well as posterior cingulate cortex and precuneus. However, FDG uptake remains preserved in the sensorimotor and visual cortices even in the advanced stage of the disease. Contrast between relatively preserved and decreased areas of FDG uptake is a clue to the diagnosis of AD.

Several amyloid-specific PET tracers (11C-labeled PiB agent, 18F-labeled PiB [Fultemetamol], 18F-Florbetapir, 18F-Florbetaben) are now in phase 3 clinical trials and may soon become available for clinical use. PiB binds to the insoluble fibrillary Aβ with high affinity, but not to amorphous amyloid plaques and NFTs. Increased cortical binding is seen in patients with AD compared to age-matched healthy controls (Figure 10.3).

Normal cortical binding in healthy controls is ≤1.5 times the cerebellum, the reference structure. Increased cortical binding can also be seen in some of the elderly controls (about 10% in patients below the age of 70 years and about 30–40% at the age of 80 years). APOE4 is a genetic risk factor for increased uptake of PiB. Patients diagnosed with MCI (prodromal AD) and increased binding have a high risk of progressing to AD with manifest dementia, whereas patients with low/negative PiB binding seldom develop dementia. Increased PiB uptake is most prominently seen in the frontal cortex (1.94-fold), striatum (1.74-fold), parietal cortex (1.71-fold), occipital cortex (1.54-fold), and temporal cortex (1.52-fold) compared to the age-matched controls. Equivalent PiB uptake is seen in areas of brain that demonstrate relatively maintained FDG uptake (primary sensorimotor cortex, subcortical white matter).

10.4.1.2 Vascular Dementia

Vascular dementia (VaD) is the second most common cause of dementia after AD. According to the National Institute of Neurological Disorders and Stroke and Association Internationale pour la Recherche et l'Enseignement en Neurosciences (NINDS-AIREN) criteria, VaD is defined as dementia with a decline in memory and intellectual ability that causes impaired functioning of daily living

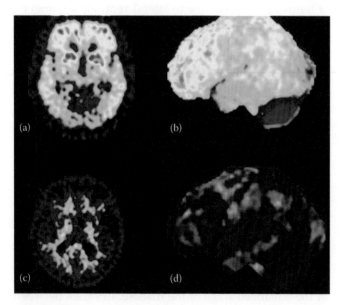

FIGURE 10.3
Alzheimer's disease (AD). Intense uptake of amyloid-specific tracer (Pittsburg[PiB]) predominantly in the frontal and parietal regions on axial image (a) as well as on surface projection (b) in a patient with clinical diagnosis of AD. Normal PiB uptake in healthy control is demonstrated in (c) and (d). (Courtesy of Prof. Alexander Drzezga, Technical University of Munich, Germany.)

associated with objective evidence of cerebrovascular disease. Most importantly, there is a temporal relationship between the cerebrovascular insult and the onset of dementia (Table 10.3).

VaD may be subclassified as dementia secondary to large vessel disease or dementia secondary to small vessel disease. Dementias associated with microhemorrhages are also sometimes included under VaD.

10.4.1.2.1 Dementia Secondary to Large Vessel Disease

Dementia secondary to large vessel disease is associated with multiple infarcts of the major arterial territories of the brain (anterior coroidal artery, middle coroidal artery, posterior cerebral artery, superior cerebellar artery, posterior inferior cerebellar artery, and anterior inferior cerebellar artery) or strategic infarction in areas such as the angular gyrus, thalamus, and basal forebrain.

10.4.1.2.2 Dementia Secondary to Small Vessel Ischemic Disease

Small vessel disease involves the innumerable perforating arteries supplying the subcortical structures (the basal ganglia, cerebral white matter, and the brain stem) and long medullary arteries supplying the deep cerebral white matter (centrum semiovale, corona radiata). Dementia secondary to small vessel disease can be due to a multitude of small vessel pathologies: ischemia, amyloid angiopathy, and cerebral autosomal dominant arteriopathy with subcortical infarct and leukoencephalopathy (CADASIL) or cerebral autosomal recessive arteriopathy with subcortical infarct and leukoencephalopathy (CARASIL) (described in detail in Section 10.4.1.2.4).

The incidence of small vessel ischemic disease increases exponentially after the age of 65. Small vessel ischemic disease manifests as lacunar infarction as well as white matter disease (WMD). WMD is the descriptive term used to describe T2/FLAIR signal hyperintensities in white matter of different locations. WMD is variably known in the literature as microangiopathic disease, leukoaraiosis, and small vessel disease. The exact pathophysiologic basis of these changes is poorly understood. Several hypotheses have been stated. Currently, the major emphasis is on endothelial dysfunction. Other hypotheses include arteriosclerosis and microscopic blood–brain barrier breakdown allowing macromolecules and toxic materials to migrate into the arterial wall (further damaging the arterial wall and narrowing the arterial lumen), interstitial space, and brain parenchyma. The vascular narrowing leads to ischemic injury, which manifests either as completed small vascular infarction (lacunar infarcts and microinfarcts),

TABLE 10.3

NINDS-AIREN Criteria for Probable VaD

Criteria	Description
1. Dementia	Cognitive decline with deterioration of memory and intellectual ability that causes impaired functioning of daily living
2. Objective evidence of cerebrovascular disease	Presence of any one of the following: (i) History of cerebrovascular disease (ii) Focal clinical signs (iii) Imaging evidence (either from CT or MRI) prior cerebrovascular insult
3. Evidence of temporal relationship with point 1 and 2	With any one of the three: (i) Onset of dementia within 3 months of stroke (ii) Abrupt deterioration of the cognitive functions (iii) Fluctuating stepwise progression of the of cognitive decline

persistent hypoperfusion-induced chronic ischemia of deep cerebral white matter (WMD), or a combination of the two.

Lacunar infarcts or lacunas are small infarcts less than 15 mm in diameter, but can range from 3 to 20 mm. They are typically located in the basal ganglia, internal capsule, thalamus, pons, corona radiata, and centrum semiovale. Lacunar infarcts can be detected both by CT and MRI with MRI being more sensitive and specific than CT. Lacunar infarcts are seen as sharply marginated round or oval cavities. In the chronic stage, lacunar infarcts are hypoattenuating on CT scans and hyperintense on T2/FLAIR. An enlarged perivascular (VR) space is the most common mimic of a lacunar infarct. It is often difficult to differentiate the two based on imaging. However, lesions smaller than 1–2 mm, distributed symmetrically in the basal ganglia, and hypointense on FLAIR are more likely to be enlarged perivascular spaces than lacunar infarcts.

WMD consists of noncavitated lesions. Their size can range from a few millimeters to confluent involvement of the entire deep cerebral white matter, usually sparing of the subcortical U fibers. Several risk factors have been identified. Some of the most important associated risk factors include Afro-Caribbean ancestry, history of hypertension (the most important modifiable risk factor), smoking, and vitamin B12 deficiency. However, WMD occurs in otherwise completely healthy patients as a manifestation of normal aging. The severity of dementia in patients with small vessel ischemic disease correlates better with cortical atrophy rather than WMD. Nonetheless, numerous studies have associated WMD with cognitive decline. WMD lesions are seen as bilaterally symmetrical or asymmetrical areas of hypoattenuation on CT and hyperintensity on T2/FLAIR MRI in the periventricular or deep cerebral white matter. These lesions can easily be distinguished from large artery infarcts by their nonvascular territory distribution, lack of well-defined margins, lack of

wedge shape, lack of cortical involvement, and lack of associated encephalomalacia.

10.4.1.2.3 Cerebral Amyloid Angiopathy

Cerebral Amyloid Angiopathy (CAA) is recognized as a major cause of spontaneous lobar hemorrhage in the elderly. CAA is also associated with a high prevalence of small vessel ischemic disease, occult cerebral microhemorrhages, and cognitive impairment. It rarely occurs before 60 years, but there is progressively increasing incidence after the age of 65. CAA is present in nearly all brains with AD. This may suggest a common amyloid-based pathogenesis of the disease. However, despite the close molecular relationship between the two diseases, CAA is a clinically distinct entity from AD. The characteristic pathophysiologic manifestation of CAA is deposition of Aβ peptide in the media and adventitia of small and medium size cortical and leptomeningeal vessels, with preferential involvement of occipital regions. Arteries supplying the basal ganglia and posterior fossa are relatively spared. There is fibrinoid degeneration, necrosis, and end-vessel microaneurysm formation. Microaneurysm rupture can result in microhemorrhages or classic large lobar hematoma. As the involved arteries are either cortical or leptomeningeal, the hemorrhages are typically lobar, affecting the brain periphery, as opposed to hemorrhagic strokes that predominantly occur in the basal ganglia, may extend into the ventricles, but rarely extend into the extra-axial compartment. The exact pathophysiologic mechanism of CAA is not clear but is related to *APP* gene mutation and with specific alleles (ε2 and ε4) of the *Apo-E* gene.

Microbleeds are not visualized on CT. These are best detected on MRI using susceptibility-weighted imaging and gradient recalled echo MRI sequences. Clinicoradiologic diagnosis of CAA can be definite CAA, probable CAA, and possible CAA (Boston criteria) based on histopathology, age of presentation, and characteristic hemorrhage pattern on MRI (Figure 10.4) [8].

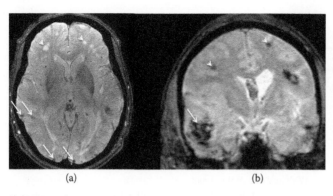

(a)   (b)

FIGURE 10.4
Cerebral amyloid angiopathy. (a) Susceptibility-weighted image demonstrates numerous minute areas of signal void predominantly in the cortical and juxtra-cortical areas secondary to local magnetic inhomogeneity due to cerebral amyloid angiopathy-related microhemorrhages (arrows). Multifocal white matter diseases (arrowhead) are also seen. (b) Coronal gradient echo image on a different patient demonstrates microhemorrhages (arrowheads) as well as areas of macrohemorrhage (arrow).

10.4.1.2.4 CADASIL

Cerebral autosomal-dominant arteriopathy with subcortical infarcts and leukoencephalopathy (CADASIL) is an autosomal dominant disease resulting from mutations of the gene encoding the transmembrane receptor NOTCH 3, located on chromosome 19. Classic presentation of CADASIL includes the following clinical symptoms: subcortical ischemic events (60%–85%), cognitive impairment (up to 60%), migraine with aura (20%–40%), mood disorder and apathy (20%), seizures (5%–10%), and motor abnormalities [9,10].

Microscopic examination reveals changes typical of chronic small vessel arteriopathy involving penetrating cerebral and leptomeningeal arteries, diffuse myelin pallor, and rarefication of hemispheric white matter predominantly in the centrum semiovale and periventricular regions.

Neuroimaging is crucial in diagnosis of CADASIL. MRI changes usually precede the onset of clinical symptoms by 10–15 years. The earliest age at which MRI changes are evident is still unknown, but the mean age at detection of MRI changes is 30 years and MRI abnormalities are present in all patients carrying the mutation after the age of 35 years. The most common MRI abnormality is punctate areas of T2/FLAIR changes in the periventricular and centrum semiovale white matter, which with time enlarges and becomes confluent and involves the external capsule and white matter of anterior temporal lobes. WMD of the anterior temporal lobe is highly suggestive of CADASIL (Figure 10.5). Lacunar infarcts of varying sizes, shapes, and numbers are seen in the areas of T2 changes and increase in number with time. Diffusion imaging may demonstrate focal or multifocal diffusion restriction. Microbleeds can be seen in up to 69% of patients with paramagnetic susceptibility-sensitive sequences (SWI, GRE).

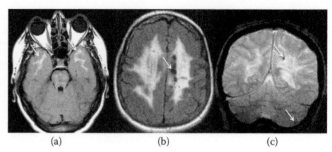

(a)   (b)   (c)

FIGURE 10.5
CADASIL. (a) Increased signal in the anterior temporal lobe white matter (arrows) on the axial fluid-attenuated inversion recovery (FLAIR) mage, classic finding of CADASIL. (b) Confluent areas of white matter hyperintensity in the centrum semiovale on FLAIR sequence, a common associated finding. There is also cyst formation (arrow) due to severe white matter disease. (c) On coronal gradient echo image of the same patient demonstrates, numerous areas signal void (arrows) due to local microhemorrhage-related magnetic inhomogeneity in the gray–white junction as well as in the cerebellum.

These MRI techniques should be routinely implemented in the evaluation of dementia patients. Prominent VR spaces, predominantly in the basal ganglia, are another common finding. Although imaging can be highly suggestive of CADSIL, genetic testing for mutation of the NOTCH3 exons is the gold standard for diagnosis of CADASIL with 100% specificity and almost 100% sensitivity. Genetic testing should be performed in patients with typical presentations in combination with neuroimaging findings or positive family history, particularly in the absence of hypertension.

Another genetic form of ischemic, nonhypertensive, cerebral small vessel disease, CARASIL, has recently been described with clinical, imaging, and histopathological findings similar to CADASIL. CARASIL is secondary to single gene mutation of HTRA1 gene on chromosome 10q. Premature baldness is a unique clinical presentation of this subtype.

10.4.1.3 Dementia with Lewy Body

Dementia with Lewy Body (DLB) is increasingly diagnosed and may be the second most common (nonvascular) cause of dementia after AD. DLB accounts for about 10%–22% of all dementia patients. Like AD, DLB is a disease of older age occurring after 65 years with a strong predilection for male patients. Most cases of DLB are sporadic. However, familial DLB cases have been reported associated with mutation of the α-synuclein (SNCA) gene. In addition to dementia, distinctive clinical features of DLB include visual hallucination, parkinsonism, cognitive fluctuations, and autonomic dysfunction. By definition, probable DLB is characterized by dementia associated with two of the following three features: (1) fluctuating cognition/level of consciousness, (2) visual hallucinations, and (3) spontaneous parkinsonian motor signs. Other suggestive clinical features include rapid eye movement sleep disorders (e.g., vivid dreams), neuroleptic sensitivity, and low dopamine transporter (DaT) in the basal ganglia as evidenced by single-photon emission computed tomography (SPECT) or PET studies.

DLB is one of the synucleinopathies. The histopathological hallmark of DLB is the Lewy body. Lewy bodies are round, eosinophilic, intracytoplasmic inclusions with a dense core surrounded by a halo. These inclusions primarily consist of SNCA. Lewy bodies are found in the hippocampus and amygdala, anterior cingulate cortex and neocortices. Like AD, amyloid plaques are also present in most patients with DLB. However, NFTs are uncommon.

Conventional neuroimaging offers little specificity for diagnosis of DLB. Although CT and MRI may show atrophy, the patterns of atrophy associated with DLB have not been well established. The absence of hippocampal/medial temporal lobe atrophy in DLB helps to differentiate the disease from AD.

Measurement of cerebral glucose metabolism by FDG offers typical metabolic abnormalities that help to diagnose DLB. In DLB, there is characteristic hypoperfusion and hypometabolism in the occipital lobes, especially in visual cortex. This feature can help distinguish DLB from AD, in which the visual cortex metabolism is relatively spared.

10.4.1.4 Frontotemporal Degeneration

Frontotemporal degeneration (FTD), formerly referred to as Pick's disease, is a group of overlapping clinical syndromes characterized by focal degeneration of frontal and/or temporal lobes. It is associated with a variety of neurodegenerative processes and genetic mutations. FTD is the third most common cause of dementia after AD and DLB. The typical age of onset between 45 and 65 years is earlier than other forms of dementia, though cases have been reported outside this range. The incidence in men and women is equal.

As with other forms of cortical dementia, the presentation is insidious. Based on the clinical presentations, FTD is classified into three distinct types: (1) behavioral-variant FTD (bv-FTD), (2) symantic dementia, and (3) syndrome of progressive nonfluent aphasia.

10.4.1.4.1 Behavioral-Variant Frontotemporal Degeneration

bv-FTD is the most common variant of FTD and accounts for one-half to two-thirds of all cases. This variant is male-predominant, has the earliest average age of onset (<60 years), has a strong association with motor neuron disease, and has the most rapidly progressive course of all the three variants. It predominantly involves frontal lobe structures. Depending on specific area of frontal lobe degeneration, patients with bv-FTD may be disinhibited (orbitofrontal degeneration), apathetic (anterior cingulate involvement), or dysexecutive (dorsolateral prefrontal degeneration).

10.4.1.4.2 Symantic Dementia

Symantic dementia (SD) is secondary to predominantly anterior temporal lobe degeneration It accounts for 20% or less of all FTDs, has an average age of onset <60 years, and has the slowest rate of progression of all of the FTDs. Typically, the disease begins with asymmetric involvement of the temporal lobe, more frequently involving the left side. If the dominant anterior temporal lobe is predominantly involved, patients present with word finding difficulty (anomia) or word recognition. If the nondominant anterior temporal lobe is predominantly involved, patients present with prosopagnosia (difficulty recognizing familiar faces) or difficulty in understanding emotions in others.

10.4.1.4.3 Progressive Nonfluent Aphasia

Progressive nonfluent aphasia (PNFA) is secondary to predominant involvement of perisylvian areas and is characterized by breakdown in spontaneous speech and difficulty in understanding language. Unlike bv-FTD, these patients recognize their language deficits.

FTD has three distinct types of immunocytochemistry signatures. The most common pattern is a ubiquitin positive and tau negative pattern, which accounts more than 60% of all FTDs. The most common ubiquitin protein is TDP-43.

Neuroimaging findings may support the diagnosis of FTD, but are not in themselves diagnostic. Structural imaging (CT and MRI) is required to exclude any other structural disease. CT and MRI may be normal early in the course of the disease. With time, there is progressive atrophy of the frontal and/or temporal lobes. Specific patterns of atrophy have been associated with the clinical syndrome in about 50%–70% of patients. As described earlier, bifrontal atrophy is typically seen in bv-FTD, prominent, marked anterior temporal lobe atrophy is characteristic of SD and predominantly left-sided perisylvian atrophy is seen in PNFA (Figures 10.6 through 10.8). Unlike the symmetric volume loss in the temporal lobes in AD, in SD the temporal lobe volume loss is often asymmetric. There is also a distinct anteroposterior gradient in the severity of volume loss (with the temporal pole more severely affected than more posterior temporal lobe) [11].

Glucose metabolism also varies widely between different subtypes of FTD without any specific pattern for each subtype. On FDG-PET, the classic abnormality is hypometabolism predominantly affecting the frontal lobes. Asymmetric bilateral frontal and temporal lobe involvement is also common. Glucose uptake remains preserved in the primary sensorimotor cortex, like AD.

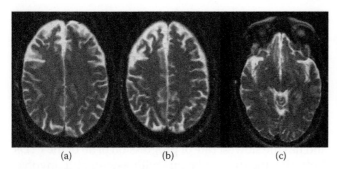

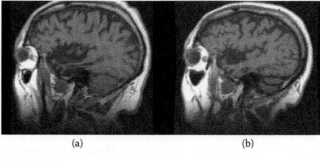

FIGURE 10.6

Behavioral-variant frontotemporal degeneration (bv-FTD). Asymmetric frontal lobe predominant atrophy with relative sparing of temporal lobes on these axial T2-weighted sequences at different levels (a, b, and c) in a patient with clinical diagnosis of bv-FTD.

FIGURE 10.8

Progressive nonfluent aphasia. Bilateral perisylvian atrophy, more severe on the left side (a) compared to the right side (b) on the parasagittal noncontrasted T1-weighted sequence in a patient with clinical pattern of symantic dementia type of frontotemporal degeneration.

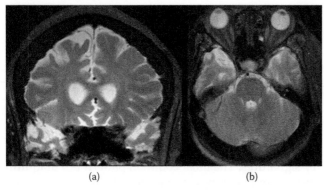

FIGURE 10.7

Symantic dementia (SD). Bilateral asymmetric temporal lobe atrophy, predominantly involving the right side on this coronal (a) and axial (b) T2-weighted sequences in a patient with clinical pattern of (SD) type of frontotemporal degeneration.

10.4.1.5 Dementia Associated with Systemic Diseases

It is extremely important to consider systemic causes of dementia in the evaluation of dementia since dementias secondary to systemic diseases are often treatable, unlike NDDs. In clinical practice, systemic causes of dementia are routinely ruled out before disease-specific workup for NDDs begins. Potentially treatable causes of dementia include nutritional deficiencies (Wernicke–Korsakoff syndrome, pellagra, vitamin B12 deficiency), chronic drug intoxication (alcohol abuse), and metabolic (hypothyroidism, Cushing's disease, chronic hepatic failure) and pseudodementia of depression. Other treatable causes of dementia include chronic subdural hematoma, frontal lobe tumor, paraneoplastic limbic encephalitis, neurosyphillis, and other chronic meningitis, including superficial siderosis (which may be a marker for CAA). Routine serum chemistry, CSF analysis, electroencephalogram (EEG), CT, and MRI are routinely performed in the workup of dementia.

10.4.2 Neurodegenerative Diseases with Predominant Cognitive and Other Neurological Symptoms

10.4.2.1 Huntington Disease

Huntington disease (HD) is a progressive, fatal, neurodegenerative disorder caused by CAG trinucleotide repeat expansion of the *HTT* gene on chromosome 4 and inherited in an autosomal dominant manner with age-dependent penetrance. As a resultant of this expansion, there is an abnormally long polyglutamine repeat in the huntingtin protein, which alters the pattern of protein folding resulting in aggregation of the protein within the nuclei similar to many other NDDs. Although these aggregates are found in cortex and subcortical structures including the striatum, atrophy is predominant in the striatum for unknown reasons.

Prevalence of HD is 4–10 per 100,000 in the Western world. Mean age of presentation is 40 years. Although there is no unique set of symptoms to indicate HD, chorea, dystonia, bradykinesia, and incoordination are usual initial presentation. Many patients also present with cognitive decline and psychiatric disturbances.

HD causes progressive brain atrophy, particularly severe degeneration of caudate nucleus that begins in the tail of the caudate and gradually progress to affect the most dorsal medial aspect. Eventually, the caudate atrophies to a paper-thin layer of gliotic tissue. This gives the "box car" appearance of the frontal horns on CT or MRI (Figure 10.9).

Striatal atrophy is readily seen on CT, although much better seen on MRI. There may be coexistent diffuse cerebral atrophy. In patients harboring the mutation, progressive destruction of the caudate head is evidenced by progressively decreased uptake of FDG-PET and increased bicaudate ratio (minimum intercaudate distance divided by the brain width

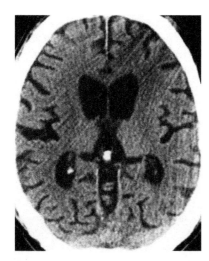

FIGURE 10.9
Huntington disease. Axial computed tomography scan demonstrate bilateral atrophy of the head of the caudate nucleus giving the "boxcar" appearance of the frontal horn.

along the same line). In addition to the atrophy, there is also abnormally increased T2 signal at the caudate head.

10.4.2.2 CADASIL

CADASIL has been discussed in detail in Section 10.4.1.2.4.

10.4.2.3 Prion Diseases

Prion diseases comprise a group of very rare rapidly progressing NDDs that affect both humans and animals. The most notable feature of this disease is the potential for transmission between human and animals. On histopathology, there are characteristic spongiform brain changes (presence of small vacuoles in the neuropil) with neuronal loss, glial proliferation, and striking absence of inflammatory response.

The transmissible agent of prion disease comprises an abnormal isoform (PrP^{Sc}, Sc stands for scrapie isoform) of a normal cell surface protein (PrP^C) of unknown function coded by a prion protein (*PRNP*) gene on chromosome 20p. The normal PrP^C isoform has a highly organized three-dimensional ultrastructure consisting of alpha helices. These alpha helices are replaced by a β-pleated sheet in the abnormal PrP^{Sc} isoform, which resists normal proteolysis. These abnormal proteins then accumulate as synaptic plaques. Nonplaque depositions also occur. It is hypothesized that misfolded protein acts as a template that encourages conversion of the normal ultrastructure of the

TABLE 10.4

Classification of Human Prion Disease

Human Prion Diseases
Creutzfeldt–Jakob disease
Sporadic CJD (sCJD)
Variant CJD (vCJD)
Iatrogenic CJD
Dural graft associated CJD
Growth hormone associated CJD
Blood transfusion associated CJD
Inherited prion diseases
Gerstmann–Straussler–Scheinker syndrome
Fatal familial insomnia
Kuru

host protein into the wild isoform that is found in diseased condition.

There are several forms of the human prion diseases, Creutzfeldt–Jakob disease (CJD), Gerstmann–Straussler–Scheinker syndrome, fatal familial insomnia, and Kuru (Table 10.4).

Although there is considerable heterogeneity of the clinical picture of the human prion diseases, there are a number of core features. All are associated with cognitive decline at some stage of the disease, which characteristically is very rapid. Memory, speech, and executive functions are often involved early in the course of the disease. Neurological signs and symptoms secondary to involvement of multiple functionally and neurochemically different components in the central nervous system are often the first clues in favor of prion disease over other more common types of dementia.

10.4.2.3.1 Creutzfeldt–Jakob Disease

CJD is the most common type of human prion disease presenting with dementia. This is a rare disease with an annual incidence of 0.25–2 cases per million population. CJD can be sporadic (sCJD), familial (fCJD), iatrogenic (iCJD), and variant (vCJD). The vast majority of cases are sporadic (85%–95%), whereas 5%–15% are familial. iCJD accounts for less than 1% of cases. Iatrogenic modes of transmission include administration of cadaveric growth hormone, dural graft transplant, corneal transplant, liver transplant, and use of contaminated neurosurgical equipment. Cadaveric growth hormone use and dural grafting comprise the vast majority of cases of iCJD. Transfusion-related CJD has phenotype similar to the vCJD. vCJD is rare and is linked to bovine spongiform encephalopathy and is discussed separately.

10.4.2.3.1.1 Sporadic Creutzfeldt–Jakob Disease

Most patients with CJD are between the ages of 40 and 80. The classic clinical triad is rapidly progressive dementia (in almost all patients), myoclonic jerks (90%), and periodic bi- or triphasic sharp-wave complexes on EEG (up to 95%). Extrapyramidal symptoms and cerebellar manifestations occur in up to two-thirds of the patients.

MRI is highly sensitive and specific for the diagnosis of CJD. Although hypodensity in the basal ganglia and occipital lobes can be seen on CT in advanced CJD, CT is not the optimal modality to evaluate this patient group except to exclude structural causes that might have similar clinical manifestations. MRI demonstrates increased T2 and FLAIR signal most commonly in the caudate head, putamen, globus pallidus, thalamus, and cerebral and cerebellar cortices (Figure 10.10). Even though there is diffuse cortical involvement, the primary sensorimotor cortex is almost always spared even in late stage of the disease (Figure 10.11). Diffusion-weighted imaging is far more sensitive (91%–92% sensitive) and more specific (94%–95% specific) than the T2/FLAIR changes but is not necessarily observed in all involved areas.

Diffusion restriction can be seen as early as 1 month after onset of clinical symptoms and can precede T2/FLAIR changes by as much as 6 months. Diffusion restriction can disappear in later stage of the disease when atrophy ensues. Specific MRI abnormalities may vary with the clinical syndrome and molecular subtypes of sCJD. As there is absence of inflammation, involved areas do not demonstrate contrast enhancement.

CSF detection of 14-3-3 protein is a useful marker of CJD with variable sensitivity and specificity. A positive result should be considered adjunctive rather than being absolutely specific for CJD. A negative result does not preclude the disease. New diagnostic criteria have been established based on clinical and imaging findings, as described in Table 10.5.

10.4.2.3.1.2 Variant Creutzfeldt–Jakob Disease

Since the first description of the "new variant" CJD, there has been intense interest in this entity because of epidemiologic as well as social concerns, particularly because of its link to bovine spongiform encephalopathy.

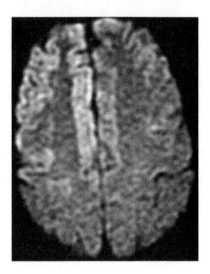

FIGURE 10.11

Another typical imaging appearance of sporadic Creutzfeldt–Jakob disease. Diffusion restriction involving the only cortical tissue of the frontal lobe, predominately on the right side on this diffusion-weighted images. These high-intensity areas showed low apparent diffusion coefficient (ADC) value on ADC map (not shown).

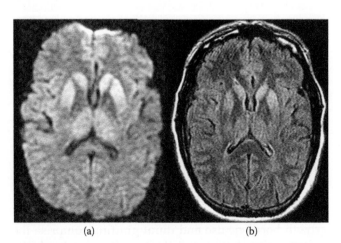

(a)   (b)

FIGURE 10.10

Typical imaging appearance of sporadic Creutzfeldt–Jakob disease. Bilateral symmetrical diffusion restriction (a) and increased signal on axial fluid-attenuated inversion recovery sequence (b) in basal ganglia and thalamus.

TABLE 10.5

MRI-CJD Consortium Criteria for Diagnosis of CJD

Clinical signs (<2 years)
Dementia
Cerebellar or visual symptoms
Pyramidal or extrapyramidal signs
Akinetic mutism
Tests
Periodic bi- or triphasic sharp waves on EEG
14-3-3 Protein in CSF
High DWI or FLAIR signal in caudate and putamen or at least two cortical regions:
Temporal
Parietal
Occipital
Probable CJD
Two clinical signs and at least one positive test
Possible CJD
Two clinical signs that are <2 years duration

The striking feature of vCJD is the early age of the patients at the time of diagnosis (mean age 29). Presentation usually includes behavioral or psychiatric disturbances, and in some cases sensory symptoms. There is no change in the *PRNP* gene in this condition; however, the three-dimensional structure of PrP^{Sc} protein is strikingly stereotypical rather than heterogeneous, as seen in sCJD. A distinct histopathological signature of vCJD is the presence of amyloid plaques. Unlike sCJD, detection of 14-3-3 protein in the CSF is not a sensitive marker of the disease. On MRI, there is distinct high signal on FLAIR in the medial pulvinar and dorsomedial thalamus (inverted hockey stick sign), which is 78% sensitive and 100% specific. DWI is less sensitive for vCJD than for sCJD.

Other rapidly progressive dementias that can have MRI findings similar to CJD include Bartonella and Wernicke's encephalopathy. These patients' MRI scans may also reveal DWI hyperintensity in the deep gray matter.

10.4.3 Neurodegenerative Diseases with Predominant Motor Symptoms (Predominant Subcortical Involvement)

10.4.3.1 Neurodegenerative Diseases with Abnormalities of Posture and Movement

In general, degenerative disorders with abnormalities of posture and movement also have a nondescript onset and gradual progression. Most cases are sporadic but a familial variant is not uncommonly seen. Broadly, degenerative parkinsonian disorders are classified as synuclenopathies or taopathies based on molecular profiles, as described in Table 10.6.

10.4.3.1.1 Parkinson Disease

Parkinson disease (PD) is a neurodegenerative disorder of the pars compacta of the substantia nigra and is recognized as one of the most common neurologic disorders, affecting approximately 1% of individuals older than 60 years. There are two major neuropathologic findings: the loss of pigmented dopaminergic neurons in the substantia nigra and the presence of SNCA containing Lewy bodies, eosinophilic proteinaceous cytoplasmic

TABLE 10.6

Classification of Parkinsonian Disorders Based on Molecular Pathology

Synucleinopathies
Parkinson disease with dementia
Dementia with Lewy body disease
Multiple system atrophy
Taopathies
Progressive supranuclear palsy
Corticobasal degeneration

inclusion bodies in the surviving cells. Most cases of idiopathic PD are believed to be due to a combination of genetic and environmental factors.

Symptoms of PD typically start insidiously, emerging slowly over weeks or months, with tremor being the most common initial symptom. Classic signs of PD include resting tremor, rigidity, bradykinesia, and postural instability. Clinically, PD can be diagnosed by an experienced neurologist with positive predictive value of 76%–98.6%.

With a classical clinical picture, there is really no role for neuroimaging. CT and MRI are performed to rule out secondary causes of PD [12]. In the early stages of PD, both CT and MRI can be either normal or show age-related changes. As disease progresses, mild cortical atrophy involving hippocampal and frontal structures may occur. In advanced stages of the disease, there may be signal drop in the substantia nigra compared to the normal population on heme-sensitive sequences [13].

Both SPECT- and PET-based ligands that target the dopaminergic system have recently become available and can diagnose PD confidently. ^{123}Ioflupane is the only FDA approved SPECT ligand available in the United States for clinical use. There are several other SPECT and PET ligands being tested in phase II or phase III clinical trials. ^{123}Ioflupane binds exclusively to the DaT in dopaminergic neurons. In normal patients, there is intense uptake of this ligand in the striatum and the image appears as bilateral "comma"-shaped striatum. In PD, there is preferentially decreased binding of this ligand to the posterolateral aspect of the striatum secondary to loss of dopaminergic neurons. The image appears as a symmetric or asymmetric "truncated comma" or even "full-stop"-shaped uptake. Imaging targeting the dopaminergic system can also be completely normal-appearing in patients with florid clinical signs of PD, which is termed as scans without evidence of dopaminergic dysfunction [14]. Many of these patients are ultimately diagnosed with essential or dystonic tremor.

10.4.3.1.2 Parkinson Plus Syndrome

Parkinson plus syndrome (PPS) includes three distinct disease types: progressive supranuclear palsy (PSP), multiple system atrophy (MSA), and corticobasal degeneration (CBD). All three diseases are frequently confused with classic PD. In fact, up to 30% of the pathologically proved PPS are initially diagnosed as PD. However, there are a few clinical features that raise the concern for PPS as described in Table 10.7.

Accurate differentiation between PD and PPS is critically important because (a) treatment such as levodopa and deep brain stimulators are generally ineffective in PPS and (b) life expectancy is much lower in PPS compared to PD.

TABLE 10.7

Subtype-Specific Clinical Features of Parkinson Plus Syndromes

Clinical Features	Suggestive of
Young onset Dysautonomia Laryngeal stridor Forward or lateral trunk flexion	MSA
Cerebellar signs	MSA-C (see below)
Axial rigidity Vertical gaze palsy	PSP
Alien limb phenomenon	CBD
Myoclonus	MSA, CBD
Poor response to levodopa	PSP, MSA, CBD
Early cognitive impairment	CBD, PSP
Pyramidal signs	CBD, MSA-C
Rapid progression (wheelchair bound in <10 years)	MSA, PSP

10.4.3.1.2.1 Progressive Supranuclear Palsy

Steele, Richardson, and Olszewski first described the clinicopathological features of PSP. Unsteadiness of gait and (frequently backward) falls within the first year of symptom onset are the presenting features in most cases. Parkinsonian features are often present, resulting in a misdiagnosis of PD. Resting tremor and cerebellar signs are strikingly absent. However, occulomotor abnormalities are common, and vertical supranuclear opthalmoparesis and cognitive impairment are prominent features of PSP. Pseudobalbar symptoms such as dysarthria or dysphagia are not uncommon.

There is loss of neurons and gliosis in the periaqueductal gray matter, superior colliculus, subthalamic nucleus, red nucleus, pallidum, dentate nucleus, pretectal and vestibular nuclei, and to some extent in the oculomotor nucleus. PSP shares histologic features of tauopathies such as CBD. NFTs and aggregations/inclusions of hyperphosphorylated tau proteins in the subcortical structures are the histologic hallmark of the disease. In contradistinction to the cortical paired helical filaments of the NFTs in AD, the filaments in PSP are subcortical, single, and straight.

Generalized brain atrophy is commonly observed in patients with PSP, especially in the frontal lobes. The characteristic finding is predominant atrophy of midbrain (superior colliculus, red nucleus), which is best seen as "mouse ear," "Mickey Mouse" sign, or "morning glory" sign on an axial MRI, and "hummingbird" sign or sign of "penguin silhouette" (in which atrophy of the midbrain tegmentum and the normal pons resemble a lateral view of a standing penguin) on midline sagittal MRI (Figures 10.12 and 10.13).

Several measurements of midbrain atrophy have been proposed for diagnosis of PSP. The most sensitive and

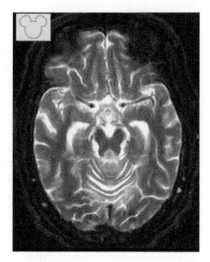

FIGURE 10.12
Progressive supranuclear palsy. Severe selective atrophy of the midbrain tegmentum with relative preservation of the tectum and cerebral peduncles gives the appearance of "mouse ear" on this axial T2-weighted image. Drawing of mouse ear in the inset.

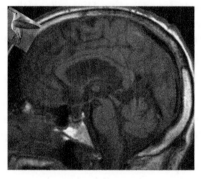

FIGURE 10.13
Progressive supranuclear palsy. Atrophy of the mid-brain tegmentum with relative preservation of the pons leads to appearance of head of the hummingbird, "hummingbird sign," or silhouette of penguin, "penguin sign," on this mid-sagittal T1-weighted sequence. The hummingbird is in the inset.

specific method is calculation of MR parkinsonism index, which is calculated by ratio of pontine-to-midbrain area on the mid sagittal plane multiplied by ratio of middle cerebellar peduncle (MCP) to superior cerebellar peduncle width on the parasagittal view that best exposes the MCP between the pons and the cerebellum [15]. This index has 100% sensitivity, 100% specificity, and 100% positive predictive value in discriminating PSP from PD or MSA with median value of 19.42 [15].

Like PD, there is reduced binding in striatal structures on radionuclide scans labeling dopamine uptake transporter. This imaging modality cannot differentiate between PD and PSP. FDG-PET studies demonstrate nonspecific reduced glucose metabolism in the caudate nucleus, putamen, thalamus, pons, and cerebral cortex with maintained metabolism in the cerebellum.

10.4.3.1.2.2 Multisystem Atrophy

Multisystem atrophy is a neurodegenerative disorder characterized by cerebellar, autonomic, and corticospinal dysfunction in addition to the symptoms of parkinsonism. Pathologically, MSA is characterized by striatonigral and olivopontocerebellar degeneration and SNCA-containing cytoplasmic inclusion bodies in glial cells. There is a consensus guideline for diagnosis and classification of MSA. Details of the criteria are outside the scope of this chapter and can be found in elsewhere [16]. Diagnosis of MSA can be definite, probable, or possible based on histopathology, age of onset, and clinical presentation. Based on the clinical presentation, MSA is classified as MSA with predominant parkinsonism (MSA-P) or MSA with predominant cerebellar ataxia (MSA-C). MSA-P includes former diagnostic subtypes striatonigral degeneration and Shy–Drager syndrome while MSA-C includes former sporadic olivopontocerebellar degeneration.

Autonomic dysfunction is usually the earliest signs of both MSA-P and MSA-C. Genitourinary symptoms are frequent initial presenting signs in women and early erectile dysfunction is invariable in men. Orthostatic hypotension is also common. Akinesia, bradykinesia, and rigidity are prominent in MSA-P and are usually evident in later stages of the MSA-C as well. Cerebellar dysfunction is predominant in MSA-C with gait and limb ataxia being the predominant signs.

CT is not very helpful for diagnosis of MSA. In the late stages of MSA-C, there is nonspecific volume loss of posterior fossa structures. Specific MRI signs suggestive of MSA-C include hyperintense putamen rim sign with or without hypointensity in the dorsolateral part of the putamen, pontine volume loss, the "hot-cross-bun" sign (cruciform pontine hyperintensity on axial T2-weighted images reflecting loss of myelinated transverse pontocerebellar fibers and pontine raphe neurons, but sparing the corticospinal tracts and pontine tegmentum), cerebellar volume loss, and T2 hyperintensity in the MCP (Figure 10.14).

Putaminal abnormalities seem to appear more often and earlier in MSA-P than MSA-C, and conversely infratentorial abnormalities seem to appear more often and earlier in MSA-C than in MSA-P. Specificity of the above-mentioned abnormalities compared to PD and healthy controls is considered quite high, whereas sensitivity especially in the early disease stages seems to be insufficient [17,18]. Advanced MRI techniques such as voxel-based morphometry, diffusion imaging, and spectroscopic imaging can also be helpful in differentiating PD from the PPS [19].

There is reduced glucose metabolism in the caudate, putamen, cerebellum, brain stem, and frontal and temporal lobes on FDG-PET.

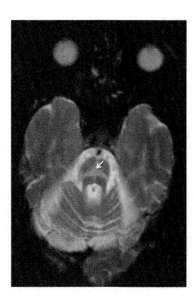

FIGURE 10.14
"Hot-cross-bun" sign in multiple system atrophy. Cruciform pontine hyperintensity on axial T2-weighted images (arrow) reflecting loss of myelinated transverse pontocerebellar fibers and pontine raphe neurons, but sparing the corticospinal tracts and pontine tegmentum.

10.4.3.1.2.3 Corticobasal-Ganglionic Degeneration

Corticobasal-ganglionic degeneration (CBD) is a NDD characterized by unilateral or asymmetric parkinsonian symptoms (rigidity, bradykinesia, akinesia, gait difficulties) as well as cortical and corticospinal tract symptoms. It affects men and women nearly equally, and the age of onset is usually in the sixth decade of life. There is characteristic absence of resting tremor [20]. Cortical symptoms include graphesthesia and loss of stereognosis. Corticospinal tract symptoms include weakness, spasticity, and hyperreflexia. Perhaps, the most striking characteristic deficit in CBD is the "alien limb phenomenon" [20], in which one of the patient's limbs moves in a semipurposeful autonomous way. The best predictors of CBD are limb dystonia, ideomotor apraxia, myoclonus, and asymmetric akinetic-rigid syndrome with late onset of gait or balance disturbances. CBD is another tauopathy and is histologically characterized by corticodentatonigral degeneration with neuronal achromasia [21].

Imaging studies are not specific for this disease. The CT scan may be normal. MRI may reveal asymmetric brain volume loss, usually in the frontal or parietal lobes. In SPECT and PET scan, there is asymmetrically reduced blood flow and metabolism in the frontal, parietal, and temporal lobes. FDG-PET studies have demonstrated significantly reduced cerebral glucose metabolism in the hemisphere contralateral to the clinically most affected side.

10.4.3.2 Neurodegeneration with Brain Iron Accumulation

Iron accumulates in specific brain areas (putamen, dentate nucleus, red nucleus) as a feature of normal aging. However, there are a few genetic diseases associated with pathological iron accumulation in the basal ganglia structures, particularly the globus pallidus and commonly present with extrapyramidal symptoms. This group of diseases is known as neurodegeneration with brain iron accumulation (NBIA). The two most common diseases in this category are pantothenate kinase-associated neurodegeneration (PKAN) and PLA2G6-associated neurodegenration (PLAN) [22]. In addition to these two diseases, several other mutations have been identified that cause excessive brain iron accumulation and similar presentations. However, detailed description of these entities is beyond the scope of this chapter.

10.4.3.2.1 Pantothenate Kinase-Associated Neurodegeneration

The most common disease in the NBIA group is PKAN, which accounts for about 50% of cases of NBIA [23]. This disease was previously known as Hallervorden–Spatz disease. This disease is autosomal recessive and is the result of a mutation in the pantothenate kinase 2 (*PKAN2*) gene in chromosome 20p, which codes for coenzyme A. The classic presentation of this disease is gait and postural difficulty, typically in children 3–6 years of age. In addition to these, both pyramidal and extrapyramidal signs are common. Prominent oro-mandibular dystonia is characteristic sign. The condition has a progressive course and affected children are wheelchair bound within a few years. Patients with an atypical variant of this disease present in adulthood (in 20s and 30s) instead of early in childhood. Unilateral dystonic tremor and focal arm dystonia are the typical presentation of this atypical variety.

Microscopically, iron accumulation is present mostly in the ferric (Fe^{3+}) form as well as ferrous (Fe^{2+}) form in the globus pallidus in a perivascular pattern. In addition, iron-laden macrophages and astrocytes are also seen with little inflammatory response.

In most of the cases of the PKAN, there is a specific imaging pattern on MRI corresponding to the excessive iron accumulation in the globus pallidus. On the T2, T2*, and other susceptibility-sensitive sequences, there is moderate to severe symmetrical hypointensity in the globus pallidus with a central focus of hyperintensity giving the classic appearance of "eye-of-the-tiger" sign (Figure 10.15).

CT scan findings are nonspecific. There may be hypoattenuation in the globus pallidus. Unlike

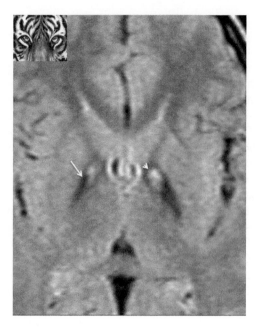

FIGURE 10.15
Pantothenate kinase-associated neurodegeneration. Transverse fluid-attenuated inversion recovery image depicts a low-signal-intensity ring (arrow) surrounding a central high-signal-intensity region (arrowhead) in the medial aspect of the globus pallidus, producing an "eye-of-the-tiger" appearance. Face of the tiger in the inset.

Parkinson diseases, there is normal uptake of the tracer on DaT scan [24].

10.4.3.2.2 PLA2G6-Associated Neurodegenration

PLAN is the second most common form of NBIA and is due to mutation of the *PLA2G6* gene on chromosome 22q. Similar to PKAN, this disease also has age-dependent differences in clinical presentation. Early onset cases have infantile neuroaxonal dystrophy characterized by progressive cognitive and motor decline, pyramidal and cerebellar signs, and visual disturbances secondary to optic atrophy. If the disease onset is later in life, there is an atypical presentation, which includes parkinsonian features mixed with pyramidal signs, eye-movement abnormalities, and cognitive decline. Unlike the infantile variant, there are no cerebellar symptoms.

In the infantile variant of the disease, there is predominant cerebellar atrophy, which is absent in the adult variant. With time, patients develop hypointensity in the globus pallidus on the T2 and susceptibility-sensitive sequences. The imaging appearance is different from PKAN as the central pallidal hyperintensity is absent (absent eye-of-the-tiger sign). MRI exams of some patients appear completely normal without any evidence of excessive iron accumulation.

10.4.3.3 Familial Idiopathic Basal Ganglionic Calcification

Familial idiopathic basal ganglionic calcification, previously known as Fahr's disease, is a rare autosomal dominant neurodegenerative disorder of unknown cause characterized by extensive calcification of the basal ganglionic structures in the absence of systemic calcium metabolic disorder. Both sporadic and familial presentations have been documented in literature. Patients with this disease usually present with cognitive decline, deterioration of motor functions, pyramidal signs, seizures, dysarthria, and headache. The disease can also present as classic parkinsonism with masklike facies, bradykinesia, shuffling gait, and classic "pill-rolling" finger movement. Usual presentation is around middle age.

The most common site of calcification is the globus pallidus. Other predominant areas are putamen, caudate nuclei, thalamus, dentate nucleus, and deep cerebral white matter.

10.4.3.4 Neurodegeneration with Abnormal Movement Disorder as a Part of Systemic Disorders

10.4.3.4.1 Hepatolenticular Degeneration (Wilson Disease)

Wilson disease is a rare autosomal recessive inherited disorder of copper metabolism due to mutation of the *ATP7B* gene on chromosome 13q resulting in impaired incorporation of copper into ceruloplasmin and excretion of excess copper into bile is impaired. There is excessive absorption of copper from the small intestine and decreased excretion of copper by the liver. This results in excessive deposition of copper in the liver, brain, and other tissues. The classic neurologic presentation of the disease is parkinsonian symptoms including tremor of the limb or head and generalized slowness of movement in the third or fourth decade of life. A characteristic clinical feature of Wilson disease is the tendency for the motor disorders to be concentrated in the bulbar musculature and to spread caudally, which is different from PD. Early in the course of the disease, when all of the symptoms are not florid, the most reliable diagnostic finding is >200 μg copper/g of dry liver tissue determined by liver biopsy. Later in the disease course corneal "Kayser–Fleischer rings" becomes increasingly evident. Low ceruloplasmin level along with "Kayser–Fleischer rings" and neurologic signs are highly suggestive of the diagnosis.

MRI findings include bilateral symmetric areas of T2 hyperintensity in the putamen (most commonly involved), head of the caudate nucleus, and ventrolateral nucleus of thalamus [25]. The pons is the second most common site of involvement and also shows increased T2 signal that may be ventral, dorsal, or throughout the entire pons [25]. Diffusion restriction is often present in the above mentioned areas in the earlier stages of the disease [25]. In some cases, globus pallidus may be spared.

10.4.4 Neurodegenerative Diseases with Predominant Gait Disturbances

10.4.4.1 Autosomal Dominant Cerebellar Ataxias

Autosomal dominant cerebellar ataxias (ADCAs) are a heterogeneous group of disorders with prominent, progressive cerebellar involvement. These are associated with trinucleotide repeat expansion and are inherited in an autosomal dominant manner with variable penetrance. These are commonly named as spinocerebellar ataxias (SCAs), further classified with an attached number corresponding to order to which each genetic mutation has been identified. About 60% of ADCAs are familial and less than one-quarter of cases are of sporadic onset. The length of the trinucleotide repeats expansion determines the age of onset of the disease in an inverse manner.

All subtypes of SCAs present with progressive cerebellar ataxia. Even though the cerebellum and spinal cord are primarily involved in these syndromes, the cortex and basal ganglia are also involved. Oculomotor abnormalities (SCA 1, 2, 3), retinopathy (SCA 7), seizures (SCA 10), and cognitive and behavioral symptoms (SCA 17) have also been described in different subtypes.

Cerebellar vermian atrophy is the imaging hallmark of ADCA and is often the only notable change in cerebellum. Pontine atrophy predominates in SCA 1, SCA 2, and SCA 7. Predominant cerebellar atrophy without involvement of brain stem is prominent feature of SCA 5 and SCA 11.

10.4.4.2 Fredriech's Ataxia

Fredriech's ataxia (FA) is the prototype of all forms of progressive SCA and accounts for about half of all cases of hereditary ataxias. FA is caused by GAA trinucleotide repeat expansion of the *FXN* gene, most commonly in the first intron, on chromosome 9. It is inherited in an autosomal recessive manner. The *FXN* gene encodes frataxin, a protein essential for proper mitochondrial functioning.

Ataxia is almost always the initial symptom. Earliest presentation includes difficulties in standing steadily and running. Upper extremity symptoms and speech difficulty occur later in the disease. Cardiomyopathy is found in more than half of the patients, and many patients die as a result of cardiac arrhythmia and congestive heart failure. Diabetes mellitus also occurs more frequently in these patients compared to the general population, with 10% of the patients developing diabetes mellitus. Impaired glucose tolerance is seen in another 10% of FA patients. Vision impairment, hearing loss, scoliosis, and high-arched foot are other manifestations of the disease. On neurological examination, there are cerebellar signs (nystagmus, truncal ataxia, dysarthria, dysmetria), pyramidal signs (absent deep tendon reflexes, extensor plantar response, distal weakness), and dorsal column signs (loss of vibration and proprioceptive sensation).

On CT and MRI, there is predominant atrophy of the cerebellum as well as cervical spinal cord.

10.4.4.3 Normal Pressure Hydrocephalus

Normal pressure hydrocephalus (NPH) is a clinical syndrome characterized by subcortical dementia, urinary incontinence, and "magnetic" or apraxic gait. NPH is frequently misdiagnosed as parkinsonian dementia syndrome in early stage of the disease. NPH is primarily a clinical diagnosis. Initial presentation with gait abnormality and dementia of <2 years are associated with a better surgical outcome. CT or MRI typically shows ventriculomegaly as defined by modified Evan's index (maximum width of the frontal horn divided by transverse intracranial width from one inner table to the other at the same level) of >0.31. Ventriculomegaly is out of proportion to the degree of sulcal prominence. Other imaging signs that have been described in NPH include prominent flow void at the aqueduct and third ventricle on T2 and FLAIR MRI, thinning of the corpus callosum on sagittal images, and rounding of the frontal horns.

10.4.5 Neurodegenerative Diseases with Only Motor Symptoms

10.4.5.1 Motor System Diseases

Motor system diseases are a group of neurodegenerative disorders involving motor neurons of the motor cortex, brain stem, and spinal cord, which manifest clinically by muscular weakness, muscle atrophy, and corticospinal signs (spasticity, hyperreflexia, fasciculation, etc.) in varying combinations. The key concept in this group of diseases is absence of any sensory symptoms. Several diseases have been classified under this group.

10.4.5.1.1 Amyotrophic Lateral Sclerosis

ALS is the most common of the motor system diseases. Patients usually present in the fifth decade of age and

men are twice as commonly affected as women. This disease can be familial in up to 10% of the cases and is inherited in an autosomal dominant manner. SOD1 mutation accounts for 10% of the disease. The earliest presentation is weakness in the distal part of the limb and cramping (fasciculation). Initial symptoms may affect only one limb. With time, other limbs are similarly involved. With the progression of the disease, the classic clinical picture of ALS gradually sets in, which includes atrophic weakness and spasticity of the limbs, fasciculation, and hyperreflexia without any sensory symptoms. There is a recently described association between ALS and FTD and is estimated to involve as many as 10%–15% of patients with FTD.

The neuropathology of ALS is characterized by the loss of both upper and lower motor neurons with astrocytic gliosis. There are ubiquitin-containing intraneuronal inclusion bodies. The extent of corticospinal tract involvement varies between patients. Pathological changes may be observed from the subcortical white matter in the motor cortex to all the way down to the spinal cord.

On MRI, some but not all, patients show increased signal on T2-weighted/FLAIR sequences as well as diffusion restriction along the corticospinal tracts extending from the subcortical white matter through the internal capsule down to the medulla and in the spinal cord (Figures 10.16 and 10.17).

There may be associated atrophy and T2 hypointensity in the motor cortex secondary to iron deposition. These features are not evident on CT. The anterior and lateral portion of the spinal cord may be atrophic

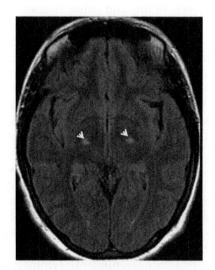

FIGURE 10.16
Amyotrophic lateral sclerosis. Bilateral symmetric hyperintensity on axial fluid-attenuated inversion recovery sequence in the motor tracts (arrowhead) at the level of posterior limb of internal capsule.

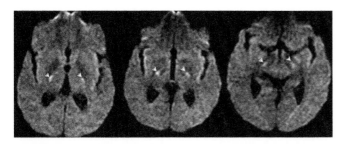

FIGURE 10.17
Amyotrophic lateral sclerosis. Bilateral focal hyperintensities (arrowheads) on axial diffusion-weighted images along the motor tracts at three different levels, which were associated with low apparent diffusion coefficient value (not shown).

because of the degeneration of motor neurons of the anterior horn as well as descending corticospinal tracts. Diffusion tensor imaging can be particularly helpful to identify the disease in the earlier stage, demonstrating loss of fractional anisotropy in the degenerating white matter tracts.

10.4.5.1.2 Progressive Muscular Atrophy

This disease is characterized by weakness and atrophy without associated corticospinal tract symptoms. Like ALS it affects men more frequently than women. The disease is slowly progressive and has a more benign course than ALS. Like ALS, initial presentation is weakness of the distal group of muscles. Proximal muscle weakness is usually late manifestation. The disease can manifest as progressive spinal muscular atrophy when degeneration predominates in the lower motor neurons of the spinal cord without involving upper motor neurons. Predominant weakness and atrophy of the muscles supplied by the brain stem nuclei is known as progressive bulbar palsy.

10.4.5.1.3 Primary Lateral Sclerosis

Primary lateral sclerosis (PLS) is another variant of motor system disease characterized by isolated degeneration of upper motor neurons only (corticospinal and corticobulbar neurons) with sparing of lower motor neurons. PLS has imaging manifestations similar to ALS.

10.4.5.2 Heredofamilial Forms of Progressive Muscular Atrophy

This is a diverse group of neurodegenerative disorders prevalent in children, often of inherited type. Several types have been described. Infantile spinomuscular atrophy (SMA type I, Wardnig–Hoffman disease) is the most common type. It has the earliest onset and most rapidly fatal course. Though alert and conscious, afflicted newborns are weak, hypotonic,

and lack stretch reflexes. Death ensues in the first year. Other types are chronic childhood SMA (SMA II), juvenile SMA (SMA III, Kugelberg–Welander disease), X-linked bulbospinal muscular atrophy (Kennedy syndrome), and progressive bulbar palsy of childhood or Fazio–Londe syndrome.

References

1. Przedborski, S, Vila, M, Jackson-Lewis, V. Neurodegeneration: What is it and where are we? *J Clin Invest* 2003; 111: 3–10.
2. Blennow, K, de Leon, MJ, Zetterberg, H. Alzheimer's disease. *Lancet* 2006; 368: 387–403.
3. Dubois, B, Feldman, HH, Jacova, C et al. Revising the definition of Alzheimer's disease: A new lexicon. *Lancet Neurol* 2010; 9: 1118–1127.
4. Urs, R, Potter, E, Barker, W et al. Visual rating system for assessing magnetic resonance images: a tool in the diagnosis of mild cognitive impairment and Alzheimer disease. *J Comput Assist Tomogr* 2009; 33: 73–78.
5. Duara, R, Loewenstein, DA, Potter, E et al. Medial temporal lobe atrophy on MRI scans and the diagnosis of Alzheimer disease. *Neurology* 2008; 71: 1986–1992.
6. Giesel, FL, Hahn, HK, Thomann, PA et al. Temporal horn index and volume of medial temporal lobe atrophy using a new semiautomated method for rapid and precise assessment. *AJNR Am J Neuroradiol* 2006; 27: 1454–1458.
7. Killiany, RJ, Hyman, BT, Gomez-Isla, T et al. MRI measures of entorhinal cortex vs hippocampus in preclinical AD. *Neurology* 2002; 58: 1188–1196.
8. Smith, SD, Eskey, CJ. Hemorrhagic stroke. *Radiol Clin North Am* 2011; 49: 27–45.
9. Chabriat, H, Joutel, A, Dichgans, M, Tournier-Lasserve, E, Bousser, MG. Cadasil. *Lancet Neurol* 2009; 8: 643–653.
10. Herve, D, Chabriat, H. Cadasil. *J Geriatr Psychiatry Neurol* 2010; 23: 269–276.
11. Chan, D, Fox, NC, Scahill, RI et al. Patterns of temporal lobe atrophy in semantic dementia and Alzheimer's disease. *Ann Neurol* 2001; 49: 433–442.
12. Chahine, LM, Stern, MB. Diagnostic markers for Parkinson's disease. *Curr Opin Neurol* 2011; 24: 309–317.
13. Gorell, JM, Ordidge, RJ, Brown, GG, Deniau, JC, Buderer, NM, Helpern, JA. Increased iron-related MRI contrast in the substantia nigra in Parkinson's disease. *Neurology* 1995; 45: 1138–1143.
14. Kagi, G, Bhatia, KP, Tolosa, E. The role of DAT-SPECT in movement disorders. *J Neurol Neurosurg Psychiatry* 2010; 81: 5–12.
15. Quattrone, A, Nicoletti, G, Messina, D et al. MR imaging index for differentiation of progressive supranuclear palsy from Parkinson disease and the Parkinson variant of multiple system atrophy. *Radiology* 2008; 246: 214–221.

16. Gilman, S, Wenning, GK, Low, PA et al. Second consensus statement on the diagnosis of multiple system atrophy. *Neurology* 2008; 71: 670–676.

17. Horimoto, Y, Aiba, I, Yasuda, T et al. Longitudinal MRI study of multiple system atrophy—When do the findings appear, and what is the course? *J Neurol* 2002; 249: 847–854.

18. Lee, EA, Cho, HI, Kim, SS, Lee, WY. Comparison of magnetic resonance imaging in subtypes of multiple system atrophy. *Parkinsonism Relat Disord* 2004; 10: 363–368.

19. Hotter, A, Esterhammer, R, Schocke, MF, Seppi, K. Potential of advanced MR imaging techniques in the differential diagnosis of parkinsonism. *Mov Disord* 2009; 24 (Suppl 2): S711–S720.

20. Scarmeas, N, Chin, SS, Marder, K. Cortical basal ganglionic degeneration. *Sci Aging Knowledge Environ* 2001; 2001: dn1.

21. Rebeiz, JJ, Kolodny, EH, Richardson, EP, Jr. Corticodentatonigral degeneration with neuronal achromasia. *Arch Neurol* 1968; 18: 20–33.

22. Schneider, SA, Hardy, J, Bhatia, KP. Syndromes of neurodegeneration with brain iron accumulation (NBIA): An update on clinical presentations, histological and genetic underpinnings, and treatment considerations. *Mov Disord* 2012; 27: 42–53.

23. Gregory, A, Polster, BJ, Hayflick, SJ. Clinical and genetic delineation of neurodegeneration with brain iron accumulation. *J Med Genet* 2009; 46: 73–80.

24. Cossu, G, Cella, C, Melis, M et al. [123I]FP-CIT SPECT findings in two patients with Hallervorden-Spatz disease with homozygous mutation in PANK2 gene. *Neurology* 2005; 64, 167–168.

25. King, AD, Walshe, JM, Kendall, BE et al. Cranial MR imaging in Wilson's disease. *AJR Am J Roentgenol* 1996; 167: 1579–1584.

26. Hegde, AN, Mohan, S, Lath, N, Lim, CC. Differential diagnosis for bilateral abnormalities of the basal ganglia and thalamus. *Radiographics* 2011; 31: 5–30.

11

Central Nervous System Infection

Asim K. Bag, Shehanaz Ellika, and Surjith Vattoth

CONTENTS

11.1 Introduction

Despite the revolutionizing advances in antibiotic therapy, infectious diseases continue to be one of the most prevalent diseases worldwide, particularly in tropical countries. Central nervous system (CNS) infections are unique because they can rapidly become fatal if they are not diagnosed and treated early.

Although clinical presentation and cerebrospinal fluid (CSF) cytology suggest infection of the CNS, neuroimaging plays a crucial role in confirming as well as localizing an infection early in the course of diseases. Due to its ready availability, computed tomography (CT) still has a role in the evaluation of patients with clinical concerns of CNS infection, particularly in emergency settings. However, magnetic resonance imaging (MRI) undoubtedly is the investigation of choice in the evaluation of CNS infection. Most of the time, it is possible to confidently diagnose CNS infection based on MRI.

Although CNS is protected by meninges and the blood–brain barrier (BBB), it is more vulnerable to infectious agents than any other tissue due to the lack of a true lymphatic system, little resistance to infection offered by the subarachnoid space, and the fact that CSF facilitates the spread of infection over the brain and spinal cord and into the ventricles [1]. Numerous organisms can cause CNS infection: viruses, bacteria, fungi, and even parasites. Different etiologic organisms have different epidemiologies and clinical and imaging manifestations. This chapter is organized according to the causes of infection.

11.2 Pediatric Infection

The manifestations of CNS infection on imaging studies are similar in children and adults; however, the epidemiologies and the causative organisms are different. Congenital infection has unique imaging manifestations and complications.

11.2.1 Congenital Intracranial Infections

Congenital intracranial infections can be transmitted during intrauterine life transplacentally or during passage through an infected birth. The main infections are often designated by the acronym "TORCH," where T stands for toxoplasmosis, O for others (such as syphilis and human immunodeficiency virus [HIV]), R for rubella, C for cytomegalovirus (CMV), and H for herpes simplex virus (HSV).

Fetuses and neonates mount different biological responses to infection compared with older children or adults with less intense host defense responses [2]. Fetal/neonatal infection is characterized by less marked or even absent inflammatory reaction. As a general rule, infections occurring in the first two weeks of intrauterine life lead to spontaneous abortion. Insults occurring during 16–20 weeks of gestation, while the CNS is actively developing, will result in congenital brain malformations involving abnormalities of neuronal proliferation and migration. Infections occurring in the third trimester manifest as destructive lesions [2].

11.2.1.1 Cytomegalovirus Infection

Congenital CMV infection is one of the most common congenital viral infections in the world and is the most common intrauterine infection in the United States. Fetal infection occurs transplacentally and is common in women who experience primary infection during pregnancy. Approximately 7%–10% of neonates with CMV infection exhibit symptoms of cytomegalic inclusion disease such as microcephaly, hepatosplenomegaly, thrombocytopenic purpura, hearing loss, and intracranial calcifications. Fetuses that are infected at a younger gestational age generally have a poorer outcome than those infected at a later stage of development, and infections that occur postnatally are less severe.

Diagnosis of congenital CMV infection is established by detecting CMV in the urine or saliva during the first 3 weeks of life by using cell culture or polymerase chain reaction or by detecting CMV-specific immunoglobulin (Ig) M (IgM) in the serum of neonates [2].

Imaging findings of congenital CMV infection include intracranial calcification (Figure 11.1), ventriculomegaly, white matter myelination abnormalities (Figure 11.2), and neuronal migrational disorders (Figure 11.3).

The severity of degree of brain destruction depends on the gestational age at which CMV infects the brain. Fetuses infected during the first half of the second trimester have agyria or lissencephaly with thin cortex, cerebellar hypoplasia, delayed myelination, marked ventriculomegaly, germinal zone cysts, and significant periventricular calcification (Figure 11.3).

Those fetuses infected later in the second trimester have polymicrogyria, impaired myelination, less ventricular dilatation, and less prominent cerebellar hypoplasia. Fetuses infected in the third trimester have normal gyral patterns, mild ventricular dilation, and mild damage to periventricular or subcortical white matter with scattered periventricular calcification or hemorrhage.

Intracranial calcification is the most commonly reported imaging finding of congenital CMV infection, occurring in 34%–70% of patients. CT is very

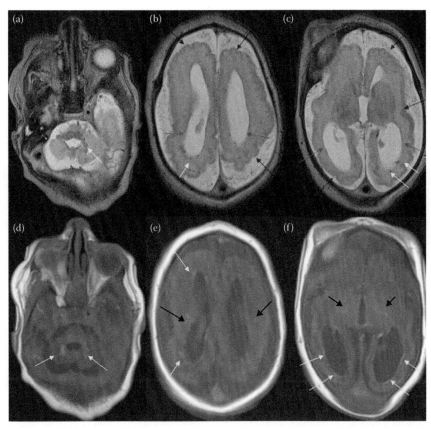

FIGURE 11.1
Congenital cytomegalovirus (CMV) infection in a 3-day-old presumed to be due to early second trimester infection: axial T2 (a–c) and T1-weighted (d–f) images demonstrate enlarged lateral ventricles (red arrows), extensive periventricular calcifications (yellow arrows), and scattered parenchymal calcifications (blue arrows). Calcifications appear hypointense on T2-weighted sequences and hyperintense on T1-weighted images. The T2-weighted sequences also better demonstrate the polymicrogyria involving almost the entire cerebral cortex (purple arrows). The cerebellum is hypoplastic and shows evidence of dysplasia.

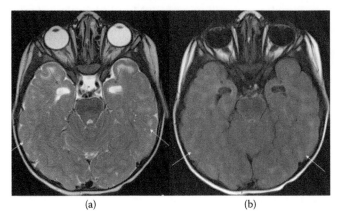

　　　　　(a)　　　　　　　　　　　　　(b)

FIGURE 11.2
Congenital CMV infection and white matter disease: axial T2-weighted (a) and fluid attenuation inversion recovery (FLAIR) (b) images demonstrate anterior temporal lobe cysts (red arrows) and patchy areas of T2 prolongation in subcortical white matter (yellow arrows).

sensitive for depicting and localizing intracranial calcification, although calcification can also be identified on MRI and ultrasound. Calcification occurs in periventricular regions (most common location), basal ganglia, and brain parenchyma. Calcifications in basal ganglia and brain parenchyma in congenital CMV are characteristically faint and punctate unlike calcifications due to other infectious processes, which tend to be more florid [3].

White matter involvement may appear either as a reduction in its volume due to the lack of formation or as areas of T2 prolongation related to impaired myelination and/or destruction. A distinct pattern of white matter abnormality in asymptomatic patients with congenital CMV infection has been described involving the deep white matter, often sparing immediate periventricular and subcortical white matter, with the largest lesions often in the parietal lobes [4]. White matter abnormalities of the anterior temporal lobe can show cystic changes with the enlargement of anterior temporal horn (Figure 11.2). Lissencephaly, pachygyria, and diffuse or focal polymicrogyria are the most common (10% of patients with congenital CMV infection) migrational abnormalities, and they are easily identified on MRI (Figures 11.1 and 11.3).

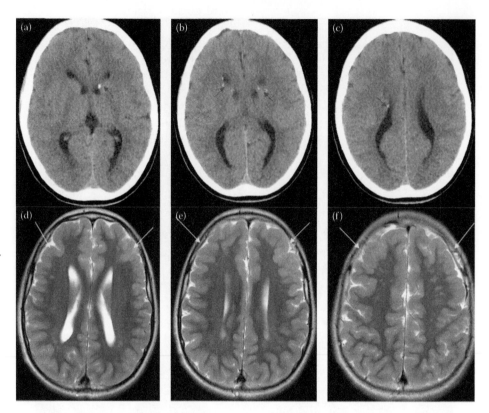

FIGURE 11.3
Congenital CMV infection in an 8-year-old male child: axial computed tomography (CT) images (a–c) show scattered foci of periventricular calcification (red arrows). In patients with congenital CMV infection, calcification may be subtle, unilateral, and less chunky than that associated with other entities. Axial T2-weighted images (d–f) show polymicrogyria involving the frontal lobes of the cerebral hemispheres (yellow arrows).

Although sensorineural hearing loss is common in children with congenital CMV infection and is seen in 10%–15% of infected infants who were symptomatic at birth, no abnormality of inner ear structures has been detected on currently available imaging modalities, indicating that abnormalities responsible for sensorineural hearing loss in congenital CMV infection are beyond the resolution of currently available imaging modalities.

11.2.1.2 Congenital Toxoplasmosis

Congenital toxoplasmosis is acquired in utero by transplacental passage of *Toxoplasma gondii*, and its likelihood and severity are closely related to the time of maternal infection.

Toxoplasmosis is the second most common TORCH infection, after CMV. Its clinical manifestations resemble those of congenital CMV infection and consist of purpuric rash, thrombocytopenia, elevated serum transaminases, and hyperbilirubinemia. However, in contrast to CMV, macrocephaly (a sign of intrauterine hydrocephalus), and chorioretinitis (a potential cause of blindness) are much more common in infants with congenital toxoplasmosis. Diagnosis is made by detecting *Toxoplasma gondii*–specific IgM or IgA in the infants' serum. The spectrum of severity of brain involvement in congenital toxoplasmosis ranges from mild (with only a few periventricular calcifications and mild atrophy) to severe (showing marked, diffuse cerebral calcifications and destructive parenchymal lesions) (Figure 11.4).

Calcifications in congenital toxoplasmosis are diffuse and involve the basal ganglia, thalami, periventricular parenchyma, and cerebral cortex. As a general rule, the intracranial calcifications in congenital toxoplasmosis tend to be more peripheral than the calcifications of CMV infection, which are more typically periventricular. If infection occurs before 20 weeks of gestation, severe ventricular dilatation, areas of porencephaly, and extensive calcifications (particularly in the basal ganglia) are noted. If infection occurs between 20 and 30 weeks of gestation, less severe ventricular dilatation and intracranial calcifications are demonstrated. After the 30th week of gestation, minimal periventricular and intracerebral calcifications with rare ventricular dilatation is noted.

Ventricular dilatation in congenital toxoplasmosis is typically a disproportionate dilatation of the posterior portions of lateral ventricles with respect to the frontal

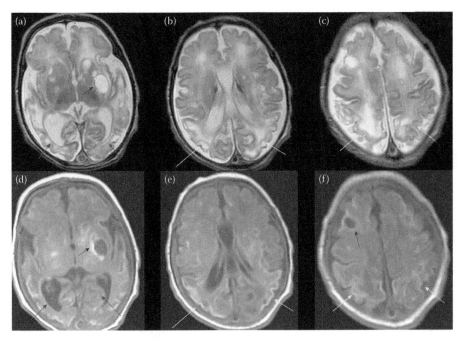

FIGURE 11.4
Congenital toxoplasmosis in a 17-day-old neonate: axial T2 (a–c) and axial precontrast T1-weighted (d–f) images demonstrate ventricular enlargement mainly in the posterior portions (red arrows) with multiple cystic foci showing peripheral calcification (blue arrows). Multiple areas of cortical calcifications are also noted (yellow arrows).

horns, secondary to prevalent white matter destruction in these regions (Figure 11.4).

11.2.1.3 Congenital/Neonatal Herpes Simplex Encephalitis

Unlike most other congenital TORCH infections, neonatal herpes simplex infection is usually acquired during passage of the fetus through an infected birth canal; ascending and transplacental infections are much less common. It is estimated that approximately 85% of neonatal herpes infections are acquired peripartum, 10% are acquired postnatally, and 5% are acquired in utero as part of the TORCH complex of congenital infections.

The vast majority of congenital herpes virus infections (about 75%–90%) are caused by herpes simplex type 2 (HSV2) unlike postnatal herpes infection, which is caused by herpes simplex type 1 (HSV1). Neonatal herpes infections can be mucocutaneous (skin, eye, mouth without CNS involvement), disseminated (with or without CNS involvement), or encephalitic. As many as one-third of neonates with herpes infection can have disease limited only to the CNS. However, some degree of CNS involvement develops in two-thirds of patients infected with herpes. Disseminated disease is characterized by neurological symptoms, such as lethargy, stupor, irritability, and seizures (often focal), progressing to coma. In addition, hepatomegaly, hyperbilirubinemia, and bleeding may occur. The outcome is poor. Any infant with a

CSF study suggestive of encephalitis (i.e., pleocytosis and elevated protein) should be considered to have herpes simplex encephalitis until proven otherwise. Although the virus can be isolated from CSF through HSV-PCR (PCR refers to polymerase chain reaction) studies, PCR is negative in 25% of infants. Therefore, a negative result should be interpreted with caution. If there is a clinical suspicion for HSV meningoencephalitis, acyclovir should be administered empirically until the results of the second PCR are known [2].

CT usually is positive in the more advanced stages of the disease. The most common CT findings are widespread areas of hypodensity predominantly in the white matter as a result of edema or necrosis in the involved areas of the brain. Neonatal HSV encephalitis typically is a more diffuse process than the adult form caused by HSV1. A gyriform pattern of enhancement and prolonged cortical retention of contrast on CT scans has also been reported. CT findings early in the disease have been shown to be poor predictors of clinical outcome.

MRI is the study of choice in neonates with suspected herpes encephalitis. In the early stages of infection, diffusion-weighted imaging (DWI) plays an important role in depicting early cellular host response, which appears as high signal intensity on DWI and a low value on an apparent diffusion coefficient (ADC) map, even when conventional MRI sequences are normal. After 1–2 days, CT and MRI show patchy, multifocal areas of abnormality (hypodense on CT, hypointensity on T1-weighted

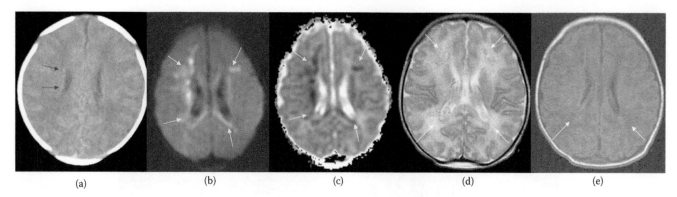

(a)   (b)   (c)   (d)   (e)

FIGURE 11.5
Congenital herpes infection: a 12-day-old neonate with herpes simplex encephalitis is shown in the figure. Axial CT image (a) demonstrates small punctate foci of hyperdensity in the periventricular location (red arrows). Axial diffusion-weighted images (b) and axial apparent diffusion coefficient (ADC) maps (c) demonstrate foci of restricted diffusion in periventricular white matter with the involvement of corpus callosum (yellow arrows). Axial T2 (d) and T1-weighted (e) sequences demonstrate the foci of T1 and T2 shortening in periventricular white matter consistent with hemorrhage (white arrows). The images also demonstrate the multifocality of brain parenchymal involvement in neonatal herpes encephalitis.

images, and hyperintensity on T2-weighted images) affecting gray and white matter, which progress over the next several days. Hemorrhage is a common finding and is seen in two-thirds of the patients with neonatal herpes encephalitis (Figure 11.5).

Contrast enhancement occurs early in a meningeal pattern. Finally, severe, diffuse cerebral atrophy with cortical thinning; multicystic encephalomalacia; and large, diffuse dystrophic calcifications develop in the periventricular regions and the cerebral cortex.

11.2.1.4 Congenital Rubella

Congenital rubella is caused by transplacental passage of HSV and has largely disappeared from the United States and other developed countries after the widespread use of vaccination. The earlier in pregnancy the maternal infection occurs, the greater the frequency and severity of the congenital infection. Compared to congenital toxoplasmosis or CMV infections, infants with congenital rubella have less frequent hepatosplenomegaly and jaundice but high incidence of cataracts and congenital heart disease (typically patent ductus arteriosus).

The imaging appearance of CNS infection depends on the time of the intrauterine infection. Early infection results in congenital anomalies, whereas late infection produces nonspecific generalized edema, gliosis, or loss of brain tissue. CT shows ventriculomegaly, multifocal regions of hypodensity in cerebral white matter along with periventricular, basal ganglia and cortical calcifications and cysts. In the most severe cases, brain destruction and microcephaly are observed. Cortical calcifications occur because the virus tends to preferentially destroy the deep cortical layers.

MRI findings include delayed myelination, multifocal areas of T2 hyperintensity resulting from insufficient

production of oligodendroglia, foci of parenchymal necrosis ventriculitis, and ventriculomegaly.

11.2.1.5 Congenital Human Immunodeficiency Virus

The transmission of HIV from infected pregnant women to their fetuses may occur transplacentally (especially during the second or third trimester), during passage through an infected birth canal, or by ingestion of maternal blood. Fetal infection accounts for 25% of cases and parturitional infection for the remaining 75% [5]. Postnatal infection due to the transmission of HIV by breast-feeding is estimated to be about 15%–30% of mothers with HIV infection [6]. Greater than 90% of pediatric AIDS is secondary to congenital infection via maternal–fetal transmission [7]. Infants with vertical transmission of HIV infection can become symptomatic after the third month of life, manifesting with hepatomegaly, lymphadenopathy, failure to thrive, interstitial pneumonitis, opportunistic infections, or neurologic disease. With HIV-associated neurologic disease, either a progressive or a static encephalopathy may occur. Acute neurological deterioration may be secondary to stroke, bacterial infections, opportunistic infections (with *Toxoplasma gondii*, CMV, varicella zoster virus [VZV], *Mycobacterium tuberculosis*, fungi, and JC virus), or neoplasm.

HIV infection in infants can be confirmed with serial serum PCR assays. The most common intracranial findings on imaging studies are atrophy and calcification of basal ganglia and subcortical white matter. Calcification is seen only in patients who were infected in utero, and children with the highest viral loads have the most marked calcifications on CT. Cerebral atrophy is usually progressive on serial MRI examinations and correlates well with histopathological changes.

Both intracranial neoplasms and opportunistic infections are rare in congenital HIV-infected infants, as opposed to adults [2]. The most common intracranial neoplasm is lymphoma, typically involving the basal ganglia and thalami, whereas CMV and progressive multifocal leukoencephalopathy (PML) are the most common forms of infectious diseases [2]. Intracranial hemorrhage and infarction are uncommon complications of pediatric AIDS, occurring in about 1.3% of children and occurring secondary to severe immune thrombocytopenia and aneurysmal arteriopathy. Aneurysmal arteriopathy primarily involves large vessels and seems to be a common cause of infarction in these patients (Figure 11.6) [8].

11.2.1.6 Differential Diagnosis of Congenital TORCH Infections

Many different disorders can mimic congenital TORCH infections, especially genetic diseases [1,2]. The MRI appearance of polymicrogyria seen with congenital CMV infection must be differentiated from classic lissencephaly and cobblestone complex [2]. CMV infection late in the gestational age is characterized by patchy (in less severe cases) to confluent (in severe cases) abnormal myelination, which may resemble metabolic leukodystrophies. Aicardi–Goutieres syndrome (pseudo-TORCH syndrome), a genetic disorder, can produce intracranial calcifications and leucoencephalopathy and be confused for congenital TORCH infections; however, CSF analysis will show increased lymphocyte counts in patients with Aicardi–Goutieres syndrome. Tuberous sclerosis complex (TSC) produces periventricular calcifications, which could be mistaken for congenital CMV infections; however, TSC is also associated with cortical tubers and pathognomonic skin manifestations.

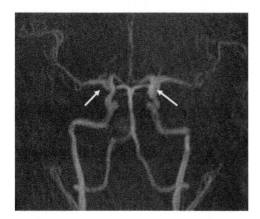

FIGURE 11.6
Human immunodeficiency virus (HIV) vasculopathy: MR angiopathy demonstrates fusiform dilatation of supraclinoid internal carotid arteries (white arrows) consistent with HIV vasculopathy.

11.2.2 Meningitis

The term "meningitis" indicates an inflammatory process involving the dura mater, leptomeninges, and CSF within the subarachnoid spaces. The term "meningoencephalitis" is used when the underlying brain parenchyma is also involved. Bacterial meningitis is the most common infectious process in the pediatric age group; etiologic agents vary with the age of patients, as do clinical presentations. In uncomplicated meningitis, the exudative inflammatory response and microorganisms are confined to the CSF and pia-arachnoid. Mechanisms of infection include direct implantation (penetrating injury), propagation of infection from a parameningeal site (sinusitis, mastoiditis), hematogenous dissemination (seeding of the choroid plexus or leptomeninges), and spread along the peripheral nervous system. In neonates, various gram-positive and gram-negative organisms including *Streptococcus agalactiae*, *Escherichia coli*, *Staphylococcus* sp., *Listeria monocytogenes*, and *Pseudomonas* sp. cause bacterial meningitis [9]. *Streptococcus pneumoniae* and *Neisseria meningitidis* account for the majority of cases of CNS infection in immunized infants, children, and adolescents. In unimmunized children, *Haemophilus influenzae* type B (Hib) occurs more commonly in patients with sickle cell anemia, asplenia, and HIV infections. Non–b subtypes of *Haemophilus influenzae* have emerged as clinically important agents causing meningitis among healthy or immunocompromised children in regions with compulsory immunization against *Haemophilus influenzae* [10]. Common organisms are *Streptococcus pneumoniae* and *Neisseria menigitidis* in adults and *Listeria monocytogenes*, *Streptococcus pneumoniae*, *Neisseria meningitidis*, and gram-negative bacilli in the elderly (see Table 11.1).

Typically, the diagnosis of pyogenic meningitis is made clinically. Neuroimaging is indicated if the clinical diagnosis is unclear, there is failure in responding

TABLE 11.1

Meningitis: Etiology

A. Acute pyogenic

Neonates: Group B streptococcus, *Escherichia coli*, *Enterobacter*, *Citrobacter*
Infants: *Streptococcus pneumoniae*, *Neisseria meningitidis*
Children: *N. meningitidis*
Adults: *S. pneumoniae*, *N. meningitidis*, GBS
Elderly: *Listeria monocytogenes*, *S. pneumoniae*, *N. meningitidis*, gram-negative bacilli

B. Acute lymphocytic

Enteroviruses (echo, coxsackie)

C. Chronic infectious

TB, fungal (cryptococcosis, coccidioidomycosis)

D. Chronic noninfectious

Sarcoidosis, rheumatoid, Wegener granulomatosis, histiocytosis

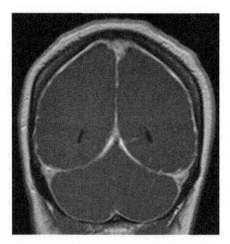

FIGURE 11.7
Pachymeningitis: coronal gadolinium (Gd)-enhanced T1W magnetic resonance imaging (MRI) showing pachymeningeal enhancement in a patient with benign intracranial hypotension. Note that the diffuse thick dural enhancement along the outer aspect of the brain at the convexities and dural reflections including falx and tentorium, and does not extend into the sulci.

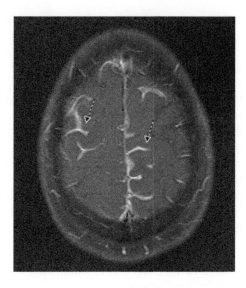

FIGURE 11.8
Leptomeningitis: axial Gd-enhanced T1W MRI showing leptomeningeal enhancement in a patient with meningitis. Note that the thin, delicate pia-arachnoid enhancement extends into the sulci (arrows).

to appropriate therapy, neurologic deterioration occurs, signs and symptoms of raised intracranial pressure develop, or persistent seizures or focal neurological deficits develop.

Although CT and MRI are the principal imaging tools for evaluating meningitis, diagnosis is based on clinical findings and CSF evaluation. The major role of imaging is to detect complications of meningitis. Although MRI is the most sensitive imaging method in detection of brain involvement in cases of infectious disease, CT is often used as the first examination, particularly in emergency situations. CT or even MRI may be normal in uncomplicated cases of meningitis and, thus, a negative CT scan or MRI does not rule out meningitis. Effaced cisterns due to subarachnoid exudates and meningeal enhancement are the primary imaging finding. Mild ventricular enlargement is common. Subtle fluid attenuation inversion recovery (FLAIR) sulcal hyperintensity (secondary to excess white blood cells [WBCs], proteinaceous exudates in the sulci) is nonspecific but suggestive of meningitis. Utilizing 3D FLAIR technique helps to eliminate the high-signal-intensity artifacts within the CSF space [11]. Contrast-enhanced FLAIR, specifically delayed postcontrast FLAIR acquisition, is even more sensitive in detecting leptomeningeal enhancement than conventional postcontrast T1-weighted images [12].

In bacterial meningitis enhancement typically involves cerebral convexities (Figure 11.7), whereas in granulomatous meningitis enhancement of the basal meninges/cisterns is more typical. Meningeal enhancement occurs in two patterns depending on which layers of the meninges are involved, pachymeninges versus leptomeninges.

Pachymeningeal (thick meninges, which is the dura) enhancement occurs along the outer aspect of the brain at the convexities or along dural reflections, does not extend into sulci, is thick, and occasionally has a nodular pattern. The pattern signifies subdural or epidural space involvement and is seen in granulomatous disease, metastasis or extramedullary hematopoesis, and intracranial hypotension in addition to infectious pachymeningitis (Figure 11.7).

Leptomeningeal (skinny meninges, which is the pia and the arachnoid) enhancement extends into sulci and cisterns and shows a thin, delicate pattern (Figure 11.8). The pattern signifies subarachnoid space infection. Leptomeningeal enhancement of a similar type is also seen in cryptococcosis, sarcoidosis, hemorrhage, or meningeal carcinomatosis [13].

11.2.2.1 Complications of Meningitis

11.2.2.1.1 Epidural Abscess, Subdural Effusions, and Empyemas

Sterile subdural effusions, common in children less than 1 year of age, mirror CSF on CT and MRI. They are particularly common in *Haemophilus influenzae* meningitis (Figure 11.9).

With the widespread use of *Haemophilus influenzae* vaccine, effusion is more common with infections caused by group B streptococcus, *Escherichia coli*, *Streptococcus pneumoniae*, *Neisseria meningitides*, and non–type b encapsulated *Haemophilus influenzae*.

Empyemas are serious but uncommon complications of bacterial meningitis and can be subdural (Figure 11.10)

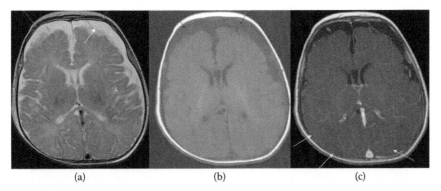

FIGURE 11.9
A 9-month-old child with meningitis and sterile subdural effusions: axial T2-weighted image (a), precontrast T1 (b), and postcontrast T1-weighted (c) images demonstrating frontal subdural fluid collections isointense to cerebral spinal fluid (CSF) (red arrows). A thick hypointense membrane is seen on the T2-weighted images in the left frontal region (white arrows). Postcontrast T1-weighted images demonstrate lepto-meningeal enhancement (yellow arrows).

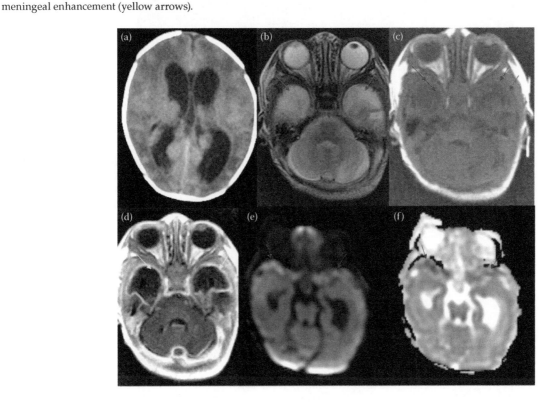

FIGURE 11.10
Subdural empyema complicating meningitis: axial noncontrast CT (a) in a premature 23-day-old male child demonstrating hydrocephalus. Axial T2 (b) and precontrast T1-weighted (c) images show subdural collections anterior to the temporal lobes (red arrows), which demonstrate peripheral enhancement (yellow arrows) on the postcontrast T1-weighed images (d) and restricted diffusion (blue arrows) (e, f) suggesting thick viscous pus in subdural empyemas.

or epidural (Figure 11.11). Unlike subdural effusion, subdural empyema demonstrates restricted diffusion on DWI (Figures 11.9 and 11.10).

11.2.2.1.2 Choroid Plexitis and Ventriculitis

Choroid plexitis and ventriculitis are the initial stages of infection, due to arrival of pathogens to the choroid plexuses and colonization of the ependymal lining and CSF. These two stages are difficult to separate from a neuroimaging perspective.

CT and MRI show a characteristic triad composed of choroid plexus engorgement, ependymal enhancement, and intraventricular debris layered in the dependent portion of ventricles (which demonstrates restricted diffusion on DWI) (Figure 11.12).

Hydrocephalus is commonly associated with choroid plexitis and ventriculitis, usually due to reduced CSF absorption [1]. Periventricular edema, seen on both CT scan and MRI, can be a consequence of unbalanced CSF dynamics but may herald the

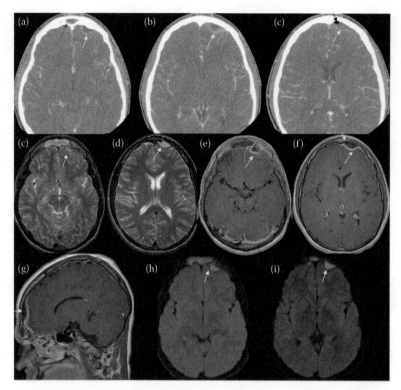

FIGURE 11.11
Epidural empyema secondary to frontal sinusitis: axial postcontrast CT images (a–c) demonstrate the opacification of the frontal sinus (red arrow) with associated left frontal epidural abscess (yellow arrows). A small focus of air is noted in the epidural abscess (black arrows). Axial T2 (c, d) and postcontrast T1-weighted axial (e, f) and sagittal (g) images again demonstrate frontal sinusitis and left frontal epidural abscess. The epidural abscess shows decreased diffusivity in the abscess (yellow arrows) and the frontal sinus (red arrows) on diffusion-weighted images (h, i).

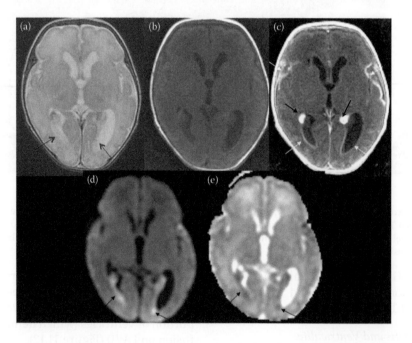

FIGURE 11.12
Ventriculitis/choroid plexitis secondary to *Escherichia coli* meningitis: axial T2-weighted image (a) demonstrates the enlargement of lateral ventricles and dependent debris in the occipital horns of the lateral ventricles (red arrows). Precontrast (b) and postcontrast (c) T1-weighted images demonstrate enhancement of the ependymal lining (yellow arrows) with congestion of the choroid glomi, which are adhered to the walls of the ventricles (blue arrows). Bilateral leptomeningeal enhancement along the sylvian fissures (white arrows) is also noted. Diffusion-weighted image (d) and ADC map (e) demonstrate decreased diffusivity in the occipital horns consistent with viscous, purulent material (black arrows).

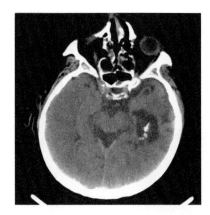

FIGURE 11.13
Trapped ventricle: axial nonenhanced CT scan (NECT) shows trapped temporal horn of the left lateral ventricle due to remote meningitis/ventriculitis sequelae. Note the subependymal calcifications hanging down from its roof into the lumen due to healed infection.

necrosis of periventricular white matter, related either to the obstruction of subependymal and periventricular veins or to endotoxins, lipopolysaccharides from gram-negative bacteria, teichoic acid from gram-positive organisms, and cytokine-induced inflammation produced by the bacteria. The exudates and inflammatory scarring due to ependymitis may block the ventricular outflow or CSF reabsorption in arachnoid granulations and produce hydrocephalus. Sometimes, one ventricle or a horn of a ventricle can be focally dilated due to scarring at its connection with the rest of the ventricular system (trapped ventricle) (Figure 11.13).

11.2.2.1.3 Hydrocephalus

Communicating hydrocephalus is the most common complication of meningitis. It is usually related to impaired CSF flow and resorption caused by the presence of an inflammatory exudate at the level of subarachnoid spaces and arachnoid villi [1]. Obstructive hydrocephalus may occur due to exudative obstruction of the aqueduct or fourth ventricular outlet foramina.

11.2.2.1.4 Venous Thrombosis

Venous thrombosis is an uncommon complication of meningitis and occurs especially in cases of superimposed dehydration. In the acute phase when the clot is dense, it may be detected on CT as high density in the sinuses on noncontrast images (Figure 11.14). Contrast scans demonstrate the "empty delta" sign with the less dense thrombus surrounded by the enhancing dural coverings (Figure 11.15).

On MRI, the appearance of sinus thrombus strongly depends on the age of the clot. Acute thrombus demonstrates the absence of the normal flow void, which is better seen as an isointensity on T1-weighted images. The classical T1 hyperintensity (subacute thrombus) is seen after a few days.

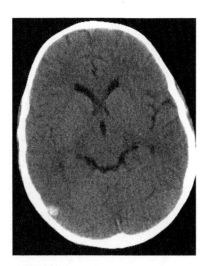

FIGURE 11.14
Venous sinus thrombosis: axial noncontrast CT image demonstrating high density in the right transverse sinus.

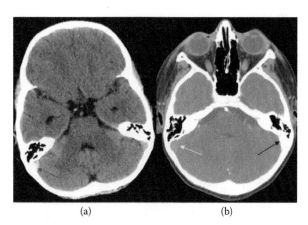

(a)   (b)

FIGURE 11.15
Empty delta sign: axial noncontrast CT image (a) demonstrates hyperdense right sigmoid sinus (red arrow). CT venogram axial source image (b) shows a filling defect in the right sigmoid sinus (yellow arrow) compared with normal left sigmoid sinus (black arrow).

Venous thrombosis may be complicated by venous infarctions, which tend to involve the cerebral cortex and subjacent white matter as well as the central white matter and basal ganglia. On CT, venous infarcts are usually poorly marginated, with hypoattenuation or mixed attenuation areas involving the cortex and adjacent subcortical white matter. Low attenuation is probably due to localized edema, whereas high attenuation is due to hemorrhage (Figure 11.16).

Around 25% of venous infarcts are hemorrhagic and range from petechial hemorrhages within edematous brain parenchyma to large subcortical hematomas.

Different MR venography techniques are very useful in the diagnosis of venous sinus thrombosis. CT venography is comparable to MR venography but is less desirable in the pediatric population due to ionizing radiation (Figure 11.17).

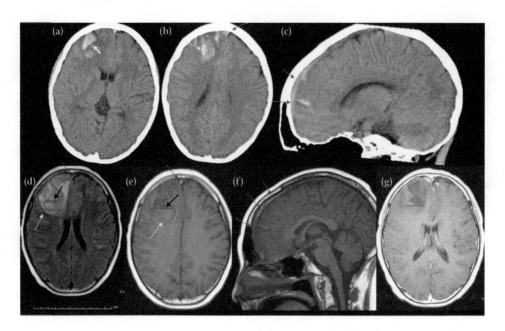

FIGURE 11.16

Thrombosis of anterior superior sagittal sinus with an associated hemorrhagic venous infarct: axial noncontrast CT images (a, b) demonstrate hyperdensity in the anterior part of the superior sagittal sinus (red arrows) with associated hemorrhagic venous infarct in the right frontal lobe (yellow arrows). Sagittal CT reconstruction (c) again demonstrates hyperdensity in the anterior one-third of sagittal sinus (red arrows). Axial FLAIR (d), precontrast axial T1 (e), and sagittal T1-weighted (f) images showing hyperintensity in the anterior part of the SSS (red arrows) with hemorrhagic infarct in the right frontal lobe with associated fluid levels (blue arrows). Postcontrast axial T1-weighted image (g) demonstrating a filling defect in the anterior part of the superior sagittal sinus (yellow arrows).

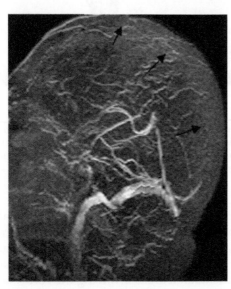

FIGURE 11.17

Superior sagittal sinus thrombosis: a sagittal reconstructed image of magnetic resonance venogram shows superior sagittal sinus thrombosis (arrows). Arterial and venous thromboses are potential complications of meningitis.

11.2.2.1.5 Arterial Infarcts

Arterial infarcts are due to arteritis, which is secondary to involvement of perivascular spaces and subsequent involvement of the arterial wall. Arteritis may result in arterial infarcts involving either large or small vessels.

CT or MRI shows either large cortical infarction, due to major vessel involvement, or multiple lacunar-type infarcts in the distribution of perforating vessels in the brain stem, basal ganglia, and white matter vessels (Figure 11.18). The lacunar-type infarcts are seen frequently with group B streptococcus, *Streptococcus pneumoniae*, and *Escherichia coli* meningitis (Figure 11.19) [2].

11.2.3 Cerebritis and Brain Abscess

Cerebritis/abscess is caused by bacteria entering the CNS through hematogenous spread from distant infection or generalized sepsis, by extension from contiguous infection, by direct traumatic implantation, or in association with cardiopulmonary malfunction. With hematogenous seeding, abscesses are typically multiple and involves gray–white junction of the brain as a result of dramatic change of arterial diameters at this location, encouraging the settling of infectious emboli. The middle cerebral artery (MCA) territory is most commonly involved. Cerebritis is the earliest stage of purulent brain infection, and it may resolve or evolve to frank abscess formation if not treated appropriately. It is very important to differentiate cerebritis from brain abscess as antibiotics are preferred over surgical drainage to treat cerebritis, whereas surgical drainage is preferred to treat brain abscess [2].

Cerebritis is seen as an area of decreased attenuation on CT, T1 hypointensity, and T2 hyperintensity

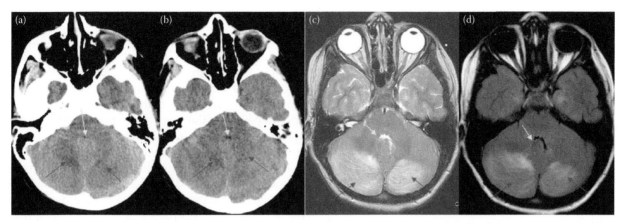

FIGURE 11.18
Post-varicella cerebellitis in an 8-year-old boy: axial noncontrast CT images (a, b) showing hypodensities in the cerebellar hemispheres bilaterally (red arrows) with effacement of the fourth ventricle (yellow arrows). Axial T2-weighted image (c) and axial FLAIR image (d) demonstrate areas of T2 prolongation involving the cortex of both the cerebellar hemispheres (red arrows). The cerebellum has a swollen appearance, and the fourth ventricle is effaced (yellow arrows).

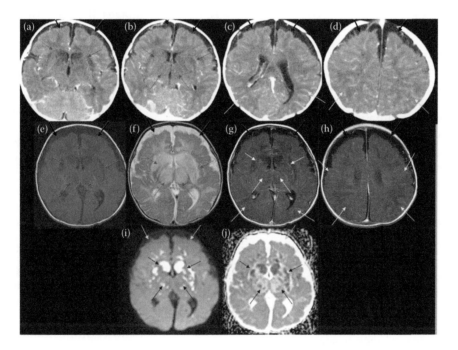

FIGURE 11.19
A 3-year-old with pneumococcal meningitis and perforator arterial infarcts: axial contrast-enhanced CT (CECT) images (a–d) demonstrate basal ganglia and thalamic hypoattenuation (red arrows), leptomeningeal enhancement (yellow arrows), and subdural fluid collections (blue arrows). Corresponding axial T1 (e) and T2-weighted (f) images demonstrate T1 and T2 prolongation in the basal ganglia and thalami (red arrows) with subdural fluid collections (blue arrows). Postcontrast T1-weighted images (g, h) demonstrate patchy enhancement in the basal ganglia (white arrows) and diffuse leptomeningeal enhancement along the convexities (yellow arrows). Axial diffusion-weighted images (i) and axial ADC maps (j) demonstrate decreased diffusivity in the basal ganglia and thalami (black arrows). No restricted diffusion is seen within the extra-axial spaces to suggest subdural empyemas (green arrows).

with ill-defined heterogeneous enhancement on post-contrast scans. Unlike in older children and adults, brain abscesses in neonates and infants are caused by gram-negative bacteria, are relatively large and often multiple, are typically without a well-defined capsule (favors their rapid enlargement), and typically originate in the periventricular white matter in contrast to gray–white junction. The bacteria most commonly implicated in pediatric cerebral abscesses are gram-negative organisms, especially *Citrobacter* sp., Enterobacteriaceae, and *Proteus* sp., especially in very young patients [14]. Other causes include microaerophilic or anaerobic streptococci, *Staphylococcus aureus*, pneumococcus, and occasionally *Haemophilus influenzae*. *Mycobacterium tuberculosis*, actinomycosis, parasitic infestations, and fungal infections rarely cause CNS abscess. Sinus infections and mastoiditis are important causes of cerebral abscess, and septic thrombophlebitis is implicated as the primary event leading to eventual abscess formation. The source of an abscess often dictates its location, number of lesions, and most likely causative agent. Cerebral abscesses that complicate sinusitis are typically adjacent to the infected sinus. Cerebral abscess in the setting of complicated mastoid disease often involves the posterior temporal lobe or cerebellum. In addition, cerebellar and posterior fossa abscesses can also be associated with occipital dermal sinus tracts.

Similar to adults, there are four stages of evolution of brain abscesses in the pediatric population: (1) early cerebritis, (2) late cerebritis, (3) early capsule formation, and (4) late capsule formation. Histopathology and imaging appearance are described in detail in the adult brain abscess section in Section 11.3.1.

11.2.4 Neurotuberculosis

Neurotuberculosis represents 1% of all tuberculosis and 10%–15% of all extrapulmonary tuberculosis cases, most (>40%) of which are in children. Neurotuberculosis is seen with a higher frequency in HIV patients and occurs from hematogenous dissemination of infection from distant active sites such as lung, bone, lymph nodes, and gastrointestinal or genitourinary tract. Bacilli usually lodge in highly vascular areas of brain such as cortex, subcortical white matter as well as in the meninges.

11.2.4.1 Tuberculous Meningitis

Tuberculous meningitis constitutes 70%–80% of all patients with neurotuberculosis and results from the rupture of small tuberculomas in the cortex or leptomeninges. In tuberculous meningitis, gelatinous exudates fill basal cisterns and may be visible as mild hyperdensity on unenhanced CT scans. Contrast enhancement of basal meninges is seen with extension into ambient, sylvian, and prepontine cisterns, around the optic chiasm, and over the surface of the cerebral and cerebellar hemispheres. Hydrocephalus due to blockage of subarachnoid spaces is seen in 45%–87% of cases at the time of diagnosis. On MRI, unenhanced T1-weighted as well as FLAIR images show higher signals than normal CSF in the basal cisterns with diffuse meningeal enhancement in the basal cisterns on the postgadolinium scans. The basal exudates may be overlooked on T2-weighted sequences due to the high intensity of CSF. Vascular involvement due to either secondary extension of arachnoiditis to vessels or direct vessel invasion may cause infarctions particularly involving the basal ganglia and thalami [15].

11.2.4.2 Parenchymal Tuberculomas

Brain parenchymal granulomas (i.e., tuberculomas) are of variable sizes with/without being associated with tuberculous meningitis. Tuberculomas can be single (especially if they are infratentorial) or multiple (particularly if they are supratentorial). The imaging appearance depends on the stage of evolution. Central necrosis appears to be hypodense, whereas granulomatous tissue shows a higher density on CT scan.

Tuberculous cerebritis demonstrates circumscribed hypodensity with ill-defined enhancement on CT scan. The degree of enhancement is variable depending on the amount of inflammatory hypervascularity, reactive neovascularity, and BBB breakage.

Noncaseating tuberculous granulomas (i.e., hard tubercles) appear on CT as isodense or slightly hyperdense lesions surrounded by edema [1]. On T1-weighted images they are iso- to hypointense, whereas on T2-weighted images they are hypo- to hyperintense. Marked nodular enhancement is seen after contrast administration, on both CT and MRI.

Caseating tuberculous granulomas (i.e., soft tubercles) appear as isodense lesions on CT, sometimes with hypodense margins. Enhancement is absent within the central caseation and there is strong enhancement at the periphery, producing a typical ring-enhancing appearance. A variable degree of white matter edema surrounds the lesion. On T1-weighted MRI images they appear as iso- to hypointense lesions, whereas on T2-weighted images they are hypointense with a central dot-like hyperintensity (corresponding to caseating necrosis), surrounded by edema. Marked ring enhancement is also seen after gadolinium administration.

Disseminated tuberculosis is characterized by the diffuse infiltration of brain by small granulomas appearing as multiple hypointense to hyperintense lesions without a central high signal and surrounded by edema on T2-weighted images. Intense nodular enhancement is seen after contrast administration.

11.2.4.3 Tuberculous Abscess

Tuberculous abscesses are rare manifestations of neurotuberculosis, seen most commonly in the immunocompromised population. Tuberculous abscesses are larger than granulomas and elicit more vasogenic edema. They result from liquefactive breakdown of caseated tuberculomas. On CT scans, they show a hypoattenuating center with hyperattenuating margins. On MRI, T1-weighted images show the center of the abscess to be hypointense and its wall to be slightly hyperintense. On T2-weighted images, the center is hyperintense and the wall hypointense. Peripheral ring enhancement is seen after contrast administration. Proton MR spectroscopy

(MRS) of a tuberculous abscess demonstrates choline, lactate, and broad lipid peaks. Proton MRS allows differentiation from untreated bacterial abscesses, which show peaks of amino acids, but not from treated bacterial abscesses or neoplasms.

11.2.5 Viral Infections

Viral infections of CNS may cause a wide spectrum of diseases, including meningitis, acute encephalitis and encephalomyelitis, postinfectious encephalitis, and subacute encephalitides. Encephalitis refers to diffuse brain disease caused by viruses, whereas cerebritis refers to focal bacterial infection; the two terms should not be used interchangeably. The term meningoencephalitis is also used as most viral infections of the brain are accompanied by the involvement of meninges, causing associated aseptic meningitis. The most common cause of viral meningitis is enterovirus, and imaging studies are usually normal. The most common causative organisms for encephalitis are herpes viruses, although other viruses, such as enterovirus, arbovirus, and rubella, may also be involved. Acute para-/postinfectious encephalitides or acute disseminated encephalomyelitis (ADEM) occurs late in the course of a viral disease or after a vaccination and are pathologically characterized by perivascular cuffing and demyelination, in the absence of the virus within the brain, suggesting an immunological pathogenesis. Subacute and chronic encephalitides are characterized by the prolonged duration of disease, which lasts for months or years, and the most common ones are subacute sclerosing panencephalitis (SSPE) and Rasmussen encephalitis. Early in the course of viral encephalitis, essentially all viruses result in an increase in water content of the affected region of the brain and imaging reflects this pathological finding and demonstrates low density on CT and T1 and T2 prolongation on MRI. Early in the course of disease, DWI may show abnormalities more clearly than conventional imaging sequences. A few of the acute and chronic viral infections with fairly specific clinical or radiographic features are discussed in Section 11.2.5.1.

11.2.5.1 Acute Encephalitis

11.2.5.1.1 Herpes Simplex Encephalitis

Unlike in neonates and congenital HSV infection, the majority of herpetic encephalitides in older children and adolescents are caused by HSV type 1. Either primary infection or reactivation of a preexisting infection may cause encephalitis. The diagnosis is made by demonstration of HSV DNA in serum or CSF. HSV encephalitis is a necrotizing hemorrhagic meningoencephalitis, usually involving the temporal lobes.

CT scans are typically normal in the first few days of disease. The earliest CT findings are poorly defined areas of low density with mild mass effects in the temporal lobes. Both the cortex and the subjacent white matter are involved. Small hyperdense foci secondary to hemorrhages may be occasionally seen within the damaged tissue. Gyriform enhancement may be seen after contrast administration, and enhancement is seen only after the appearance of hypodense areas on CT scans. MRI is more sensitive than CT and is the gold standard in diagnostic imaging of HSV encephalitis. DWI shows restricted diffusion before any other abnormality is detected on other sequences. In young infants who have primary CNS involvement rather than reactivation of latent herpes simplex encephalitis, the involvement is predominantly in the cerebral hemispheres with involvement of both cortex and white matter. In older children and adolescents, infection is usually a reactivation of latent HSV infection in the trigeminal ganglion and the areas commonly involved are regions of the limbic system.

DWI shows restricted diffusion early in the disease, and findings persist for approximately one week. Conventional morphologic MRI shows T1 hypointensity and T2 hyperintensity in the temporal lobe, insular cortex, orbital surface of the frontal lobe, and cingulate gyrus. Hemorrhages are not uncommonly seen in the cortex and subcortical white matter in the first week, which are best demonstrated on heme-sensitive sequences (susceptibility-weighted imaging and gradient echo imaging). After gadolinium administration, there is a variable degree of enhancement, predominantly involving the pial and cortical surfaces with a typical gyriform pattern.

11.2.5.1.2 Varicella Zoster Encephalitis

CNS complications of varicella affect less than 0.1% of children with chicken pox and include acute cerebellitis, encephalitis, and vasculitis, and these complications represent vascular involvement by the virus [16]. Acute cerebellitis occurs in a few days to two weeks after the exanthema, usually resolving after a few weeks or months. Imaging findings include diffuse cerebellar swelling and bilateral, symmetrical areas of hypodensity on CT and T1 hypointensity and T2 hyperintensity on MRI, with preferential involvement of the gray matter of cerebellar hemispheres (Figure 11.19).

Multifocal leukoencephalopathy, secondary to small-vessel vasculitis, is another pattern of VZV encephalitis. Delayed onset of neurological deficits 1–4 months after chicken pox or herpes zoster infection may rarely occur probably due to VZV vasculitis involving the large vessels.

MRI commonly shows basal ganglia infarction (usually unilateral) with variable involvement of the cerebral cortex in MCA distribution. MR angiography, CT angiography, and/or catheter angiography may appear normal or show a narrowing of the distal internal carotid artery and proximal segments of the anterior cerebral artery or middle cerebral artery.

11.2.5.1.3 Epstein–Barr Virus

Epstein–Barr virus (EBV) accounts for approximately 5% of acute encephalitis in children. Meningitis, transverse myelitis, Guillain–Barre syndrome, and cranial neuropathies have also been described in association with EBV infection. Imaging findings may be normal or demonstrate hypodensity on CT with T1 hypointensity and T2 hyperintensity in the cerebral cortex, subcortical white matter, thalami, basal ganglia, and occasionally the brain stem and cerebellum. EBV has an affinity for the deep cerebral nuclei, and thus the presence of T2 hyperintensity in basal ganglia and thalami should raise suspicion for EBV encephalitis in the correct clinical setting.

11.2.5.1.4 Influenza-Associated Encephalitis/ Encephalopathy

Acute encephalitis/encephalopathy is an uncommon complication of influenza virus infection. It is still unclear whether CNS involvement is caused by direct invasion by the virus or by an immune-mediated process. Transient splenial lesions with T2 hyperintensity and reduced diffusion have been described (Figure 11.20).

Differential diagnoses for splenial reversible lesions include infections with rotavirus, measles virus, mumps virus, HHV-6, *Salmonella* spp., and *Escherichia coli*-associated hemolytic uremic syndrome; noninfectious causes include diffuse axonal injury, multiple sclerosis, epilepsy, hypoxic ischemic injury, and antiepileptic drugs.

11.2.5.1.5 Arthropod-Borne Viruses

Arthropod-borne viruses are considered "arboviruses" due to their arthropod-borne mode of transmission. The important arboviruses include alphavirus (importantly, eastern equine encephalitis virus and western equine encephalitis virus), flavivirus (importantly, Japanese encephalitis virus and St. Louis encephalitis virus), bunyavirus (LaCrosse encephalitis and California encephalitis viruses), and reovirus (Colorado tick fever virus). Imaging findings in arbovirus infections are diverse. Japanese encephalitis demonstrates T2 hyperintensity and diffusion restriction in the thalami, corpus striatum, cerebral cortex, brain stem, cerebellum, and occasionally white matter (Figure 11.21) [2].

11.2.5.2 Chronic Encephalitis

A few viral agents are associated with "slow infections" and include measles virus (causing SSPE), enterovirus, and JC polyoma virus.

11.2.5.2.1 Subacute Sclerosing Panencephalitis

SSPE is a slow virus infection, occurring several years after a primary measles infection and resulting from a

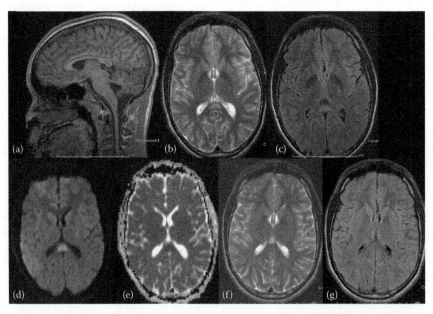

FIGURE 11.20
Reversible splenial lesions associated with influenza encephalitis: sagittal T1-weighted image (a) shows swelling and hypointensity of the splenium of corpus callosum. Axial T2 (b) and FLAIR (c) images demonstrate T2 prolongation in the splenium. Diffusion-weighted image (d) and ADC map (e) show reduced diffusivity in the region of signal abnormality. Follow-up T2 (f) and FLAIR (g) images taken one year later demonstrate complete resolution of the signal abnormality.

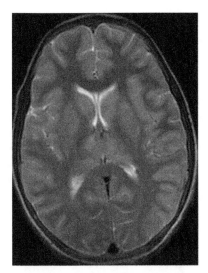

FIGURE 11.21
Japanese encephalitis: bilateral symmetrical T2 hyperintensity in the thalami in Japanese encephalitis. (Case courtesy of Dr. Shilpa Shanke, King Edward Memorial Hospital, Mumbai, India.)

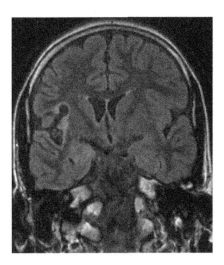

FIGURE 11.22
Rasmussen's encephalitis: coronal FLAIR image demonstrates moderate atrophy of the right frontotemporal regions with associated areas of gliosis. The right lateral ventricle shows mild ex vacuo dilatation.

persistent measles virus, characterized by a defective genomic RNA. After the introduction of measles vaccination, SSPE has almost been eradicated in developed countries. MRI is the modality of choice for imaging SSPE. Early in the course of disease, CT usually is normal. Eventually, diffuse atrophy with multifocal areas of hypoattenuation in subcortical and periventricular white matter is demonstrated. Imaging appearances of SSPE on MRI has distinct patterns based on the stage of the disease. In the early stage (the first 3–4 months after clinical signs and symptoms), imaging studies usually are normal. Later on, patients develop focal, patchy, and asymmetrical T2 hyperintensity in the cerebral cortex and subcortical white matter (predominantly in the parietal and temporal lobes). In the most advanced stage, there are T2 hyperintensities in the brain stem and periventricular white matter associated with diffuse atrophic changes. MRS may demonstrate decreased *N*-acetyl aspartate (NAA) (severe neuronal loss), an increase in myoinositol (active gliosis) and choline (demyelination or inflammation), and the presence of a lactate peak (macrophagic infiltration).

11.2.5.2.2 Rasmussen Encephalitis

Rasmussen encephalitis is characterized by seizures, progressive hemiplegia, and progressive psychomotor retardation and is one of the causes of intractable epilepsy in childhood. The most common pattern of seizures is partial motor seizures.

The etiology and physiopathology of this encephalitis are not well understood. The main hypotheses suggest a viral infection (such as CMV, HSV, EBV, or slow virus) or an autoimmune disease related to autoantibodies to the Glu R3 protein of glutamate receptors [17].

Imaging performed soon after the onset of disease may be normal. On CT, cerebral swelling with focal hypoattenuation has been described as the earliest imaging finding. As the disease evolves, T2 hyperintensity in the cerebral cortex and subcortical white matter is noted with subsequent progressive cortical atrophy, either focal or hemispheric, with predominant involvement of the frontal or frontotemporal lobes. Progressive T2 hyperintensity and atrophy of the ipsilateral basal ganglia is seen in 65% of affected patients (Figure 11.22).

Proton MRS may be positive earlier than conventional MRI and shows a decreased NAA peak and increased concentrations of choline, myoinositol, and lactate. An MR spectrum acquired with short echo times (TE = 35 milliseconds) demonstrates elevated glutamine/glutamate, probably secondary to neurotransmitter release from the nearly continuous seizure activity.

11.3 Infection in Adults

As mentioned in Section 11.2.3, imaging manifestation of CNS infection closely mimics imaging patterns of pediatric CNS infection; only the epidemiology is different. Similar to the evaluation of pediatric CNS infection, neuroimaging plays a crucial role in the management of adult infection. Adult CNS infection will also be discussed based on etiologic organisms.

11.3.1 Bacterial Infection

11.3.1.1 Intra-Axial Infection

Intra-axial infection classically manifests as cerebritis, which ultimately evolves to brain abscess. Cerebritis and brain abscess most commonly occur in the supratentorial compartment, but up to 14% cases are infratentorial in location. The frontal and parietal lobes are most commonly affected. The location is usually the gray–white junction in cases of hematogenous dissemination of infection. Multiple lesions are seen in septic emboli. Involvement of the inferior aspects of frontal and temporal lobes may be due to the direct spread of infection from adjacent sinusitis and otomastoiditis, respectively. There are four phases in the evolution of pyogenic parenchymal infections—early cerebritis (3–5 days), late cerebritis (4–5 days to 10–14 days), early capsule (beginning at about 2 weeks), and late capsule (which may last several weeks or months) stages—and then the resolving abscess [18].

11.3.1.1.1 Early Cerebritis

In this stage, the infection is focal but not yet localized. Nonenhanced CT (NECT) scan images show an ill-defined, hypodense, usually gray–white-junction lesion with mass effect. Contrast-enhanced CT (CECT) scan may show mild patchy enhancement. On T1W MRI it is seen as a poorly marginated, mixed hypointense or isointense mass, and T2W/FLAIR images show an ill-defined hyperintense mass. Post gadolinium administration, T1W contrast-enhanced images (post Gd T1) show patchy enhancement. DWI shows patchy areas of diffusion restriction (increased signal on DWI and low value on ADC map) in cerebritis and abscess.

11.3.1.1.2 Late Cerebritis

In this stage, the infection becomes more established as small necrotic zones coalesce. NECT shows central low density area, peripheral edema, and increased mass effect. CECT shows irregular rim enhancement that fills in on delayed images. On T1W MRI the lesion has a hypointense center, and on T2W images the center is hyperintense. The edema characteristically becomes very marked in this stage with mass effect (Figure 11.23).

Post Gd T1 shows intense, irregular rim enhancement. DWI shows diffusion restriction in cerebritis and abscess (Figure 11.24).

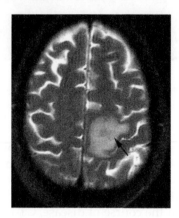

FIGURE 11.23
Axial T2W MRI showing the hyperintense center of late cerebritis (arrow): no definite T2 capsule has been formed. Note the significant perilesional edema.

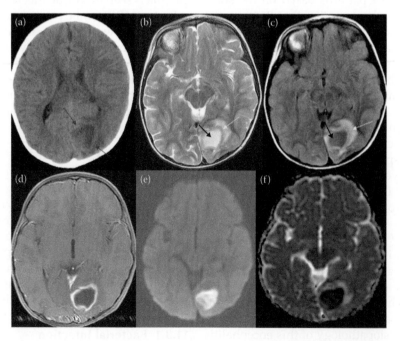

FIGURE 11.24
Cerebral abscess: axial noncontrast CT (a) shows an ill-defined low attenuation lesion in the left occipital lobe (red arrows). Axial T2 (b) and FLAIR (c) demonstrate central pus (blue arrows) and peripheral hypointense abscess wall (yellow arrows). There is surrounding vasogenic edema. Postcontrast T1-weighted image (d) demonstrates peripheral enhancement of the abscess capsule. Axial diffusion-weighted image (e) and ADC map (f) demonstrate decreased diffusivity.

11.3.1.1.3 *Early Capsule*

In this stage, a collagen/reticulin capsule surrounds the core of liquefied necrotic debris/pus and the edema progressively subsides as the capsule matures. NECT shows a hypodense mass with moderate vasogenic edema and mass effect. CECT shows a low-density center with a distinct, thin enhancing rim. On T1W MRI, the lesion has a hypointense center with an isointense to hyperintense rim (Figure 11.25).

On T2W images, the center is hyperintense with a hypointense rim due to collagen, hemorrhage, or paramagnetic free radicals (Figure 11.26).

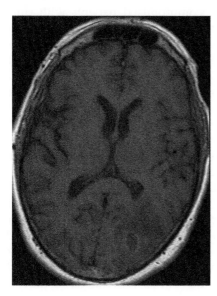

FIGURE 11.25
Brain abscess: axial T1W MRI shows a left parieto-occipital lobe abscess in early capsule stage with a hypointense center and a hyperintense rim.

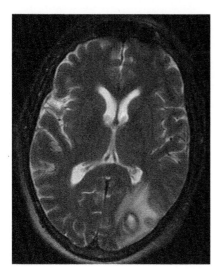

FIGURE 11.26
Brain abscess: axial T2W MRI shows the same abscess as in Figure 11.7 with a hyperintense center and a hypointense rim.

Post Gd T1 shows a well-defined, thin-walled enhancing rim. The capsule is thickest near the cortex (because this side is more vascularized and mounts more intense host response) and thinnest near ependyma in 50% of cases (Figure 11.27).

Unlike the late cerebritis stage, this stage does not show central contrast enhancement as it is centrally occupied by pus. Diffusion-weighted images show diffusion restriction within the abscess core due to a complex mixture of proteins, inflammatory cells, cellular debris, and bacteria in high-viscosity pus.

11.3.1.1.4 *Late Capsule*

In this stage, the cavity shrinks and the capsule thickens. The well-formed capsule has an inner inflammatory layer of granulation tissue and macrophages, a middle collagenous layer, and an outer gliotic layer. The edema and the mass effect diminish further. Daughter abscesses may be identified usually along the deep medial margin of the abscess.

11.3.1.1.5 *Resolving Abscess*

Edema subsides, T2 hypointense rim resolves, and the diffusion restriction resolves with an increase in central ADC value (shows hyperintense appearance in ADC images). The enhancement resolves last. Small ring-/punctate-enhancing focus may persist for months.

11.3.1.1.6 *Intra-Axial Infection by Rare Organisms*

Some bacterial pathogens like *Listeria monocytogenes* and *Citrobacter* infections have characteristic imaging

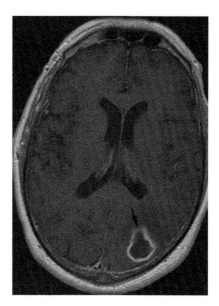

FIGURE 11.27
Brain abscess: axial Gd-enhanced T1W MRI shows a well-defined, thin-walled enhancing rim of the abscess. The capsule is thickest near the cortex where it is well vascularized and thinnest toward the ependymal aspect (arrow).

findings. *Listeria monocytogenes*, which is an anaerobic gram-positive bacillus, usually affects immunocompromised hosts and produces rhombencephalitis [19]. *Citrobacter*, a gram-negative bacterium that is the cause of 5% of neonatal meningitis and 80% of neonatal brain abscesses, produces multiple large cystic white matter lesions, pneumocephalus, and square-shaped abscesses with dot-like foci of septal enhancement [20].

11.3.1.1.7 Differential Diagnosis of Ring-Enhancing Lesions

Table 11.2 enumerates the various causes of ring-enhancing lesions in CT and MRI. It is important to note that approximately 50% of brain abscesses have a ring, which is thinner toward the inner ependymal aspect whereas a break in the ring in case of demyelination occurs toward the outer aspect (Figure 11.28).

TABLE 11.2

Ring-Enhancing Lesions

Common
- Primary brain tumors like anaplastic astrocytoma
- Metastatic brain tumors
- Abscess: thinner ring toward ependyma
- Granuloma
- Resolving hematoma
- Infarct

Less common
- Thrombosed AV malformation
- Demyelinating disease (MS): broken ring toward cortex

Uncommon
- Thrombosed aneurysm
- Primary CNS lymphoma in AIDS

T1 and T2 signal characteristics of varying stages of blood in evolving hematomas may help to differentiate them from abscesses. Thrombosed aneurysms and vascular malformations may also demonstrate ring enhancement, but the continuity with blood vessels will help to identify these lesions (Figure 11.29).

Infarcts, especially those in basal ganglia and thalami, may produce ring enhancement in the subacute stage, but the gyriform enhancement in other areas of infarct in the same arterial distribution helps to differentiate from abscess. CNS lymphoma usually is not centrally necrotic and the T2WI shows central hypointensity, but it could show a central necrotic fluid signal in immunocompromised patients with ring enhancement. Radionuclide single photon emission CT (SPECT) imaging with thallium helps to differentiate between the two by showing uptake in lymphoma but not in abscess. Differentiating a primary or metastatic tumor from an abscess is further described in Section 11.3.1.1.8.

11.3.1.1.8 Differentiating Tumors from Abscesses

As mentioned earlier, tumors and pyogenic abscesses may have similar ring enhancements on postcontrast images. Differentiating between these two entities is extremely important, as their management is entirely different. Assessing the wall characteristics can help to differentiate a tumor from an abscess. The abscess wall can be hyperintense in T1WI and hypointense in T2WI, whereas the reverse is often true for tumors. The enhancing abscess wall is typically uniform and thin, but it is thick and nodular in a tumor. The abscess wall facing the cortex may be thicker than the wall facing the ventricle as described. No such gradient is seen in tumors. Enhancement outside or inside a capsule suggests a tumor. The walls of various types of cystic or necrotic brain tumors show significantly

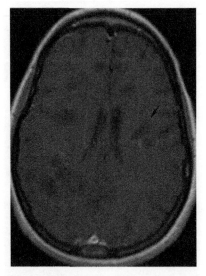

FIGURE 11.28
Active demyelination: axial Gd-enhanced T1W MRI shows multiple ring-enhancing lesions of active demyelination. Note the broken ring appearance with the break toward the outer aspect (arrow), a contrasting feature with the ring enhancement of abscess, where the ring is thinnest toward the inner aspect.

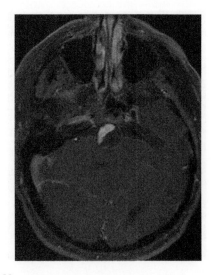

FIGURE 11.29
Thrombosed aneurysm: axial Gd-enhanced T1W MRI shows a ring-enhancing partially thrombosed basilar artery aneurysm.

greater values of diffusion restriction with lower ADCs relative to those of abscess walls. Perfusion imaging shows increased values of relative cerebral blood volume (rCBV) in tumors. The mean rCBV ratios of peripheral walls of various types of cystic or necrotic brain tumors relative to normal white matter are significantly higher (2.90+/−0.62) than the mean rCBV ratio (0.45+/−0.11) of pyogenic cerebral abscess walls [21]. The presence of elevated amino acid resonance peaks in a cyst wall on MRS suggests an abscess.

Diffusion restriction of the necrotic pus filled center can differentiate abscesses from low-grade tumors but not from highly cellular tumors like glioblastoma multiforme (GBM) or lymphoma, which also restrict diffusion due to their central cellular contents. However, the degree of restriction in the core of an abscess usually is significantly higher than that in a tumor.

MRS shows elevated amino acids and metabolic breakdown products like alanine, succinate, acetate, and lactate in bacterial abscesses. The peaks for amino acids leucine, isoleucine, and valine are at 0.9 ppm; alanine at 1.48 ppm; acetate at 1.92 ppm; and succinate at 2.41 ppm. Associated reduction to absence of NAA, creatine, and choline may be seen. Tuberculous abscesses show high lipid and lactate but usually no elevated amino acids or other peaks in contrast to bacterial abscesses. The α,α-trehalose peak is specific for *Cryptococcus* abscesses, the peaks of which occur at 3.77–3.85 and 5.19 ppm [22].

11.3.1.1.9 Septic Emboli

Patients with valvular heart disease, cyanotic heart disease, and intravenous drug abuse are at risk for septic emboli. Multiple bilateral peripheral infarcts/abscesses can be seen, which have both cytotoxic and vasogenic edemas. Large infarcts can occur if the embolic material occludes major arterial branches (Figure 11.30).

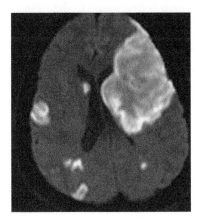

FIGURE 11.30
Septic emboli: axial diffusion-weighted imaging (DWI) shows multiple septic emboli producing diffusion restriction bilaterally in a patient with aortic valve endocarditis. The left anterior middle cerebral artery (MCA) territory infarct is due to a large anterior MCA branch occlusion due to a septic embolus.

Complications include the formation of mycotic aneurysms.

11.3.1.1.10 Mycotic Aneurysms

The name mycotic aneurysm was coined in 1885 by Osler to describe aneurysms associated with bacterial endocarditis as they had fresh fungus vegetation appearance. But caution is needed when interpreting the term "mycotic aneurysm" as bacteria rather than fungi cause the majority of mycotic aneurysms. Infection of the arterial wall focally destroys it, leading to contained rupture and pseudoaneurysm formation. The wall of the aneurysm consists of compressed perivascular tissue, hematoma, and fibroinflammatory tissue [23]. They tend to be fusiform and peripheral, and they are not always at vascular bifurcations. It is noted that 70% are solitary and one-third occurs more centrally, which are indistinguishable from more classic "berry" aneurysms [24]. Arterial stenosis or occlusion adjacent to an aneurysm, a rapid change in aneurysm morphology, or the presence of other similar aneurysms should favor the diagnosis of mycotic aneurysm [25]. The possibility of an infected aneurysm (a more favored term than mycotic aneurysm) should be considered in a patient with atypical peripheral intracerebral hemorrhage and known systemic infection.

11.3.1.2 Extra-Axial Infection

11.3.1.2.1 Subdural Empyema/Abscess

Sterile subdural effusion is the most common extra-axial collection in meningitis cases, which may be due to dural irritation by infected fluid in adjacent subarachnoid space fluid. Subdural effusion follows CSF density in CT and signal in MRI, but an infected subdural empyema is of higher density and signal than CSF. Empyema in the subdural space is a neurosurgical emergency with a mortality of 10%–15%, whereas epidural empyema may occasionally have an indolent course, as the dura functions as a barrier between infection and brain.

Sinusitis is a common cause of supratentorial epidural/subdural empyema, and otomastoiditis is common in infratentorial empyema. The subdural collections are concavo-convex (crescentic) in shape and lie along the convexities, interhemispheric fissure, or tentorium. The empyema margins enhance and the pus within them restricts diffusion, which helps to differentiate subdural empyema from effusion (Figure 11.31).

Associated brain edema is common [26].

11.3.1.2.2 Epidural Empyema/Abscess

Like epidural hematoma, epidural empyema is also biconvex (lentiform) in shape and may cross the midline (Figure 11.32).

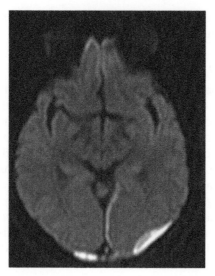

FIGURE 11.31
Axial DWI shows left temporo-occipital convexity and posterior parafalcine diffusion-restricting empyemas. Note that the subdural collections do not cross midline or dural reflections. The right para-sagittal extra-axial diffusion-restricting empyema is actually the most inferior aspect of the epidural abscess shown in Figure 11.10.

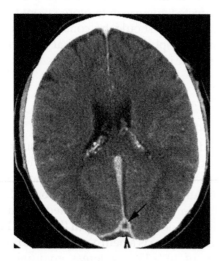

FIGURE 11.32
Empty delta sign: axial CECT shows a parieto-occipital epidural abscess crossing the midline (arrowhead). Note that there is associated superior sagittal sinus thrombosis, which is seen as an empty delta sign of the sinus (arrow). The thin left parafalcine subdural fluid cannot be differentiated from a simple subdural effusion in CT, but it was proved to be a diffusion-restricting subdural empyema in MRI, as shown in Figure 11.15.

This is in contrast to subdural space collection, which is concavo-convex and follows dural reflections rather than crossing the midline. Also note that the epidural collection does not cross suture lines, whereas subdural does. The contents appear isodense to hyperdense to CSF on CT and hyperintense to CSF on MRI and restrict diffusion. The displaced dura appears as a hypointense line along the deep margin of collection on both T1WI and T2WI, and the dural margins enhance intensely.

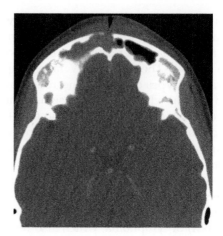

FIGURE 11.33
Axial CECT shows a case of Pott's puffy tumor, frontal sinusitis, and osteomyelitis with the infection breaking through the anterior sinus wall (arrow) and producing a boggy soft-tissue swelling.

11.3.1.2.3 Pott's Puffy Tumor

"Pott's puffy tumor," first described by Sir Percival Potts, is a complication of acute sinusitis, usually of the frontal sinus or mastoid sinus. The condition is more common in adolescents and is usually caused by streptococcus, *Haemophilus influenzae, Staphylococcus* sp., or *Klebsiella* sp. The infection erodes through the wall of the sinus and forms a subperiosteal abscess that can later break into the soft tissues (Figure 11.33).

It can be associated with the intracranial extension of infection with meningitis, epidural abscess, subdural empyema, or brain abscess [27].

11.3.1.3 Tuberculosis

CNS tuberculosis has a pattern of involvement and imaging appearances similar to those of childhood neurotuberculosis, which is discussed in detail in Section 11.2.4.

11.3.1.4 Lyme Disease

Lyme disease is caused by *Borrelia burgdorferi*. It is transmitted to humans by the bite of infected black-legged ixodid ticks. This is a multisystem disease prevalent worldwide. There are several stages of the disease primarily affecting skin, joints, heart, and nervous system.

CNS symptoms appear in about 15%–20% of patients. The most common early neurologic manifestations include meningitis, meningoencephalitis, cranial neuropathy (facial nerve is most commonly involved), and radiculoneuritis. Late neurologic manifestations are aseptic meningitis and encephalitis; they occur years after the initial skin infection.

The imaging of patients with CNS Lyme disease often returns negative results. Characteristic findings include bilateral periventricular/subcortical T2 hyperintense lesions without any mass effect. Involved segments of the cranial nerves appear thickened and enhanced [28].

11.3.1.5 Syphilis

Syphilis is a sexually transmitted disease caused by *Treponema pallidum*. The incidence of syphilis including neurosyphilis has increased dramatically with the prevalence of AIDS. It is noted that 5%–10% of primary syphilis patients develop neurosyphilis.

Although neurosyphilis can occur at any stage of the disease, it usually occurs late in the course of the disease. CNS involvement is most often asymptomatic even with positive CSF tests. Symptomatic neurosyphilis can be menigovascular or parenchymal or a mixed presentation of these two. Ocular and otologic involvement, meningitis, and polyradiculopathy may also occur.

There is no specific imaging signature for neurosyphilis. Meningovascular disease can produce small as well as arterial territory infarcts. Depending on the stage of evolution of arterial territory infarcts, imaging appearances vary in both CT and MRI.

11.3.2 Human Immunodeficiency Virus and Related Infection

HIV is a human retrovirus that causes AIDS. About 65 million people have been infected with this deadly virus and more than 25 million people have died from this disease since its inception in 1981. The disease is widely prevalent in Africa where more than 64% of HIV-infected people reside. The introduction of highly active antiretroviral therapy (HAART) has decreased the overall incidence of this infection and has substantially increased the survival after AIDS diagnosis. Although CNS opportunistic infections have decreased dramatically, HIV associated neurocognitive disorder (HAND) remains the most prevalent form of CNS manifestation today.

HIV is a neurotrophic virus that infects CNS soon after exposure, probably through infected monocytes and lymphocytes that cross BBB easily. Although neurons are not directly infected by HIV, they can be injured via indirect mechanisms that manifest as a cognitive impairment. In the absence of opportunistic infections, HIV causes encephalopathy, myelopathy, peripheral neuropathy, and myopathy. Neurologic complications arise from not only direct infection of neurons by HIV but also opportunistic infections and neoplasm and drug-related complications. The development of neurologic manifestations depends on a variety of factors including therapy with HAART and the status of host immune function. The blood level of CD4+ lymphocyte is a good predictor of host immune response, and a CD4+ cell count < 200 cells/μL predisposes patients to opportunistic CNS infection.

11.3.2.1 Human Immunodeficiency Virus Associated with Neurocognitive Disorder

HAND is the most common neurologic manifestation in AIDS patients; it was previously referred to as AIDS dementia complex or subacute encephalitis. HAND is related to the viral infection of the CNS. The proportion of individuals with cognitive impairment by the disease has not changed over the past two decades, even with HAART. Current estimates find that nearly 50% of HIV patients in the United Sates demonstrate some degree of cognitive impairment compared to age- and sex-matched controls [29]. Clinical manifestations of HAND have been classified according to the degree of neurocognitive dysfunctions as normal cognition, asymptomatic neurocognitive impairment, mild neurocognitive disorder, and HIV-associated dementia. Clinicopathologically, HAND is related to subacute encephalitis with HIV-infected multinucleated giant cells. Multinucleated giant cells are located in the cortex, basal ganglia, and/or white matter.

Although MRI is better than CT in depicting HIV-induced changes in the brain, conventional MRI sequences do not demonstrate any abnormality in the earliest stage of the disease. Cortical atrophy with passive enlargement of CSF spaces the most common imaging finding in the early stages. Periventricular white matter hyperintensity without any mass effect is seen in the later stages of the disease. There is no enhancement of the white matter lesions, and the disease can sometimes be confused with periventricular microangioparhic changes or even progressive multifocal leukoencephalopathy (PML). Treatment with HAART reduces CSF viral loads and white matter hyperintensity. Diffusion tensor imaging has also been used variably to demonstrate white matter injury in AIDS patients.

MRS can be complementary to structural MRI. A reduction of NAA, a normal neuronal marker, is evident in the early onset of infection, even in asymptomatic individuals. This decline is greater in symptomatic compared with asymptomatic patients. High choline, a cell membrane metabolic marker, is also seen in patients with HIV infection, even in asymptomatic patients.

11.3.2.2 Opportunistic Infections in Human Immunodeficiency Virus

11.3.2.2.1 Toxoplasmosis

CNS toxoplasmosis, the most common cause of CNS space-occupying lesions in AIDS patients, favors basal ganglia and jusxtacortical areas. Multifocal involvement is much more common; solitary lesions occur only in one-third of cases. Solitary involvement is seen only

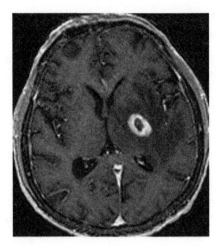

FIGURE 11.34
Axial Gd-enhanced T1W MRI of toxoplasmosis shows a left basal ganglia ring-enhancing lesion with an eccentric nodular focus of enhancement anteriorly (eccentric target sign).

in one-third of cases. CT scans show multiple isodense to hypodense lesions in the basal ganglia and at gray–white interfaces. MRI shows isointense to hypointense signals on T1WI and hypointense signals on T2WI with a nonnecrotic center, which is characteristic and more common. The center can become T2 hyperintense when it is necrotic. DWI shows diffusion restriction. Ring enhancement with eccentric nodular enhancement, the "eccentric target sign," is relatively specific for the diagnosis (Figure 11.34).

Lymphoma can exactly mimic CNS toxoplasmosis, and both of them have heterogenous ring enhancement, low rCBV on MRI perfusion imaging. Diffusion restriction is seen at the periphery of a lymphoma, which sometime can also be seen in CNS toxoplasmosis. The best imaging modality to differentiate between the two is [201]thallium SPECT scan, which shows uptake in lymphoma but not in toxoplasmosis [30]. Table 11.3 shows the features that differentiate toxoplasmosis from lymphoma.

11.3.2.2.2 Cryptococcosis

Cryptococcosis is the most common cause of meningitis in HIV-positive patients and is the most common fungal infection in AIDS. The spectrum of radiologic findings ranges from basilar meningitis to intraparenchymal lesions (Figure 11.35).

Parenchymal lesions include parenchymal enhancing mass lesions called cryptococcomas (cryptococcal abscess), dilated perivascular Virchow–Robin spaces with nonenhancing gelatinous pseudocysts (distended with cryptococcus and mucoid material, but no inflammatory infiltrate as BBB is not disrupted here) (Figure 11.36), and rarely military or leptomeningeal enhancing nodules (granulomas) [31].

TABLE 11.3

Toxoplasmosis versus Lymphoma

	Toxoplasmosis	Lymphoma
Basal ganglia involvement	Yes	Yes
Juxtacortical involvement	Commonly	Less frequent
More than three lesions	Commonly	Less frequent
Enhancing rim	Thin with eccentric nodule	Thick
Edema	Marked	Moderate
NECT	Hypodense	Hyperdense
T2W MRI	Hypointense	Hypointense
T2 hyperintense center	Yes	Yes
Diffusion restriction	Yes	Yes
rCBV in perfusion MRI	Low	Low
Thallium uptake	No	Yes

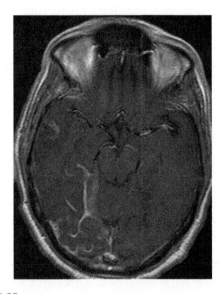

FIGURE 11.35
Cryptococcosis: axial Gd-enhanced T1W MRI shows leptomeningeal enhancement in cryptococcal meningitis.

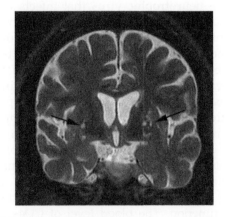

FIGURE 11.36
Cryptococcosis: coronal T2WI shows bilateral basal ganglia gelatinous pseudocysts of cryptococcosis along the perivascular Virchow–Robin spaces (arrows).

Obstructive hydrocephalus may occur as a complication. The dilated perivascular spaces/gelatinous pseudocysts are usually seen along the basal ganglia and thalami, but they may be seen in brain stem, cerebellum, or cerebral hemispheres. On CT scans, they appear as hypodense foci in the basal ganglia regions that usually follow CSF density. They follow CSF on T2WI as well but may be hyperintense on FLAIR and proton density images, they do not enhance usually, and there is no edema or mass effect. The degree of enhancement depends on the host immune status. Immune reconstitution inflammatory syndrome (IRIS) should be considered in HIV-positive patients who were recently started on HAART and shows increased nodular meningeal or subependymal enhancement and increase in size of the gelatinous pseudocysts. Other common conditions that are unmasked in IRIS are tuberculosis and PML [32].

11.3.2.2.3 Progressive Multifocal Leukoencephalopathy

PML is a demyelinating disease caused by the reactivation of JC virus in HIV-infected patients. Before the introduction of HAART, PML affected 3%–7% of patients with HIV infection and was the cause of up to 18% of fatal CNS infections. HAART has significantly reduced the incidence of PML and has significantly increased 1-year survival. However, PML is still the second most common cause of all AIDS-related deaths [33].

Unlike many other opportunistic infections, PML occurs early in the course of AIDS even with CD4+ cell count >200/µL and can also occur in patients receiving HAART. The pathogenesis of PML can be divided into three distinct phases: (1) phase of clinically unapparent infection, (2) phase of latent peripheral infection, and (3) finally phase of reactivation and dissemination. In the final phase, oligodendrocytes are infected, which leads to demyelination of the neuron, the dominant histopathologic finding. The histopathologic hallmark of PML is lytic infection of the oligodendrocytes associated with swollen "bizarre astrocytes" and notable absence of inflammatory response.

Clinical symptoms and signs of PML are nonspecific. PML can be the initial AIDS-defining illness in up to 25% of cases. Clinical presentations depend on the areas of the brain infected by the virus. Common clinical symptoms include extremity weakness, cognitive deficits, speech and visual abnormalities, ataxia, seizure, and headache.

PML has classic neuroimaging signatures. In the correct clinical context, PML can be diagnosed confidently with neuroimaging. Even though CT can detect PML-induced changes, MRI is the diagnostic modality of choice. On CT, there is confluent hypodensity in subcortical white matter sparing the adjacent cortex (Figure 11.37).

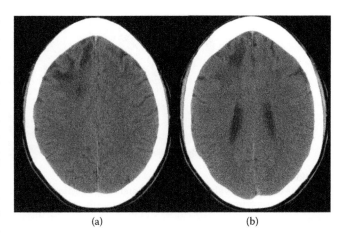
(a)   (b)

FIGURE 11.37
Progressive multifocal leukoencephalopathy (PML): noncontrast CT scan of brain at two different levels (a and b) demonstrates hypodensity in the subcortical u-fibers in the right frontal lobe with sparing of the adjacent cortex. Note: absence of mass effect also a subtle involvement in the left frontal region.

Even with striking abnormality, there is noticeable absence of any mass effect or any enhancement on postcontrast images.

MRI appearances of PML include single or multifocal T2/FLAIR hyperintense lesions in the subcortical white matter predominantly involving the frontal and parietal lobes. Middle cerebellar peduncle is another most commonly involved site with frequent extension of a lesion into the adjacent brain stem as well as cerebellum (Figure 11.38).

Characteristic appearances include T1 hypointense and T2 hyperintense white matter lesions involving the subcortical white matter with notable sparing of the adjacent cortex. Lesions typically are focal at the earlier stages of the disease, which enlarge and become confluent as the disease progresses (Figure 11.39).

There is no mass effect. In fact, there may be associated atrophy in later stages. The advancing edge of the lesion may show hyperintensity on T1-weighted images secondary to lipid-laden macrophages as well as diffusion restriction on diffusion-weighted images [33]. Characteristically, PML lesions do not enhance with contrast.

However, faint enhancement can be seen at the advancing edge in patients treated with HAART secondary to inflammatory response associated with IRIS.

11.3.2.2.4 Other Infections in Acquired Immunodeficiency Syndrome

In AIDS patients, there is also a higher incidence of CNS infection with CMV, tuberculosis, and syphilis. In addition to this, AIDS patients are subject to the same category of infections occurring in immunocompetent patients. These infections should always be considered in the correct clinical and imaging context.

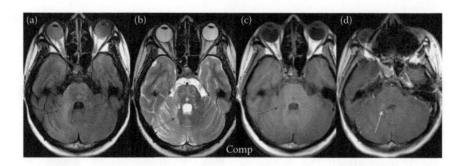

FIGURE 11.38

A 12-year-old female with congenital HIV and PML infection: axial FLAIR (a), axial T2 (b), and precontrast T1-weighted (c) images demonstrating asymmetric primary white matter changes mostly in the right half of the pons, right middle cerebellar peduncle, and right cerebellum (red arrows). A high signal is noted on T2 and FLAIR images with discrete contrast enhancement on postcontrast T1-weighted (d) images (yellow arrow) with no mass effect.

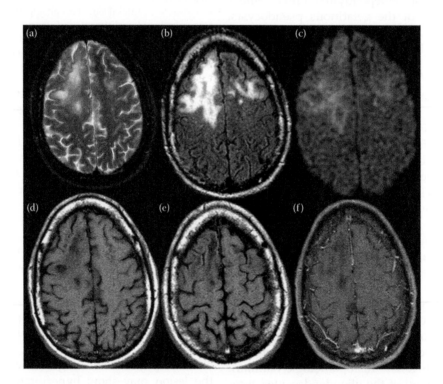

FIGURE 11.39

PML: (a) a T2-weighted image demonstrates subcortical T2 hyperintensity with a maintained cortical ribbon. Note the subtle T2 hyperintensity in the left frontal lobe from a second earlier stage lesion. On FLAIR sequence, the abnormal signal is seen much better, particularly the left frontal lobe lesion. On diffusion-weighted sequence (c), there is a thin rim of diffusion restriction along the posterior advancing edge in both the lesions. On precontrast T1-weighted sequences (d, e), there is prominent T1 hypointensity at the core of the lesion. Note the absent mass effect. On postcontrast T1-weighted sequence (f), there is no enhancement of lesions.

11.3.3 Other Viral Infections

11.3.3.1 Herpes Simplex Encephalitis

HSV type 1 is the causative agent of 95% of herpetic encephalitis and the most common cause of fatal sporadic encephalitis, which accounts for up to 20% of all encephalitis cases.

Clinical presentation and imaging appearances of HSV1 infection are similar to those of the pediatric acute HSV1 infection, as described in Section 11.2.5.1.1.

11.3.3.2 Other Herpetic Infections

Other herpetic infections like varicella, Epstein–Barr, and CMV also has clinical and imaging profiles similar to those of the pediatric infection.

11.3.4 Infection by Parasites

11.3.4.1 Neurocysticercosis

Neurocysticercosis (NCC) is caused by pork tapeworm *Taenia solium* larvae. It is transmitted by the consumption of their eggs in contaminated food or water; they form primary larvae called "oncospheres" in the human gastrointestinal (GI) tract, which then migrate to the brain and develop into the secondary larvae called cysticerci producing NCC. Humans are the intermediate host in this case. Sometimes humans may be a definitive host infected with the tapeworm by consuming undercooked pork with viable larvae, which attach themselves to the human GI tract.

There are four stages of NCC, namely, "vesicle," "colloid vesicle," "granular nodule," and "calcified nodule" stages. The vesicular stage has the larva with its fluid-containing bladder. The fluid is clear and seen as a round CSF-like cyst with a mural nodule (scolex) on imaging. There is no edema (Figure 11.40).

In the colloid vesicle stage, the larva dies, the cystic fluid becomes turbid, cysts begin to shrink, and metabolic products lead to inflammation. Cysts appear hyperintense to CSF with ring enhancement and perilesional edema (Figure 11.41).

By the granular nodule stage, cysts shrink with wall thickening. In this stage, cysts appear isodense on CT scan, isointense on T1WI, and isointense to hypointense on T2WI with nodular or microring enhancement. Edema decreases, but it is not completely resolved. The calcified nodule stage is when lesions completely calcify, without edema or mass effect (Figure 11.42).

Racemose (grape-like) NCC, characterized by abnormal, large growth of cystic membrane without scolex, predominantly occurs in basal cisterns or ventricles (Figure 11.43). It is rare in the brain parenchyma because brain parenchyma does not allow enough room for the growth of large cysts [34].

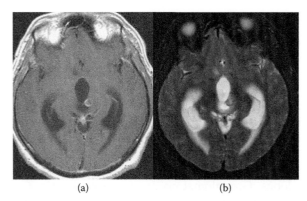

(a)   (b)

FIGURE 11.41
Colloid vesicle stage of NCC: axial Gd-enhanced T1W MRI (a) shows a ring-enhancing lesion of the colloid vesicle stage of NCC with an enhancing scolex in the left lateral wall of the third ventricle/thalamus, producing obstructive hydrocephalus. Axial T2WI (b) shows that there is significant edema around the lesion.

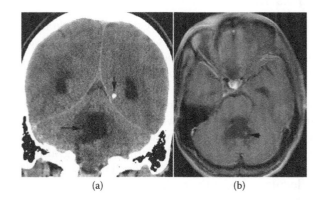

(a)   (b)

FIGURE 11.42
Colloid vesicle of NCC: coronal CECT (a) shows a calcified nodule (vertical arrow) stage of NCC. Also note a cyst (horizontal arrow) occupying the fourth ventricle. Axial Gd-enhanced T1W MRI (b) shows that the cyst in the fourth ventricle is a colloid vesicle of NCC with an enhancing scolex (arrowhead).

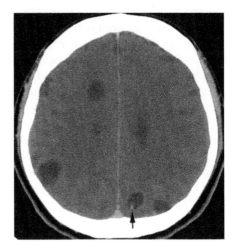

FIGURE 11.40
Axial CECT shows multiple cystic lesions of the vesicular stage of neurocysticercosis (NCC). The hyperdense scolex (arrow) helps to suggest the diagnosis. Note that there is no significant edema or ring enhancement.

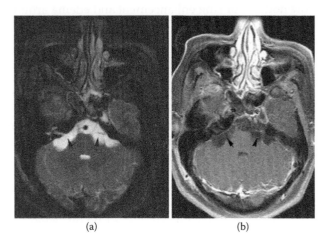

(a)   (b)

FIGURE 11.43
Racemose (grape-like) NCC: axial T2WI (a) and axial Gd-enhanced T1W MRI (b) show racemose (grape-like) NCC in the basal cisterns characterized by abnormal, large growth of cystic membrane without scolex.

11.3.4.2 Amebic Disease

Free-living amebae like Entamoeba *histolytica* can cause meningoencephalitis, which primarily affects the meninges, cortex, and deep gray matter. A history of travel to endemic areas is an extremely important clue. Lesions can be hemorrhagic and can sometimes mimic metastasis. Primary amebic meningoencephalitis (PAM) is caused by *Naegleria fowleri*, and it affects the leptomeninges and cisterns, most prominently in the region of the olfactory bulb and frontal and temporal lobes. Granulomatous amebic encephalitis (GAE), which produces ring-enhancing lesions and gyriform enhancement, is usually caused by *Acanthameba* species or rarely caused by *Balamuthia mandrillaris* and *Sappinia diploidea* [35].

11.3.4.3 Hydatid Disease

Hydatid cysts occur due to infections with *Echinococcus granulosus* and *Echinococcus multilocularis* or *alveolaris* species of tapeworms. Dog is the definitive host and sheep the intermediate host. Humans become an accidental intermediate host due to either contact with the infested definitive host or consumption of contaminated food. CNS involvement is typically seen in a child or young adult who resides or has travelled to endemic areas. Typical Echinococcus granulosus lesions are usually is seen as very large, noncalcified, unilocular cysts in the parietal lobe, without pericystic edema or enhancement of the cyst wall. The germinal membrane of the cyst can be sometimes detached and seen as a membrane floating in the cyst and hydatid sand in the dependent position of the cyst. *Echinococcus multilocularis* or *alveolaris* presents as a multilocular large cyst or clusters of cysts. The small irregular cysts show nodular or ring enhancement and edema around the lesions [36].

11.3.4.4 Cerebral Malaria

Different plasmodium species cause malaria. *Plasmodium falciparum* has the most virulent clinical course and can involve CNS. Malarial parasites infect the red blood corpuscles, which sequester in the microvasculature and produce infarcts and hemorrhage, typically involving basal ganglia and thalami. On CT, there is hypodensity in the deep nuclear structures, basal ganglia, and thalami.

MRI shows multiple infarcts restricting diffusion and hemorrhagic foci blooming in gradient echo images involving the cortex and basal ganglia, especially the thalami. Deep white matter and cerebellum can also be involved (Figure 11.44). Diffuse brain edema may also occur [37].

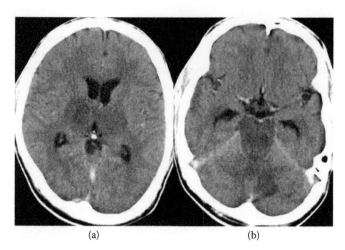

(a)   (b)

FIGURE 11.44
Cerebral malaria: CECT scan demonstrates bilateral symmetrical hypodensity in the basal ganglia, thalami, and brain stem secondary to vascular insult in the artery supplying these areas. (Courtesy of Dr. Shilpa Sankhe, King Edward Memorial Hospital, Mumbai, India.)

11.3.5 Infection by Fungi

11.3.5.1 Aspergillosis

Aspergillus fumigatus infection usually occurs in immunodeficiency due to neutropenia, steroids, or chronic granulomatous disease rather than in AIDS. It could be due to hematogenous or direct spread from fungal sinusitis, which can have a rapidly fatal course with high mortality (up to 50%). Vasculitis of the perforating arteries can lead to acute infarction or hemorrhage in basal ganglia, thalami, brain stem, and sometimes corpus callosum, which should strongly suggest the diagnosis. Aspergillus can extend into the brain tissue, resulting in an infectious cerebritis or abscess; meningeal disease is less common as the fungal hyphae are too large to cross the microvasculature supplying the meninges. Skull base and orbital involvement can lead to cranial nerve palsies and visual impairment. Dural enhancement adjacent to the enhancing lesions of infected paranasal sinuses, calvaria, and optic nerves can occur [38]. The prominence of ring enhancement of the abscess may be related to immune status. The abscesses restrict diffusion. A study has shown that diffusion restriction occurs in the projections and walls of the fungal abscess, whereas the abscess core does not exhibit reduced diffusion; this is a contrasting feature to pyogenic and tuberculous abscesses, which showed low ADC of the wall and the cavity [39].

11.3.5.2 Mucormycosis

Mucormycosis is caused by one of the mucoraceal fungi, including *Absidia*, *Mucor*, and *Rhizopus*. Rhinocerebral mucormycosis is the most common form, and it typically develops in diabetic or immunocompromised

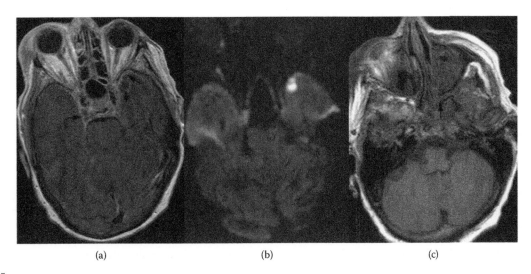

(a)   (b)   (c)

FIGURE 11.45

Axial Gd-enhanced T1W MRI (a) shows a left anteroinferior temporal pole ring-enhancing abscess (vertical short arrow) and adjacent dural enhancement (oblique arrow). Also note the right cavernous sinus filling defect due to cavernous sinus thrombosis in this patient with invasive fungal infection. Axial DWI (b) shows diffusion restriction within the left temporal lobe abscess. Axial T1WI without fat suppression shows obliteration of the left pterygopalatine fossa and retromaxillary fat with fungal soft tissue and also the involvement of the left masticator space and bilateral maxillary sinuses. Note the corresponding normal T1 hyperintense fat on the right side.

patients on corticosteroids, intravenous drug abusers, or individuals with profound neutropenia. It presents as an acute fulminant infection, which is often rapidly fatal when the saprophytic spores are converted into hyphae and become invasive, spreading through the paranasal sinuses into the brain, orbits, and cavernous sinuses. Vascular invasion with vasculitis, occlusion, pseudoaneurysm formation, or infarction can occur. Fungal cerebritis and abscess can also be observed (Figure 11.45).

A chronic form of mucormycosis also exists in addition to this classic fulminant type [40]. The constant features of invasive mucormycosis occur irrespective of the body site of infection, infarction, or hemorrhage [41].

11.3.6 Infection by Prion Particles

Please refer to Section 10.4.2.3 in Chapter 10 on neurodegenerative diseases.

References

1. Tortori-Donati P, Rossi A, and Biancheri R. Infectious diseases. In: Paolo Tortori-Donati AR, Raybaud C, Biancheri R, eds. *Pediatric Neuroradiology*, Vol. 1. Berlin Heidelberg: Springer; 2005:469–542.
2. Barkovich AJ. *Pediatric Neuroimaging*. 5th ed. Philadelphia: Lippincott Williams & Wilkins; 2011.
3. Fink KR, Thapa MM, Ishak GE, and Pruthi S. Neuroimaging of pediatric central nervous system cytomegalovirus infection. *Radiographics* 2010; 30: 1779–1796.
4. van der Knaap MS, Vermeulen G, Barkhof F, Hart AA, Loeber JG, and Weel JF. Pattern of white matter abnormalities at MR imaging: use of polymerase chain reaction testing of Guthrie cards to link pattern with congenital cytomegalovirus infection. *Radiology* 2004; 230: 529–536.
5. Volpe JJ. *Neurology of the Newborn*. 5th ed. Philadelphia: Saunders; 2008.
6. WHO. AIDS eoidemic update. In *World Health Organization*. World Health Organization, Geneva; 2002 Dec , https://www.unaids.org/en/media/unaids/contentassets/dataimport/publications/irc-pub03/epiupdate2002_en.pdf (accessed March 20, 2013).
7. CDC. In *HIV/AIDS Surveillance Rep.* (C. f. D. C. a. Prevention, ed.), Vol. 8. 1996:1–33, http://www.cdc.gov/hiv/topics/surveillance/resources/reports/pdf/hasr1202.pdf (accessed March 20, 2013).
8. Shah SS, Zimmerman RA, Rorke LB, and Vezina LG. Cerebrovascular complications of HIV in children. *AJNR Am J Neuroradiol* 1996; 17: 1913–1917.
9. Hamada S, Vearncombe M, McGeer A, and Shah PS. Neonatal group B streptococcal disease: incidence, presentation, and mortality. *J Matern Fetal Neonatal Med* 2008; 21: 53–57.
10. Chavez-Bueno S and McCracken GH, Jr. Bacterial meningitis in children. *Pediatr Clin North Am* 2005; 52: 795–810, vii.
11. Lummel N, Schoepf V, Burke M, Brueckmann H, and Linn J. 3D fluid-attenuated inversion recovery imaging: reduced CSF artifacts and enhanced sensitivity and specificity for subarachnoid hemorrhage. *AJNR Am J Neuroradiol* 2011; 32: 2054–2060.
12. Kremer S, Abu Eid M, Bierry G, Bogorin A, Koob M, Dietemann JL, and Fruehlich S. Accuracy of delayed postcontrast FLAIR MR imaging for the diagnosis of leptomeningeal infectious or tumoral diseases. *J Neuroradiol* 2006; 33: 285–291.

13. Smirniotopoulos JG, Murphy FM, Rushing EJ, Rees JH, and Schroeder JW. Patterns of contrast enhancement in the brain and meninges. *Radiographics* 2007; 27: 525–551.

14. Patrick CC and Kaplan SL. Current concepts in the pathogenesis and management of brain abscesses in children. *Pediatr Clin North Am* 1988; 35: 625–636.

15. Gupta RK, Gupta S, Singh D, Sharma B, Kohli A, and Gujral RB. MR imaging and angiography in tuberculous meningitis. *Neuroradiology* 1994; 36: 87–92.

16. Johnson R and Milbourn PE. Central nervous system manifestations of chickenpox. *Can Med Assoc J* 1970; 102: 831–834.

17. Rogers SW, Andrews PI, Gahring LC, Whisenand T, Cauley K, Crain B, Hughes TE, Heinemann SF, and McNamara JO. Autoantibodies to glutamate receptor GluR3 in Rasmussen's encephalitis. *Science* 1994; 265: 648–651.

18. Enzmann DR, Britt RH, and Yeager AS. Experimental brain abscess evolution: computed tomographic and neuropathologic correlation. *Radiology* 1979; 133: 113–122.

19. Alper G, Knepper L, and Kanal E. MR findings in listerial rhombencephalitis. *AJNR Am J Neuroradiol* 1996; 17: 593–596.

20. Hedlund GL. Citrobacter meningitis. In: Salzman KL, Barkovich AJ, Osborn AG, eds. *Diagnostic Imaging: Brain*. Philadelphia: Amirsys; 2010:20–23.

21. Chan JH, Tsui EY, Chau LF, Chow KY, Chan MS, Yuen MK, Chan TL, Cheng WK, and Wong KP. Discrimination of an infected brain tumor from a cerebral abscess by combined MR perfusion and diffusion imaging. *Comput Med Imaging Graph* 2002; 26: 19–23.

22. Himmelreich U, Dzendrowskyj TE, Allen C, Dowd S, Malik R, Shehan BP, Russell P, Mountford CE, and Sorrell TC. Cryptococcomas distinguished from gliomas with MR spectroscopy: an experimental rat and cell culture study. *Radiology* 2001; 220: 122–128.

23. Gonda RL, Jr, Gutierrez OH, and Azodo MV. Mycotic aneurysms of the aorta: radiologic features. *Radiology* 1988; 168: 343–346.

24. Corr P, Wright M, and Handler LC. Endocarditis-related cerebral aneurysms: radiologic changes with treatment. *AJNR Am J Neuroradiol* 1995; 16: 745–748.

25. Chapot R, Houdart E, Saint-Maurice JP, Aymard A, Mounayer C, Lot G, and Merland J J. Endovascular treatment of cerebral mycotic aneurysms. *Radiology* 2002; 222: 389–396.

26. Greenlee JE. Subdural empyema. *Curr Treat Options Neurol* 2003; 5: 13–22.

27. Masterson L and Leong P. Pott's puffy tumour: a forgotten complication of frontal sinus disease. *Oral Maxillofac Surg* 2009; 13: 115–117.

28. Saremi F, Helmy M, Farzin S, Zee CS, and Go JL. MRI of cranial nerve enhancement. *AJR Am J Roentgenol* 2005; 185: 1487–1497.

29. Clifford DB. HIV-associated neurocognitive disease continues in the antiretroviral era. *Top HIV Med* 2008; 16: 94–98.

30. Lorberboym M, Estok L, Machac J, Germano I, Sacher M, Feldman R, Wallach F, and Dorfman D. Rapid differential diagnosis of cerebral toxoplasmosis and primary central nervous system lymphoma by thallium-201 SPECT. *J Nucl Med* 1996; 37: 1150–1154.

31. Mathews VP, Alo PL, Glass JD, Kumar AJ, and McArthur JC. AIDS-related CNS cryptococcosis: radiologic-pathologic correlation. *AJNR Am J Neuroradiol* 1992; 13: 1477–1486.

32. Biagetti C, Nicola M, Borderi M, Pavoni M, Tampellini L, Verucchi G, and Chiodo F. Paradoxical immune reconstitution inflammatory syndrome associated with previous Cryptococcus neoformans infection in an HIV-positive patient requiring neurosurgical intervention. *New Microbiol* 2009; 32: 209–212.

33. Bag AK, Cure JK, Chapman PR, Roberson GH, and Shah R. JC virus infection of the brain. *AJNR Am J Neuroradiol* 2010; 31: 1564–1576.

34. Kim SW, Kim MK, Oh SM, and Park SH. Racemose cysticercosis in the cerebellar hemisphere. *J Korean Neurosurg Soc* 2010; 48: 59–61.

35. Sarica FB, Tufan K, Cekinmez M, Erdogan B, and Altinors MN. A rare but fatal case of granulomatous amebic encephalitis with brain abscess: the first case reported from Turkey. *Turk Neurosurg* 2009; 19: 256–259.

36. Wani NA, Kosar TL, Khan AQ, and Ahmad SS. Multidetector-row computed tomography in cerebral hydatid cyst. *J Neurosci Rural Pract* 2010; 1: 112–114.

37. Nickerson JP, Tong KA, and Raghavan R. Imaging cerebral malaria with a susceptibility-weighted MR sequence. *AJNR Am J Neuroradiol* 2009; 30: e85–86.

38. Ashdown BC, Tien RD, and Felsberg GJ. Aspergillosis of the brain and paranasal sinuses in immunocompromised patients: CT and MR imaging findings. *AJR Am J Roentgenol* 1994; 162: 155–159.

39. Luthra G, Parihar A, Nath K, Jaiswal S, Prasad KN, Husain N, Husain M, Singh S, Behari S, and Gupta RK. Comparative evaluation of fungal, tubercular, and pyogenic brain abscesses with conventional and diffusion MR imaging and proton MR spectroscopy. *AJNR Am J Neuroradiol* 2007; 28: 1332–1338.

40. Rumboldt Z and Castillo M. Indolent intracranial mucormycosis: case report. *AJNR Am J Neuroradiol* 2002; 23: 932–934.

41. Horger M, Hebart H, Schimmel H, Vogel M, Brodoefel H, Oechsle K, Hahn U, Mittelbronn M, Bethge W, and Claussen CD. Disseminated mucormycosis in haematological patients: CT and MRI findings with pathological correlation. *Br J Radiol* 2006; 79: e88–95.

12

Head Trauma

Eytan Raz and Pier Luigi Di Paolo

CONTENTS

12.1 Introduction

Traumatic brain injury (TBI) is one of the most common causes of morbidity and mortality in the Western world. Each year in the United States alone, more than two million people sustain a head trauma, and 10% of these injuries are fatal [1]. Ten percent of survivors experience neurological deficits of varying degrees [2]. It is estimated that as many as 5.3 million people in the United States are living with disability related to TBI, approximately 2% of the population. The leading cause of TBI is injury related to falls, followed by motor vehicle or traffic collisions, and any cause of being "struck by or against" [3].

Classification of the clinical severity of TBI is based on the Glasgow Coma Scale (GCS) (Table 12.1) [4]. The GCS is a neurological scale that allows recording of the level of consciousness through assessment of eye, motor, and verbal responses. The severity distribution is approximately 80% mild (GCS score of 13–15), 10% moderate (GCS score of 12–9), and 10% severe (GCS scores of 8 or less). It is known that patients with the same GCS score can have extremely different outcomes: duration of posttraumatic amnesia and loss of consciousness are other important clinical factors when establishing the severity of TBI (Table 12.2).

The role of neuroimaging in head trauma is well established. According to the ACR appropriateness criteria, there is general consensus that patients with moderate or high risk for intracranial injury should have a head computed tomography (CT done early [5]. CT is the best modality because it is widely available, fast, and highly accurate in the detection of skull fractures and intracranial hemorrhage; moreover, life support and monitoring equipment can be fitted in the CT room without restrictions, and generally, there are no contraindications to emergency patient scanning. There is more discordance regarding patients with GCS > 13, and head CT has been proposed as a screening tool in this population, as well due to the low cost and wide availability of CT. The use of the New Orleans criteria [6] establishes that a head CT should be performed in patients with GCS of 15 if there is a risk factor such as headache, vomiting, drug or alcohol intoxication, patient older than 60, short-term memory deficit, physical findings of supraclavicular trauma, and/or seizure; use of these criteria allows a sensitivity of 100% of identification of a brain lesion [6].

TABLE 12.1

Glasgow Coma Scale

Eye Opening	Verbal Response	Motor Response
Opens spontaneously 4	Normal conversation 5	Normal 6
Opens to voice 3	Disoriented conversation 4	Localizes pain 5
Opens to pain 2	Inappropriate words 3	Withdraws from pain 4
None 1	Incomprehensible sounds 2	Decorticate posturing 3
	None 1	Decerebrate posturing 2
		None 1

TABLE 12.2

Severity of Traumatic Brain Injury

	Mild	Moderate	Severe
GCS	3–8	9–12	13–15
PTA	<1 day	>1 to < 7 days	>7 days
LOC	0–30 minutes	>30 minutes to <24 hours	>24 hours

CT also has a role in case of clinical deterioration by detecting delayed hematoma or cerebral edema [7] and in setting of subacute or chronic head injury for detecting atrophy, hydrocephalus, encephalomalacia, and chronic subdural hematoma (SDH). Magnetic resonance imaging (MRI) is more sensitive than CT in few occasions. MRI enables the detection of the different stages of hemorrhage, although it is not as sensitive as CT for hyperacute hemorrhage and subarachnoid hemorrhage (SAH). MRI is more sensitive than CT for identification of diffuse axonal injury (DAI) and in evaluating presence of ischemia, which can be a secondary injury related to trauma. Notably, skull films have little to no role in the setting of acute trauma; their use is appropriate only for the detection of radiopaque foreign bodies.

12.2 How to Read a Head CT for Trauma

The role of imaging in head trauma is paramount both for the diagnosis and evaluation of the extent of damage and in determining the appropriate therapy. CT is very fast and sensitive enough for the entities expected after trauma, such as skull fractures and intracranial hemorrhages. Treatable neurosurgical lesions are easily diagnosed with CT. When evaluating a CT for head trauma, it is suggested to start with evaluation of scout

view, followed by evaluation of four windows, soft tissue, bone, brain, and subdural windows, which should be preferably scrolled in this order. The soft tissue window allows having an idea of the location and the intensity of the impact. The bone window is useful to evaluate the presence of fractures; care must be taken not to misinterpret sutures for fractures (the sutures of the calvarium and skull base are symmetric) and to pay particular attention to particular areas such as the temporal bone, the ossicles, skull base, the occipital condyles, and the incompletely visualized vertebrae. In the brain window, we evaluate the symmetry with particular attention to the gray–white matter interface and the basal ganglia, which should be well defined; the sites of subcutaneous swelling or fractures seen in the prior windows should be further evaluated with maximal attention; particular attention must be paid to evaluate the presence of hemorrhages with particular care to SAH, which can be easily missed if subtle; also frequent sites of contusion such as the basal frontal lobes and the basal temporal lobes at the level of the petrous ridges should be carefully scrutinized. It is suggested to terminate the evaluation of the brain with a subdural window (width 200, level 70), similar to the soft tissue window, to evaluate the convexity along the edges of the intracranial cavity.

12.3 Classification of Injury

TBI may be divided in to two types: primary injury, the direct result of trauma to the head, and secondary injury, which arise as complications of primary lesions. Secondary injuries are potentially preventable, whereas primary injuries, by definition, have already occurred by the time the patient first presents (Table 12.3). TBI can be further divided according to location (intraaxial or extra-axial) and mechanism (blunt/closed and penetrating/open).

12.3.1 Skull Fractures

Skull fractures are a common finding in cranial trauma. The presence of a skull fracture is not necessarily significant clinically and the absence of a skull fracture does not exclude a brain injury *per se*: that is the reason why it is not necessary to perform skull x-rays to diagnose fractures [8,9]. Skull fractures are common in the parietal, frontal, and occipital regions although they may also affect the skull base. There are three types of fractures: linear, depressed, and basilar fractures. Linear fractures are the most common, are usually caused by

TABLE 12.3

Imaging Classification of Traumatic Brain Injury

Primary Injury	Secondary Injury
Extra-axial injury	**Acute**
Skull fracture	Diffuse cerebral swelling
Epidural hematoma	Brain herniation
Subdural hematoma	Infarction
Subarachnoid hemorrhage	Infection
Intraventricular hemorrhage	**Chronic**
Intra-axial injury	Hydrocephalus
Diffuse axonal injury	Encephalomalacia
Cerebral contusion	Cerebrospinal fluid leak
Intraparenchymal hematoma	Leptomeningeal cyst
Vascular injury	
Dissection	
Carotid-cavernous fistula	
Arteriovenous dural fistula	
Pseudoaneurysm	

lesser forces, and are frequently isolated, without any subjacent brain injury (Figure 12.1). Extra attention must be paid in order not to confuse calvarial fractures with cranial sutures and synchondroses and vice versa [10]; review of bone window in the three planes and three-dimensional (3D) reconstructions can also add sensitivity for evaluation of linear fractures (Figure 12.2) [11].

Depressed fractures arise from blunt force trauma, are typically comminuted with inwardly displaced broken bone, and are commonly associated with underlying brain injury (Figure 12.3). Associate infection occurs in up to 10% of cases, with high morbidity (high frequency of epilepsy) and high mortality. Depressed skull fractures may require neurosurgical evaluation to elevate the fracture and remove bone fragments if the depressed fracture is greater than the thickness of the cranium or if there is evidence of dural penetration, associated intracranial hematoma, pneumocephalus, or gross cosmetic deformity [12] (Figures 12.4 and 12.5).

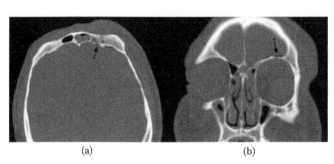

(a)   (b)

FIGURE 12.1
Patient with a left orbital roof fracture. The fracture violates the inner table (arrow, a) and communicates with the intracranial space, being associated with few small intracranial locules of air (arrow, b).

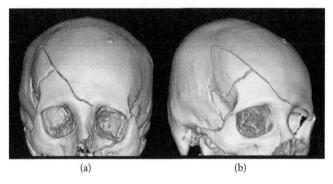

(a)   (b)

FIGURE 12.2
Thirty-six-year-old patient presenting to the emergency department after hitting the steering wheel in a motor vehicle accident. Three-dimensional surface rendered images demonstrating the extension of the skull fracture. Notice also the left maxillary sinus wall and orbit fractures.

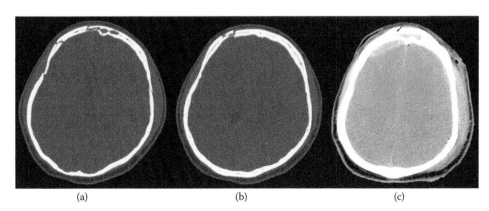

(a)   (b)   (c)

FIGURE 12.3
Same patient of Figure 12.2. Thirty-six-year-old patient presenting to the emergency department after hitting the steering wheel in a motor vehicle accident. Unenhanced head CT in the bone (a, b) and brain (c) windows demonstrates a fracture involving the anterior aspect of the frontal bone, associated with an underlying epidural hematoma (visible in Figure 12.3c).

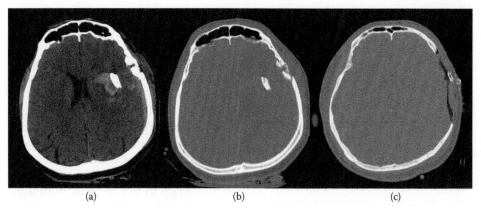

FIGURE 12.4
Depressed fracture. Unenhanced CT with brain (a) and bone (b) windows demonstrating a severely depressed comminuted fracture involving the left calvarium. The inner bone fragment is displaced medially and is associated with subdural, subarachnoid, and intraparenchymal hemorrhage. The severity of the findings necessitated surgical intervention (postoperative CT, c) with debridement and removal of the inner fragment and craniectomy.

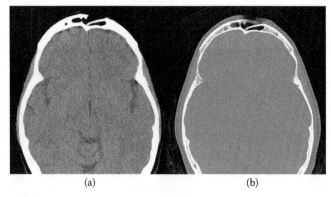

FIGURE 12.5
Frontal sinus fracture. CT with brain (a) and bone (b) windows demonstrates the presence of a superficial depressed fracture involving the left frontal sinus, in continuity with the superficial laceration. The inner aspect of the frontal sinus is unremarkable, without subjacent brain involvement.

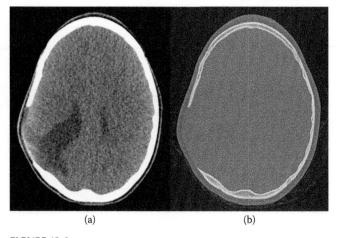

FIGURE 12.6
Three-year-old patient with history of trauma. Unenhanced CT with brain (a) and bone (b) windows demonstrates a splaying of the bone edges with an associated underlying encephalomalacia and volume loss. This is consistent with a leptomeningeal cyst.

Basilar fractures occur through the skull base and are very rare and sometimes difficult to detect. When a basilar fracture is seen, a computed tomography angiography (CTA) is recommended to evaluate internal carotid arteries.

Diastatic skull fracture occurs when the fracture causes widening of the suture; it is more common when the sutures are not yet fused, such as in children. In adults, it typically affects the lambdoid suture, which is a suture that does not fuse until old age.

Growing skull fracture is a kind of fracture seen most commonly in children and happens when there is dural tear with development of a cerebrospinal fluid (CSF)-filled collection in the fracture and progressive enlargement of the fracture margins caused by CSF pulsations [13]. This is also termed leptomeningeal cyst and typically occurs in the base of the skull (Figure 12.6).

12.3.2 Epidural Hematoma

The epidural space is the potential space located between the inner table of the skull and the dura, which represents the functional periosteum of the inner table of the skull. The epidural hemorrhage often occurs in the temporoparietal region in the so-called Marchant zone (90% of the cases), typically occurring when a fracture crosses the vascular territory of the middle meningeal artery or vein (Figure 12.7). When there is tearing of these vessels, the blood moves in the epidural space resulting in the epidural hematoma [14]. The dura is tightly adherent to the inner table of the skull at cranial sutures and this is the reason why the extension of the epidural hematoma tends to be limited across the sutures, although exceptions are common [11] (Figure 12.8). Clinically, after

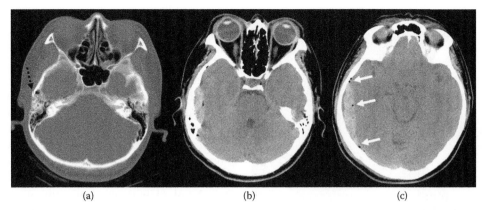

FIGURE 12.7
Epidural hematoma. There is a nondisplaced fracture of the petrous portion of the right temporal bone (black arrow, a) with a subjacent extra-axial collection consistent with an acute epidural hematoma (b, c). Notice the presence of few small air bubbles (arrows, c), related to the involvement of the mastoid air cells.

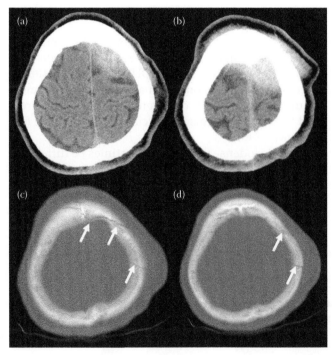

FIGURE 12.8
Epidural hematoma, exception. Patient with a bifrontal nondisplaced calvarial fracture (arrows, c, d) that crosses the coronal suture on the left and extends into the left parietal calvarium. There is associated high left frontal convexity and parasagittal extra-axial hyperattenuated collection (a, b) consistent with an acute epidural hematoma. Sometimes, epidural hematoma can cross the sutures.

the injury, there may be a lucid interval, defined as a temporary improvement in the patient's condition after the injury, followed by deterioration; 50% of patients with epidural hematoma experience the lucid interval. Epidural hematomas are usually biconvex hyperdense CT collection: the shape is related to the firm attachment of the dura to the skull. Epidural hematoma can

sometimes contain different components, showing the "swirl sign," which is a bad prognostic sign, representing an active component of bleeding within a chronic hematoma [15]. The active component is isodense to the brain and represents actively extravasating unclotted blood, while the chronic component is the hyperdense epidural hematoma [11,16]. Chronic epidural hematomas are low density with peripheral enhancement and may often lose the biconvex shape. They have to be differentiated from other epidural lesions such as tumors (Figure 12.9). The venous epidural hematoma occurs most frequently in the middle cranial fossa in the pediatric population and carries a lower morbidity than arterial epidural hematomas [17].

12.3.3 Subdural Hematoma

Between the dura and the underlying arachnoid, there is a potential space named subdural space, which usually contains a minimal amount of fluid similar to CSF and is traversed by bridging cortical veins; hemorrhage can insinuate in this subdural space, constituting the SDH. SDHs are caused by rupture of bridging veins, which, from the cerebral convexities, traverse the subarachnoid space to reach the dural sinuses. The entry point of these veins into the dural sinus is fixed; with trauma, the rotational motion of the brain causes the shearing of the bridging veins, which eventually tear in the subdural portion that is the weakest part due to the lack of arachnoid trabeculae sheathing [11].

In elderly patients, the cerebral atrophy allows for increased movement between the brain parenchyma and the calvarium, resulting in an increased incidence of SDHs. Acute SDH has a high mortality rate up to 40%. With SDH, as with the epidural hematoma, a lucid clinical interval may be seen, which can last up to few days.

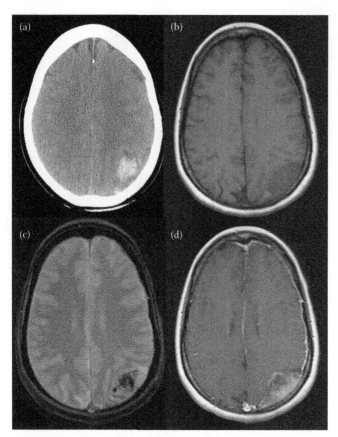

FIGURE 12.9
Hemorrhagic meningioma. Thirty-one-year-old female undergoes CT for trauma (a), which demonstrates an intracranial parietal extra-axial hemorrhage with atypical features, but possibly related to an epidural hematoma. The atypical features and the lack of overlying calvarial fractures prompted the further evaluation with an MRI: unenhanced T1 (b), gradient-echo (c), and post-contrast T1 (d) demonstrate an enhancing hemorrhagic extra-axial mass, which was removed and was hemorrhagic meningioma.

On CT, the acute SDH appears as a hyperdense, homogeneous, crescent-shaped extra-axial collection (Figure 12.10). The hematoma can be variably thick. In patients with anemia, the hematoma can be isodense [16]. Most SDHs are supratentorial and are located along the convexity. SDHs are frequently seen along the whole hemispheric convexity from the anterior falx to the posterior falx cerebri (Figure 12.11). They are also frequently seen along the falx and tentorium (Figure 12.10), contrary to the epidural hematoma, which, by definition, cannot be located along these meningeal structures. Subacute and chronic SDHs may be concave, simulating epidural hematomas, and are associated with peripheral enhancement caused by the vascularization of the subdural membrane. This vascularization is formed by vessels without tight junctions, which can easily leak resulting in repeated bleeding within the hematoma. SDHs can thus be very heterogeneous due to these repeated episodic bleedings that result in compartments separated by septations [18]. Chronic SDH can also be seen without history of head trauma, in elderly patients with coagulopathy (Figure 12.12). SDHs have to be differentiated from other lesions such as empyema or tumors (Figure 12.13). Also, in children, presence of different aged SDHs should raise suspicion of child abuse (see Section 12.3.10).

Bilateral isodense SDHs can sometimes be difficult to call because they can be very thin and symmetric. In order not to be misled, the sulcal size has to be carefully evaluated and the gray–white matter interface should be scrutinized to determine if it is buckled inward [19].

Rarely, SDH can be the presentation of an aneurysm rupture, even without associated SAH [20].

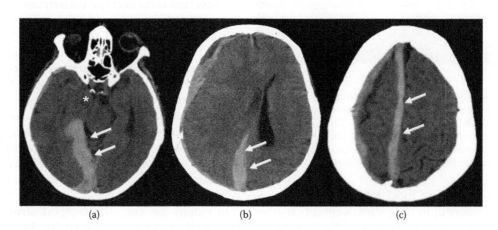

    (a)   (b)   (c)

FIGURE 12.10
Sixty-five-year-old patient presenting to the emergency department for altered mental status one day after a minor trauma. Unenhanced CT demonstrates extensive subdural acute hemorrhage seen layering over the right tentorium cerebelli (arrows, a), along the falx cerebri (arrows, b, c), and along the right convexity. There is extensive right hemispheric cerebral edema. There is marked leftward midline shift measuring with effacement of the right lateral ventricle. There is also medialization of the right uncus (asterisk, a) with effacement of right basilar cisterns compatible with transtentorial herniation.

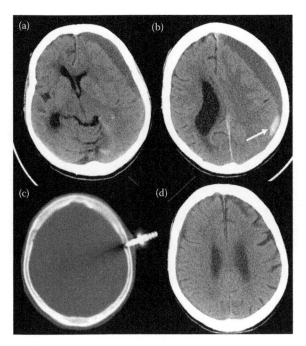

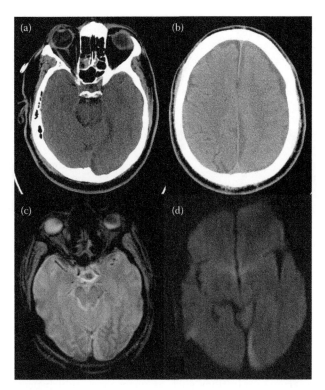

FIGURE 12.11

Acute on chronic subdural hematoma. There is a large left frontoparietal extra-axial collection associated mass effect and left to right midline shift (a, b). It is compatible with a subdural hematoma, demonstrating attenuation slightly higher than that of cerebrospinal fluid. A small hyperdense component in the posterior aspect represents a region of acute hemorrhage within the chronic subdural hematoma (arrow, b). A subdural evacuation port system (SEPS) was placed (c). Follow-up CT performed 1 month after removal of the SEPS (d), demonstrating resolution of the subdural collection.

FIGURE 12.13

Empyema mimicking a subdural hematoma. Patient presenting with fever, sepsis, and altered mental status. Unenhanced CT (a, b) demonstrates a subdural low-attenuated collection along the tentorium cerebelli, falx cerebri, and left convexity. Given the clinical history, a subdural empyema was considered and an MRI was recommended. MRI of the brain with gradient-echo (c) and diffusion weighted images (d) demonstrates the lack of susceptibility within the collection and the diffusion restriction, compatible with purulent collection.

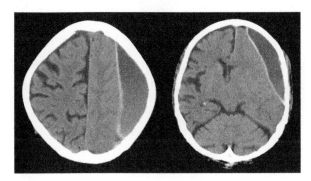

FIGURE 12.12

Chronic subdural hematoma. Crescent-shaped extra-axial collection, crossing the sutures, is seen along the left convexity, compatible with a chronic subdural hematoma. There is subjacent mass effect. Most subdural hematomas are supratentorial along the convexity.

12.3.4 Subarachnoid and Intraventricular Hemorrhage

Often after trauma, a small amount of subarachnoid and intraventricular hemorrhage is present and can be very subtle. SAH in trauma results from injury to small cortical veins traversing the subarachnoid space or from subdural or intraparenchymal hematomas, which extend through the subarachnoid space (Figure 12.14) [11,16]. In

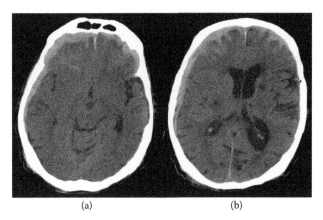

(a)   (b)

FIGURE 12.14

Traumatic subarachnoid hemorrhage. Patient is victim of a motor vehicle accident. Subdural hemorrhage is noticed, associated with peripheral subarachnoid hemorrhage in the bilateral frontal sulci.

neither case, the volume of hemorrhage is comparable to that faced in aneurysmal SAH. Another difference is that typically aneurysmal SAH is located in the suprasellar, ambiens, middle cerebral artery cistern, and interhemispheric fissure (Figure 12.15), while traumatic SAH is

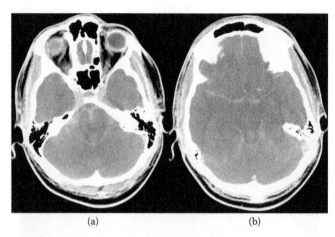

FIGURE 12.15
Aneurysmal subarachnoid hemorrhage. Patient with a ruptured posterior communicating aneurysm. Subarachnoid hemorrhage is noticed in the cistern, ambiens cistern, middle cerebral arteries cisterns, and Sylvian fissures.

located peripherally. To further evaluate a suspected SAH, a CTA is an optimal imaging technique, with very high sensitivity and specificity [21]. SAH is associated with secondary complications such as vasospasm, which brings to ischemic infarction; communicating hydrocephalus, related to the engorgement of the arachnoid villi with phagocytized blood cells and impaired absorption of CSF.

In the setting of brain trauma, there is a mimicker of SAH, called the pseudo-SAH [22]: the diffuse brain swelling compresses the sulci with secondary engorgement and dilation of small pial vessels in the subarachnoid space, which appear hyperdense on CT, mimicking a SAH.

12.3.5 Contusion

Cortical contusion is the most common parenchymal injury. Contusions occur on the gyral surface with possible extension to the subjacent white matter. Pathologically they are characterized by petechial hemorrhage, due to the high vascularity of the gray matter, with surrounding edema. Rarely the hemorrhage can extend also superficially toward the subarachnoid space [16].

The contusion occurring at the site of the impact is called coup contusion, whereas a contrecoup injury is located 180° from the site of impact (Figure 12.16). Contusions are more probable to occur where the bone is irregular and presents roughened edges, such as in the anterior cranial fossa where the frontal lobe may be contused by sliding on the cribriform plate, along the petrous ridges and in the greater sphenoid wings where the inferior temporal lobe is prone to contusions. A particular kind of contusion is the gliding contusion, typically happening in the superior parasagittal frontal lobes. A contusion can also occur if the brain hits against the falx or the tentorium (Figure 12.17). Half of

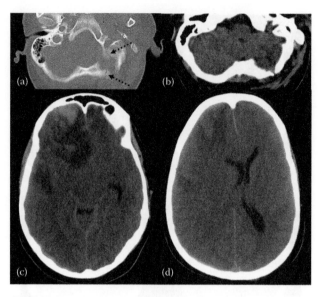

FIGURE 12.16
Coup contrecoup injury. Left occipital trauma with a linear occipital bone fracture (arrows, a), a small left cerebellar contusion (b), and a right large frontal contralateral contrecoup type contusion. Within the right frontal contusion, there are multiple areas of hemorrhage. There is a significant amount of global edema with effacement of the expected sulcal pattern and right to left midline shift with complete effacement of the third ventricle (c) and significant effacement of the right lateral ventricle (d).

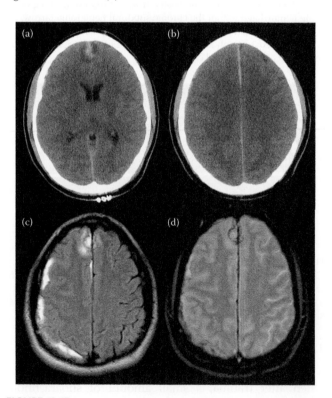

FIGURE 12.17
Contusion along the falx cerebri. Patient with rotational trauma demonstrates a hyperdense contusion focus in the bilateral anterior medial aspect of the frontal lobes, adjacent to the falx cerebri as seen on the CT (a, b) and on the MRI (FLAIR, c, and gradient-echo, d). This happens when the brain hurts against the falx.

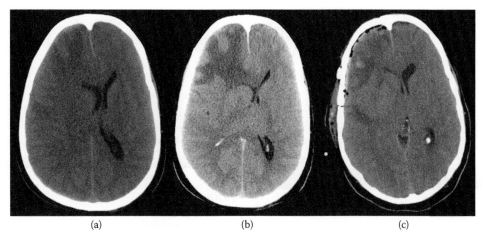

FIGURE 12.18
Increased edema after trauma. Same patient of Figure 12.16. Baseline (a) and follow-up CT images performed 2 days after trauma (b) demonstrate the increased edema and increased mass effect, which have developed in the right frontal region, surrounding the right frontal contusion. This prompted the need for surgical evacuation (postop CT, c).

contusions are hyperdense on CT, rounded, superficial at the level of the gyri, with mass effect and surrounding edema. Contusions are more conspicuous on MRI, especially when they are not hemorrhagic; MRI also has a higher sensitivity for detection of contusions in the basal frontal and temporal lobes, very common sites as previously noted, very obvious using coronal sequences [23]. The edema may increase for several days after the trauma, contributing to an increase in the intracranial pressure (Figure 12.18). After recovery, the lesion shrinks leading to the formation of encephalomalacia with gliosis (Figure 12.19).

12.3.6 Diffuse Axonal Injury

DAI is a type of TBI commonly associated with loss of consciousness and vegetative state. DAI is a shearing injury that develops when the skull undergoes a rapid rotation, causing some parts of the brain to accelerate or decelerate faster than other regions; this results in axonal stretching, edema, and axonal injury [24]. Some anatomical structures are electively involved in case of DAI: the gray–white junction, because the fibers have different environment and hence different inertial force; the body and the splenium of the corpus callosum, which hit the falx cerebri during the movement of the brain; and the dorsolateral midbrain, where the superior cerebellar peduncles are located, in relation to the contact with the tentorial notch. CT is not sensitive to DAI and CT can often be normal in these patients (Figure 12.20); CT is positive only when hemorrhages are present together with the DAI. In these cases, CT shows small regions of hyperattenuation surrounded by a small amount of edema in the above-mentioned locations. But since DAI is often (80% of the times) nonhemorrhagic, DAI is one

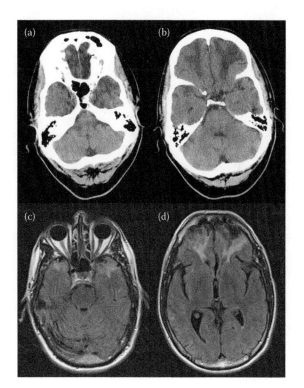

FIGURE 12.19
Chronic traumatic brain injury. Patient with a history of brain trauma 8 years before this scan was acquired. CT scan (a, b) demonstrates extensive low-attenuation changes involving the frontal basal cortex and subcortical white matter with associated volume loss. Similar changes are noted in the temporal poles (a). The findings are compatible with posttraumatic encephalomalacia. FLAIR images from an MRI (c, d), which confirms the above-mentioned findings.

of the few brain traumatic conditions for which MRI is recommended over CT [25] (Figure 12.20); gradient-echo sequence is the most sensitive to evaluate hemorrhagic foci (Figure 12.21).

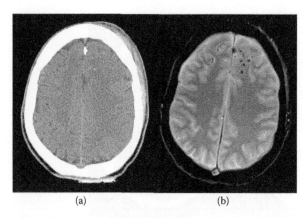

(a)   (b)

FIGURE 12.20
Low sensitivity of CT for DAI. Patient in coma after a major trauma. CT (a) demonstrates soft tissue swelling in the left frontal region and some small foci of hyperdensity within the left frontal lobe. MRI (gradient-echo, b) demonstrates multiple additional foci of susceptibility, more conspicuous compared to the CT.

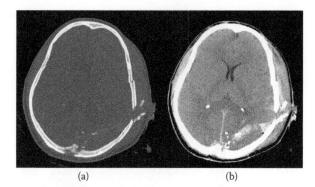

(a)   (b)

FIGURE 12.22
Penetrating injury, CT in bone (a) and brain (b) window. Patient victim of a gunshot. The entry wound is in the left medial parietal region and the exit wound is in the left lateral parietal region. Notice the hemorrhage along the bullet tract.

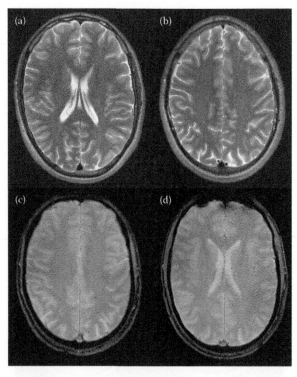

FIGURE 12.21
Gradient-echo to visualize hemorrhagic foci. Patient with DAI and multiple hemorrhagic foci within the brain parenchyma not visible on T2 (a, b) but visualized on the gradient-echo sequence as multiple small black dots (c, d).

12.3.7 Penetrating Injuries

Penetrating injuries are associated with bullets, stab wounds, or bone fragments. This results in a laceration of the brain with high morbidity and mortality (Figure 12.22). The best clinical predictor of outcome is the GCS at admission. If the penetrating injury involves the head and neck, many vital structures

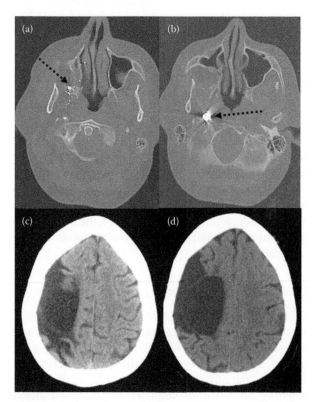

FIGURE 12.23
Internal carotid artery injury and brain ischemic infarction caused by a gunshot injury. CT with bone window at the level of skull base (a, b) and CT of the brain (c, d) without contrast. There is a bullet in the region of the carotid space (arrow, b) just inferior to the skull base, at the level of the C1 segment of the internal carotid artery. Bullet fragments through the pterygoid muscles are also noticed (arrow, a). Extensive encephalomalacia in the right frontal and parietal lobes (c, d) in the distribution of the right middle cerebral artery is related to the prior internal carotid artery traumatic vascular injury and subsequent ischemic infarction.

may be compromised (Figures 12.23 and 12.24). Focal neurologic sign after a neck penetrating injury should suggest a stroke and a CTA should be performed. CT is undoubtedly the best option in these types of patients

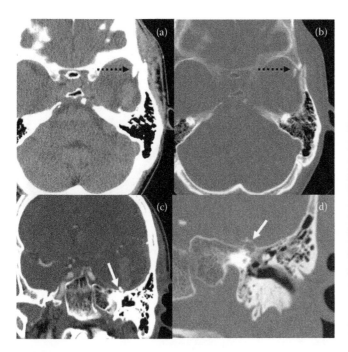

FIGURE 12.24
Knife penetrating injury. Patient with a knife injury presenting with left facial nerve palsy. Knife penetrating injury was through the left middle cranial fossa (arrows in the entry point, a, b) to the left geniculate ganglion. (c, d) The destruction of the bone covering the geniculate ganglion is well seen (arrow pointing to the fracture through the geniculate ganglion).

since it can determine the location and shape of the foreign body [26]. In the event of penetrating injury, the risk of infection should be encountered [27].

12.3.8 Vascular Traumatic Injury

Arterial dissection in the setting of trauma is usually extracranial and caused by a fracture through the carotid canal at the base of the skull (internal carotid artery) and a cervical fracture through the transverse foramina (vertebral artery). Sometimes the dissection can be intracranial, in this case most commonly involving the supraclinoid internal carotid artery. The bifurcation of the anterior cerebral artery in pericallosal and callosomarginal arteries is a highly vulnerable site to vascular injury because of the anatomic relationship with the anterior aspect of the falx cerebri (Figure 12.25) [28].

Traumatic intracranial aneurysms are usually pseudoaneurysm (false aneurysms), in which there is rupture of the layers of the wall of the artery with the surrounding hematoma preventing blood extravasation (Figure 12.26) [29]. Most of traumatic intracranial pseudoaneurysms are located in the anterior circulation, although the posterior circulation can also be affected [30]; the intracranial compartment into which the hemorrhage occurs depends on the location of the segment

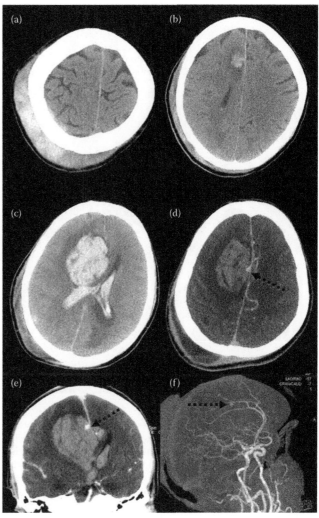

FIGURE 12.25
Posttraumatic pseudoaneurysm. Baseline CT scan (a, b) after trauma demonstrates a right parietal soft tissue swelling and scalp hematoma associated with a contrecoup contusion in the right medial frontal lobe adjacent to the falx cerebri. Ten days later, the patient's status worsens suddenly and a CT (c) demonstrates a large intraparenchymal hemorrhage together with intraventricular hemorrhage. CTA (source images, d, e; maximum intensity projection [MIP] reconstruction, f) demonstrates the relationship of the hematoma with an aneurysm (arrows, d through f) of the pericallosal artery.

of the vessel involved and can hence be extradural (middle meningeal artery) or subarachnoid. The risk of hemorrhage in traumatic pseudoaneurysms is around 20%, and the peak incidence of rupture is 2 weeks after trauma [31].

Another potential vascular complication of head trauma is the carotid cavernous fistula (CCF), which is a pathologic communication between the internal carotid artery and the cavernous sinus. The trauma-related CCF is usually a direct communication, while the indirect type, in which dural branches communicate with the cavernous sinus, is related to other etiologies, such as hypertension, collagen vascular

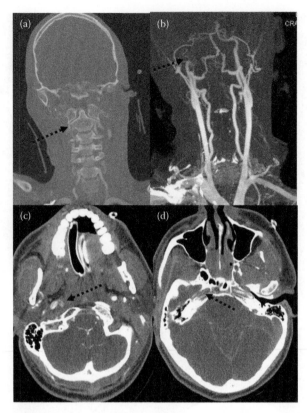

FIGURE 12.26
Posttraumatic internal carotid artery occlusion. Patient status after a motor vehicle accident with a vertebral fracture (arrow, a). There is a right internal carotid artery occlusion associated in the distal cervical segment (arrow, b) and hematoma in the carotid space (arrow, c). No flow is seen in the intracranial petrous segment of the right invasive coronary angiography (ICA) (arrow, d).

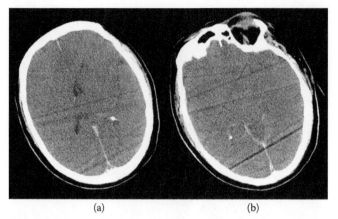

(a) (b)

FIGURE 12.27
Diffuse brain edema, CT. Brain-dead patient after a severe car crash. Notice the diffuse brain swelling (a, b) with no discernible sulci and cistern (b) and with slit-like ventricle (b). There is also diffuse loss of gray–white differentiation.

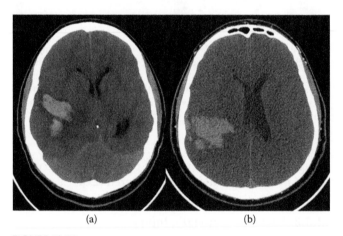

(a) (b)

FIGURE 12.28
Brain death seen on CT. Brain-dead patient with a large intraparenchymal hematoma (a, b). Notice the diffuse brain swelling with loss of gray–white differentiation and the reversal sign in the cerebellum (a), which appears relatively hyperdense compared to the supratentorial brain parenchyma.

disease, or atherosclerosis. Clinically, a CCF manifests with pulsating exophthalmos, orbital bruit, motility disturbance, chemosis, glaucoma, and ultimately vision loss. Notably, CCF is a treatable entity, with endovascular embolization or surgical therapy. CT/CTA findings include proptosis with enlargement of the extraocular muscle and enlargement of the superior ophthalmic vein. The enlargement of the cavernous sinus is sometimes seen. With the use of CTA, the early opacification of the cavernous sinus can be appreciated during the arterial phase. CTA is particularly useful in treatment planning by precisely identifying the location of the fistula relative to surrounding anatomical structures.

12.3.9 Brain Death

Brain death is the worst possible complication of head trauma. Brain death is defined as the complete irreversible cessation of brain function. CT findings include diffuse cerebral edema, swollen gyri, and the reversal

sign. The reversal sign is characterized by reversal of the gray–white matter densities and relatively increased density of the thalami, brainstem, and/or cerebellum (Figures 12.27 and 12.28) [32]. One of the only possible surgical therapies in patient with severe brain edema after trauma is a decompressive craniectomy (Figure 12.29). The absence of cerebral blood flow, which is caused by the increased intracranial pressure and is accepted as a sign of brain death, is classically demonstrated with digital subtraction angiography, although recently the role of CTA has been better defined (Figure 12.30) [33]. The most sensitive accurate CTA criteria for establishing brain death have been described by Frampas et al. with a simplified 4-point score [34]. To use these criteria, three acquisitions have to be performed.

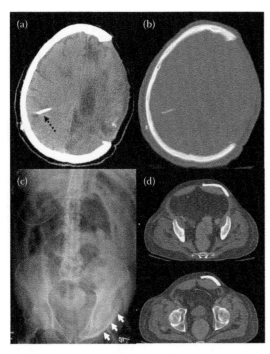

FIGURE 12.29
Decompressive craniectomy in traumatic brain swelling. This patient had a decompressive craniectomy performed in his left hemisphere due to the swelling developed after a severe trauma related to a motor vehicle accident. Notice the intracranial pressure monitoring device on the right (arrow, a). The skull flap is stored in the abdominal wall subcutaneous tissue to maintain its viability and sterility, as seen both on the abdominal x-ray (c, arrows point to the skull flap) and on the abdominal CT (axial images, d, notice the skull flap in the abdominal subcutaneous tissue).

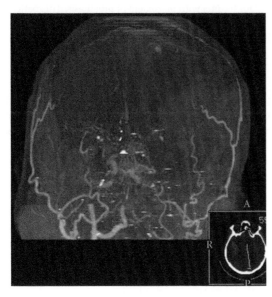

FIGURE 12.30
Brain death seen on CTA. Same patient of Figure 12.28. Brain-dead patient with a large intraparenchymal hematoma. A CTA was done to prove the brain death. CTA demonstrates the lack of flow within the intracranial compartment with preservation of the opacification of the external carotid arteries.

[1] First scan precontrast, followed by contrast injection (IV nonionic contrast medium, 120 mL; concentration 300 mg/mL with a rate = 3 mL/s using a 18G needle.). [2] Second scan with a 20 seconds delay. [3] Third scan with 60 seconds delay. The first scan serves as baseline, and the second scan is to evaluate the opacification of superficial temporal arteries to confirm correct injection. The third scan is the one on which the intracranial vessels, in particular the cortical branches of the two middle cerebral arteries and the two internal cerebral veins, should be assessed for the opacification.

12.3.10 Nonaccidental Trauma

Nonaccidental trauma is the radiology term for child abuse. Attention should be drawn to skull fractures, which, in this setting, result from contact injury. Fractures are usually depressed, cross the midline, are bilateral, and involve the occiput. Shaken baby syndrome is a triad of SDH, retinal hemorrhage, and brain edema caused by intentional shaking, which is often fatal and can cause severe brain damage (Figure 12.31). There is often little evidence of external injury. Retinal hemorrhages are intraretinal or preretinal; the SDHs are often interhemispheric and of different ages. Interhemispheric SDHs are an early and specific finding in Shaken Baby Syndrome [35]. Strangulation can cause hypoxia, producing distinctive CT findings (Figure 12.32): loss of gray–white matter differentiation, diffuse hypodensity of the cortex with frequent preservation of the basal ganglia and cerebellum (white cerebellum sign). Other than being helpful for the diagnosis, imaging provides evidence for potential forensic investigation [36,37].

12.3.11 Orbital Trauma

For orbital trauma, CT is the modality of choice. A useful approach to evaluate the orbit is to start anteriorly and progress posteriorly: first examine the soft tissue, the anterior chamber, and the position of the lens and evaluate the globe including the posterior segment; after that examine the bony orbit for fractures and evaluate for foreign bodies, vessels, and optic nerve; always look for associated intracranial injury. Signs of orbital injury are soft tissue swelling around the region of the trauma: it is around those regions where a fracture can be identified [38]. The location of the fracture is key in the description of orbital trauma. The most common orbital fracture is the blowout fracture, which is caused by a blunt injury directed to the orbit with force being dissipated by a fracture of the surrounding bone, usually the medial orbital wall or the orbital floor. In fractures of the orbital floor, special

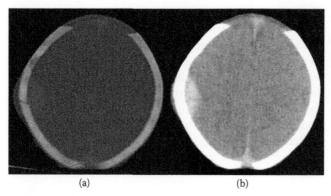

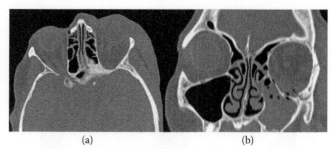

FIGURE 12.31

Child with parietal fracture and underlying epidural hematoma. Unenhanced CT with bone (a) and brain windows (b) demonstrates a fracture of the right parietal bone with a subjacent epidural hematoma.

FIGURE 12.33

Orbital trauma. Patient was punched in the region of the left eye. There is extensive soft tissue swelling and hematoma in the left temporal region with proptosis seen on the axial image (a). The coronal reconstruction (b) demonstrates a fracture of the left orbital floor, associated with intraorbital hematoma, orbital emphysema, and opacification of the left maxillary sinus. In this kind of fracture, attention must be drawn to the inferior rectus muscle to identify entrapment.

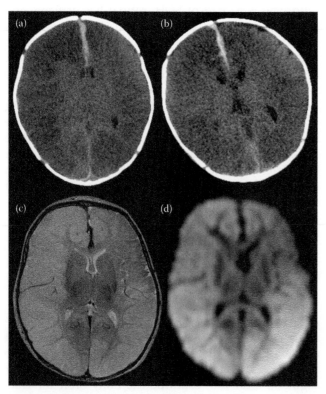

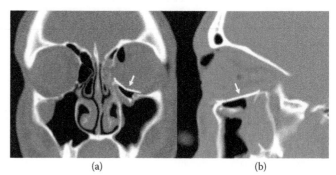

FIGURE 12.34

Orbital floor trauma with placement of prosthesis. This patient had a fracture of the orbital floor and was surgically treated with placement of a prosthesis (arrows, a, b).

FIGURE 12.32

Child abuse, CT, and MRI. Seven-week-old infant status post-strangulation. Unenhanced CT (a, b) demonstrates interhemishperic subdural hematoma (early and specific finding of nonaccidental trauma) extensive bilateral loss of the gray–white matter differentiation and diffuse sulcal effacement indicating diffuse hypoxic/ischemic brain injury, indicating strangulation. There is relative sparing of the basal ganglia and a few portions of both cerebral hemispheres. Subdural hemorrhage is noted in the interhemispheric fissure and subarachnoid hemorrhage in the medial right frontal sulcus. MRI with T2 (c) and diffusion weighted imaging (d) sequences demonstrates the cortical swelling with diffusion restriction, thus confirming the hypoxic-ischemic injury.

attention must be drawn to the inferior rectus muscle to identify entrapment (Figure 12.33). For fractures of the orbital floor, plating is a recognized therapeutic option, which can be accomplished using different materials (Figure 12.34). When the medial wall of the orbit is fractured, typically the lamina papyracea is involved. Findings associated with fracture include retro-orbital hematoma, subperiosteal hematoma, or muscle entrapment (Figure 12.35).

In traumatic hyphema, CT images may show increased attenuation in the anterior chamber, with a decreased volume of the anterior chamber, compared to that of the contralateral normal globe [38].

In case of an open-globe injury, CT findings include a change in globe contour, intraocular air, or intraocular foreign bodies. Chronic appearance of an open-globe injury can appear as a shrunken calcified "lump," also known as phthisis bulbi.

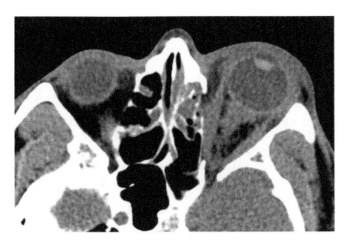

FIGURE 12.35
Retrobulbar hematoma. CT in a patient with orbital trauma demonstrates a retro-orbital hematoma just posteriorly to the left globe in the region of the optic nerve.

12.4 Summary

This chapter described the different types of intracranial injuries that can be seen in patients after head trauma. CT is the most useful technique for initial evaluation of head trauma patients, although MRI should be considered in some particular cases.

References

1. Corrigan JD, Selassie AW, Orman JAL. The epidemiology of traumatic brain injury. *J Head Trauma Rehabil* 2010; 25: 72–80.
2. Gentry LR. Imaging of closed head injury. *Radiology* 1994; 191: 1–17.
3. Brown AW, Elovic EP, Kothari S, Flanagan SR, Kwasnica C. Congenital and acquired brain injury. 1. Epidemiology, pathophysiology, prognostication, innovative treatments, and prevention. *Arch Phys Med Rehabil* 2008; 89: S3–S8.
4. Teasdale G, Jennett B. Assessment of coma and impaired consciousness. A practical scale. *Lancet* 1974; 2: 81–84.
5. Davis PC, Drayer BP, Anderson RE, Braffman B, Deck MD, Hasso AN et al. Head trauma. American college of radiology. ACR appropriateness criteria. *Radiology* 2000; 215 (Suppl): 507–524.
6. Haydel MJ, Preston CA, Mills TJ, Luber S, Blaudeau E, DeBlieux PM. Indications for computed tomography in patients with minor head injury. *N Engl J Med* 2000; 343: 100–105.
7. Stein SC, Spettell C, Young G, Ross SE. Delayed and progressive brain injury in closed-head trauma: radiological demonstration. *Neurosurgery* 1993; 32: 25–30; discussion 30–21.
8. Mogbo KI, Slovis TL, Canady AI, Allasio DJ, Arfken CL. Appropriate imaging in children with skull fractures and suspicion of abuse. *Radiology* 1998; 208: 521–524.
9. Lloyd DA, Carty H, Patterson M, Butcher CK, Roe D. Predictive value of skull radiography for intracranial injury in children with blunt head injury. *Lancet* 1997; 349: 821–824.
10. Sanchez T, Stewart D, Walvick M, Swischuk L. Skull fracture vs. accessory sutures: how can we tell the difference? *Emerg Radiol* 2010; 17: 413–418.
11. Kubal WS. Updated imaging of traumatic brain injury. *Radiol Clin North Am* 2012; 50: 15–41.
12. Bullock MR, Chesnut R, Ghajar J, Gordon D, Hartl R, Newell DW et al. Surgical management of depressed cranial fractures. *Neurosurgery* 2006; 58: S56–S60; discussion Si–Siv.
13. Ciurea AV, Gorgan MR, Tascu A, Sandu AM, Rizea RE. Traumatic brain injury in infants and toddlers, 0–3 years old. *J Med Life* 2011; 4: 234–243.
14. Merino-deVillasante J, Taveras JM. Computerized tomography (CT) in acute head trauma. *AJR Am J Roentgenol* 1976; 126: 765–778.
15. Al-Nakshabandi NA. The swirl sign. *Radiology* 2001; 218: 433.
16. Provenzale J. CT and MR imaging of acute cranial trauma. *Emerg Radiol* 2007; 14: 1–12.
17. Gean AD, Fischbein NJ, Purcell DD, Aiken AH, Manley GT, Stiver SI. Benign anterior temporal epidural hematoma: indolent lesion with a characteristic CT imaging appearance after blunt head trauma. *Radiology* 2010; 257: 212–218.
18. Hellwig D, Kuhn TJ, Bauer BL, List-Hellwig E. Endoscopic treatment of septated chronic subdural hematoma. *Surg Neurol* 1996; 45: 272–277.
19. Penchet G, Loiseau H, Castel JP. Chronic bilateral subdural hematomas. *Neurochirurgie* 1998; 44: 247–252.
20. Gilad R, Fatterpekar GM, Johnson DM, Patel AB. Migrating subdural hematoma without subarachnoid hemorrhage in the case of a patient with a ruptured aneurysm in the intrasellar anterior communicating artery. *Am J Neuroradiol* 2007; 28: 2014–2016.
21. Lu L, Zhang LJ, Poon CS, Wu SY, Zhou CS, Luo S, Wang M, Lu GM. Digital subtraction CT angiography for detection of intracranial aneurysms: comparison with three-dimensional digital subtraction angiography. *Radiology* 2012; 262: 605–612.
22. Yuzawa H, Higano S, Mugikura S, Umetsu A, Murata T, Nakagawa A, Koyama A, Takahashi S. Pseudo-subarachnoid hemorrhage found in patients with postresuscitation encephalopathy: characteristics of CT findings and clinical importance. *Am J Neuroradiol* 2008; 29: 1544–1549.
23. Hähnel S, Stippich C, Weber I, Darm H, Schill T, Jost J et al. Prevalence of cerebral microhemorrhages in amateur boxers as detected by 3T MR imaging. *Am J Neuroradiol* 2008; 29: 388–391.
24. Li X-Y, Feng D-F. Diffuse axonal injury: novel insights into detection and treatment. *J Clin Neurosci* 2009; 16: 614–619.

25. You JS, Kim SW, Lee HS, Chung SP. Use of diffusion-weighted MRI in the emergency department for unconscious trauma patients with negative brain CT. *Emerg Med J* 2010; 27: 131–132.
26. Provenzale JM. Imaging of traumatic brain injury: a review of the recent medical literature. *Am J Roentgenol* 2010; 194: 16–19.
27. Wellwood J, Alcantara A, Michael DB. Neurotrauma: the role of CT angiogram. *Neurol Res* 2002; 24 (Suppl 1): S13–S16.
28. Soria ED, Paroski MW, Schamann ME. Traumatic aneurysms of cerebral vessels: a case study and review of the literature. *Angiology* 1988; 39: 609–615.
29. Acosta C, Williams PE, Clark K. Traumatic aneurysms of the cerebral vessels. *J Neurosurg* 1972; 36: 531–536.
30. Nakstad P, Nornes H, Hauge HN. Traumatic aneurysms of the pericallosal arteries. *Neuroradiology* 1986; 28: 335–338.
31. Cohen JE, Gomori JM, Segal R et al. Results of endovascular treatment of traumatic intracranial aneurysms. *Neurosurgery* 2008; 63: 476–485; discussion 485–486.
32. Han BK, Towbin RB, De Courten-Myers G, McLaurin RL, Ball WS. Reversal sign on CT: effect of anoxic/ischemic cerebral injury in children. *Am J Neuroradiol* 1989; 10: 1191–1198.
33. Wijdicks EFM. The case against confirmatory tests for determining brain death in adults. *Neurology* 2010; 75: 77–83.
34. Frampas E, Videcoq M, de Kerviler E, Ricolfi F, Kuoch V, Mourey F et al. CT angiography for brain death diagnosis. *Am J Neuroradiol* 2009; 30: 1566–1570.
35. Oehmichen M, Meissner C, Saternus K-S. Fall or shaken: traumatic brain injury in children caused by falls or abuse at home—a review on biomechanics and diagnosis. *Neuropediatrics* 2005; 36: 240–245.
36. Hoskote A, Richards P, Anslow P, McShane T. Subdural haematoma and non-accidental head injury in children. *Childs Nerv Syst* 2002; 18: 311–317.
37. Jaspan T, Griffiths PD, McConachie NS, Punt JAG. Neuroimaging for non-accidental head injury in childhood: a proposed protocol. *Clin Radiol* 2003; 58: 44–53.
38. Kubal WS. Imaging of orbital trauma. *Radiographics* 2008; 28: 1729–1739.

Section III

Cardiovascular System

13

Coronary Artery Imaging

Robert Donnino and Monvadi B. Srichai

CONTENTS

13.1 Introduction

Coronary artery disease (CAD) is one of the leading causes of morbidity and mortality throughout the world [1]. Detection of the presence and extent of CAD has become an integral part of the clinical care and management for patients with known or suspected CAD. Directly imaging the coronary arteries poses unique challenges for imaging technology, because of their relatively small size (1–5 mm in diameter) and constant motion. In the 1980s, electron beam computed tomography (EBCT) was employed to perform cardiac studies (most notably coronary calcium scoring). While EBCT was well suited to imaging coronary arteries, given its excellent temporal resolution, the relatively high cost and limited use (primarily cardiac studies) led to the widespread replacement of EBCT by multi-detector computed tomography (MDCT). This chapter focuses primarily on MDCT; as

in current practice, EBCT is used less frequently. Since the development of the first MDCT in the late 1990s, this technology has evolved to make noninvasive imaging of the coronary arteries feasible and reliable, and coronary computed tomography angiography (CCTA) continues to play an increasingly important role in clinical practice.

13.2 Technological Considerations

Technological advancement of computed tomography (CT) for coronary imaging has been very rapid over the past decade and continues to evolve at a rapid pace. Significant advances have been made to both improve image quality and reduce patient radiation exposure. It is important to note that MDCT systems and their capabilities vary significantly depending on the manufacturer, model, and other factors. Although some notable features of certain scanners are mentioned, in-depth discussion and comparison of available technologies are not covered in this chapter.

13.2.1 Electrocardiographic Gating

Because of the constant motion of the coronary arteries, electrocardiographic (ECG) gating is required for all coronary CT imaging. ECG synchronization is generally achieved by detection of the R wave on the ECG signal (Figure 13.1). The "R-R interval" is the time between

consecutive R waves (i.e., QRS complexes). Timing of image acquisition or image reconstructions is often expressed as a percent of this interval (e.g., 50% of the R-R interval would be half way between two consecutive R waves). Alternatively, the timing may be expressed as the actual delay time (e.g., "450 ms" would be 450 ms after the R wave and "–450 ms" would be 450 ms before the R wave). ECG gating usually employs one of two types of gating techniques: (1) retrospective or (2) prospective gating.

For retrospective gating (Figure 13.2), image acquisition is achieved through conventional spiral imaging with simultaneous recording of the ECG over several heartbeats (usually 6–10 beats). The pitch is often set very low, depending on the heart rate. Images can then be reconstructed retrospectively, at one or more phases of the cardiac cycle (i.e., of the R-R interval). Since image acquisition is performed throughout the R-R interval, reconstructions can be made at any phase of the cardiac cycle. The cardiac phase or phases least affected by cardiac motion artifact can then be chosen for image interpretation.

When prospective triggering is used, the data acquisition is triggered by a prespecified time or phase of the cardiac cycle and is often performed in conjunction with step and shoot (axial) scan mode over several heartbeats (Figure 13.3). This acquisition can be done at a single phase of the cardiac cycle (e.g., 75% of the R-R interval) or across a range of phases (e.g., 60%–80%

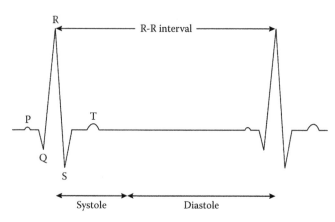

FIGURE 13.1
Basic ECG tracing.

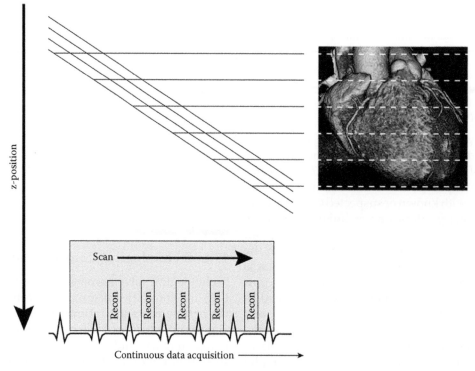

FIGURE 13.2
Retrospective gating with helical scan acquisition and image reconstruction (Recon) relative to ECG tracing.

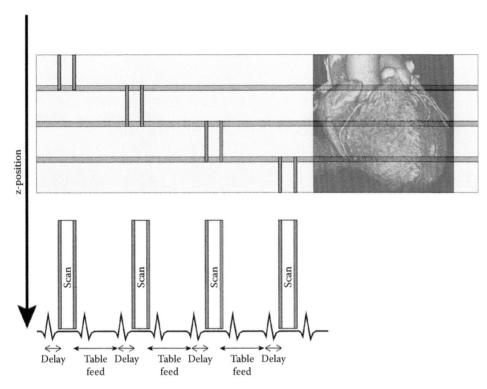

FIGURE 13.3
Prospective triggering with axial, step and shoot, scan acquisition, and corresponding image reconstruction. Scan indicates the minimum acquisition time needed to generate an image (half the gantry rotation time). The gray bars on either side indicate the addition of "padding" to the scan acquisition.

of the R-R interval) sometimes denoted as "padding" (Figure 13.3). The interval that is set for acquisition is typically in mid-to-late diastole, as coronary motion artifact is most prominent outside of these time frames (although this may not be the case at higher heart rates, as discussed in Section 13.2.6). The disadvantage of this technique is that the image reconstructions are limited to the prespecified phase (or range of phases) of the cardiac cycle. Also, with this more limited dataset, it is often impossible to compensate for an arrhythmia (e.g., an unexpected premature beat) that may occur during acquisition, although some scanner models have developed specific algorithms to compensate for arrhythmias. Finally, functional data such as the left ventricular ejection fraction is usually not possible when prospective gating is used. The advantage of prospective gating, however, is the significant reduction in radiation exposure that is achieved with this technique, particularly when very little or no padding is used [2–4].

13.2.2 Temporal Resolution

Temporal resolution refers to the amount of time necessary to acquire enough data to generate an image. Temporal resolution is less of a concern when imaging a stationary object or organ. When imaging the constantly moving coronary arteries, however, excellent temporal resolution is necessary to avoid blurring of the images. For MDCT, temporal resolution is largely dependent on the rotation speed of the gantry; however, other imaging parameters are also important. A gantry rotation of 180° is necessary to produce a complete two-dimensional (2D) image (using standard half-scan reconstruction). Thus, an estimate of temporal resolution for most scanners is simply the amount of time needed for the gantry to rotate half of a complete rotation (e.g., 175 ms for a scanner with a 350-ms gantry rotation time). The utilization of multicycle reconstruction can significantly improve the effective temporal resolution by merging the datasets from several different heartbeats to create a single image (Figure 13.4). This strategy, however, is susceptible to image artifacts from slight beat-to-beat changes in cardiac position, even when ECG gating is employed. Dual-source scanners use two sets of sources and detector rows positioned at 90° angles to each other within the gantry. Both of these sources acquire images simultaneously, allowing complete images to be reconstructed after only a 90° rotation of the gantry. This improves the effective temporal resolution of the scanner to one-fourth of the gantry rotation time (e.g., 75–83 ms for gantry rotations of 300–330 ms).

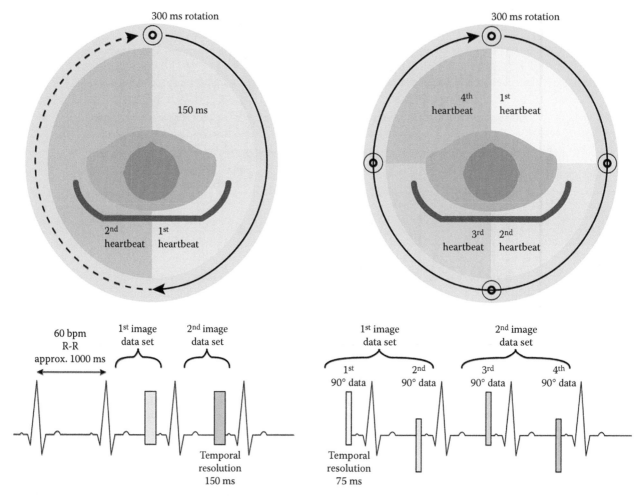

FIGURE 13.4
Single (left) and multisegment (right) reconstruction schemes.

13.2.3 Heart Rate

Given the limitations of temporal resolution with CT, patient heart rates of less than 60–65 beats/min are usually recommended for optimal image quality (for single-source systems). If necessary, temporary reduction of the heart rate is usually achieved by the administration of beta-adrenergic blocking agents (or calcium channel blockers), given to the patient before the scan. While institutional algorithms vary, it is reasonable to administer beta-blockers (e.g., 50–100 mg metoprolol tartrate) at least one hour before the scan for patients with heart rates >65–70 beats/min. For higher heart rates, some protocols include an initial dose 12 hours before the scan, with a second dose 1 hour prior. If the heart rate remains >65 beats/min at the time of the study, additional beta-blocker can be given intravenously (e.g., 5 mg intravenous metoprolol every five minutes). If any rate control agent is administered intravenously, patients should first be placed on a cardiac monitor, and blood pressures should be checked before each administration. While generally well tolerated, patients should be screened for potential contraindications such as a known allergic reaction or significant bronchospastic disease before administration. Because beta-blockers can exacerbate bronchospasm, patients with significant bronchospastic disease (e.g., asthma) can be given a calcium channel blocker (e.g., diltiazem) as an alternative. Beta-blockers and calcium channel blockers have the added advantage of being able to suppress ectopic beats (e.g., premature ventricular contractions) that can affect image quality; however, adequate suppression does not always occur. Both of these agents should be used with caution in patients with low blood pressure (e.g., systolic <100 mm Hg) or acutely ill patients (e.g., those with decompensated heart failure or severe aortic valve insufficiency).

It is important to keep in mind that patients' heart rates will change with breath-holding. Before the intravenous administration of agents for heart rate control, a "practice" breath-hold should be performed to evaluate the heart rate during full inspiration. Although the heart rate will usually decrease (by up to 5–10 beats/min or more), this is not consistent, and it may actually increase in some patients. Also important to note is that the heart rate generally increases slightly after the administration of sublingual nitroglycerin and may increase further as the contrast injection begins. Therefore, a goal heart rate just before the scan (e.g., 60 beats/min) should be approximately 5 beats/min slower than the desired heart rate for the scan.

13.2.4 Spatial Resolution

Spatial resolution is the minimum distance needed to view two objects as separate objects. Since small coronary arteries and branch vessels can measure less than 2 mm in diameter, spatial resolution is important for visualization of both vessel lumen and atherosclerotic plaques. Current generation MDCT scanners can acquire images with a slice thickness as thin as 0.5 mm and can generate nearly isotropic voxels as small as 0.35 × 0.35 × 0.35 mm. Isotropic voxels allow for image manipulation in multiple planes with minimal image distortion. Nitrates (e.g., sublingual nitroglycerin) are usually administered just before the scan for coronary vasodilatation providing optimal vessel visualization. Nitrates may cause transient hypotension but are generally well tolerated when administered in the supine position. Before administration, patients should have blood pressure monitoring. Nitrates also commonly cause a mild headache that is self-limiting. Patients should be appropriately screened for any contraindications such as a known allergic reaction or the recent use of phosphodiesterase inhibitors (e.g., sildenafil). Nitrates should be given cautiously to patients with low blood pressure (e.g., systolic <100 mm Hg), especially if given with concomitant beta-blocker administration.

13.2.5 Contrast Administration

Administration of intravenous iodinated contrast is necessary for CCTA; however, it is not used for coronary calcium scoring. For CCTA, contrast agents with high iodine concentrations are recommended for the high contrast-to-noise ratio necessary for optimal image quality [5]. Nonionic agents are also advantageous to avoid subtle heart rate alterations during image acquisition. Depending on individual manufacturers, models, and protocols, contrast rates range from 4 to 7 mL/s and total contrast volumes usually range from 50 to 120 mL. Dual-head pumps allow for the injection of saline (40–50 mL) immediately following the contrast injection (at the same rate as the contrast injection) to maximize contrast enhancement of the coronary arteries (Figure 13.5). If some opacification of the right heart is desired, a mixture of contrast and saline may be substituted for saline or triphasic injections may be employed (e.g., contrast, followed by contrast/saline mixture, followed by saline) (Figure 13.6).

With the short scan times in CCTA, accurate timing of the contrast agent is essential. One of two methods

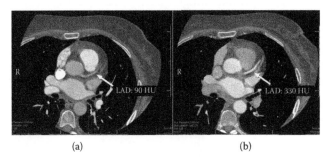

(a)   (b)

FIGURE 13.5
Example of poor (a) and good (b) contrast opacification of the coronary artery.

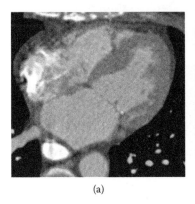 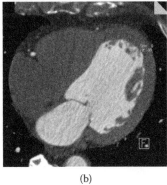 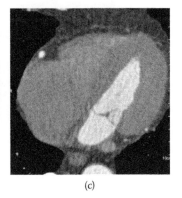

(a)   (b)   (c)

FIGURE 13.6
Examples of different contrast administration protocols. (a) With single-phase contrast-only protocols, mixing of high-attenuation contrast with unopacified blood in the right atrium often causes streak artifact that may impair visualization of the right coronary artery. (b) With dual-phase contrast-saline protocols, lack of contrast in the right heart improves evaluation of the right coronary artery, but limits evaluation of the right-sided heart structures. (c) With triple-phase contrast-saline protocols, low-attenuation contrast in the right heart allows for visualization of right heart structures without corresponding streak artifact often noted with single-phase protocols.

for contrast timing is recommended for coronary studies. Using the "bolus tracking" method, sample images are taken every 1–2 seconds at a region of interest (e.g., ascending or descending aorta) during the contrast injection. When enhancement in the region of interest reaches a prespecified level (e.g., 180 HU), the scanner is automatically triggered to begin scanning. The "test bolus" method involves injecting a small amount of contrast (e.g., 10 mL) intravenously while sampling images every 1–2 seconds in the region of interest (e.g., ascending aorta) to determine the time of peak enhancement. This time is then used for the full contrast injection, usually with an additional 2–3-second delay for the contrast to reach to coronary arteries, when the ascending aorta is used as the region of interest.

13.2.6 Postprocessing

Image reconstruction is a necessary step, converting raw data into viewable images. This can be done in a semiautomated manner, but initial set-up protocols and occasionally individual adjustments need to be made for optimal image quality. One goal of reconstruction is to process images from the cardiac phase with the least amount of motion or other artifact. Typically, images from mid-diastole, usually 70%–75% of the R-R interval, yield the best images for evaluation (depending slightly on the scanner manufacturer)

(Figure 13.7). Sometimes, however, optimal images may be found at end systole (approximately 35%–40% of the R-R interval), particularly of the right coronary artery (RCA). These end-systolic images are often optimal when heart rates are relatively high (e.g., >70 beats/min) [6–8]. At times, more than one phase may be necessary for optimal evaluation of different coronary arteries (e.g., end-systolic phase for the right coronary and mid-diastolic phase for the left coronary system) or even for different segments of a given artery. Most vendors have automatic algorithms that reconstruct images at the optimal phase for evaluation. These algorithms are not always accurate, however, and reconstructions at additional phases should be made manually if image quality is suboptimal because of motion artifact.

For coronary evaluation, field of view of the reconstructions should be generally limited to the smallest diameter possible that includes the cardiac structures. With the spatial resolution of most scanners at 0.4–0.5 mm, field of view should be reconstructed at no more than 20–25 cm for optimal viewing (assuming a standard 512 × 512 matrix is used) (Figure 13.8). Axial slice thickness is generally set at the thinnest slices possible. In patients with increased image noise (e.g., obese patients), however, using slightly thicker slice widths may produce better image quality.

The reconstruction convolution kernel can be adjusted to improve the "sharpness" of the image. Softer kernels

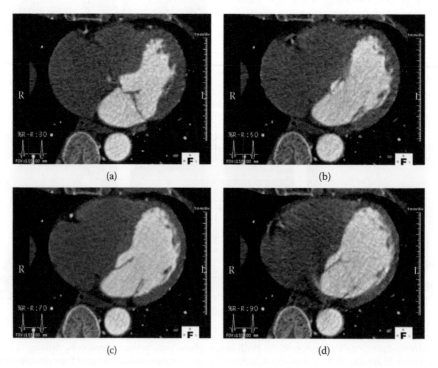

(a) (b)

(c) (d)

FIGURE 13.7
Image reconstruction at different phases of the cardiac cycle including (a) 30%, (b) 50%, (c) 70%, and (d) 90% phases. The 70% phase represents the best phase for interpretation given the least amount of motion in the right coronary artery.

will minimize noise and may be ideal for obese patients, but with lower spatial resolution. Sharper kernels improve spatial resolution, but with increased image noise. Images with extensive calcification and/or intracoronary stents may be better visualized at sharper kernels (Figure 13.9).

Finally, artifact from inconsistent ECG gating or the presence of an ectopic beat during the scan can cause misregistration artifact and render images unevaluable or give the false impression that there is a vessel stenosis. Most manufacturers offer ECG editing functions that can minimize this artifact through manual manipulation or "rejection" of the abnormal beats. This may not be possible if prospective ECG gating is used.

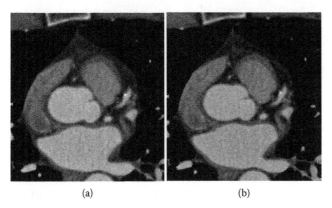

(a)   (b)

FIGURE 13.8
Comparison between (a) large field-of-view and (b) small field-of-view reconstructions with 512 × 512 matrix. There is demonstrable improvement in the spatial resolution with the small field-of-view reconstruction compared with the large field-of-view reconstruction (zoomed to demonstrate similar structures).

13.2.7 Image Interpretation

Evaluation of coronary calcium scores is done in a semi-automated manner, which differs between software packages, but usually involves the transaxial images with little or no additional reformations (Figure 13.10).

Evaluation of the coronaries on CCTA requires image manipulation and significantly greater skill on the part of the interpreter. Given the nonlinear nature of the coronary arteries and eccentric presence of coronary plaques, visualizing the arteries and plaques from different planes are often essential for accurate image interpretation. Isotropic voxels allow for the multiplanar reformation (MPR) with minimal image distortion. Most processing software will display three orthogonal views simultaneously, allowing manual manipulation for optimal view of each coronary segment. Curved MPR images are often created by an automated or semi-automated algorithm. These images often display the entire coronary vessel in a single 2D image, with the ability to rotate the artery around a focal point. This view is often helpful for interpretation; however, the curved reformation can cause artificial vessel distortion and may inaccurately track the vessel centerline. Abnormalities or suspected artifact seen on these reformations can be confirmed through transaxial and/or manually manipulated straight MPR (Figure 13.10).

Maximum-intensity projections (MIP) are created using thicker sections and can be helpful to visualize a longer segment of a vessel or to reduce the appearance of image noise. Because there is a loss of image information with thicker sections, lesions detected using MIP should be further evaluated using MPR. Three-dimensional (3D) volume rendered images of the coronaries or whole

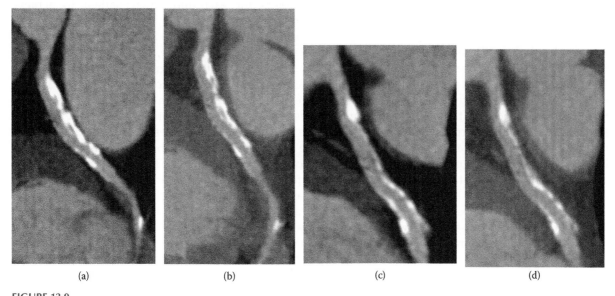

(a)   (b)   (c)   (d)

FIGURE 13.9
(a, c) Medium-soft and (b, d) medium sharp reconstruction kernels demonstrate slightly decreased blooming artifact with the calcified plaques using the sharper reconstruction kernel.

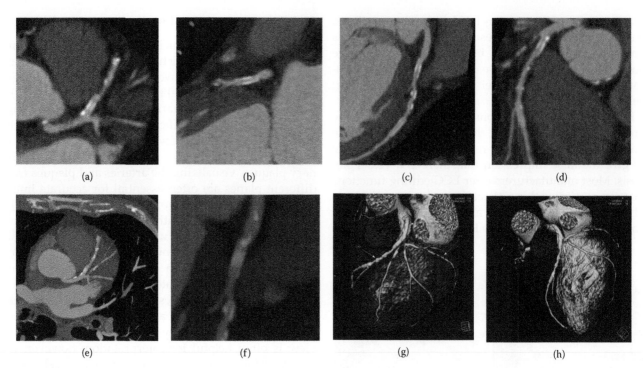

FIGURE 13.10
Different image postprocessing techniques used in the evaluation of coronary arteries including (a, b) straight multiplanar reformations, (c, d) curved multiplanar reformations, (e, f) thin maximum-intensity projection reformations, and (g, h) 3D volume rendered techniques.

heart with the exclusion of surrounding structures such as bones, lung tissue, and extracardiac vessels can be generated as well (Figure 13.10). These images may be helpful when interpreting structural relationships such as vessel course in complicated cases (e.g., congenital anomalies or coronary bypass grafts). These surface renderings should not be used for estimation of vessel stenosis.

13.2.8 Radiation Exposure

The exposure to ionizing radiation during CT imaging and its potential effects on the body have received a great deal of attention in recent years. This has been particularly so for CCTA. Although the true effect of low-level ionizing radiation on the body is difficult to assess [9], several recent reports estimate a significant cancer risk because of radiation exposure from CCTA [10]. With the expansion of the use of CCTA, it is critical for the operator to take steps to reduce radiation dose.

Many different strategies have been employed to reduce the radiation exposure associated with CCTA [11]. One obvious way to reduce radiation exposure is to reduce the number of unnecessary studies being performed. While patient care must be individualized, current recommendations serve as an important guide for appropriate patient selection [12]. Some dose reduction strategies are specific to certain manufacturers

and models while others are more broadly applicable. While limiting the radiation exposure may diminish image quality, any viable dose reduction strategy must not compromise the high diagnostic capabilities of CCTA. Thus, a strategy to lower radiation dose as much as possible but still maintain diagnostic images is essential. Many dose reduction strategies require careful attention of the operator to adjust the scan parameters for each individual patient to achieve this goal. A prime example is the gating mode used. As described in Section 13.2.1, gating can be either retrospective or prospective, with prospective gating exposing the patient to a significantly lower radiation dose. Because of the limitations of prospective gating, however, retrospective gating may be desired or necessary. When retrospective gating is employed, dose modulation techniques should be used. With dose modulation, the scan operator sets the range of the cardiac cycle (i.e., the R-R interval) during which the tube will be running at full power. During the remainder of the cardiac cycle, the tube current is significantly reduced (e.g., by approximately 80%). This allows maximal image quality during a time when the coronaries can be assessed with the least amount of motion artifact (typically between mid-to-late diastole, as discussed in Section 13.2.6). During the remainder of the cardiac cycle, the image quality is significantly diminished; however, it is of sufficient quality to evaluate left ventricular wall motion and ejection fraction.

Another important strategy employed to reduce radiation exposure is the use of reduced tube voltage. For CCTA, the tube voltage is most commonly set at 120 kV. Since radiation dose is proportional to the square of the tube potential, a reduction to 100 kV will reduce the radiation dose by approximately 30% [13]. While this will increase image noise (and reduce signal-to-noise ratio), multiple studies have shown this to provide adequate image quality in nonobese patients [14,15]. Many labs use specific cutoffs for body weight and/or body mass index (e.g., ≤28 or ≤30 kg/m²) to determine when to reduce the voltage to 100 kV, although ideal cutoffs may differ between labs because of differences in scanner type and other parameters. Further reduction of voltage to 80 kV in nonobese patients has been studied experimentally and warrants further investigation [16,17]. Tube current can also be adjusted based on patient size, with higher current necessary for larger patients. Many scanners now offer automatic, dynamic exposure control, which adjusts the current based on the changing tissue density throughout the scan length. Based on information from the topogram images, the system will increase or decrease the current for more or less dense tissue, respectively. These automated adjustments can reduce radiation dose up to 20% in thoracic studies [18].

Reducing scan length (in the z-direction) will also minimize radiation exposure. The minimum length necessary to cover the coronary arteries should always be used. If a noncontrast scan is performed for coronary calcium before the CCTA, the images can be used to visualize the coronaries arteries and shorten the length of the CCTA to the minimum necessary. Patients with coronary bypass grafts involving an internal mammary artery will be exposed to higher radiation doses because of longer scan lengths.

Two additional dose reduction strategies are worth mentioning briefly; however, they are available only for specific, newer generation scanners. First, 320-detector row volume scanners can acquire whole heart imaging in a single heartbeat and can lower the effective radiation exposure by up to 90% [19]. Newer generation dual-source scanners employ a very high pitch (up to 3.4) acquisition technique, made possible by the high temporal resolution of these scanners. These scans can also reduce radiation exposure by over 90% and can acquire diagnostic images of the coronary arteries at less than 1 mSv in nonobese patients [20–22].

Postprocessing techniques are being developed to improve image quality and reduce noise, to allow for diagnostic image acquisition at lower tube potential and current. Iterative reconstruction algorithms differ between scanner and software developers but hold promise for the future [23–25].

Women are at higher risk for potential consequences of cancer development because of breast exposure. The routine use of breast shields for reducing radiation exposure in CCTA remains controversial. Studies using breast shields for CCTA are lacking, and shields may increase image noise. Thus, the above-outlined radiation-lowering techniques are generally favored over routine breast shield use [11]; however, continued investigation is certainly warranted [26,27]. Younger patients are also at higher risk for cancer development because of the potential long length of time necessary for a malignancy to develop after radiation exposure, as well as the higher rate of cell division in young patients. In the pediatric population, other modalities, such as ultrasound or cardiac magnetic resonance imaging (MRI), should be considered as an alternative to CT if possible, especially if repeat testing is anticipated.

13.3 Coronary Anatomy

The anatomy of the coronary arterial tree varies in different individuals and may not precisely follow typical descriptions. Only a small number of common variants will be mentioned. Most commonly, two coronary arteries arise from the aortic sinuses (or sinuses of Valsalva): the RCA from the right aortic sinus and the left main coronary artery (also known as the left coronary artery) from the left aortic sinus (Figures 13.11 through 13.15). The left main artery is typically large in caliber (4–5 mm) and is variable in length (usually from 1 to 20 mm) as it bifurcates into the left anterior descending (LAD) and left circumflex (LCX) arteries. In approximately 15% of individuals, a third branch occurs at this site and is referred to as the ramus intermedius (Figure 13.14). Recommended guidelines for coronary anatomy

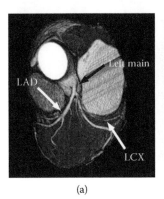 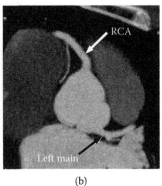

(a)   (b)

FIGURE 13.11
The left main coronary artery on a 3D volume rendered image (a), and a maximal intensity projection image (b).

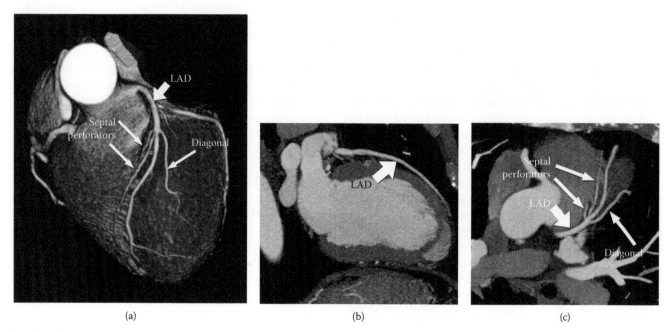

(a)   (b)   (c)

FIGURE 13.12
The left anterior descending artery with branch arteries on a 3D volume rendered image (a), and maximal intensity projection images (b, c).

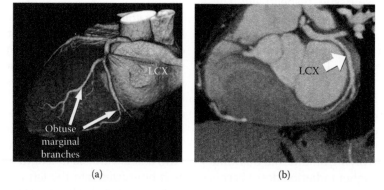

(a)   (b)

FIGURE 13.13
The left circumflex artery with branch arteries on a 3D volume rendered image (a), and a maximal intensity projection image (b).

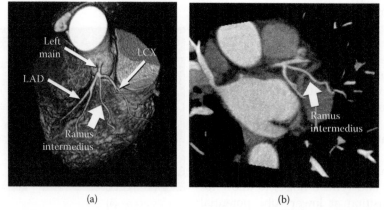

(a)   (b)

FIGURE 13.14
The ramus intermedius on a 3D volume rendered image (a), and a maximal intensity projection image (b).

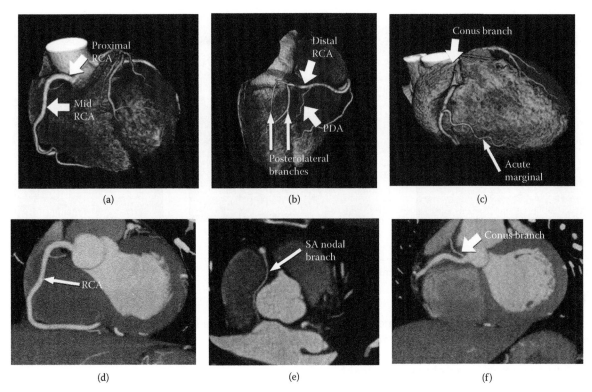

FIGURE 13.15
The right coronary artery with branch arteries on a 3D volume rendered images (a through c), and maximal intensity projection images (d through f).

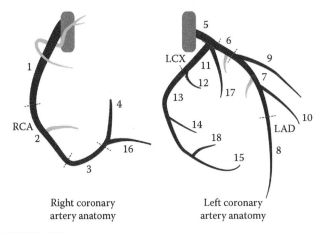

FIGURE 13.16
Standard coronary segmentation scheme.

segmental nomenclature for CCTA [28] (Figure 13.16) have been adapted almost identically from the American Heart Association model standardized previously for invasive angiography [29].

With its long course and branch vessels, the blood supply from LAD subtends a large area of the LV. The LAD courses anteriorly between the left and right ventricles in the interventricular groove and continues to follow in this course to the apex of the heart (Figure 13.12). Several

branch vessels arise from the LAD. Diagonal branches arise from the LAD and course laterally across the anterior and anterolateral segments of the left ventricle. The number of diagonal branches is variable (usually 1–4) and are ordered "first," "second," and so on, starting with the most proximal branch. The size of each diagonal is also quite variable, and frequently, one or more diagonal branches are too small in caliber for accurate plaque evaluation by CCTA. Also arising from the LAD are several septal perforator branches. These arteries course medially and dive into the interventricular septum that they subtend. These branches are frequently too small for CCTA evaluation. For anatomical nomenclature, the LAD is usually divided into three segments (proximal, mid, and distal). The proximal segment extends from the origin to the first diagonal or first septal branch (whichever is more proximal). The remaining length of the LAD can be split in half to describe the mid and distal segments. A portion of the LAD may take an intramuscular course into the myocardium, a so-called myocardial bridge, in up to 26%–58% of patients [30–32]. While bridges are frequently incidental, they may cause ischemia in rare cases, and they should be recognized and reported when present [33].

Arising from the left main bifurcation (or trifurcation), the LCX courses laterally and along the left atrioventricular groove, between the left atrium and the

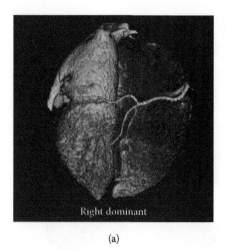

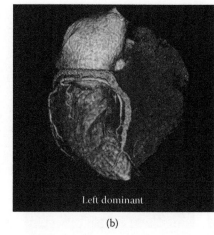

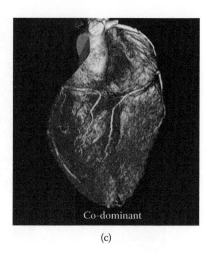

(a)   (b)   (c)

FIGURE 13.17
(a) Right dominant, (b) left dominant, and (c) codominant coronary systems.

LV (Figure 13.13). Obtuse marginal branches, varying in size and number (usually 1–3), arise from the LCX and course anteriorly to supply the lateral wall of the LV. It is not uncommon for an obtuse marginal branch to be larger in caliber than the LCX, distal to its origin. Standard nomenclature divides the LCX into proximal and distal segments with the origin of first obtuse marginal used as the dividing point.

The RCA courses along the right atrioventricular groove giving rise to several branch arteries (Figure 13.15). The first branch artery is usually the conus branch, which is small in caliber and supplies the right ventricular outflow tract; however, this branch may originate as a separate ostium from the aorta in up to 35% of patients [34]. In nearly 60% of patients, the sinoatrial branch, also small in caliber, arises from the RCA (in the remaining patients, the origin is from the LCX). The RCA also gives rise to right ventricular branches, the largest of which is called the acute marginal branch. Approximately 85% of patients exhibit so-called right dominant branching pattern of the RCA. In this pattern, the RCA continues around the lateral aspect of the heart to the posterior interventricular groove and branches to give rise to the posterior descending artery and the posterolateral arteries, supplying the posterior and posterolateral segments of the LV, respectively. Approximately 8% of patients exhibit left dominance, where both of these arteries branch from the LCX. The remaining 7% of patients exhibit codominance in which the supply to this region of the LV is shared between the RCA and LCX [35] (Figure 13.17). In cases of left dominance, the RCA may be quite small in caliber and is typically much shorter in length compared with right dominant anatomy. In a right dominant anatomy, standard nomenclature for the RCA segments is the proximal, mid, and distal segments. The two dividing points are the acute

margins of the heart (i.e., the acute angles of the RCA) (Figure 13.15).

13.4 Clinical Applications of Coronary Computed Tomography

13.4.1 Calcium Scoring

Calcification of the coronary arteries is a pathologic process caused by atherosclerotic disease [36]. The extent of calcification is associated with the total amount of coronary atherosclerosis. Coronary calcification is only weakly correlated to the degree of stenosis, however, and is not clinically reliable for determining the degree of arterial obstruction [37,38]. Thus, measuring the total amount of coronary calcification is an excellent surrogate for the amount of total coronary atherosclerotic burden but should not be used to estimate arterial stenosis.

Coronary calcification is measured using noncontrast, ECG-gated images. Typically, the images are obtained with 120 kV at a slice thickness of 3 mm using prospective ECG gating. Most commercially available postprocessing software packages allow relatively simple, semiautomated techniques for the identification and quantification of calcium (Figure 13.18). The presence of coronary calcification is usually defined as pixels with signal density >130 HU within the coronary arterial bed. The interpreter should be careful not to include noncoronary calcification such as mitral annular, aortic, and pericardial calcifications (Figure 13.19). A commonly used scoring system is the Agatston calcium score, which is derived from the total area of each plaque (i.e., number

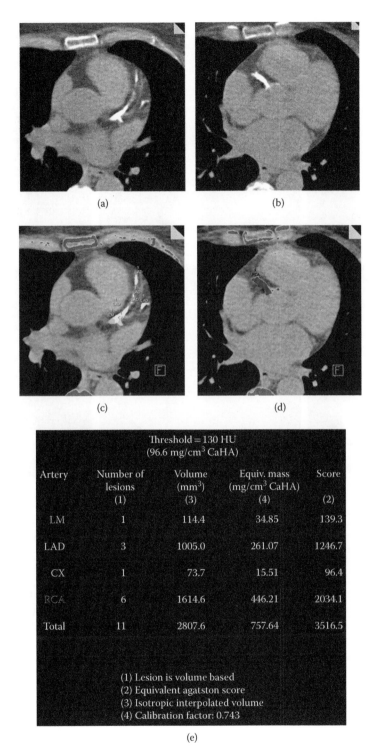

Threshold = 130 HU (96.6 mg/cm^3 CaHA)				
Artery	Number of lesions (1)	Volume (mm^3) (3)	Equiv. mass (mg/cm^3 CaHA) (4)	Score (2)
LM	1	114.4	34.85	139.3
LAD	3	1005.0	261.07	1246.7
CX	1	73.7	15.51	96.4
RCA	6	1614.6	446.21	2034.1
Total	11	2807.6	757.64	3516.5

(1) Lesion is volume based
(2) Equivalent agatston score
(3) Isotropic interpolated volume
(4) Calibration factor: 0.743

(e)

FIGURE 13.18
Example of a calcium score as performed on noncontrast, axial images (a, b) with color-coded calcium identified by a semi-automated process (c, d). A computer-generated summary report of coronary calcium is typically produced (e).

of pixels), multiplied by a factor of 1–4, based on the peak attenuation found in each plaque, and summed for all slices [39]. A calcium volumetric score or an absolute calcium mass can also be used [40,41]. Scan reproducibility is very good, although motion artifact can cause an overestimation or underestimation of calcium. Either MDCT or EBCT can be used for calcium scoring. The better temporal resolution of EBCT makes it less susceptible to motion artifact; however, correlation between MDCT and EBCT is fairly good.

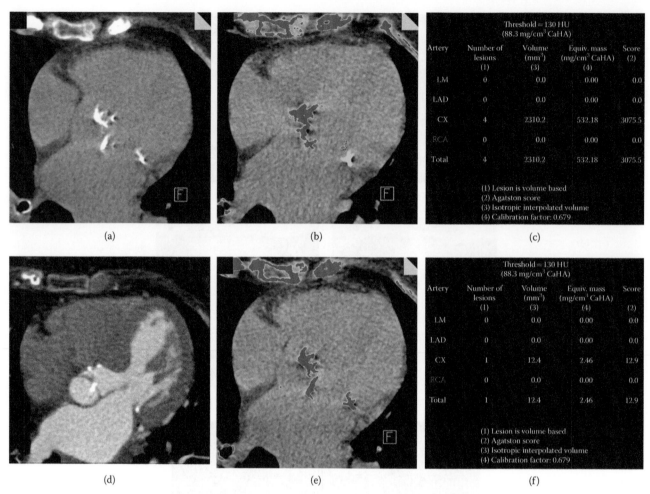

FIGURE 13.19
Demonstration of difficulty with distinguishing between coronary calcification and mitral annular calcification on a noncontrast (a, b) compared to a contrast study (d). Accidental inclusion of the mitral annular calcification, depicted by blue coloring (b) can lead to an erroneously high calcium score (c) when compared with the correct measurement (e, f).

As a surrogate for atherosclerotic burden, a patient's calcium score is a strong predictor of future adverse cardiovascular events (e.g., myocardial infarction) and overall mortality. Although strongly associated with age and less strongly with other traditional cardiovascular risk factors, calcium scores have independent predictive value beyond a patient's age and known risk factors. This has been demonstrated in large studies, in both men and women and across multiple ethnicities [42–45]. In appropriately selected patients, a calcium score can help risk stratify intermediate-risk patients as high or low risk for future cardiovascular events. This determination may lead to the initiation or intensification of various treatments (e.g., cholesterol lowering agents). Importantly, this test is not recommended for those at very low or high cardiovascular risk, but instead those in the low to intermediate risk group, as they are most likely to benefit from the findings [46]. It should be noted that,

while ample evidence exists to show the ability of a coronary calcium score (CCS) to aid in risk stratification, the strategy of adjusting treatment based on this result has not been extensively investigated. The change in calcium score in response to treatment is controversial, and repeat follow-up studies are not recommended for this purpose.

In addition to its clinical use as a standalone test, a coronary calcium scan is usually obtained just before most CCTA scans as well. Obtaining a coronary calcium scan can allow for further narrowing of the scan range of the CCTA, thus lowering radiation exposure of the CCTA scan. Also, extensive coronary calcification can cause significant attenuation and image artifacts and may limit evaluation of the coronary arteries. This raises the risk of the CCTA scan being nondiagnostic, and the decision on whether to proceed with a CCTA must be made for all patients with extensive coronary calcium. While some institutions will not proceed with the CCTA if calcium score exceeds a certain threshold (usually in the range of 600–1000), there is no universal agreement on specific cutoff values, and the decision to proceed is usually made by the performing and/or referring physicians.

13.4.2 Coronary Computed Tomography Angiography

More than 10 years ago, early reports confirmed the potential use of MDCT coronary angiography [47]. These initial studies used early generation MDCT scanners and scans were limited by several factors including very long breath-hold times (up to 40 seconds), poor temporal resolution, and suboptimal image quality. About 37% of coronary segments on these early scans were considered not assessable [48]. With rapid improvements in spatial and temporal resolution, MDCT has recently emerged as an accurate and reliable modality for evaluation of the coronary arteries. Using 64-detector MDCT and higher, a large and growing

body of literature from both single- and multicenter studies supports the accuracy of this technology for the detection of coronary plaques and the resulting degree of coronary stenosis [49–51]. To determine the accuracy, CCTA is most frequently compared to conventional invasive angiography as the gold standard of coronary artery imaging. Conventional angiography has both better temporal and spatial resolution than CCTA. It is important to note, however, that conventional angiography only images the lumen of the artery and cannot directly visualize plaque or identify plaque that has been remodeled outside of the lumen (Figure 13.20). Most comparison studies have focused on the ability of CCTA to identify obstructive plaque from nonobstructive plaque, usually defined by a plaque causing at least 50% luminal narrowing or stenosis. The performance characteristics of CCTA vary from study to study depending on many factors including the patient population studied, type of hardware/software used, interpreter experience, and so on. Nonetheless, most studies have demonstrated good sensitivity and specificity,

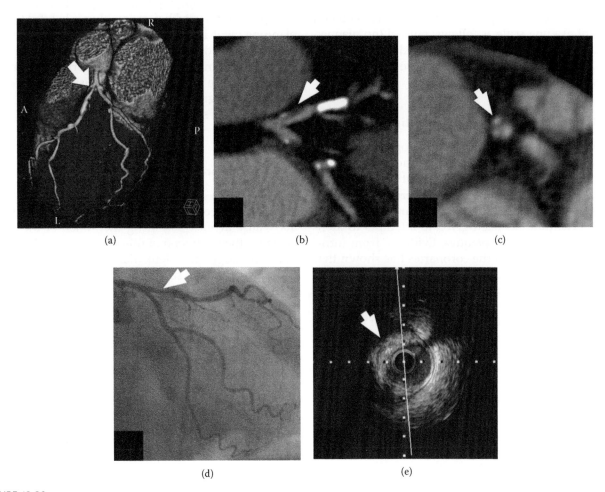

(a)   (b)   (c)

(d)   (e)

FIGURE 13.20
Example of patient with mixed plaque associated with positive remodeling and moderate stenosis on (a–c) CT coronary angiogram with corresponding (d) x-ray angiogram and (e) intravascular ultrasound images.

with particularly high negative predictive values. This indicates that CCTA is an excellent test for "ruling out" obstructive disease [49,51,52]. On the other hand, positive predictive values have been more modest, indicating that when plaques are present, CCTA is susceptible to overestimating the degree of stenosis compared to conventional angiography [50–52]. This, in part, has led to the recommendation of using CCTA to evaluate patients with low to intermediate risk of obstructive disease. Patients with known obstructive CAD or those at very high risk for obstructive CAD (e.g., those with typical angina or myocardial infarction) are generally better suited for other imaging such as invasive angiography. Likewise, CCTA is not recommended for screening patients who are at low risk for obstructive CAD without cardiac symptoms [46].

Reporting the degree of lumen stenosis caused by plaque is essential and is often the most important value reported in a CCTA. The manner in which this gets reported, however, varies significantly between institutions. Grading stenosis can be quantitative, semiquantitative, or descriptive. Recent guidelines by the Society of Cardiovascular Computed Tomography recommend a 6-point grading scale as follows: normal (no plaque/stenosis), minimal (<25% stenosis), mild (25%–49% stenosis), moderate (50%–69% stenosis), severe (70%–99% stenosis), or occluded [28].

13.4.3 Coronary Plaques Characteristics

Coronary plaques are complex, heterogeneous structures. While the presence of these plaques are widespread throughout the general population (increasing significantly with age), only a small percentage lead to coronary events (e.g., myocardial infarction). A great deal of attention has been given to attempts to identify these "vulnerable" plaques. Evidence from intravascular ultrasound of the coronaries has shown that plaques with certain characteristic components, such as necrotic cores, are more likely to cause future coronary events [53]. The high spatial and contrast resolution of CCTA allows for the identification of different plaque components or plaque types based on the degree of enhancement. Motoyama and colleagues have shown that low-attenuation plaques (density <30 HU) have been associated with a significant increase in risk for future coronary events, regardless of the degree of lumen stenosis [54,55]. This group has also demonstrated an increased risk of coronary events in those plaques that exhibit positive remodeling [54,55] (Figures 13.20 and 13.21).

Confirmation of these findings with additional studies is warranted and should help clarify the role of plaque type by CCTA in clinical care. When reporting coronary plaques, reporting the plaque type as one of following three is recommended: (1) calcified, (2) noncalcified, and (3) mixed (both calcified and noncalcified components).

13.4.4 Coronary Artery Bypass Grafts

Coronary artery bypass grafts can be imaged using CCTA with high accuracy [56,57]. In fact, grafts may be better visualized than native coronaries. This is because of their often larger diameters (for saphenous vein grafts) and the relative lack of motion depending on graft location and course (Figure 13.22). However, there are potential caveats to graft evaluation. Surgical clips cause artifact that may obscure the view of the graft for a short segment or segments. The point of anastomosis of the graft with the native artery may also be difficult to assess because of small distal artery caliber or motion of the heart at this location. Nonetheless, several published reports show excellent performance of CCTA for evaluation of bypass grafts, with exceptionally high negative predictive values [56,57]. Knowledge of number of type of bypass grafts used before imaging is helpful for scan planning, as it is important to include the entire graft from origin to distal anastomosis within the scan field. In particular, internal mammary artery grafts require imaging of the entire thorax for visualization of the graft from origin to distal anastomosis (Figure 13.22). This increased scan length will increase patient radiation exposure.

13.4.5 Intracoronary Stents

Intracoronary stents are frequently used to treat obstructive coronary lesions. Their presence of CCTA may cause artifact obscuring the lumen of the vessel; however, the likelihood of this greatly depends on stent size. The larger the stent diameter, the higher is the likelihood that the segment will be evaluable (Figure 13.23). More specifically, coronary segments with stents of at least 3.0 mm in diameter can usually be evaluated. Segments with stents of 2.5 mm or less may be evaluable but with less reliability [58]. Additionally, overlapping stents may cause further beam hardening artifact and may obscure lumen evaluation even at 3.0 mm diameter. Minimizing motion artifact and adjusting the reconstruction kernel (see Section 13.2.6) may improve evaluation of a coronary segment with a stent present.

13.4.6 Coronary Anomalies

Anomalous coronary arteries are not rare, being present in approximately 1% of the population [59]. Coronary anomalies are traditionally classified depending on

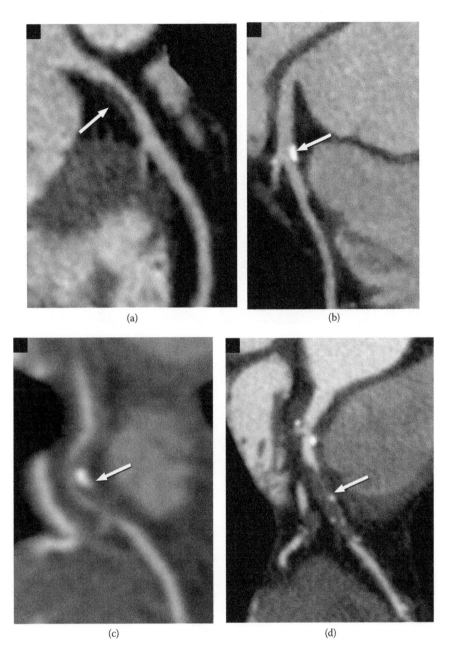

FIGURE 13.21
Examples of (a) noncalcified, (b) calcified, and (c, d) mixed calcified and noncalcified plaques with occlusion.

whether there is an anomaly of origin and course, intrinsic coronary anatomy or coronary termination. While many different anomalous variants have been described, some are much more common than others. Although still poorly understood, the prognosis and clinical significance of these anomalies range from completely benign to life-threatening [59,60]. Although cardiac catheterization has traditionally been used for characterization of coronary artery anomalies, the complex 3D nature of these anomalies often require wide field-of-view 3D imaging techniques such as CCTA or coronary magnetic resonance angiography for full delineation of the anatomic origin and course of the coronary arteries in addition to their relationship with surrounding intraluminal and extraluminal structures. In particular, with anomalies of coronary origin, descriptive information on location origin, angle of takeoff (e.g., from the aorta), and any vessel stenosis or abnormal shape is also important. In the subset of patients with an anomalous origin of the LAD from the right coronary cusp, the presence of an intramural course within the wall of the aorta has been linked to clinical symptoms

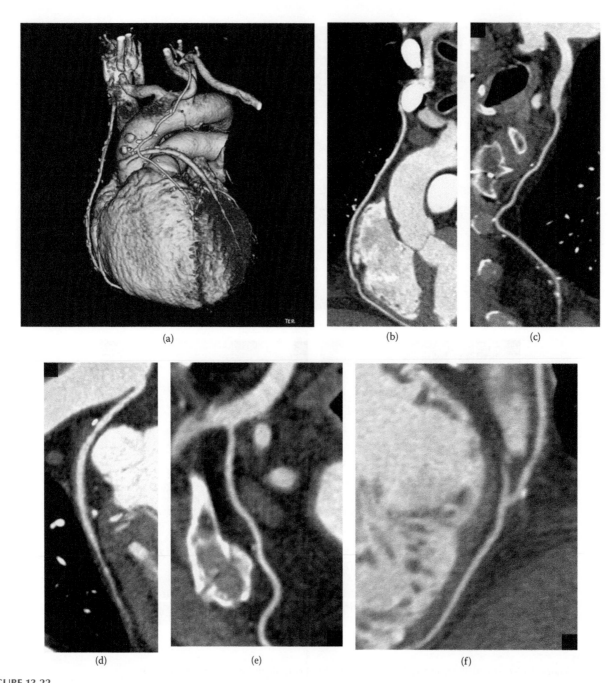

FIGURE 13.22
(a) Patient with five-vessel coronary artery bypass grafting including in situ left internal mammary artery graft to left anterior descending artery, in situ right internal mammary artery grafted to the right coronary artery, saphenous vein grafted to the diagonal branch, and two additional saphenous vein grafts that are occluded (b–d). Curved multiplanar reformations can demonstrate the grafts in their entire length including evaluation of the (e) proximal and (f) distal anastomotic sites.

and sudden death [61] (Figure 13.24). CCTA evidence of this intramural course is characterized by an acute angle takeoff from the aorta and a slit-like appearance of the vessel [62].

Cardiac MRI, if available, can also be used for characterization of coronary anomalies. Cardiac MRI has the disadvantage of lower spatial resolution, but avoids the concern of ionizing radiation. This may be particularly desirable in the pediatric population and in very young adults. In these populations, however, coronary plaque may not be a concern and may thus allow for the use of low dose radiation protocols on CCTA to significantly reduce patient radiation exposure.

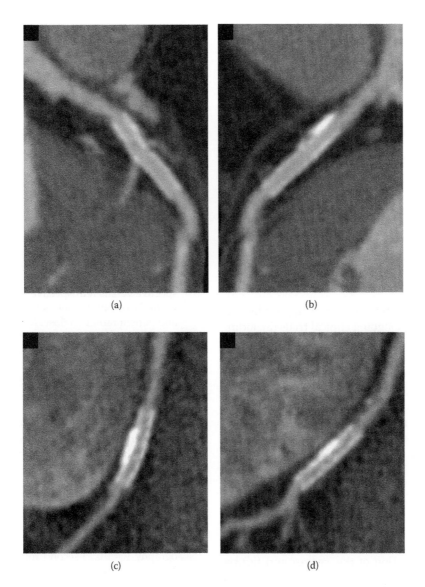

(a)   (b)

(c)   (d)

FIGURE 13.23
Examples of (a, b) large 3.5-mm stent in the proximal left anterior descending artery and (c, d) smaller 2.5-mm stent in the distal right coronary artery.

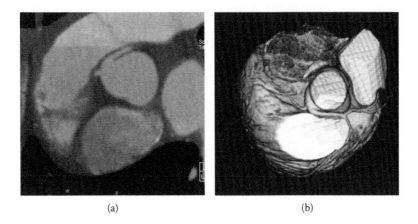

(a)   (b)

FIGURE 13.24
Anomalous left coronary artery from the right coronary sinus demonstrating an interarterial course on maximal intensity projection images (a, c), 3D volume rendered (b) and 3D endoscopic shaded surface display image showing the vessel origins from "inside" the aorta.

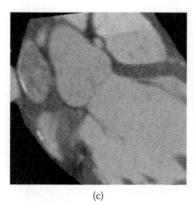
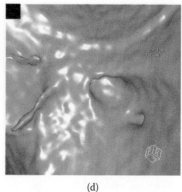

(c)   (d)

FIGURE 13.24   (*Continued*)

13.5 Future Directions

Both CCTA technology and its clinical application are evolving at a rapid pace. Ongoing clinical trials (including the "PROMISE" and "RESCUE" trials) will be among the largest cardiac imaging trials in history and we are sure to gain valuable insights from their results. Institutions and operators that perform CCTA should stay abreast of changing technology and clinical guidelines to optimize patient care by minimizing radiation exposure, maximizing image quality, and screening out inappropriate referrals.

Acknowledgments

We gratefully acknowledge Martha Helmers for her hard work with preparation of the images and figures for this chapter. Dr. Srichai was supported by grant number K12HS019473 from the Agency for Healthcare Research and Quality during this project. The content is solely the responsibility of the authors and does not necessarily represent the official views of the Agency for Healthcare Research and Quality.

References

1. Mendis S, Puska P, Norrving B (eds.). *Global Atlas on Cardiovascular Disease Prevention and Control.* Geneva: World Health Organization; 2011.
2. Earls JP. How to use a prospective gated technique for cardiac CT. *J Cardiovasc Comput Tomogr.* 2009; 3: 45–51.
3. Scheffel H, Alkadhi H, Leschka S, Plass A, Desbiolles L, Guber I, Krauss T, Gruenenfelder J, Genoni M, Luescher TF et al. Low-dose CT coronary angiography in the step-and-shoot mode: Diagnostic performance. *Heart.* 2008; 94: 1132–1137.
4. Shuman WP, Branch KR, May JM, Mitsumori LM, Lockhart DW, Dubinsky TJ, Warren BH, Caldwell JH. Prospective versus retrospective ECG gating for 64-detector CT of the coronary arteries: Comparison of image quality and patient radiation dose. *Radiology.* 2008; 248: 431–437.
5. Abbara S, Arbab-Zadeh A, Callister TQ, Desai MY, Mamuya W, Thomson L, Weigold WG. SCCT guidelines for performance of coronary computed tomographic angiography: A report of the society of cardiovascular computed tomography guidelines committee. *J Cardiovasc Comput Tomogr.* 2009; 3: 190–204.
6. Husmann L, Leschka S, Desbiolles L, Schepis T, Gaemperli O, Seifert B, Cattin P, Frauenfelder T, Flohr TG, Marincek B et al. Coronary artery motion and cardiac phases: Dependency on heart rate—implications for CT image reconstruction. *Radiology.* 2007; 245: 567–576.
7. Wintersperger BJ, Nikolaou K, von Ziegler F, Johnson T, Rist C, Leber A, Flohr T, Knez A, Reiser MF, Becker CR. Image quality, motion artifacts, and reconstruction timing of 64-slice coronary computed tomography angiography with 0.33-second rotation speed. *Invest Radiol.* 2006; 41: 436–442.
8. Nagatani Y, Takahashi M, Takazakura R, Nitta N, Murata K, Ushio N, Matsuo S, Yamamoto T, Horie M. Multidetector-row computed tomography coronary angiography: Optimization of image reconstruction phase according to the heart rate. *Circ J.* 2007; 71: 112–121.
9. Gerber TC, Carr JJ, Arai AE, Dixon RL, Ferrari VA, Gomes AS, Heller GV, McCollough CH, McNitt-Gray MF, Mettler FA et al. Ionizing radiation in cardiac imaging: A science advisory from the American heart association committee on cardiac imaging of the council on clinical cardiology and committee on cardiovascular imaging and intervention of the council on cardiovascular radiology and intervention. *Circulation.* 2009; 119: 1056–1065.
10. Einstein AJ, Henzlova MJ, Rajagopalan S. Estimating risk of cancer associated with radiation exposure from 64-slice computed tomography coronary angiography. *JAMA.* 2007; 298: 317–323.
11. Halliburton SS, Abbara S, Chen MY, Gentry R, Mahesh M, Raff GL, Shaw LJ, Hausleiter J. SCCT guidelines on radiation dose and dose-optimization strategies in cardiovascular CT. *J Cardiovasc Comput Tomogr.* 2011; 5: 198–224.

12. Taylor AJ, Cerqueira M, Hodgson JM, Mark D, Min J, O'Gara P, Rubin GD. ACCF/SCCT/ACR/AHA/ASE/ASNC/NASCI/SCAI/SCMR 2010 appropriate use criteria for cardiac computed tomography. A report of the American College of Cardiology Foundation appropriate use criteria task force, the Society of Cardiovascular Computed Tomography, the American College of Radiology, the American Heart Association, the American Society Of Echocardiography, the American Society Of Nuclear Cardiology, the North American Society for Cardiovascular Imaging, the Society for Cardiovascular Angiography and Interventions, and the Society for Cardiovascular Magnetic Resonance. *Circulation*. 2010; 122: e525–e555.

13. Bischoff B, Hein F, Meyer T, Hadamitzky M, Martinoff S, Schomig A, Hausleiter J. Impact of a reduced tube voltage on CT angiography and radiation dose: Results of the PROTECTION I study. *JACC Cardiovasc Imaging*. 2009; 2: 940–946.

14. Blankstein R, Bolen MA, Pale R, Murphy MK, Shah AB, Bezerra HG, Sarwar A, Rogers IS, Hoffmann U, Abbara S et al. Use of 100 kV versus 120 kV in cardiac dual source computed tomography: Effect on radiation dose and image quality. *Int J Cardiovasc Imaging*. 2011; 27: 579–586.

15. Feuchtner GM, Jodocy D, Klauser A, Haberfellner B, Aglan I, Spoeck A, Hiehs S, Soegner P, Jaschke W. Radiation dose reduction by using 100-kV tube voltage in cardiac 64-slice computed tomography: A comparative study. *Eur J Radiol*. 2010; 75: e51–e56.

16. Wang D, Hu XH, Zhang SZ, Wu RZ, Xie SS, Chen B, Zhang QW. Image quality and dose performance of 80 kV low dose scan protocol in high-pitch spiral coronary CT angiography: Feasibility study. *Int J Cardiovasc Imaging*. 2011; 28: 415–423.

17. LaBounty TM, Leipsic J, Poulter R, Wood D, Johnson M, Srichai MB, Cury RC, Heilbron B, Hague C, Lin FY et al. Coronary CT angiography of patients with a normal body mass index using 80 kVp versus 100 kVp: A prospective, multicenter, multivendor randomized trial. *AJR Am J Roentgenol*. 2011; 197: W860–W867.

18. Mulkens TH, Bellinck P, Baeyaert M, Ghysen D, Van Dijck X, Mussen E, Venstermans C, Termote JL. Use of an automatic exposure control mechanism for dose optimization in multi-detector row ct examinations: Clinical evaluation. *Radiology*. 2005; 237: 213–223.

19. Einstein AJ, Elliston CD, Arai AE, Chen MY, Mather R, Pearson GD, Delapaz RL, Nickoloff E, Dutta A, Brenner DJ. Radiation dose from single-heartbeat coronary CT angiography performed with a 320-detector row volume scanner. *Radiology*. 2010; 254: 698–706.

20. Achenbach S, Marwan M, Ropers D, Schepis T, Pflederer T, Anders K, Kuettner A, Daniel WG, Uder M, Lell MM. Coronary computed tomography angiography with a consistent dose below 1 mSv using prospectively electrocardiogram-triggered high-pitch spiral acquisition. *Eur Heart J*. 2010; 31: 340–346.

21. Achenbach S, Marwan M, Schepis T, Pflederer T, Bruder H, Allmendinger T, Petersilka M, Anders K, Lell M, Kuettner A et al. High-pitch spiral acquisition: A new scan mode for coronary CT angiography. *J Cardiovasc Comput Tomogr*. 2009; 3: 117–121.

22. Hausleiter J, Bischoff B, Hein F, Meyer T, Hadamitzky M, Thierfelder C, Allmendinger T, Flohr TG, Schomig A, Martinoff S. Feasibility of dual-source cardiac CT angiography with high-pitch scan protocols. *J Cardiovasc Comput Tomogr*. 2009; 3: 236–242.

23. Gosling O, Loader R, Venables P, Roobottom C, Rowles N, Bellenger N, Morgan-Hughes G. A comparison of radiation doses between state-of-the-art multislice CT coronary angiography with iterative reconstruction, multislice CT coronary angiography with standard filtered back-projection and invasive diagnostic coronary angiography. *Heart*. 2010; 96: 922–926.

24. Leipsic J, Labounty TM, Heilbron B, Min JK, Mancini GB, Lin FY, Taylor C, Dunning A, Earls JP. Estimated radiation dose reduction using adaptive statistical iterative reconstruction in coronary CT angiography: The ERASIR study. *AJR Am J Roentgenol*. 2010; 195: 655–660.

25. Leipsic J, Labounty TM, Heilbron B, Min JK, Mancini GB, Lin FY, Taylor C, Dunning A, Earls JP. Adaptive statistical iterative reconstruction: Assessment of image noise and image quality in coronary CT angiography. *AJR Am J Roentgenol*. 2010; 195: 649–654.

26. Parker MS, Kelleher NM, Hoots JA, Chung JK, Fatouros PP, Benedict SH. Absorbed radiation dose of the female breast during diagnostic multidetector chest CT and dose reduction with a tungsten-antimony composite breast shield: Preliminary results. *Clin Radiol*. 2008; 63: 278–288.

27. Yilmaz MH, Albayram S, Yasar D, Ozer H, Adaletli I, Selcuk D, Akman C, Altug A. Female breast radiation exposure during thorax multidetector computed tomography and the effectiveness of bismuth breast shield to reduce breast radiation dose. *J Comput Assist Tomogr*. 2007; 31: 138–142.

28. Raff GL, Abidov A, Achenbach S, Berman DS, Boxt LM, Budoff MJ, Cheng V, DeFrance T, Hellinger JC, Karlsberg RP. SCCT guidelines for the interpretation and reporting of coronary computed tomographic angiography. *J Cardiovasc Comput Tomogr*. 2009; 3: 122–136.

29. Austen WG, Edwards JE, Frye RL, Gensini GG, Gott VL, Griffith LS, McGoon DC, Murphy ML, Roe BB. A reporting system on patients evaluated for coronary artery disease. Report of the Ad Hoc Committee for Grading of Coronary Artery Disease, Council on Cardiovascular Surgery, American Heart Association. *Circulation*. 1975; 51: 5–40.

30. Zeina AR, Odeh M, Blinder J, Rosenschein U, Barmeir E. Myocardial bridge: Evaluation on MDCT. *AJR Am J Roentgenol*. 2007; 188: 1069–1073.

31. Leschka S, Koepfli P, Husmann L, Plass A, Vachenauer R, Gaemperli O, Schepis T, Genoni M, Marincek B, Eberli FR et al. Myocardial bridging: Depiction rate and morphology at ct coronary angiography—comparison with conventional coronary angiography. *Radiology*. 2008; 246: 754–762.

32. Kim PJ, Hur G, Kim SY, Namgung J, Hong SW, Kim YH, Lee WR. Frequency of myocardial bridges and dynamic compression of epicardial coronary arteries: A comparison between computed tomography and invasive coronary angiography. *Circulation*. 2009; 119: 1408–1416.

33. Mohlenkamp S, Hort W, Ge J, Erbel R. Update on myocardial bridging. *Circulation*. 2002; 106: 2616–2622.

34. O'Brien JP, Srichai MB, Hecht EM, Kim DC, Jacobs JE. Anatomy of the heart at multidetector CT: What the radiologist needs to know. *Radiographics*. 2007; 27: 1569–1582.

35. Miller S. Normal angiographic anatomy and measurements. *Cardiac Angiography*. Boston, MA: Little, Brown; 1984: 51–71.

36. Wexler L, Brundage B, Crouse J, Detrano R, Fuster V, Maddahi J, Rumberger J, Stanford W, White R, Taubert K. Coronary artery calcification: Pathophysiology, epidemiology, imaging methods, and clinical implications. A statement for health professionals from the American Heart Association. Writing group. *Circulation*. 1996; 94: 1175–1192.

37. Gottlieb I, Miller JM, Arbab-Zadeh A, Dewey M, Clouse ME, Sara L, Niinuma H, Bush DE, Paul N, Vavere AL et al. The absence of coronary calcification does not exclude obstructive coronary artery disease or the need for revascularization in patients referred for conventional coronary angiography. *J Am Coll Cardiol*. 2010; 55: 627–634.

38. Detrano R, Hsiai T, Wang S, Puentes G, Fallavollita J, Shields P, Stanford W, Wolfkiel C, Georgiou D, Budoff M et al. Prognostic value of coronary calcification and angiographic stenoses in patients undergoing coronary angiography. *J Am Coll Cardiol*. 1996; 27: 285–290.

39. Agatston AS, Janowitz WR, Hildner FJ, Zusmer NR, Viamonte M, Jr., Detrano R. Quantification of coronary artery calcium using ultrafast computed tomography. *J Am Coll Cardiol*. 1990; 15: 827–832.

40. Callister TQ, Cooil B, Raya SP, Lippolis NJ, Russo DJ, Raggi P. Coronary artery disease: Improved reproducibility of calcium scoring with an electron-beam ct volumetric method. *Radiology*. 1998; 208: 807–814.

41. Hong C, Bae KT, Pilgram TK. Coronary artery calcium: Accuracy and reproducibility of measurements with multi-detector row CT—assessment of effects of different thresholds and quantification methods. *Radiology*. 2003; 227: 795–801.

42. Detrano R, Guerci AD, Carr JJ, Bild DE, Burke G, Folsom AR, Liu K, Shea S, Szklo M, Bluemke DA et al. Coronary calcium as a predictor of coronary events in four racial or ethnic groups. *N Engl J Med*. 2008; 358: 1336–1345.

43. Arad Y, Goodman KJ, Roth M, Newstein D, Guerci AD. Coronary calcification, coronary disease risk factors, C-reactive protein, and atherosclerotic cardiovascular disease events: The St. Francis Heart Study. *J Am Coll Cardiol*. 2005; 46: 158–165.

44. Greenland P, LaBree L, Azen SP, Doherty TM, Detrano RC. Coronary artery calcium score combined with Framingham score for risk prediction in asymptomatic individuals. *JAMA*. 2004; 291: 210–215.

45. LaMonte MJ, FitzGerald SJ, Church TS, Barlow CE, Radford NB, Levine BD, Pippin JJ, Gibbons LW, Blair SN, Nichaman MZ. Coronary artery calcium score and coronary heart disease events in a large cohort of asymptomatic men and women. *Am J Epidemiol*. 2005; 162: 421–429.

46. Greenland P, Alpert JS, Beller GA, Benjamin EJ, Budoff MJ, Fayad ZA, Foster E, Hlatky MA, Hodgson JM, Kushner FG et al. 2010 ACCF/AHA guideline for assessment of cardiovascular risk in asymptomatic adults: A report of the American College of Cardiology Foundation/American Heart Association Task Force on practice guidelines. *Circulation*. 2010; 122: e584–e636.

47. Achenbach S, Ulzheimer S, Baum U, Kachelriess M, Ropers D, Giesler T, Bautz W, Daniel WG, Kalender WA, Moshage W. Noninvasive coronary angiography by retrospectively ECG-gated multislice spiral ct. *Circulation*. 2000; 102: 2823–2828.

48. Nieman K, Oudkerk M, Rensing BJ, van Ooijen P, Munne A, van Geuns RJ, de Feyter PJ. Coronary angiography with multi-slice computed tomography. *Lancet*. 2001; 357: 599–603.

49. Meijboom WB, Meijs MF, Schuijf JD, Cramer MJ, Mollet NR, van Mieghem CA, Nieman K, van Werkhoven JM, Pundziute G, Weustink AC et al Diagnostic accuracy of 64-slice computed tomography coronary angiography: A prospective, multicenter, multivendor study. *J Am Coll Cardiol*. 2008; 52: 2135–2144.

50. Miller JM, Rochitte CE, Dewey M, Arbab-Zadeh A, Niinuma H, Gottlieb I, Paul N, Clouse ME, Shapiro EP, Hoe J et al. Diagnostic performance of coronary angiography by 64-row CT. *N Engl J Med*. 2008; 359: 2324–2336.

51. Budoff MJ, Dowe D, Jollis JG, Gitter M, Sutherland J, Halamert E, Scherer M, Bellinger R, Martin A, Benton R et al. Diagnostic performance of 64-multidetector row coronary computed tomographic angiography for evaluation of coronary artery stenosis in individuals without known coronary artery disease: Results from the prospective multicenter accuracy (assessment by coronary computed tomographic angiography of individuals undergoing invasive coronary angiography) trial. *J Am Coll Cardiol*. 2008; 52: 1724–1732.

52. Mowatt G, Cook JA, Hillis GS, Walker S, Fraser C, Jia X, Waugh N. 64-slice computed tomography angiography in the diagnosis and assessment of coronary artery disease: Systematic review and meta-analysis. *Heart*. 2008; 94: 1386–1393.

53. Narula J, Finn AV, Demaria AN. Picking plaques that pop. *J Am Coll Cardiol*. 2005; 45: 1970–1973.

54. Motoyama S, Kondo T, Sarai M, Sugiura A, Harigaya H, Sato T, Inoue K, Okumura M, Ishii J, Anno H et al. Multislice computed tomographic characteristics of coronary lesions in acute coronary syndromes. *J Am Coll Cardiol*. 2007; 50: 319–326.

55. Motoyama S, Sarai M, Harigaya H, Anno H, Inoue K, Hara T, Naruse H, Ishii J, Hishida H, Wong ND et al. Computed tomographic angiography characteristics of atherosclerotic plaques subsequently resulting in acute coronary syndrome. *J Am Coll Cardiol*. 2009; 54: 49–57.

56. Weustink AC, Nieman K, Pugliese F, Mollet NR, Meijboom WB, van Mieghem C, ten Kate GJ, Cademartiri F, Krestin GP, de Feyter PJ. Diagnostic accuracy of computed tomography angiography in patients after bypass grafting: Comparison with invasive coronary angiography. *JACC Cardiovasc Imaging*. 2009; 2: 816–824.

57. Hamon M, Lepage O, Malagutti P, Riddell JW, Morello R, Agostini D. Diagnostic performance of 16- and 64-section spiral CT for coronary artery bypass graft assessment: Meta-analysis. *Radiology.* 2008; 247: 679–686.

58. Pugliese F, Weustink AC, Van Mieghem C, Alberghina F, Otsuka M, Meijboom WB, van Pelt N, Mollet NR, Cademartiri F, Krestin GP et al. Dual source coronary computed tomography angiography for detecting in-stent restenosis. *Heart.* 2008; 94: 848–854.

59. Angelini P, Velasco JA, Flamm S. Coronary anomalies: Incidence, pathophysiology, and clinical relevance. *Circulation.* 2002; 105: 2449–2454.

60. Angelini P. Coronary artery anomalies—current clinical issues: Definitions, classification, incidence, clinical relevance, and treatment guidelines. *Tex Heart Inst J.* 2002; 29: 271–278.

61. Cheitlin MD, De Castro CM, McAllister HA. Sudden death as a complication of anomalous left coronary origin from the anterior sinus of valsalva, a not-so-minor congenital anomaly. *Circulation.* 1974; 50: 780–787.

62. Miller JA, Anavekar NS, El Yaman MM, Burkhart HM, Miller AJ, Julsrud PR. Computed tomographic angiography identification of intramural segments in anomalous coronary arteries with interarterial course. *Int J Cardiovasc Imaging.* 2011; 28(6): 1525–1532.

14

Cardiovascular CT Imaging of Valvular Structure and Myocardial Perfusion: Anatomic and Functional CT Data for the Planning of Cardiovascular Procedures

Kheng-Thye Ho and Paul Schoenhagen

CONTENTS

14.1 Introduction

Over the last several years, computed tomography (CT) has become an established imaging modality for multiple cardiovascular indications, including aortic disease, pulmonary artery disease, and structural heart disease. As described in other chapters of the book, a particular well-studied area has been coronary CT angiography (CTA). Based on data from multicenter trials and meta-analysis, the role of CTA is well understood and documented in appropriateness criteria.

Simultaneously, novel innovative applications of CT have evolved, specifically related to planning of interventional procedures, including transcatheter valvular procedures and percutaneous coronary intervention (PCI). Based on the 3D data obtained with CT, it plays an important role for *anatomic* guidance in the context of these less-invasive procedures. Additional *functional* cardiac assessment can further add information in specific clinical situations. In the context of planning of valvular and coronary interventions, assessment of valve function and fractional flow reserve (FFR)/myocardial perfusion allows the evaluation of lesion significance. However, the clinical impact of imaging on subsequent treatment decision and outcome is not well understood.

In this chapter, we will discuss two important examples: imaging of valvular structure in the context of transcatheter valvular intervention and myocardial perfusion imaging (MPI) in the context of coronary artery disease (CAD)/PCI.

14.1.1 Technological Consideration for CT Imaging

14.1.1.1 Scanner Technology

The use of advanced cardiovascular 3D anatomic and functional CT imaging has become possible due to scanner generations with fast gantry rotation time, dual-source technology, and large number of detector rows arranged with narrow collimated widths [1,2]. Data covering the entire heart, synchronized to the heartbeat, are acquired within a single breath-hold. Scanners with extended anatomical coverage along the patient's long-axis or extended z-coverage (e.g., 320-row detector scanners) acquire up to 16 cm per gantry rotation and can cover the entire heart in one rotation [1]. A 360° rotation of the x-ray tube (gantry) requires between 270 and 350 ms with state-of-the-art scanners and determines the temporal resolution. The best temporal resolution (75 ms) can be achieved using dual-tube technology [2]. Recent developments with dual-source technology allow low-dose, high-pitch cardiac imaging for coronary and valvular imaging [3]. In patient with low heart rate, spiral CT scans can be acquired using pitch values up to 3.2, acquiring data from the entire heart during the diastolic phase of a single heartbeat. Using dual-source scanner, dynamic MPI can be performed using a shuttle mode, with rapid alternation between myocardial regions [4].

Images are reconstructed with slice thickness ranging from 0.5 to 3 mm depending on the specific cardiac application. Spatial resolution in the axial image plane is typically 0.5 mm × 0.5 mm.

Because of the extensive and rapid motion of valvular structures during the cardiac cycle, use of state-of-the-art scanners (at a minimum 64-slice technology) is critical for imaging of valvular structures and myocardial perfusion. Imaging of valvular structures and myocardial perfusion often requires advanced protocols with superior spatial and temporal resolution. Such protocols are associated with increased radiation exposure, which must be justified for individual patients [5].

14.1.1.2 Axial (Sequential) and Helical (Spiral) Acquisition Modes

For most cardiovascular indications, imaging is synchronized to the cardiac cycle. This is necessary to focus data acquisition/reconstruction on a period in the cardiac cycle with minimal motion (and subsequently reduce motion artifact) and in order to align blocks of images from subsequent gantry rotations with limited z-coverage (and subsequently avoid "step" artifacts). Synchronization can be performed with different modes of data acquisition. The two basic approaches are axial (sequential, "step and shoot") and helical (spiral) imaging.

In the axial acquisition mode, data are acquired during rotation of the gantry around a stationary patient [6]. Data acquisition is prospectively triggered by electrocardiogram (ECG) signal during the desired cardiac phase. If necessary to cover the anatomy of interest, the patient table is incremented to a new position between periods of data acquisition. The major advantage of the axial technique for cardiac imaging is reduced x-ray exposure because exposure occurs only during a narrow, prespecified window of the cardiac cycle (with the x-ray tube turned off for the remainder of the cardiac cycle). However, this precludes reconstruction during multiple phases of the cardiac cycle. Other potential limitations of the axial mode include increased sensitivity to arrhythmia due to prospective referencing of the ECG signal and increased examination times due to the increment of the patient table between data acquisitions. Axial imaging provides best results for patients with low and regular heart rates, but is increasingly used to reduce radiation exposure.

In the helical acquisition mode, data are acquired continuously during simultaneous rotation of the gantry and translation of the patient table, with simultaneous recording of the ECG signal. Most often, data are then retrospectively referenced to the simultaneously recorded ECG signal after the acquisition and reconstructed during one or more cardiac phases. Typically, images are initially reconstructed in a diastolic window. Because only data during a limited prespecified portion of the cardiac cycle is typically used for reconstruction, reduction of the tube current (to 4%–20% of the maximum value) outside the prespecified phase (tube current modulation) is typically used with significantly reduced radiation exposure [7–9]. Helical data acquisition permits reconstruction of overlapping slices and reconstruction during multiple cardiac phases for dynamic 4D display of cardiac and valvular motions. Advantages of the helical technique are faster anatomic coverage and less sensitivity to arrhythmia. However, the helical mode is associated with higher patient radiation doses because of continuous x-ray exposure during the entire cardiac cycle.

Alternatively, helical data acquisition can be prospectively triggered by the ECG signal. Prospectively ECG-triggered helical scanning, similar to ECG-triggered axial scanning, switches the x-ray tube on and off to acquire data from only the target cardiac phase during continuous movement of the patient table [10]. For prospective ECG-triggered, high-pitch helical imaging, data acquisition is triggered by the ECG signal to occur during a diastolic window of a single cardiac cycle [2,3]. Because of the rapid acquisition, this technique is associated with a lower radiation dose compared to retrospective ECG-gated helical imaging.

14.1.1.3 Radiation Dose and Dose Sparing Acquisition Techniques

There is concern about the rising radiation exposure from medical imaging and its potential long-term effects [11,12]. The specialized protocols used for valvular assessment and MPI are frequently associated with high levels of radiation exposure. Therefore, careful individual planning of the imaging protocol and consideration of potential alternative imaging modalities is important to control radiation exposure [5].

Balancing diagnostic yield and radiation exposure requires adjusting acquisition parameters to patient characteristics and the specific clinical question. Strategies associated with lower dose for cardiovascular CT imaging include prospectively ECG-triggered imaging techniques, tube current modulation with retrospective ECG-gated helical imaging, use of low x-ray tube voltage (e.g., 100 kVp) [13–15], and iterative reconstruction [16].

14.1.1.4 Image Reconstruction and Analysis

The acquired CT images typically undergo an initial systematic review of all cardiac and extracardiac findings and are then further processed for more focused evaluation of valvular structure and myocardial perfusion.

If images are reviewed and processed at several locations, client–server workstation models are increasingly used. Such servers provide access to multiple users (clients) at multiple locations, but the data are maintained and updated on the central server. Because image storage and data analysis take place at the server level, the system requirements of the individual user interface at the point of care are less.

There is an increasing number of software programs allowing dedicated reconstructions for visualization and also fusion of CT data with other imaging modalities, including conventional angiography. These solutions provide increasing integration of the CT data into the interventional procedure. However, it is critical to understand the potential limitations of advanced image processing to avoid misinterpretation.

14.1.1.4.1 Volume-Rendered Technique

Volume-rendered (VR) techniques assign a specific color and opacity value to every voxel inside a volume of interest (Figure 14.1). By changing the color and opacity settings, the user can interactively highlight groups of voxels for display, for example, left ventricle (LV) versus chest wall and vice versa. It is important to consider that the appearance of VR images (VRIs) is determined by the specific image settings, which can, for example, change the appearance of luminal stenosis severity. It is therefore important to analyze the VRIs in the context of the information obtained from the review of the

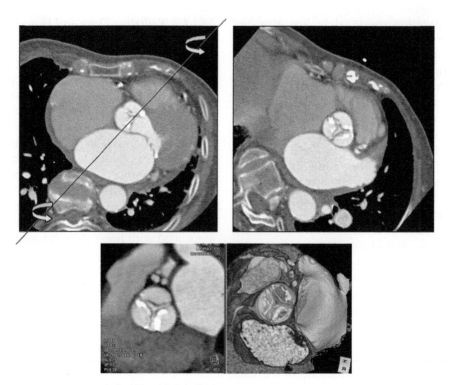

FIGURE 14.1
Axial image, multiplanar reformation (MPR), and volume-rendered image (VRI). The axial image (left upper panel) cuts obliquely through the aortic valve (AV) plane. MPR describes creation of thin cut planes through the 3D volume (right upper panel). The orientation new plane is shown by the red line. The image is now aligned with the AV plane. The VRI (right lower panel) gives a 3D impression of the AV with its calcification.

original axial images and reformatted multiplanar reformation (MPR)/maximum intensity projection images.

14.1.1.4.2 *4D Image Reconstruction*

Images acquired using a retrospectively ECG-gated helical mode can be reconstructed at multiple phases throughout the cardiac cycle (e.g., at 5% or 10% intervals). These reconstructions can subsequently be viewed as a cineloop and provide functional assessment of valvular structures with limited temporal resolution compared to echocardiography (Figure 14.2).

14.1.1.4.3 *Segmentation and Image Fusion/Coregistration*

Segmentation involves isolating the data from specific regions of interest (e.g., aorta [in the context of endovascular stenting] or the left atrium and pulmonary vein [in the context of pulmonary vein ablation]). Various segmentation techniques exist beyond manual segmentation, including threshold-based segmentation and region-growing segmentation.

An exciting area of investigation is image fusion. This can involve registration of images from two imaging modalities (e.g., CT and angiography) or of images from one imaging modality and one functional dataset (e.g., EPS electroanatomical mapping).

14.2 Imaging of Valvular Structure in the Context of Transcatheter Valvular Intervention

Imaging with echocardiography is a critical component for planning conventional surgical valvular repair/replacement. Preoperative CT imaging is used for the identification of high-risk anatomic findings, in particular for patients undergoing reoperative cardiothoracic surgery [17–20]. More recently, preoperative assessment has been used in the context of minimally invasive and robotic-assisted surgery, which are associated with decreased direct visualization and novel approaches of vascular access [21,22]. The experience with imaging for standard and minimally invasive surgical procedures demonstrates the importance of image guidance and has been the basis for use of imaging guidance for transcatheter valve procedures.

14.2.1 Transcatheter Valve Procedures

Image guidance has a significant impact on novel transcatheter valve procedures. The preoperative understanding of the valvular structures is important for

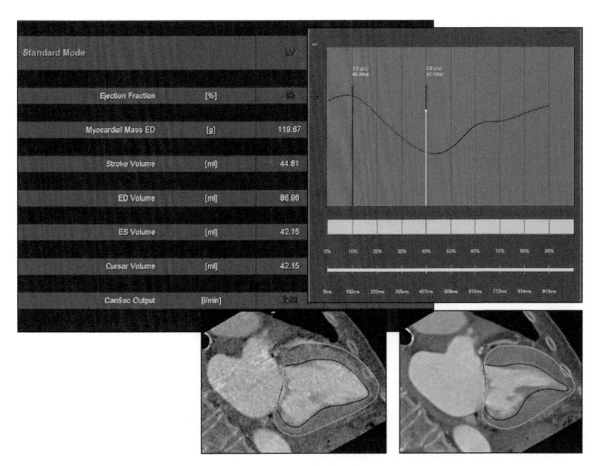

FIGURE 14.2
Calculation of left ventricular ejection fraction (LVEF). This figure demonstrates image reformation of the LV in diastole (left lower panel) and systole (right lower panel). The endocardial and epicardial contours are traced automatically providing EF and LV mass.

planning of procedural detail. The emerging experience of CT imaging in the context of aortic, mitral, and pulmonic valve procedures is described in the following paragraphs. However, there is still a lack of data evaluating the clinical impact of imaging, for example, the impact of assessment of the annulus diameter on eligibility for the procedure and choice of the device size [23]. Further evaluation in particular of 3D imaging modalities is necessary.

14.2.1.1 Transcatheter Aortic Valve Implantation

The complex anatomy of the aortic root provides the framework within which the aortic valve (AV) is suspended. Implantation of a stent/valve has complex and incompletely understood consequences for these structures and their relationships. CT imaging allows evaluation of these relationships before the procedure [23–28]. Multi-detector CT (MDCT) with 4D reconstruction also provides limited insight into the changes of root geometry throughout the cardiac cycle and allows reconstruction at specific positions in the RR interval [29] (Figures 14.3 through 14.9).

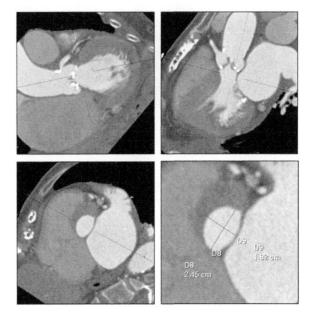

FIGURE 14.3
MPR at the level of LV outflow tract (LVOT). This figure demonstrates image reformation of the high LVOT and measurement of its elliptical dimensions.

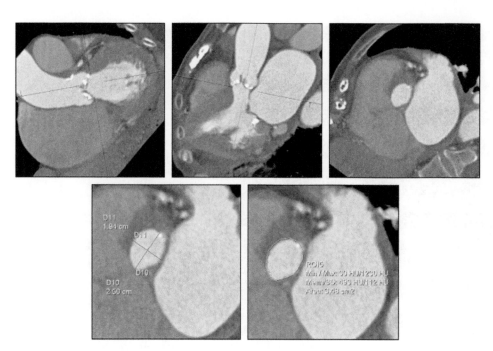

FIGURE 14.4

MPR at the level of aortic annulus. This figure demonstrates image reformation of the aortic annulus (inferior virtual basal ring) and measurement of its elliptical dimensions and area (see also Figure 14.2).

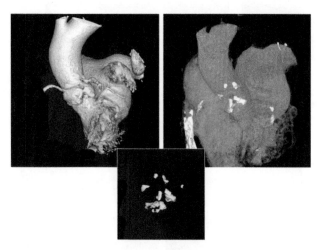

FIGURE 14.5

VRI of aortic root. This figure shows different VRIs of the aortic root, demonstrating the coronary artery ostia and the valve calcification.

The aortic annulus is the interface between the LV outflow tract and the aortic root and is defined by the hinge point/commissures of the AV leaflets (Figures 14.3 and 14.4). The commissures extend upward into the aortic root in the shape of a crown, similar to the struts of a bioprosthetic valve. In clinical imaging, the level of the annulus is defined at the lowest point of the valve hinge point (inferior virtual basal ring). Detailed 3D analysis demonstrates that this clinical defined annulus is typically elliptical [26,30,31].

Visualization of a plane at the tip of the leaflets at different phases of the cardiac cycle allows determination of the maximal opening of the AV during the cardiac cycle by planimetry (typically mid-late systole) [32]. Direct planimetry of AV area (AVA) with CT has been shown to provide reproducible results in comparison to transesophageal echocardiography and magnetic resonance imaging (MRI) (Figure 14.6) [33,34]. Similarly, planimetry of the regurgitant orifice area in patients with aortic regurgitation has been examined [35,36]. An advantage of the direct observation of the AV opening area is the ability to correlate the pattern of valve opening with leaflet anatomy. Detailed analysis allows the assessment of the location of calcification, leaflet thickening, fusion, and geometry and symmetry of the opening area [37]. Importantly, CT also allows description of the relationship of the leaflet calcification to the coronary artery ostia (Figure 14.7) [25,26,38,39]. CT also allows the prediction of 2D angiographic projections orthogonal to the AVA, simplifying the subsequent implantation of the percutaneous valve [40].

Based on emerging data, the detailed evaluation of aortic root anatomy appears important for successful deployment of the percutaneous valve prosthesis (Figure 14.8) [41–44].

14.2.1.2 Transcatheter Mitral and Pulmonic Valve Procedures

The complex anatomic structure of the mitral annulus (MA) determines valve function, but the interactions are incompletely understood [45]. 3D imaging in the context

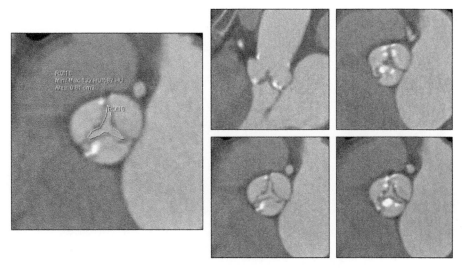

FIGURE 14.6
MPR at the level of aortic valve. This figure demonstrates image reformation at the AV with planimetry of the severely stenotic AV (left lower panel).

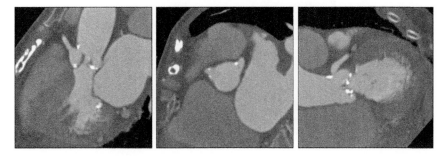

FIGURE 14.7
MPR at the level of coronary artery ostia. This figure demonstrates image reformation of the ostia of the coronary arteries. These images show the height of the coronary ostia in relationship to the valve leaflets.

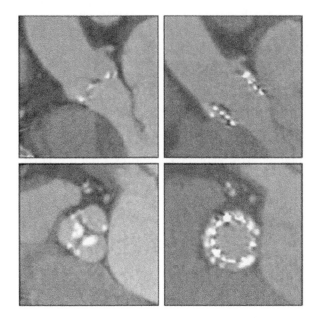

FIGURE 14.8
MPR before and after transcatheter aortic valve implantation (TAVI). This figure demonstrates image reformation of the aortic root before and after TAVI. The position of the stent valve in the root and the displacement of the calcified valve leaflets behind the struts are shown.

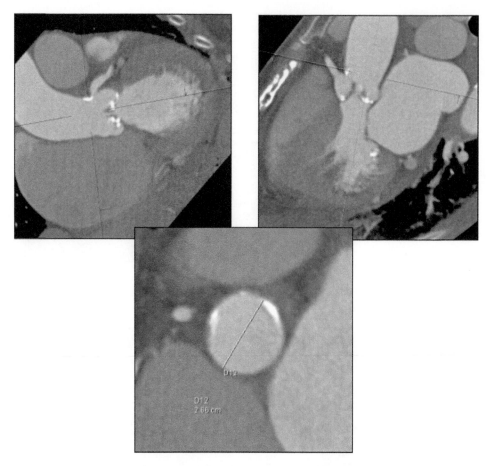

FIGURE 14.9
MPR at the level of the sinotubular junction (STJ). This figure demonstrates image reformation at the level of the STJ.

of transcatheter mitral valve procedures [46] allows a detailed understanding of the mitral valve apparatus including the MA, valve leaflets, and chordae tendineae/papillary muscles (Figures 14.10 and 14.11). Real-time 3D, full-volume acquisition with transesophageal echocardiography allows imaging of the entire annular volume including the valve over full cardiac cycles [47–51].

Using CT, assessment of the mitral valve leaflets is limited due to their rapid motion [52]. Most of the emerging CT data, therefore, describes MA anatomy (Figure 14.10). Accurate definition of MA geometry is critical for preoperative planning in the context of recently introduced transcatheter approaches for ring annuloplasty [53–55]. These devices are placed in the coronary sinus (CS), with the intention to displace the posterior mitral valve leaflet forward and reduce mitral regurgitation (MR) severity. A recent study [56] showed the feasibility of percutaneous reduction in functional MR with a novel CS-based mitral annuloplasty device in patients with heart failure and was associated with an improvement in quality of life and exercise tolerance.

The assessment of the annulus and its surrounding structures has been described with CT. The data show nonplanar shape of the MA and substantial dynamic changes of the shape, size, and motion throughout the cardiac cycle, with significant differences between healthy subjects and patients with cardiomyopathy [57].

A remaining concern is the proximity of the CS to the left circumflex coronary artery (LCx) and the potential risk of CS-based devices potentially impinging on the LCx [58]. CT studies described *in vivo* anatomical relationships between MA and CS as well as between CS and LCx (Figure 14.11) [59,60]. These data raise concern for potential coronary ischemia induced by a CS-based device and emphasize the need to evaluate the relationship between the CS/great cardiac vein and LCx is an important factor in determining the safety of CS-based devices.

Other recent applications of CT have been described in the context of valve-in-valve implantation [61].

Clinical studies describe safety, procedural success, and short-term effectiveness for transcatheter pulmonic valve replacement in patients with dysfunctional right ventricular outflow tract conduits and pulmonary regurgitation [62]. However, the current literature about

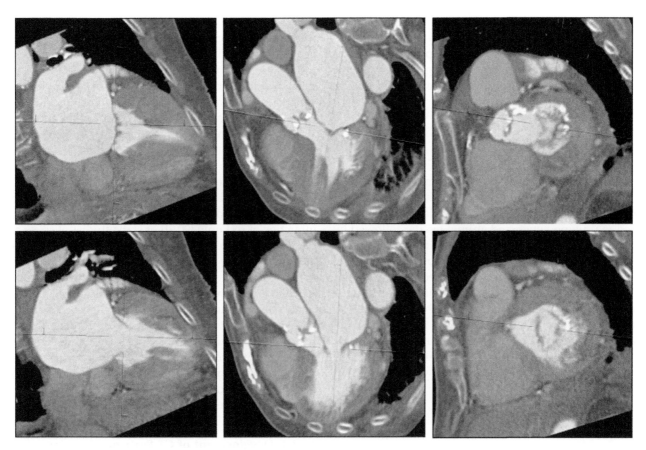

FIGURE 14.10
MPR of the mitral valve. This figure demonstrates image reformation at the level of the mitral valve. The upper images show a more systolic phase and the lower images show a more diastolic phase of the cardiac cycle.

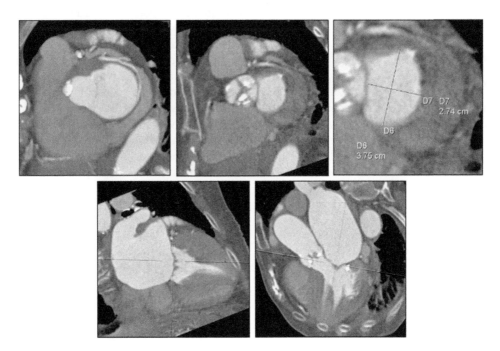

FIGURE 14.11
MPR of the coronary sinus (CS) and mitral annulus (MA). This figure demonstrates image reformation at the level of the CS (left upper panel) with its relationship to the left circumflex coronary artery (LCx). The right upper panel shows measurements of the MA.

CT imaging in the context of transcatheter pulmonic valve replacement is limited. A recent study describes implantation of a new percutaneous pulmonary valve into a dilated pulmonary trunk, using patient specific data to influence the design of the device and ensure patient safety [63].

14.2.1.3 Role of 3D Imaging for Endovascular Device Design

Beyond its value for clinical decision-making in the individual patient, 3D datasets are increasingly used for device design [64]. Traditionally, device design has relied mainly on bench and animal testing followed by human clinical trials [65]. Advances in medical imaging and computational modeling allow simulation of physiological conditions in patient-specific 3D vascular models [66]. Such models can account for the unique features of the human circulation with appropriate 3D anatomical and physiological input data to define relevant boundary conditions. This approach will allow prospective design of devices that can withstand the force variations in the cardiovascular system.

14.2.2 Other Modalities

The description of the role of C-arm CT (rotational angiography) [67–70], 3D echocardiography [71–77], and interventional cardiovascular magnetic resonance (CMR) [78–81] for real-time procedural image guidance during minimally invasive and catheter-based therapies is beyond the scope of this chapter.

14.3 CT Myocardial Perfusion Imaging

Coronary CTA allows noninvasive delineation of coronary stenoses with particular high negative predictive value (NPV) [82,83]. The positive predictive value (PPV) for significant coronary atherosclerosis is lower due to challenges in interpreting lesions with heavy calcification [82,83]. This is particularly relevant for lesions with intermediate severity and questionable clinical significance, where anatomically based strategy of coronary evaluation in general is limited [84]. For these lesions, demonstration of cardiac ischemia is important for the evaluation of the prognostic significance of a coronary plaque and is correlated with outcomes. Techniques such as nuclear cardiology derive their value from detecting and demonstrating the extent of ischemia [85,86]. There is also a need to reliably differentiate ischemia from infarction in a clinical setting. While both conditions are part of the continuum of ischemic heart disease, management strategies for ischemia or

infarction are different [85]. Moreover, ischemia and infarction may coexist in the same patient. An ideal evaluative approach to CAD incorporates anatomical information with functional data about ischemia and infarction [87]. The ability of cardiac CT to provide such functional information would significantly add to its current strengths of visualizing coronary plaques.

Up to 2009, there was little and inconsistent data regarding CT detection of myocardial perfusion, besides early experiences with electron beam CT (EBCT) [88]. Initial reports on dynamic MPI were limited to animal studies [89]. The studies conducted in humans were limited to static perfused blood volume studies of myocardial infarction at rest only [90,91] or static studies at stress and rest [92,93]. However, with the advent of new technical advances in wide-detector scanner and dual-source scanners, there is now a growing body of literature on the subject, and it is likely that the clinical technique will be well established within the next five years. This section summarizes the historical development of the field, reviews recent literature on the subject, describes the technology behind and the techniques of static and dynamic perfusion imaging, provides a suggested template for the systematic reading of CT perfusion studies, and looks into possible future developments in the field.

14.3.1 Development of CT Perfusion Imaging

The first work on evaluation of myocardial blood flow (MBF) with CT systems occurred in the 1980s, with publications measuring flow in dogs and healthy human volunteers [94–96]. These studies utilized EBCT, which has a higher temporal resolution than multislice CT (MSCT) systems. It was concluded that ultrafast CT had promise for quantifying MBF by the analysis of the first-pass effect of iodinated contrast medium on myocardial density. Significant correlation with microsphere measurements was reported, especially at lower flow rates. However, it was noted that high flow rates (greater than 2.5 mL/min/g) were underestimated with this technique. Further work in the 1990s [97] expanded on this to estimate intramyocardial vascular volume by EBCT, characterize how this volume changes during vasodilatation, and evaluated the feasibility and validity of measuring regional myocardial perfusion in human subjects. However, EBCT as a technology did not receive widespread uptake and the work while viewed as interesting did not find significant clinical utilization.

14.3.2 Animal Studies

There have been various animal studies to refine models used in CT myocardial perfusion, ranging from the use of 64-slice scanners to 128-slice dual-source scanners (Table 14.1) [89,98,99,101,102]. This parallels

TABLE 14.1
Animal Studies Evaluating CT Myocardial Perfusion

Author	Scanner	Stress Protocol	N	Population	Reference Standard	Results	Conclusion
George et al. [89]	64-Detector MDCT	Adenosine stress	8	Dogs	Microsphere MBF	Mean MBF in stenosed vs. remote territories was 1.37 ± 0.46 mL/g/min and 1.29 ± 0.48 mL/g/min at baseline and 2.54 ± 0.93 mL/g/min and 8.94 ± 5.74 mL/g/min during adenosine infusion, respectively.	Adenosine-augmented MDCT MPI provides semiquantitative measurements of myocardial perfusion during first-pass MDCT imaging in a canine model of LAD stenosis.
George et al. [98]	64-Detector MDCT	Adenosine stress	6	Dogs	Microsphere MBF	The myocardial upslope-to-LV-upslope and myocardial upslope-to-LV-max ratio correlated with MBF ($R_1 = 0.92$ and $R_2 = 0.87$) Absolute MBF derived by model-based deconvolution analysis modestly overestimated MBF compared with microsphere MBF.	Dynamic MDCT MBF measurements using upslope and model-based deconvolution methods correlate well with microsphere MBF.
Yim et al. [99]	64-Detector MDCT	–	17	Pigs	Histology 2,3,5-triphenyltetrazolium chloride (TTC) staining	The areas of perfusion deficit noted in early arterial phase images and color perfusion map (CPM) coincided exactly with the areas of poor TTC staining in 12 of 15 pigs (80%) $k = 0.736$.	CE MDCT and CPMs helpful in detecting MI.
Christian et al. [100]	64-Detector MDCT	Adenosine stress	8	Pigs	Microsphere MBF	MBF control 0.65 ± 0.28, MBF adenosine 2.6 ± 0.7 mL/min/g, $r = 0.94$.	CT first-pass MPI is feasible using a simple semiquantitative analysis, which provides reasonable estimates of MBF.
Mahnken et al. [101]	DSCT (64-slice)	Adenosine stress	10	Pigs	–	CT MBF in stenosis group was significantly lower in the poststenotic myocardium than that in the normal myocardium.	CT MBF permits quantitative whole-heart perfusion imaging. It successfully demonstrates the hemodynamic effect of high-grade coronary artery stenosis.
Bamberg et al. [102]	DSCT (128-slice)	Adenosine stress	7	Pigs	Microsphere MBF	CT MBF correlated with microsphere MBF at rest and stress. CT MBF overestimated microsphere MBF independently of adenosine stress and stenosis severity.	CT MBF at rest and stress show a valid difference, but an underestimation with microsphere MBF in pigs.

reports in human subjects utilizing 64-slice scanners and first- and second-generation dual-source scanners. Animal studies have been helpful in testing paradigms regarding scanning techniques and feasibility of protocols. They have also allowed histological correlation of infarct size with defect size, and exposure of radiation at doses which would be of concern in humans. There are issues that are much more difficult to investigate in clinical studies.

14.3.3 Human Studies

The first clinical report on perfusion imaging in the era of MDCT scanners was published in 2005 by Kurata [103] and described adenosine-stress myocardial perfusion in humans (Table 14.2). Scan parameters were as follows: retrospectively ECG gated, 912 channel detectors along the gantry and 16 channel detectors along the z-axis, tube voltage 120 kV, tube current 380 mA, scan field-of-view (FOV) 50 cm, gantry rotation 0.5 s/rotation, matrix 512 × 512, slice width 0.625 mm, and helical pitch 0.275:1. In this group of 12 patients, the agreement between CT perfusion (CTP) and nuclear perfusion was reported as 83%. The authors concluded that adenosine-stress MSCT was a potential alternative to stress myocardial perfusion scintigraphy (MPS) in the evaluation of patients with CAD. The next reports in humans using 64-slice scanners [93,107] demonstrated the presence of perfusion defects that correlated with single-photon emission CT (SPECT) and coronary angiography. However, it has been with the introduction of dual-source scanners and 320-row MDCT that the field has seen exponential development. Regarding stress CTP, there have been five studies performed on the 64-slice CT scanner [104–106, 110,111], six with the 128-slice dual-source CT (DSCT) scanner [108,109,112,113,116,114], and one with the 320-row CT scanner [115] to date. There is also an ongoing prospective multicenter trial [117,118] (CORE320) to assess the diagnostic performance of combined 320-row CTA and myocardial CTP imaging in comparison with the combination of invasive coronary angiography and SPECT MPI, the results of which will be ready in 2013. Issues that have not been resolved at this time are formal quantitation algorithms of defect size, the relative value of scans performed on dual-source 320-detector scanners and dual-energy CT (DECT) studies, the clinical value of quantitation of blood flow with dynamic perfusion imaging, and benefits over semiquantitative methods with multi-detector row CT scanners. Dual-energy scanning was preliminarily reported in 2009 and expanded on in three other studies. One of the questions has been the physiologic mechanism by which ischemic defects are detected with rest studies. To address this issue, there have been two reports of DECT with adenosine stress.

14.3.4 Dynamic and Static CPT Imaging

An understanding of the dynamics of contrast flow into and out of the myocardium from the blood pool is necessary for successful and accurate CT MPI. This knowledge also serves to elucidate the mechanism of imaging employed by different scanners.

Key to the measurement of myocardial perfusion with contrast is the accurate characterization of the arterial input function (AIF) [119]. The AIF is the input of contrast into the myocardium. In initial studies on the subject, the AIF was measured at multiple time points with dynamic imaging. This was described with electron-beam CT (EBCT), and these measurements have become the reference standard for defining the AIF [95,96,120–122].

In dynamic CTP imaging, a series of images is acquired one after another, for a preset time per image. Dynamic image acquisition is very helpful in the study of dynamic processes, such as the transit of contrast through the heart. The entire myocardium is scanned repeatedly in real time via the shuttle mode to quantify the flow of iodine-based contrast agents through the heart. This is achieved using ECG triggering. The CT scan starts prior to the intravenous injection of contrast, and the scanner produces a number of CT images prior to the arrival of the contrast bolus to the heart. The Hounsfield units (HUs) in the region of interest (myocardium) are measured sequentially. This is necessary as the mathematical models used to compute parametric maps require an input function (HU over time). The technique allows the construction of time-attenuation curves (TACs), which describe the delivery of contrast into the myocardium and its subsequent washout over time (Figure 14.12). Such curves can be plotted for a specific area of the myocardium or for the entire heart. Analytical evaluation of the TACs for each voxel of the imaged volume by dedicated algorithms yields blood flow parameters [123,124]. The shuttle mode allows the CT scanner to repeatedly image the heart, which is wider than the detector array. The scanner rapidly alternates between two table positions and acquires prospectively ECG-triggered axial images at these positions. In the case of the second-generation DSCT scanner, alternating between two table positions using a detector width of 38.4 mm with an overlap of 10% yields a coverage of 73 mm [109]. For heart rates below 63 bpm, the two table positions are imaged in consecutive heartbeats. The resulting sampling rate is one full scan every two heartbeats and one full scan every four heartbeats for heart rates exceeding 63 beats/min. Dynamic perfusion imaging requires a high-enough temporal resolution to image at stress heart rates and sufficient detector coverage to image the entire myocardium in rapid succession. The radiation exposure must also be kept reasonable. Each stress

TABLE 14.2

Human Studies Evaluating CT Myocardial Perfusion

Author	Scanner	Stress Mode	Reference	N	Population	Radiation (mSv)	Sensitivity (%)	Specificity (%)	Results	Conclusion
Kurata et al. [103]	16-Detector	Adenosine	SPECT-MPI	12	Suspected CAD	–	90	79	The agreement between MSCT and MPS was 83%.	Adenosine-stress CE-MSCT can describe both adenosine-induced myocardial ischemia and coronary artery stenoses in patients with CAD.
George et al. [93]	64-Detector, 256 detector	Adenosine	SPECT-MPI, quantitative coronary angiography (QCA)	24 (64)/16 (256)	Abnormal SPECT	16.8/21.6	81	85	The sensitivity, specificity, PPV, and NPV for the combination of CTA and CTP to detect obstructive atherosclerosis causing perfusion abnormalities was 86%, 92%, 92%, and 85% in the per-patient analysis and 79%, 91%, 75%, and 92% in the per vessel/territory analysis.	The combination of CTA and CTP can detect atherosclerosis causing perfusion abnormalities when compared with the combination of QCA and SPECT.
Blankstein et al. [104]	DSCT (64-slice)	Adenosine	Invasive angiography and SPECT defects in combination	33	Abnormal SPECT	12.7	93	74	For the detection of vessels with >50% stenosis with a corresponding SPECT perfusion abnormality, CTP had a sensitivity of 93% and a specificity of 74%.	Adenosine-stress CT can identify stress-induced myocardial perfusion defects with diagnostic accuracy comparable to SPECT, with similar radiation dose and advantage of providing information on coronary stenosis.

(Continued)

TABLE 14.2 (Continued)

Human Studies Evaluating CT Myocardial Perfusion

Author	Scanner	Stress Mode	Reference	N	Population	Radiation (mSv)	Sensitivity (%)	Specificity (%)	Results	Conclusion
Rocha-Filho et al. [105]	DSCT (64-slice)	Adenosine	QCA	34	Population at high risk of CAD	9.8	91	91	CTA alone: sensitivity 83%, specificity 71%, NPV 87%, and PPV 66%. CTA in combination with CTP: sensitivity 91%, specificity 91%, NPV 93%, and PPV 86%.	A combination protocol involving adenosine perfusion CT imaging and cardiac CTA in a dual-source technique is feasible, and CTP adds incremental value to cardiac CTA in the detection of significant CAD.
Okada et al. [106]	DSCT (64-slice)	Adenosine	SPECT-MPI	47		10.0			On a per-segment basis, CTP and SPECT-MPI demonstrated excellent correlation: Goodman–Kruskall gamma = 0.59 (stress) and 0.75 (rest). On a per-vessel basis, CTP and SPECT-MPI summed scores demonstrated good correlation: Pearson r = 0.56 or stress and 0.66 for rest. On a per-patient basis, CTP and SPECT-MPI demonstrated good correlation: Pearson r = 0.60 (stress) and 0.76 (rest).	CTP compares favorably with SPECT-MPI for detection, extent, and severity of myocardial perfusion defects at rest and stress.
Cury et al. [107]	64-Detector	Dipyridamole	QCA	26	Abnormal SPECT	Mean radiation dose 14.7 ± 3.0 (min. 11.4, max. 20.3)	88	79	Sensitivity, specificity, PPV, and NPV were 88.0%, 79.3%, 66.7%, and 93.3% for CTP.	Dipyridamole CT myocardial perfusion at rest and during stress is feasible, and results are similar to SPECT scintigraphy.

Study	CT	Stress	Standard	N	Population	Dose			Results	Conclusions
Bastarrika et al. [108]	DSCT (128-slice)	Adenosine	MRI-MPI	3	Abnormal SPECT	8.69 (stress-only imaging)	—	—	CTP images correlated with SPECT images.	CT integrative imaging of CAD with assessment of coronary stenosis, cardiac function, perfusion, and viability is possible.
Ho et al. [109]	DSCT (128-slice)	Dipyridamole	SPECT-MPI	35	Abnormal SPECT	9.2	83	78	In reversible defects, MBF was 0.65 ± 0.21 cc/cc/min and 0.63 ± 0.18 cc/cc/min at stress and rest, respectively. In fixed defects, the MBF was 0.57 ± 0.22 cc/cc/min at stress and 0.54 ± 0.23 cc/cc/min at rest, respectively. Sensitivity, specificity, PPV, and NPV was 0.83, 0.78, 0.79, and 0.82, respectively.	Vasodilator-stress CT MPI is feasible at a radiation dose similar to nuclear MPI. It identifies areas of abnormal flow reserve and infarction with a high degree of correlation to nuclear MPI as well as to stenoses detected in CTA and internal carotid artery.
Ko et al. [110]	DSCT (64-slice)	Adenosine DECT	MRI-MPI	41	Known CAD	8.6	89	78	Stress DECT had 89% sensitivity, 78% specificity, and 82% accuracy for detecting segments with reversible perfusion defects seen on strain-phase MRI, and 89% sensitivity, 76% specificity, and 83% accuracy for detecting segments with hemodynamically significant stenoses on invasive angiography.	Adenosine stress DECT can identify stress-induced myocardial perfusion defect in patients with CAD.

(Continued)

TABLE 14.2 (*Continued*)
Human Studies Evaluating CT Myocardial Perfusion

Author	Scanner	Stress Mode	Reference	N	Population	Radiation (mSv)	Sensitivity (%)	Specificity (%)	Results	Conclusion
Tamarappoo et al. [111]	DSCT (64-slice)	Adenosine	SPECT-MPI	30	Abnormal SPECT	18 ± 7.1	92	86	Extent of defect measured on stress-CT MPI correlated with that on SPECT-MPI, k = 0.71. Sensitivity, specificity, PPV, and NPV for detection of defect compared to SPECT was 92%, 86%, 71%, 96%.	Stress and reversible defects measured on CT MPI using a visual semiquantitative approach showed strong similarity with SPECT-MPI, suggesting clinical and prognostic values of CT MPI.
Weininger et al. [112]	DSCT (128-slice)	Adenosine	MRI-MPI	20	Chest pain + high likelihood CAD	12.8/15.2	93	99	Real-time perfusion CT (vs. SPECT) had 86% (84%) sensitivity, 98% (92%) specificity, 94% (88%) PPV, and 96% (92%) NPV in comparison with perfusion MRI for the detection of myocardial perfusion defects. Compared with MRI, dual-energy myocardial perfusion CT (vs. SPECT) had 93% (94%) sensitivity, 99% (98%) specificity, 92% (88%) PPV, and 96% (94%) NPV for detecting hypoperfused myocardial segments.	Myocardial perfusion CT imaging in patients with acute chest pain is clinically feasible. Compared to MRI and SPECT, both dynamic real-time perfusion CT and first-pass dual-energy perfusion CT showed good agreement for the detection of myocardial perfusion defects.

| Feuchtner et al. [113] | DSCT (128-slice) | Adenosine | MRI-MPI | 30 | Known and suspected CAD | 2.5 | 96 | 88 | The performance of stress-CTP for detection of myocardial perfusion defects compared with CMR was sensitivity, 96%; specificity, 88%; PPV, 93%; NPV, 94% (per vessel). The accuracy improved from 84% to 95% after adding stress CTP to CTA. | Adenosine-induced stress 128-slice dual-source high-pitch myocardial CTP allows for simultaneous assessment of reversible myocardial ischemia and coronary stenosis, with good diagnostic accuracy as compared with CMR and invasive angiography, at a very low radiation exposure. |
| Bamberg et al. [114] | DSCT (128-slice) | Adenosine | FFR | 36 | Known and suspected CAD | 10.0 | 93 | 87 | While the diagnostic accuracy of CT for the detection of anatomically significant coronary artery stenosis (>50%) was high, it was low for the detection of hemodynamically significant stenosis PPV 49%. With use of estimated MBF to reclassify lesions depicted with CTA, 30 of 70 (43%) coronary lesions were graded as not hemodynamically significant, which significantly increased PPV to 78%. | Dynamic CT-based stress MPI may allow detection of hemodynamically significant coronary artery stenosis. |

(Continued)

TABLE 14.2 (*Continued*)
Human Studies Evaluating CT Myocardial Perfusion

Author	Scanner	Stress Mode	Reference	N	Population	Radiation (mSv)	Sensitivity (%)	Specificity (%)	Results	Conclusion
									The presence of a coronary artery stenosis with a corresponding MBF less than 75 mL/100 mL/min had a high risk for hemodynamic significance (odds ratio 86.9; 95% confidence interval 17.6–430.4).	
Ko et al. [115]	320-Detector	Adenosine	FFR	42	Known CAD	5.3 (Stress CTP only)	76	84	CT MPI correctly identified 31/41 (76%) ischemic territories and 38/45 (84%) non-ischemic territories. Per-vessel territory sensitivity, specificity, PPV, and NPV of CTP were 76%, 84%, 82%, and 79%, respectively. The combination of a ≥50% stenosis on CTA and perfusion defect on CTP was 98% specific for ischemia, while the presence of, 50% stenosis on CTA and normal perfusion on CTP was 100% specific for the exclusion of ischemia.	CT MPI is moderately accurate in identifying perfusion defects associated with ischemia as assessed by FFR in patients considered for revascularization. In territories where CTA and CTP are concordant, CTA/CTP is highly accurate in the detection and exclusion of ischemia. This is achievable with acceptable radiation exposure using 320-row detector CT and prospective ECG gating.

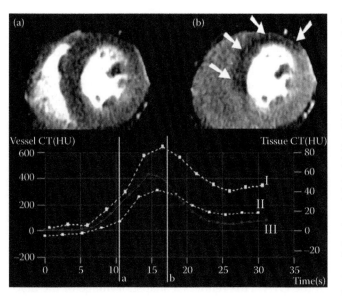

FIGURE 14.12
Dynamic computed tomography myocardial perfusion imaging time-attenuation curves (CT MPI TACs) and snapshot images. The graph shows typical TACs acquired by dynamic CT MPI and two snapshot images of the same mid-ventricular slice, corresponding to different time points of CT MPI scan. The yellow curve (I) in the graph represents the TAC in normal tissue and the gray curve (II) represents the TAC of infarcted area. The red curve (III) is the TAC of the ascending aorta. Image (a) was taken at the time point indicated by line (a) in the graph. Image (b) was taken 6 seconds later, as indicated by line (b). The variation between the images emphasized the difficulty of timing a static scan to robustly assess the extend of a perfusion defect. HU—Hounsfield unit.

or rest scan yields 10 to 15 3D volume datasets, containing the TACs for each individual voxel of the entire myocardium. A dedicated reconstruction algorithm for myocardial perfusion [101] automatically generates each CT image from low spatial frequency components from a full rotation reconstruction and high spatial frequency components from a cardiac reconstruction. This approach yields images with a high temporal resolution while maintaining CT value stability [125]. Images can be reconstructed with a slice thickness of 3 mm, an increment of 2 mm, and a medium smooth kernel (B25).

MBF is computed from the TACs contained in 4D volume datasets. Blood flow through each voxel of myocardium is computed based on the maximum slope of the TAC of this voxel [101]. This computation yields a 3D CT dataset, with the intensity values representing MBF in cubic centimeters of blood per cubic centimeter of tissue per minute instead of HUs. These quantitative 3D color maps of MBF can be analyzed visually or quantitatively and can be overlaid onto the anatomical HU CT dataset.

The alternative to dynamic multi-detector imaging is static multi-detector imaging. In a static acquisition, a single image is acquired for a preset time interval, over 5–10 seconds (Figure 14.13). Owing to the helical nature of MDCTA acquisition, direct measurement of the TACs cannot be performed. Static arterial phase CT imaging acquires a single-contrast phase. Local inhomogeneities in contrast distribution during that specific phase were

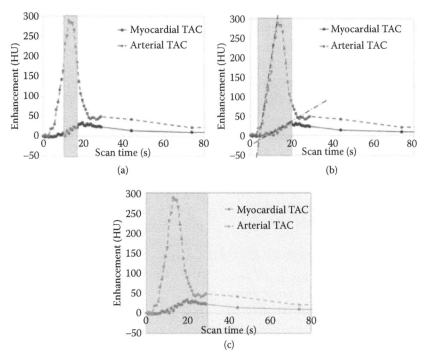

FIGURE 14.13
Scan protocol of (a) qualitative, (b) semiquantitative, and (c) quantitative myocardial CT perfusion (CTP). The gray box in each graph represents the data acquisition window with respect to the arterial and myocardial TAC after a bolus injection of contrast. The dashed line in (B) represents the upslope of each TAC.

used in earlier studies as a surrogate marker of blood flow. Arterial phase CT has been shown to demonstrate perfusion defects [89,93,104]. However, it cannot quantitate blood flow, and the difficulty in timing the scan, long duration of the scan, and inadequate temporal resolution make it hard to reproducibly capture the transient contrast distribution inhomogeneity. Past clinical CT MPI research has focused on static imaging of the myocardium because technical limitations have prevented rapid repetitive imaging that is required for dynamic perfusion imaging [93,104,126].

Recently, techniques have been described in canine models to reconstruct and extrapolate the TAC of the AIF by combining bolus-tracking and time-registered helical static MDCT image datasets [127]. This is similar in principle to the quantitation of MBF by magnetic resonance perfusion imaging using a dual-bolus approach [128,129]. In CTP imaging, bolus-tracking imaging data are used to record the early part of contrast enhancement over time. In addition, helical MDCT images can be registered to their time of acquisition and used to construct the latter portion of the AIF. The TAC of the AIF is constructed by combining bolus-tracking and time-registered helical MDCT image datasets. These calculations have been found to correlate with measurements from dynamic perfusion imaging.

In this model, the following assumptions are made regarding the behavior of the contrast used [95]:

1. Complete mixing of the contrast occurs proximal to the arrival of the contrast in the heart.

2. The volume of the contrast administered is small in comparison to the volume of the circulation.

3. The administration of the contrast is not associated with hemodynamic or physiologic changes of the circulation.

4. The CT attenuation value in the vasculature accurately reflects the concentration of the contrast.

5. The recirculation of the contrast is negligible.

6. There is no extravascular diffusion of the contrast during its first-pass circulation through the vasculature.

However, iodinated contrast agents are not hemodynamically inert and have an influence on coronary blood flow, inducing a reduction in coronary flow followed by a hyperemic response. During first pass, there is also significant diffusion of the contrast agents into the interstitial space, particularly for nonionic and low-molecular-weight compounds. The first-pass extraction of contrast is around 33% with maximal vasodilation and is substantially higher at lower flow

rates. The characterization of the AIF by this method facilitates the semiquantitative measurement of myocardial perfusion distribution imaging but does not allow full quantitation afforded by dynamic perfusion imaging. Another limitation is that the interpolation of data during the 3.6-second pause between bolus-tracking and helical CT imaging, while allowing for tube current and collimator changes, can introduce errors in the AIF characterization.

14.3.5 Clinical Myocardial CTP Imaging

14.3.5.1 Qualitative Method

Myocardial perfusion images can be acquired at the same time that a coronary CTA is performed (Figure 14.13). The timing of scanning is thus dependent on the timing of the CTA. This renders a snapshot image of the myocardial perfusion. The technique has a reasonable ability to detect infarction [130–136]. There have been some reports of the identification of ischemia [130]. The reasons resting CTP can detect ischemia are unclear. One hypothesis is that coronary vasodilation from either pre-CT scan nitroglycerin or iodinated contrast or the mild stress of having a CT scan may cause myocardial ischemia. Differentiation of infarction or ischemia using CTP will warrant further study.

The identification of hypoperfusion with this technique is completely dependent on the timing of the CTA. The signal density in the myocardium accurately reflects the relative myocardial perfusion only if the CTA is acquired during the peak myocardial contrast enhancement. However in CTA, the acquisition is timed to occur during peak arterial contrast enhancement. Contrast arrival in the ischemic or infarcted myocardium can be significantly delayed compared to that in coronary arteries.

Visual registration of density differences in coronary CTA source images is used to distinguish hypoperfused myocardium from normal myocardium [93,104]. It has the advantage that no further contrast injection and radiation exposure is required over that used for the CTA. However, myocardial defects may vary in size and intensity depending on the exact scan timing. This qualitative (or relative) technique has limitations in detecting balanced ischemia (as in cases of left-main or triple-vessel CAD).

14.3.5.2 Semiquantitative Method

In this technique, dynamic scanning of the heart is performed to cover the time between contrast arrival in the myocardium, to peak enhancement of the myocardium. The upslope of the myocardial TAC is normalized to that of the corresponding arterial TAC, measured from either the LV cavity of the aorta. In this scan, only the rising portion of the TAC is sampled. Myocardial perfusion measured in this way correlates with, but significantly underestimates, that measured by the gold standard microsphere technique [137].

The upslope technique relies on the assumption that the rate of contrast accumulation in myocardium (upslope of myocardial TAC) equals the produce of myocardial perfusion and the arterial concentration of the contrast, provided there is no venous outflow from the myocardium. The latter is unrealistic and is the likely cause of the underestimation of myocardial perfusion. The slope of the tissue enhancement curve, the time taken to reach the maximum slope, and maximum arterial enhancement are dependent on the bolus volume, the rate of injection, and the patient's cardiac output. While variations in these parameters have little impact on the deconvolution method, they can affect the slope method. The optimum bolus size and delivery rate have not been carefully studied in perfusion CT.

14.3.5.3 Quantitative Method

This provides absolute quantitation of myocardial perfusion and more accurate assessment of CAD. By performing dynamic contrast-enhanced (CE) myocardial imaging, changes in contrast enhancement of the myocardium and its input artery over time are monitored, allowing for detailed modeling of the tissue contrast distribution with time [101,109,138].

14.3.5.4 Generation of Quantitative Myocardial Perfusion Estimates

During a dynamic CE CT study, contrast is injected in a bolus fashion and the input at the arterial inlet of the heart generates a TAC. This can be depicted as a series of bolus injections of varying magnitude (Figure 14.12). The corresponding myocardial tissue response function (time–density curve) to the bolus injections (also known as the impulse residual function [IRF]) describes the change of contrast concentration in tissue with time following the ideal bolus injection. IRF is affected by tissue vascular properties such as blood volume, mean transit time, and permeability. The myocardial TAC can be considered to the superimposition of corresponding IRFs separated by infinitely small time intervals. The form of the myocardial TAC is primarily controlled by blood flow, AIF, and IRF. Mathematically, the myocardial TAC is described as equal to the product of flow and AIF "convoluted" (convolution) with the IRF [139]. The goal of quantitative myocardial CTP is to reverse the convolution, by a process called "deconvolution," to decouple the cross-effect of AIF from flow and IRF on myocardial TAC, allowing perfusion and other physiologic parameters to be estimated [140].

Deconvolution is highly sensitive to noise [141]. In practice, deconvolution is performed using certain assumptions regarding tracer kinetics. The most commonly used tracer models include the compartment model [142–144], Johnson and Wilson model, and the MMID4 (multiple path, multiple tracer, indicator dilution, 4 region) model [98,145]. Of these, the latter two are more sophisticated, are comparable, and have demonstrated similar linear correlation relationships with the gold standard microsphere technique. The Johnson and Wilson model has also been validated for human myocardial perfusion measurements [146,147].

14.3.6 Artifacts in CT Myocardial Perfusion Imaging

14.3.6.1 Beam Hardening

Beam hardening is a major limitation in MPI. This is a result of the polychromatic nature of the x-rays used in CT and the energy-dependent x-ray attenuation [148]. It occurs when x-rays pass through the objects of high density. This results in a selective attenuation of lower energy beams and increased mean energy of the residual beams. In the example of perfusion imaging, x-ray beams that have different energies pass through heart chambers filled with concentrated iodine contrast and are attenuated to different extents. X-ray photons with lower energies are preferentially removed first, resulting in the mean energies of x-rays from different views being shifted by different amounts, depending on the levels of attenuation. The inconsistency of x-ray energies between views results in error in the estimation of x-ray attenuation and produces artifacts in images that can be erroneously interpreted as perfusion defects. The artifact appears as hypoenhanced areas that mimic true perfusion defects. There are a few characteristics of such artifacts that may help in their identification. The defects are usually triangular in appearance, appear to originate from the adjacent regions of high attenuation, and do not conform to particular vascular territories [89]. Common locations include the basal inferolateral wall, due to the proximity of the descending aorta filled with contrast, and dense vertebral bodies.

14.3.6.2 Correction of Beam Hardening Artifacts

Beam hardening may be associated with dark and bright band artifacts in the perfusion images of the heart. These may manifest areas of hypoenhancement and increased enhancement in others, resulting in both false positive and false negative findings, affecting the sensitivity and specificity of the technique. It is helpful to implement beam hardening correction algorithms to improve the accuracy of CT myocardial perfusion. There are two possible beam hardening correction techniques:

1. Postreconstruction image–based method: This method works on reconstructed images, with no need for access to original raw data. Beam hardening results in high-attenuating regions of the reconstructed images. An error image is generated through a process of forward projection and filtered back projection. The beam hardening corrected image is then obtained by subtracting the original image from the error image [149]. This technique has been validated against microsphere measurements in pigs [147] and SPECT technetium-99m sestamibi in humans [138].

2. DECT: This generates simulated monochromatic images [150], thus eliminating beam hardening that arises from the polychromatic nature of x-rays. This can be performed with both the dual-source systems, equipped with two pairs of x-ray tubes and detectors (e.g., SOMATOM Definition Flash; Siemens Healthcare, Erlangen, Germany) and a CT scanner with a single x-ray tube with rapid switching capabilities between 80 and 140 kVp [151] (e.g., Discovery CT750 HD; GE Healthcare, Waukesha, WI). More investigations into both techniques are needed before wider-based use.

14.3.6.3 Patient Motion

A common source of image degradation is patient motion during the dynamic acquisition. With a dynamic image series, motion results in misalignment of the time frames leading to artifacts in MBF quantification and regional partial volume correction. Patient motion entirely within the plane of the image may be corrected by the use of image registration methods. Patient motion out of the image plane leads to the loss of data, although there may be some limited ability to track moving tissue from slice to slice in multislice studies. While it may not be possible to completely avoid motion, it can be mitigated by ensuring patient comfort, coaching of breath-holding, and minimizing the total scanning time. Even arm motion, or motion of the legs, may result in significant chest movement in the axial direction. Patient comfort and cooperation is of great importance. If despite preventive measures, patient motion is noted during the acquisition, *post hoc* motion correction algorithms can be applied, but may not always be successful. Motion artifacts may be recognized because the apparent perfusion defects do not correspond to specific vascular territories, are not associated with wall motion abnormalities, and may not be seen to persist across different phases

of the cardiac cycle. Motion may also arise from cardiac or respiratory motion. This will manifest with signs of misregistration such as blurring of cardiac margins, pulmonary vessels, cardiac trabeculae, or sternum. The reader should actively look for the above possible signs of patient motion before embarking into the details of reading the study, as motion has the potential of resulting in spurious findings. The effects of cardiac motion may be mitigated by the use of beta blockers to ensure a lower heart rate.

14.3.6.4 Cone Beam Artifacts

Cone beam artifact is a reconstruction artifact [152] and occurs more commonly in the outer detector than the inner detector rows. These are also more pronounced by the greater number of detector rows. There are algorithms to correct for these artifacts, but they may still occur and are detected by the presence of bands extending across the whole FOV.

14.3.6.5 Low Signal-to-Noise Ratio

Noise is the variability of the attenuation value between two neighboring voxels compared to the average attenuation measured in that area. To lower noise in an image, the price to pay is the high dose of radiation. One of the main determinants of noise is the number of milliampere per second produced by the x-ray tube.

Methods to reduce radiation dose may involve trade-offs in image quality (increase in noise, decrease in low-contrast resolution, etc.). It is important to remember the objective of a perfusion study is to be able to confidently identify the presence of perfusion defects. The dose used should facilitate this aim. As a rule of thumb, patients weighing between 65 and 90 kg should be scanned with 100 kV and those greater than 90–100 kg should be imaged with 120 kV. If the dose used is inadequate, it may be difficult to define defects accurately, thus defeating the goal of the study.

14.3.6.6 Radiation Dose Considerations

In a technique such as CT myocardial perfusion, adhering to the ALARA (as low as reasonably achievable) is important. Patients with CAD may expect to undergo repeated evaluations for extent and severity of ischemia or infarction over a period of years. For the technique to grow, methods to reduce dose must be established and implemented. This is an area of ongoing development. At present, quantitative techniques result in higher radiation exposure than nonquantitative techniques. The need for measurement of the entire arterial and myocardial TAC for generating absolute myocardial perfusion parameters in quantitative techniques results in a longer exposure to radiation.

14.3.7 Dose-Reduction Techniques

14.3.7.1 Iterative Reconstruction

Compared to the widely used filtered back projection algorithm, iterative reconstruction algorithms result in less image noise and improved image quality at lower radiation dose. Its implementation in the projection domain requires larger amounts of computing memory and more powerful computers. Studies have estimated that radiation dose of MPI studies can be reduced by 30%–60% [153]. All the major manufacturers have iterative reconstruction software. In this technique, the estimate of the image is used to generate forward projections, which are then compared to the actual measured projection acquired during acquisition. The difference between the forward projection and the measured projection is the error matrix, which is computed for all projections measured around 360°. Each specific iterative algorithm uses the error matrix to update the next iteration of the image and reduces the error matrix in the subsequent iteration. After a number of iterations, the estimated image becomes an accurate depiction of the object that was scanned. Iterative algorithms, unlike filtered back projection algorithms, can model many of the physical parameters and can make better use of the acquired data. This results in images with higher signal-to-noise ratio (SNR) at the same dose or in images of similar SNR at lower dose.

14.3.7.2 Postreconstruction Image Processing

Postreconstruction image processing methods can be applied together with iterative reconstruction to further reduce image noise and achieve accurate myocardial perfusion measurements in low-dose myocardial CTP scans. The image obtained with iterative reconstruction can be further subjected to processing. Examples include principal component analysis (PCA) and neighborhood smart smoothing, which work to smooth TACs temporally and spatially, respectively, in reconstructed images. Preliminary results suggest that use of both iterative reconstruction and PCA together may result in maintenance of diagnostic quality of perfusion scans with reduction of effective dose of up to eight times. More work is in progress.

14.3.7.3 Scan Length

A large-enough FOV providing an adequate scan length is an important consideration in CT myocardial perfusion studies for the following reasons:

1. Patients with established CAD often have dilated hearts. A larger FOV is necessary for the entire heart to be imaged without truncation. This also facilitates MPR of the axial images into short-axis and vertical long-axis orientations, allowing evaluation of perfusion in all orthogonal views.

2. A large detector coverage will allow myocardial perfusion assessment with a single injection of contrast, reducing risk of nephrotoxicity and arrhythmia from contrast injection [154].

At present, Toshiba's Aquilion ONE (Tokyo, Japan) has the largest FOV at 16 cm of axial coverage with 320 slices [155]. The limited scan length is compensated by other manufacturers (e.g., Siemen Healthcare's SOMATOM Definition Flash and GE Healthcare's Discovery CT750 HD) through the axial shuttle mode. The scanner rapidly alternates between two table positions and acquires prospectively ECG-triggered axial images at these positions. In the case of the DSCT scanner, alternating between two table positions using a detector width of 38.4 mm with an overlap of 10% yields a coverage of 73 mm [146]. The potential drawback of this technique is the limited sampling of the TACs. For heart rates below 63 beats/min, the two table positions are imaged in consecutive heartbeats. The resulting sampling rate is one full scan every two heartbeats and one scan every four heartbeats for heart rates exceeding 63 beats/min. Theoretically, the peak enhancement of the arterial TAC could be missed, resulting in the overestimation of myocardial perfusion. Although this was not found to be so in our experience, further investigations are needed.

14.3.8 DECT Perfusion Imaging

14.3.8.1 Principles

The energy setting (kilovoltage) of the x-ray tube determines the energy of photons in the resultant x-ray beam. Modification of the tube's potential causes an alteration of photon energy. The attenuation characteristics of iodine, soft tissue, and bone vary as a function of x-ray photon energy. A change in the photon energy results in a corresponding modification of the attenuation of the x-ray beams in the materials scanned. X-ray absorption is dependent on [1] the energy levels used (e.g., 80 and 140 kV scans of a single object results in different attenuation) and [2] the nature of the tissue scanned.

In dual-energy scanning, two x-ray sources set at different voltages result in two datasets showing different attenuation levels. With the dual-source scanners, the two datasets are simultaneously acquired in a single scan, using two x-ray sources set at different kilovolt levels. The material-specific difference in attenuation makes classification of the elementary chemical composition of the scanned tissue possible. The low kilovolt and high kilovolt datasets are then reconstructed separately, and subtraction techniques or digital manipulation can be applied directly to the reconstructed images. Ultimately, the dual-energy image is a combination of the low- and high-energy CT images. Prior to the advent of dual-source scanners, the two scans at different energy levels had to be acquired sequentially. This resulted in interscan motion artifacts, differences in contrast concentrations between scans, long scan times, and high radiation dose.

There have been reports of using DECT on a dual-source MDCT scanner to determine regional myocardial perfusion [90,126,156,157]. In a study with 35 patients [90], iodine distribution maps were determined from the image sets with different x-ray energies. The myocardial blood pool was analyzed by determining the iodine content within the myocardium on the basis of the unique x-ray absorption characteristics of this element at different kilovolt levels. The resulting color-coded "iodine map" representing the myocardial blood pool was then superimposed onto gray-scale MPR of the myocardium in short-axis and long-axis views, from which the iodine content in the voxels had been digitally subtracted to generate a virtually non-enhanced scan. In 16 patients, stress/rest SPECT was also performed. In the five patients with fixed defects, DECT correctly identified 90% of the perfusion defects, and in the 11 patients with reversible defects, DECT correctly identified 88% of the defects on a per-defect basis. It is interesting that DECT imaging at rest correlated with inducible ischemia by stress/rest SPECT; however, the physiology underlying this observation was not clearly elucidated.

Most studies with resting DECT have demonstrated higher sensitivities in the detection of infarcts, especially chronic infarcts. This is partly related to the presence of associated imaging findings such as wall thinning. The technique appears to perform best for the detection of fixed or mixed defects (sensitivity 90%–93%, specificity 70%–94%, accuracy 83%–93%), but less impressively for reversible defects (sensitivity 50%–80%, specificity 80%–90%, accuracy 80%). These findings indicate that myocardial areas of hypoattenuation in MDCT can indeed correspond to infarctions and perfusion defects at the same time. As MDCT of the heart is typically performed at rest conditions, sensitivity for perfusion defects detected with stress perfusion MRI is significantly reduced. A differentiation of recent infarctions with normal wall thickness and myocardial perfusion defects does not seem possible with the standard CE coronary angiography protocol. Sensitivity for chronic MI is high, and infarct volume and localization correlate well to findings in delayed-enhancement MRI. However, diagnostic accuracy for the assessment of myocardial perfusion defects is reduced comparing MDCT data to stress perfusion MRI, most probably because CE MDCT of the heart is typically performed at resting conditions.

To address the limitation of detecting reversible defects with resting DECT, there have also been reports with adenosine-stress DECT [9,110]. An iodine map contains a broad range of iodine concentrations within the myocardium and may be influenced by beam hardening artifacts, cardiac motion artifacts, and normalization of iodine to the areas of normal myocardial perfusion. The authors felt that adenosine-stress DECT-based iodine mapping would improve the sensitivity of the detection of hemodynamically significant stenosis causing perfusion defects. In this population of 41 patients, stress DECT had 89% sensitivity, 78% specificity, and 82% accuracy for detection of segments with reversible defects compared to stress MRI.

14.3.9 CT Myocardial Perfusion Protocols

14.3.9.1 Patient Selection and Preparation

Patients should be screened for contraindications to cardiac CT and vasodilator administration. These include allergy to iodinated contrast, abnormal renal function (serum creatinine level >200 mmol/L and not on renal dialysis), inability to follow breath-hold instructions, a history of active asthma or severe obstructive lung disease, second-degree (Mobitz Type II) or third-degree AV block without a functioning pacemaker, atrial fibrillation, an acute MI (within 48 hours), unstable coronary syndrome, and systolic blood pressure <90 mm Hg.

Patients need to avoid caffeine, methylxanthine-containing products, oral dipyridamole, theophylline, beta blockers, and metformin prior to stress testing. A single 18-gauge venula is inserted into the right antecubital vein for dipyridamole and contrast administration. ECG and heart rate are monitored by a cardiologist during the imaging procedure, and patients are evaluated clinically for signs of fluid overload for an hour after the study. For the perfusion scan, patients are instructed to hold their breath for 30 seconds. They are asked to exhale gently over a few seconds and not abruptly, if unable to maintain the breath-hold. All patients are observed for an hour after the study.

14.3.9.2 Stress–Rest and Rest–Stress Protocols

Either a stress scan can be performed first, followed by a rest scan or vice versa. The advantages of a stress–rest study are the reduction of the possibility of residual contrast in the myocardium arising from the earlier performance of a rest study. The stress study is deemed the more important of the two acquisitions, as it is more helpful in delineating the extent of abnormal flow reserve. The advantage of a rest–stress protocol is the simultaneous acquisition of the coronary CTA at the time of the rest study, thereby reducing the need of a stress study if the coronary arteries are normal.

14.3.10 Image Acquisition and Pharmacological Stress Protocol

14.3.10.1 Dynamic Perfusion Imaging

Following a topogram from the carina to just below the diaphragm, a low-dose ECG-gated scan of the entire heart is acquired. This scan is used to precisely position the range of the subsequent perfusion scan over the myocardium. Dipyridamole is then infused intravenously at a dose of 0.56 mg/kg/min over 4 minutes. Three minutes after the end of the infusion, a test-bolus scan is acquired at the level of the mid-LV after injection of 18 cc of contrast (Utravist 370®; Bayer Schering Pharma, Berlin, Germany), followed by 50 cc of saline. Immediately thereafter, stress perfusion images of the myocardium are acquired with injection of 50 cc of contrast, followed by 50 cc of saline. The scan commences 4 seconds before arrival of contrast in the LV; timing is based on the TAC from the test-bolus scan. If adenosine is used as a stress agent, it is infused at a rate of 140 μg/kg/min for 3 minutes, at which point the stress CTP scan was initiated. Adenosine injection is continued during the CT examination.

After the dipyridamole stress scan, intravenous aminophylline (1.5 mg/kg body weight) is administered over 5 minutes to reverse the effects of dipyridamole [158] (this step is not necessary if adenosine is used as it has a short half-life and its effects resolve with 10 seconds of termination of infusion). Fifteen minutes are allowed to elapse for the effects of the dipyridamole to be reversed and for the heart rate to return to baseline (in the case of adenosine, this can be shortened to a minimum of 5 minutes). If the heart rate differs by more than 30% from that during the stress scan, a second test-bolus scan is acquired. Next, rest perfusion images are acquired with the same injection protocol as the stress scan. Thereafter, a coronary CTA of the entire heart and bypass grafts, if any, is acquired after injection of 60 cc of contrast, followed by 60 cc of saline. The scan is timed to take place during the maximum attenuation seen in the TAC in the aorta in the rest perfusion scan. All injections are done at a flow rate of 5 cc/s. Contrast agent is warmed to body temperature to decrease viscosity.

14.3.10.2 Static Perfusion Imaging

14.3.10.2.1 320-Row Scanners (Aquilion ONE)

For the stress acquisition, intravenous adenosine infusion is administered as above for 5 minutes and another 60 cc of contrast is injected at 5 cc/s. Scan acquisition is timed to occur when contrast attenuation in the descending aorta reaches a predetermined threshold of 300 HU. For a 320-row detector scanner, the acquisition is performed using prospective ECG gating set at 70%–90% of the RR window. Scan parameters are as follow: 320 mm × 0.5 mm detector collimation, 120 kV tube voltage, 350–500 mA tube current, 350 ms gantry rotation time, and 350 ms scan time. With gantry rotation of 350 ms, the temporal rotation is 175 ms using half-scan reconstruction. When heart rates are more than 65 bpm, multisegment acquisition is performed over two heartbeats, with a resultant temporal resolution of 90 ms.

14.3.10.2.2 Dual-Source Scanners

Dual-source scanners can also acquire perfusion data with the ECG-synchronized high-pitch spiral mode[27] [113] or retrospective ECG gating with tube current modulation [104]. With the high-pitch spiral mode, the CT scan is triggered using "bolus-tracking technique," after 100 HU is reached in the ascending aorta. Patients hold the breath at mid-inspiration. The scan length extended from the pulmonary artery bifurcation to the apex of the heart. Prospective ECG synchronization is applied. The scan start is triggered at 60% of the RR interval, resulting in end-diastolic image acquisition from 60% to 80%. Scan parameters are slice acquisition, 2 × 128 × 0.6 mm; gantry rotation time, 280 ms; and tube potential, 100 kV if body mass index (BMI) was <30 kg/m² and 120 kV if BMI was >30 kg/m². Tube current–time product is set at 320 mA/rotation. Pitch factor is 3.4. When using retrospective ECG gating with tube current modulation, employing the 64-slice DSCT scanner (Definition; Siemens Medical Systems, Forchheim, Germany) with a gantry rotation time of 330 ms, the resulting temporal resolution is 83 ms, with a pitch factor of 0.36 [104].

14.3.10.2.3 64-Row Scanners

This has been described by various authors [103,159]. With a 64-slice scanner, imaging parameters were collimation, 32 × 0.6 mm; gantry rotation time, 330 ms; tube voltage, 120 kV; effective tube current–time product, 850 mAs; beam pitch, 0.24; and table speed, 9.2 mm per rotation. The delay between the beginning of contrast material administration and scanning was, on average, 24 seconds (range 18–32 seconds). Breath-hold scan time varied from 11 to 16 seconds.

14.3.11 Interpretation of CT Myocardial Perfusion Studies

The following describes the systematic evaluation of CT myocardial perfusion studies. As discussed, there are varying technologies and software available on different scanners for the evaluation of CTP; however, the principles of evaluation should remain the same regardless of the scanners.

14.3.11.1 Processing of Dataset and Data Quality

Most scanners have automated or semiautomated software to enable processing of a dataset. Once completed, the dataset should be evaluated for the quality of acquisition and possible artifacts. This would include vigilance regarding artifacts arising from patient movement on the table, suboptimal breath-holding during acquisition, radiodense objects such as surgical clips and wires in patients with previous bypass surgery, coronary stenting, and pacemakers or pacing leads. Such artifacts could result in spurious defects resulting in errors of interpretation. Many systems have automated motion-correction software that helps in countering the effects of breathing. Registration of datasets, in particular rest and stress datasets, is critical in facilitating the comparison of similar segments of the myocardium and allowing the quantitation of defect size. Datasets should also be evaluated for the presence of beam hardening and cone beam artifacts as previously discussed. While much has been said about reduction of radiation dose, each study must also be assessed for adequate radiation to enable suitable SNRs. For dynamic perfusion datasets, in addition to the issues listed above, the integrity of the TACs must be evaluated. The curve should start at the baseline just prior to the delivery of contrast to the myocardium (flat part of the curve). This should be followed by a steep slope (fast phase), which documents the delivery of contrast to the myocardium, followed by a peaking and subsequent tapering of the curve representing the washout of the contrast. Truncation of the curves, which indicates inappropriate timing of acquisition, must be noted as this would impact on the appropriate interpretability of the study.

14.3.11.2 Systematic Evaluation of Perfusion

The datasets should be processed so that the myocardium is displayed in the horizontal long-axis, vertical long-axis, and short-axis projections [160]. In the short axis, the myocardium should be evaluated at the apex, mid-, and basal-ventricular sections. If both rest and stress datasets are available, by convention as in nuclear studies, the stress images can be displayed above the rest images to facilitate comparison (Figure 14.14). Interpretation should start with review of the horizontal and vertical long-axis projections. This allows the reader to identify potential defects in the septum; apex; anterior, lateral, and inferior

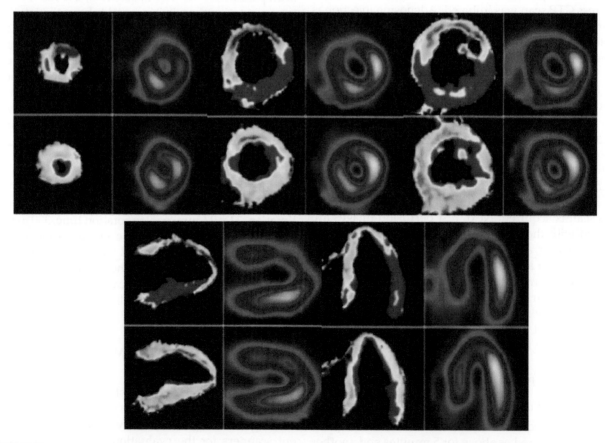

FIGURE 14.14
Display of CT myocardial perfusion images in the short-axis, vertical and horizontal long-axis views. In each view, the stress image is in the upper row and the rest image below. The corresponding nuclear perfusion image is displayed side-by-side.

walls and the territory involved and have a preliminary impression as to whether the defect represents an infarct or an area of abnormal flow reserve. With this first impression, the reader next looks at the short-axis projections moving from the apex to the base of the heart. Each defect should be assessed in both the stress and rest datasets. This sequence allows confirmation of the first impression from evaluating the horizontal and vertical long-axis images. The first reading of the dataset should be blinded as to the findings of the CTA. This allows for objectivity in assessing perfusion studies. However, with the perfusion study findings in hand, the reader should next systematically evaluate the CTA data [161]. The next step entails the integration of both perfusion and CTA results. Defects detected in the perfusion studies should be correlated with CTA findings and vice versa. These findings should also be interpreted in the light of information regarding LV ejection fraction and regional wall-motion abnormalities if available. For completeness of reporting, mention should be made to the presence of extracardiac findings, if any.

14.3.11.3 Quantitation of Perfusion Findings

14.3.11.3.1 Semiquantitative Findings

This includes measures such as the size of the defect by Bull's eye quantitation, which may be provided by automated software, and the relative extent of infarcts and reversible defects. The global LV ejection fraction also provides useful information in the evaluation of patients with CAD and should be included.

14.3.11.3.2 Quantitation of Blood Flow

These measures are available with dynamic perfusion studies and should be reported. The blood flow of at stress and rest for specific territories of the myocardium, of defects, and the flow reserve should be reported. The values of flow and corresponding flow reserve [162–166] have prognostic information and can aid in the management of patients. The flow values can also document areas of myocardial steal and identify this high-risk group of patients [109] who cannot be identified with certainty with the qualitative assessment of perfusion (Figure 14.15).

14.3.11.3.3 Differentiating Fixed from Reversible Defects

To determine whether a perfusion defect that is detected during stress is reversible or fixed (Figure 14.16), it is necessary to compare its MBF to the flow in healthy myocardium at rest [109]. If the defect is also present at rest, that is, its MBF is less than that of normal tissue at rest, it is considered a fixed defect. If the defect resolves at rest, that is, has the same MBF as normal tissue, it is considered reversible (Figure 14.17). Due to the large interindividual variation of MBF values in normal myocardium [162], there are no universal norms for MBF at rest.

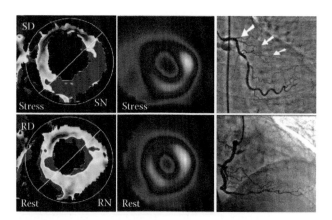

FIGURE 14.15
Reversible defect in CT MPI and nuclear MPI and invasive coronary angiography findings. Nuclear MPI (middle panels) demonstrates a large reversible defect involving the left anterior descending coronary artery (LAD) territory in the mid-ventricle, associated with poststress dilation. CT MPI (left panels) shows the same findings: during stress, the defect (SD), involving the anterior wall and septum, has a myocardial blood flow (MBF) of 0.57 cc/cc/min (blue), whereas the normal tissue (SN), that is, the inferior wall and lateral wall, has an MBF of 1.09 cc/cc/min (red). At rest, the defect (RD) resolves and has an MBF similar to that of the normal myocardium at rest (RN), 0.82 cc/cc/min and 0.81 cc/cc/min (yellow-green). The mean MBF of this area of myocardium is 0.90 cc/cc/min and 0.81 cc/cc/min at stress and rest, respectively. The reduction of MBF in the defect area at stress even below its MBF at rest demonstrates horizontal myocardial steal occurring during vasodilator stress. These findings are compatible with the angiographic findings (rightmost panels) of severe, complete occlusion of the proximal LAD (top row, white arrow) and the presence of collaterals from the LCx and right coronary artery (RCA). The absence of a perfusion defect in the LCx territory in both CT MPI and nuclear MPI suggests that there is flow reserve despite the presence of stenosis in the LCx.

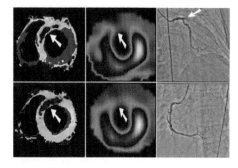

FIGURE 14.16
Fixed defect in CT myocardial perfusion and nuclear MPI and invasive coronary angiography findings. Demonstration of a fixed defect involving the anterior wall and septum on CT MPI and nuclear MPI and the corresponding occluded proximal LAD in the invasive angiography study. The infarcted area shows a severely reduced MBF of similar magnitude in both the rest and stress images (0.54 cc/cc/min and 0.56 cc/cc/min, respectively, displayed in blue). MBF of the lateral wall and inferior wall in the stress and rest images was 1.10 cc/cc/min (red) and 0.80 cc/cc/min (green), respectively. This demonstrates increased MBF during stress in myocardium supplied by LCx and RCA, but no increase in myocardium supplied by the LAD.

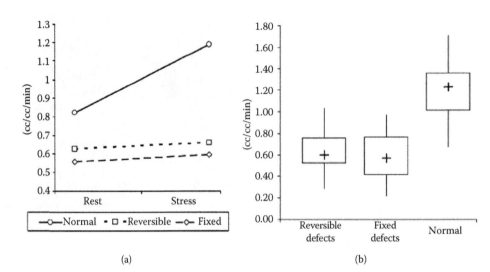

FIGURE 14.17
MBF for normal tissue, fixed and reversible defects at rest and stress. (a) MBF for normal tissue, fixed and reversible defects at rest and stress. (b) MBF for perfusion defects and normal tissue at stress. Median (cross), interquartile range (box), and mean ± 1.96 SD (whiskers).

14.3.11.3.4 Quantitation of Radiation Dose

This should be reported for the perfusion study and the CTA. It is foreseeable that as the technique becomes widely accepted, patients may have sequential studies over a period of years. The availability of dose data will be useful in the complete approach to the management.

14.4 Conclusion and Future Developments

Novel innovative applications of CT are related to planning of interventional procedures, including transcatheter valvular procedures and coronary PCI. 3D reconstructions of CT data play an important role for guidance in the context of these less-invasive procedures. In the context of planning of valvular and coronary intervention, assessment of valve function and FFR/myocardial perfusion allows the evaluation of lesion significance. While technical progress has been impressive, there is a lack of cross-modality comparison and data regarding the prognostic value of these novel applications of CT. The accumulation of such data will help establish the true clinical role, and strengths and limitations of these techniques. Eventually, evidence-based data demonstrating favorable impact on clinical outcome in controlled clinical trials are necessary.

References

1. Rybicki FJ, Otero HJ, Steigner ML et al. Initial evaluation of coronary images from 320-detector row computed tomography. *Int J Cardiovasc Imaging*. 2008;24:535–46.
2. Achenbach S, Marwan M, Ropers D et al. Coronary computed tomography angiography with a consistent dose below 1 mSv using prospectively electrocardiogram-triggered high-pitch spiral acquisition. *Eur Heart J*. 2010;31:340–6.
3. Flohr TG, Leng S, Yu L et al. Dual-source spiral CT with pitch up to 3.2 and 75 ms temporal resolution: Image reconstruction and assessment of image quality. *Med Phys*. 2009;36:5641–53.
4. Ho KT, Chua KC, Klotz E, Panknin C. Stress and rest dynamic myocardial perfusion imaging by evaluation of complete time-attenuation curves with dual-source CT. *JACC Cardiovasc Imaging*. 2010;3:811–20.
5. Halliburton SS, Schoenhagen P. Cardiovascular imaging with computed tomography: Responsible steps to balancing diagnostic yield and radiation exposure. *JACC Cardiovasc Imaging*. 2010;3:536–40.
6. Husmann L, Valenta I, Gaemperli O et al. Feasibility of low-dose coronary CT angiography: First experience with prospective ECG-gating. *Eur Heart J*. 2007;29:191–7.
7. Jakobs T, Becker CR, Ohnesorge B et al. Multislice helical CT of the heart with retrospective ECG gating: Reduction of radiation exposure by ECG-controlled tube current modulation. *Eur Radiol*. 2002;12:1081–6.
8. Leschka S, Scheffel H, Desbiolles L et al. Image quality and reconstruction intervals of dual-source CT coronary angiography: Recommendations for ECG-pulsing windowing. *Invest Radiol*. 2007;42:543–9.

9. Morin RL, Gerber TC, McCollough CH. Radiation dose in computed tomography of the heart. *Circulation.* 2003;107:917–22.

10. DeFrance T, Dubois E, Gebow D, Ramirez A, Wolf F, Feuchtner GM. Helical prospective ECG-gating in cardiac computed tomography: Radiation dose and image quality. *Int J Cardiovasc Imaging.* 2010;26:99–107.

11. Brenner DJ, Hall EJ. Computed tomography—An increasing source of radiation exposure. *N Engl J Med.* 2007;357:2277–84.

12. Einstein AJ, Henzlova MJ, Rajagopalan S. Estimating risk of cancer associated with radiation exposure from 64-slice computed tomography coronary angiography. *JAMA.* 2007;298:317–23.

13. Hausleiter J, Meyer T, Hermann F et al. Estimated radiation dose associated with cardiac CT angiography. *JAMA.* 2009;301:500–7.

14. Hausleiter J, Martinoff S, Hadamitzky M et al. Image quality and radiation exposure with a low tube voltage protocol for coronary CT angiography results of the PROTECTION II Trial. *JACC Cardiovasc Imaging.* 2010;3:1113–23.

15. Leschka S, Stolzmann P, Schmid FT et al. Low kilovoltage cardiac dual-source CT: Attenuation, noise, and radiation dose. *Eur Radiol.* 2008;18:1809–17.

16. Leipsic J, Labounty TM, Heilbron B et al. Estimated radiation dose reduction using adaptive statistical iterative reconstruction in coronary CT angiography: The ERASIR study. *AJR Am J Roentgenol.* 2010;195:655–60.

17. Gasparovic H, Rybicki FJ, Millstine J et al. Three dimensional computed tomographic imaging in planning the surgical approach for redo cardiac surgery after coronary revascularization. *Eur J Cardiothorac Surg.* 2005;28:244–9.

18. Aviram G, Sharony R, Kramer A et al. Modification of surgical planning based on cardiac multidetector computed tomography in reoperative heart surgery. *Ann Thorac Surg.* 2005;79:589–95.

19. Kamdar AR, Meadows TA, Roselli EE et al. Multidetector computed tomographic angiography in planning of reoperative cardiothoracic surgery. *Ann Thorac Surg.* 2008;85:1239–45.

20. Maluenda G, Goldstein MA, Lemesle G et al. Perioperative outcomes in reoperative cardiac surgery guided by cardiac multidetector computed tomographic angiography. *Am Heart J.* 2010;159:301–6.

21. Nifong LW, Chitwood PS, Pappas CR, Smith CR, Argenziano VA, Starnes PM. Robotic mitral valve surgery: A United States multicenter trial. *J Thorac Cardiovasc Surg.* 2005;129:1395–404.

22. Falk V, Mourgues F, Adhami L et al. Cardio navigation: Planning, simulation, and augmented reality in robotic assisted endoscopic bypass grafting. *Ann Thorac Surg.* 2005;79:2040–7.

23. Messika-Zeitoun D, Serfaty JM, Brochet E et al. Multimodal assessment of the aortic annulus diameter. Implication for transcatheter aortic valve implantation. *J Am Coll Cardiol.* 2009;2010;55:186–94.

24. Schoenhagen P, Tuzcu EM, Kapadia SR, Desai MY, Svensson LG. Three-dimensional imaging of the aortic valve and aortic root with computed tomography: New standards in an era of transcatheter valve repair/implantation. *Eur Heart J.* 2009;30:2079–86.

25. Tops LF, Wood DA, Delgado V. Noninvasive evaluation of the aortic root with multislice computed tomography: Implications for transcatheter aortic valve replacement. *J Am Coll Cardiol Imaging.* 2008;1:321–30.

26. Akhtar M, Tuzcu EM, Kapadia SR et al. Aortic root morphology in patients undergoing percutaneous aortic valve replacement. Evidence of aortic root remodeling. *J Thorac Cardiovasc Surg.* 2009;137:950–6.

27. Del Valle-Fernández R, Jelnin V, Panagopoulos G et al. A method for standardized computed tomography angiography-based measurement of aortic valvar structures. *Eur Heart J.* 2010;31:2170–8.

28. Ng ACT, Delgado V, van der Kley F et al. Comparison of aortic root dimensions and geometries before and after transcatheter aortic valve implantation by 2-and 3-dimensional transesophageal echocardiography and multislice computed tomography. *Circ Cardiovasc Imaging.* 2010;3:94–102.

29. Kazui T, Kin H, Tsuboi J, Yoshioka K, Okabayashi H, Kawazoe K. Perioperative dynamic morphological changes of the aortic annulus during aortic root remodeling with aortic annuloplasty at systolic and diastolic phases. *J Heart Valve Dis.* 2008;17:366–70.

30. Tops LF, Wood DA, Delgado V. Noninvasive evaluation of the aortic root with multislice computed tomography: Implications for transcatheter aortic valve replacement. *J Am Coll Cardiol Imaging.* 2008;1:321–30.

31. Doddamani S, Grushko MJ, Makaryus AN et al. Demonstration of left ventricular outflow tract eccentricity by 64-slice multi-detector CT. *Int J Cardiovasc Imaging.* 2009;25:175–81.

32. Willmann JK, Weishaupt D, Lachat M et al. Electrocardiographically gated multi-detector CT for assessment of valvular morphology and calcifications in aortic stenosis. *Radiology.* 2002;225:120–8.

33. Shah RG, Novaro GM, Blandon RJ, Whiteman MS, Asher CR, Kirsch J. Aortic valve area: Meta-analysis of diagnostic performance of multi-detector computed tomography for aortic valve area measurements as compared to transthoracic echocardiography. *Int J Cardiovasc Imaging.* 2009;25:601–9.

34. Feuchtner GM, Dichtl W, Friedrich GJ et al. Multislice computed tomography for detection of patients with aortic valve stenosis and quantification of severity. *J Am Coll Cardiol.* 2006;47:1410–7.

35. Alkadhi H, Desbiolles L, Husmann L et al. Aortic regurgitation: Assessment with 64-section CT. *Radiology.* 2007;245:111–21.

36. Zeb I, Mao SS, Hamirani YS et al. Central aortic valve coaptation area during diastole as seen by 64-multidetector computed tomography (MDCT). *Int J Cardiovasc Imaging.* 2010;26:947–51.

37. Morgan-Hughes GJ, Owens PE, Roobottom CA, Marshall AJ. Three dimensional volume quantification of aortic valve calcification using multislice computed tomography. *Heart.* 2003;89:1191–4.

38. Knight J, Kurtcuoglu V, Muffly K et al. Ex vivo and in vivo coronary ostial locations in humans. *Surg Radiol Anat.* 2009;31:597–604.

39. Stolzmann P, Knight J, Desbiolles L et al. Remodelling of the aortic root in severe tricuspid aortic stenosis: Implications for transcatheter aortic valve implantation. *Eur Radiol.* 2009;19:1316–23.

40. Kurra V, Kapadia SR, Tuzcu EM et al. Pre-procedural imaging of aortic root orientation and dimensions: Comparison between X-ray angiographic planar imaging and 3-dimensional multidetector row computed tomography. *JACC Cardiovasc Interv.* 2010;3:105–13.

41. John D, Buellesfeld L, Yuecel S et al. Correlation of device landing zone calcification and acute procedural success in patients undergoing transcatheter aortic valve implantations with the self-expanding corevalve prosthesis. *J Am Coll Cardiol Interv.* 2010;3:233–43.

42. Latsios G, Gerckens U, Buellesfeld L et al. 2010. "Device landing zone" calcification, assessed by MSCT, as a predictive factor for pacemaker implantation after TAVI. *Catheter Cardiovasc Interv.* 2010;76:431–9.

43. Delgado V, Ng ACT, van de Veire NR et al. Transcatheter aortic valve implantation: Role of multi-detector row computed tomography to evaluate prosthesis positioning and deployment in relation to valve function. *Eur Heart J.* 2010;8:113–23.

44. Jilaihawi H, Chin D, Spyt T et al. Prosthesis-patient mismatch after transcatheter aortic valve implantation with the Medtronic-Corevalve bioprosthesis. *Eur Heart J.* 2009;119:1034–48.

45. Van Mieghem NM, Piazza N, Anderson RH et al. Anatomy of the mitral valvular complex and its implications for transcatheter interventions for mitral regurgitation. *J Am Coll Cardiol.* 2010;56:617–26.

46. Feldman T, Kar S, Rinaldi M et al. Percutaneous mitral repair with the MitraClip system: Safety and midterm durability in the initial EVEREST (Endovascular Valve Edge-to-Edge REpair Study) cohort. *J Am Coll Cardiol.* 2009;54:686–94.

47. Dall'Agata A, Taams MA, Fioretti PM, Roelandt JR, Van Herwerden LA. Cosgrove-Edwards mitral ring dynamics measured with transesophageal three-dimensional echocardiography. *Ann Thorac Surg.* 1998;65:485–90.

48. Pai RG, Tanimoto M, Jintapakorn W, Azevedo J, Pandian NG, Shah PM. Volume-rendered three-dimensional dynamic anatomy of the mitral annulus using a transesophageal echocardiographic technique. *J Heart Valve Dis.* 1995;4:623–7.

49. Kaplan SR, Bashein G, Sheehan FH et al. Three-dimensional echocardiographic assessment of annular shape changes in the normal and regurgitant mitral valve. *Am Heart J.* 2000;139:378–87.

50. Komoda T, Hetzer R, Uyama C et al. Mitral annular function assessed by 3D imaging for mitral valve surgery. *J Heart Valve Dis.* 1994;3:483–90.

51. Levine RA, Handschumacher MD, Sanfilippo AJ et al. Three-dimensional echocardiographic reconstruction of the mitral valve, with implications for the diagnosis of mitral valve prolapse. *Circulation.* 1989;80:589–98.

52. Feuchtner GM, Alkadhi H, Karlo C et al. Cardiac CT angiography for the diagnosis of mitral valve prolapse: Comparison with echocardiography. *Radiology.* 2010;254:374–83.

53. Maselli D, Guarracino F, Chiaramonti F et al. Percutaneous mitral annuloplasty: An anatomic study of human coronary sinus and its relation with mitral valve annulus and coronary arteries. *Circulation.* 2006;114:377–80.

54. Kaye DM, Byrne M, Alferness C, Power J. Feasibility and short-term efficacy of percutaneous mitral annular reduction for the therapy of heart failure-induced mitral regurgitation. *Circulation.* 2003;108:1795–7.

55. Tops LF, Van de Veire NR, Schuijf JD et al. Noninvasive evaluation of coronary sinus anatomy and its relation to the mitral valve annulus: Implications for percutaneous mitral annuloplasty. *Circulation.* 2007;115:1426–32.

56. Schofer J, Siminiak T, Haude M et al. Percutaneous mitral annuloplasty for functional mitral regurgitation: Results of the CARILLON Mitral Annuloplasty Device European Union Study. *Circulation.* 2009;120:326–33.

57. Alkadhi H, Desbiolles L, Stolzmann P et al. Mitral annular shape, size, and motion in normals and in patients with cardiomyopathy: Evaluation with computed tomography. *Invest Radiol.* 2009;44:218–25.

58. Maselli D, Guarracino F, Chiaramonti F, Mangia F, Borelli G, Minzioni G. Percutaneous mitral annuloplasty: An anatomic study of human coronary sinus and its relation with mitral valve annulus and coronary arteries. *Circulation* 2006;114:377–80.

59. Choure AJ, Garcia MJ, Hesse B et al. In vivo analysis of the anatomical relationship of coronary sinus to mitral annulus and left circumflex coronary artery using cardiac multidetector computed tomography: Implications for percutaneous coronary sinus mitral annuloplasty. *J Am Coll Cardiol.* 2006;48:1938–45.

60. Gopal A, Shah A, Shareghi S et al. The role of cardiovascular computed tomographic angiography for coronary sinus mitral annuloplasty. *J Invasive Cardiol.* 2010;22:67–73.

61. Webb JG, Wood DA, Ye J et al. Transcatheter valve-in-valve implantation for failed bioprosthetic heart valves. *Circulation.* 2010;121:1634–6.

62. Zahn EM, Hellenbrand WE, Lock JE, McElhinney DB. Implantation of the melody transcatheter pulmonary valve in patients with a dysfunctional right ventricular outflow tract conduit early results from the US Clinical trial. *J Am Coll Cardiol.* 2009;54:1722–9.

63. Schievano S, Taylor AM, Capelli C et al. First-in-man implantation of a novel percutaneous valve: A new approach to medical device development. *Euro Interv.* 2010;5:745–50.

64. Schoenhagen P, Hill A. 2009. Transcatheter aortic valve implantation and potential role of 3D imaging. *Expert Rev Med Devices.* 2009;6:411–21.

65. Abel DB, Dehdashtian MM, Rodger ST, Smith AC, Smith LJ, Waninger MS. Evolution and future of pre-clinical testing for endovascular grafts. *J Endovasc Ther* 2006;13:649–59.

66. Zarins CK, Taylor CA. Endovascular device design in the future: Transformation from trial and error to computational design. *J Endovasc Ther.* 2009;16(Suppl 1): I12–21.

67. Tommasini G, Camerini A, Gatti A, Derchi G, Bruzzone A, Vecchio C. Panoramic coronary angiography. *J Am Coll Cardiol.* 1998;31: 871–7.

68. Garcia JA, Chen SY, Messenger JC et al. Initial clinical experience of selective coronary angiography using one prolonged injection and a 180 degrees rotational trajectory. *Catheter Cardiovasc Interv.* 2007;70:190–6.

69. Neubauer AM, Garcia JA, Messenger JC et al. Clinical feasibility of a fully automated 3D reconstruction of rotational coronary X-ray angiograms. *Circ Cardiovasc Interv.* 2010;3:71–9.

70. Schwartz JG, Neubauer AM, Fagan TE, Noordhoek NJ, Grass M, Carroll JD. Potential role of three-dimensional rotational angiography and C-arm CT for valvular repair and implantation. *Int J Cardiovasc Imaging.* 2011;27:1205–22.

71. Johri AM, Passeri JJ, Picard MH. Three dimensional echocardiography: Approaches and clinical utility. *Heart.* 2010;96:390–7.

72. Hung J, Lang R, Flachskampf F et al. 3D Echocardiography: A review of the current status and future directions. *J Am Soc Echocardiogr.* 2007;20:213–33.

73. Balzer J, Kelm M, Kühl HP. Real-time three-dimensional transoesophageal echocardiography for guidance of non-coronary interventions in the catheter laboratory. *J Echocardiogr.* 2009;10:341–9.

74. Balzer J, Kuhl H, Rassaf T et al. Real-time transesophageal three-dimensional echocardiography for guidance of percutaneous cardiac interventions: First experience. *Clin Res Cardiol.* 2008;97:565–74.

75. Bouzas-Mosquera A, Alvarez-Garcia N, Ortiz-Vazquez E, Cuenca-Castillo JJ. Role of real-time 3-dimensional transesophageal echocardiography in transcatheter aortic valve implantation. *Eur J Cardiothorac Surg.* 2009;35:909.

76. Détaint D, Lepage L, Himbert D et al. Determinants of significant paravalvular regurgitation after transcatheter aortic valve: Implantation impact of device and annulus discongruence. *JACC Cardiovasc Interv.* 2009;2:821–7.

77. Daimon M, Shiota T, Gillinov AM et al. Percutaneous mitral valve repair for chronic ischemic mitral regurgitation: A real-time three-dimensional echocardiographic study in an ovine model. *Circulation.* 2005;111:2183–9.

78. Guttman MA, Ozturk C, Raval AN et al. Interventional cardiovascular procedures guided by real-time MR imaging: An interactive interface using multiple slices, adaptive projection modes and live 3D renderings. *J Magn Reson Imaging.* 2007;26:1429–35.

79. Elgort DR, Wong EY, Hillenbrand CM, Wacker FK, Lewin JS, Duerk JL. Real-time catheter tracking and adaptive imaging. *J Magn Reson Imaging.* 2003;18:621–6.

80. Kuehne T, Yilmaz S, Meinus C. Magnetic resonance imaging-guided transcatheter implantation of a prosthetic valve in aortic valve position: Feasibility study in swine. *J Am Coll Cardiol.* 2004;44:2247–9.

81. Kim JH, Kocaturk O, Ozturk C et al. Mitral cerclage annuloplasty, a novel transcatheter treatment for secondary mitral valve regurgitation: Initial results in swine. *J Am Coll Cardiol.* 2009;54:638–51.

82. Ropers D, Rixe J, Anders K et al. Usefulness of multidetector row spiral computed tomography with 64- × 0.6-mm collimation and 330-ms rotation for the noninvasive detection of significant coronary artery stenoses. *Am J Cardiol.* 2006;97:343–8.

83. Nikolaou K, Knez A, Rist C et al. Accuracy of 64-MDCT in the diagnosis of ischemic heart disease. *AJR Am J Roentgenol* 2006;187:111–7.

84. Meijboom WB, Van Mieghem CA, van Pelt N et al. Comprehensive assessment of coronary artery stenoses: Computed tomography coronary angiography versus conventional coronary angiography and correlation with fractional flow reserve in patients with stable angina. *J Am Coll Cardiol.* 2008;52:636–43.

85. Beller GA. First annual Mario S. Verani, MD. Memorial lecture: Clinical value of myocardial perfusion imaging in coronary artery disease. *J Nucl Cardiol.* 2003;10:529–42.

86. Elhendy A, Mahoney DW, Burger KN, McCully RB, Pellikka PA. Prognostic value of exercise echocardiography in patients with classic angina pectoris. *Am J Cardiol.* 2004;94:559–63.

87. Di Carli MF, Dorbala S, Curillova Z et al. Relationship between CT coronary angiography and stress perfusion imaging in patients with suspected ischemic heart disease assessed by integrated PET-CT imaging. *J Nucl Cardiol.* 2007;14:799–809.

88. Schmermund A, Bell MR, Lerman LO, Ritman EL, Rumberger JA. Quantitative evaluation of regional myocardial perfusion using fast X-ray computed tomography. *Herz.* 1997;22:29–39.

89. George RT, Silva C, Cordeiro MA et al. Multidetector computed tomography myocardial perfusion imaging during adenosine stress. *J Am Coll Cardiol.* 2006;48:153–60.

90. Ruzsics B, Lee H, Zwerner PL, Gebregziabher M, Costello P, Schoepf UJ. Dual-energy CT of the heart for diagnosing coronary artery stenosis and myocardial ischemia-initial experience. *Eur Radiol.* 2008;18:2414–24.

91. Ruzsics B, Suranyi P, Kiss P et al. Automated multidetector computed tomography evaluation of subacutely infarcted myocardium. *J Cardiovasc Comput Tomogr.* 2008;2:26–32.

92. Blankstein R, Okada D, Rocha-Filho J, Rybicki F, Brady T, Cury R. Cardiac myocardial perfusion imaging using dual source computed tomography. *Int J Cardiovasc Imaging.* 2009;25:209–16.

93. George RT, Arbab-Zadeh A, Miller JM et al. Adenosine stress 64- and 256-row detector computed tomography angiography and perfusion imaging: A pilot study evaluating the transmural extent of perfusion abnormalities to predict atherosclerosis causing myocardial ischemia. *Circ Cardiovasc Imaging.* 2009;2:174–82.

94. Gould RG, Lipton MJ, McNamara MT, Sievers RE, Koshold S, Higgins CB. Measurement of regional myocardial blood flow in dogs by ultrafast CT. *Invest Radiol.* 1988;23:348–53.

95. Rumberger JA, Feiring AJ, Lipton MJ, Higgins CB, Ell SR, Marcus ML. Use of ultrafast computed tomography to quantitate regional myocardial perfusion: A preliminary report. *J Am Coll Cardiol.* 1987;9:59–69.

96. Wolfkiel CJ, Ferguson JL, Chomka EV et al. Measurement of myocardial blood flow by ultrafast computed tomography. *Circulation.* 1987;76:1262–73.

97. Bell MR, Lerman LO, Rumberger JA. Validation of minimally invasive measurement of myocardial perfusion using electron beam computed tomography and application in human volunteers. *Heart.* 1999;81:628–35.

98. George RT, Jerosch-Herold M, Silva C et al. Quantification of myocardial perfusion using dynamic 64-detector computed tomography. *Invest Radiol.* 2007;42:815–22.

99. Yim NY, Kim YH, Choi S et al. Multidetector-row computed tomographic evaluation of myocardial perfusion in reperfused chronic myocardial infarction: Value of color-coded perfusion map in a porcine model. *Int J Cardiovasc Imaging.* 2009;25(Suppl 1):65–74.

100. Christian TF, Frankish ML, Sisemoore JH et al. Myocardial perfusion imaging with first-pass computed tomographic imaging: Measurement of coronary flow reserve in an animal model of regional hyperemia. *J Nucl Cardiol.* 2010;17:625–30.

101. Mahnken AH, Klotz E, Pietsch H et al. Quantitative whole heart stress perfusion CT imaging as noninvasive assessment of hemodynamics in coronary artery stenosis: Preliminary animal experience. *Invest Radiol.* 2010;45:298–305.

102. Bamberg F, Hinkel R, Schwarz F et al. Accuracy of dynamic computed tomography adenosine stress myocardial perfusion imaging in estimating myocardial blood flow at various degrees of coronary artery stenosis using a porcine animal model. *Invest Radiol.* 2012;47:71–7.

103. Kurata A, Mochizuki T, Koyama Y et al. Myocardial perfusion imaging using adenosine triphosphate stress multislice spiral computed tomography: Alternative to stress myocardial perfusion scintigraphy. *Circ J.* 2005;69:550–7.

104. Blankstein R, Shturman LD, Rogers IS et al. Adenosine-induced stress myocardial perfusion imaging using dual-source cardiac computed tomography. *J Am Coll Cardiol.* 2009;54:1072–84.

105. Rocha-Filho JA, Blankstein R, Shturman LD et al. Incremental value of adenosine-induced stress myocardial perfusion imaging with dual-source CT at cardiac CT angiography. *Radiology.* 2010;254:410–9.

106. Okada DR, Ghoshhajra BB, Blankstein R et al. Direct comparison of rest and adenosine stress myocardial perfusion CT with rest and stress SPECT. *J Nucl Cardiol.* 2010;17:27–37.

107. Cury RC, Magalhaes TA, Borges AC et al. Dipyridamole stress and rest myocardial perfusion by 64-detector row computed tomography in patients with suspected coronary artery disease. *Am J Cardiol.* 2010;106:310–5.

108. Bastarrika G, Ramos-Duran L, Schoepf UJ et al. Adenosine-stress dynamic myocardial volume perfusion imaging with second generation dual-source computed tomography: Concepts and first experiences. *J Cardiovasc Comput Tomogr.* 2010; 4:127–35.

109. Ho KT, Chua KC, Klotz E, Panknin C. Stress and rest dynamic myocardial perfusion imaging by evaluation of complete time-attenuation curves with dual-source CT. *JACC Cardiovasc Imaging.* 2010; 3:811–20.

110. Ko SM, Choi JW, Song MG et al. Myocardial perfusion imaging using adenosine-induced stress dual-energy computed tomography of the heart: Comparison with cardiac magnetic resonance imaging and conventional coronary angiography. *Eur Radiol.* 2011;21:26–35.

111. Tamarappoo BK, Dey D, Nakazato R et al. Comparison of the extent and severity of myocardial perfusion defects measured by CT coronary angiography and SPECT myocardial perfusion imaging. *JACC Cardiovasc Imaging.* 2010;3:1010–9.

112. Weininger M, Schoepf UJ, Ramachandra A et al. Adenosine-stress dynamic real-time myocardial perfusion CT and adenosine-stress first-pass dual-energy myocardial perfusion CT for the assessment of acute chest pain: Initial results. *Eur J Radiol.* 2012;81:3703–10.

113. Feuchtner G, Goetti R, Plass A et al. Adenosine stress high-pitch 128-slice dual-source myocardial computed tomography perfusion for imaging of reversible myocardial ischemia: Comparison with magnetic resonance imaging. *Circ Cardiovasc Imaging.* 2011; 4:540–9.

114. Bamberg F, Becker A, Schwarz F et al. Detection of hemodynamically significant coronary artery stenosis: Incremental diagnostic value of dynamic CT-based myocardial perfusion imaging. *Radiology.* 2011;260:689–98.

115. Ko BS, Cameron JD, Meredith IT et al. Computed tomography stress myocardial perfusion imaging in patients considered for revascularization: A comparison with fractional flow reserve. *Eur Heart J.* 2012;33:67–77.

116. Bamberg F, Klotz E, Flohr T et al. Dynamic myocardial stress perfusion imaging using fast dual-source CT with alternating table positions: Initial experience. *Eur Radiol.* 2010;20:1168–73.

117. Vavere AL, Simon GG, George RT et al. Diagnostic performance of combined noninvasive coronary angiography and myocardial perfusion imaging using 320 row detector computed tomography: Design and implementation of the CORE320 multicenter, multinational diagnostic study. *J Cardiovasc Comput Tomogr.* 2011;5:370–81.

118. George RT, Arbab-Zadeh A, Cerci RJ et al. Diagnostic performance of combined noninvasive coronary angiography and myocardial perfusion imaging using 320-MDCT: The CT angiography and perfusion methods of the CORE320 multicenter multinational diagnostic study. *AJR Am J Roentgenol.* 2011;197:829–37.

119. Coulam CM, Warner HR, Wood EH, Bassingthwaighte JB. A transfer function analysis of coronary and renal circulation calculated from upstream and downstream indicator-dilution curves. *Circ Res.* 1966;19:879–90.

120. Mohlenkamp S, Behrenbeck TR, Lerman A et al. Coronary microvascular functional reserve: Quantification of long-term changes with electron-beam CT preliminary results in a porcine model. *Radiology.* 2001;221:229–36.
121. Wang T, Wu X, Chung N, Ritman EL. Myocardial blood flow estimated by synchronous, multislice, high-speed computed tomography. *IEEE Trans Med Imaging.* 1989;8:70–7.
122. Wu XS, Ewert DL, Liu YH, Ritman EL. In vivo relation of intramyocardial blood volume to myocardial perfusion. Evidence supporting microvascular site for autoregulation. *Circulation.* 1992;85:730–7.
123. Miles KA. Measurement of tissue perfusion by dynamic computed tomography. *Br J Radiol.* 1991;64:409–12.
124. Wintermark M, Maeder P, Thiran JP, Schnyder P, Meuli R. Quantitative assessment of regional cerebral blood flows by perfusion CT studies at low injection rates: A critical review of the underlying theoretical models. *Eur Radiol.* 2001;11:1220–30.
125. Bruder H, Raupach R, Klotz E, Stierstorfer K, Flohr T. Spatio-temporal filtration of dynamic CT data diffusion filters. In: *SPIE Medical Imaging 2009: Physics of Medical Imaging.* Lake Buena Vista, FL, 2009, pp. 725857–10.
126. Ruzsics B, Schwarz F, Schoepf UJ et al. Comparison of dual-energy computed tomography of the heart with single photon emission computed tomography for assessment of coronary artery stenosis and of the myocardial blood supply. *Am J Cardiol.* 2009;104:318–26.
127. George RT, Ichihara T, Lima JA, Lardo AC. A method for reconstructing the arterial input function during helical CT: Implications for myocardial perfusion distribution imaging. *Radiology.* 2010; 255:396–404.
128. Jerosch-Herold M, Wilke N, Stillman AE. Magnetic resonance quantification of the myocardial perfusion reserve with a Fermi function model for constrained deconvolution. *Med Phys.* 1998;25:73–84.
129. Christian TF, Rettmann DW, Aletras AH et al. Absolute myocardial perfusion in canines measured by using dual-bolus first-pass MR imaging. *Radiology.* 2004;232:677–84.
130. Kachenoura N, Lodato JA, Gaspar T et al. Value of multidetector computed tomography evaluation of myocardial perfusion in the assessment of ischemic heart disease: Comparison with nuclear perfusion imaging. *Eur Radiol.* 2009;19:1897–905.
131. Kachenoura N, Veronesi F, Lodato JA et al. Volumetric quantification of myocardial perfusion using analysis of multi-detector computed tomography 3D datasets: Comparison with nuclear perfusion imaging. *Eur Radiol.* 2010;20:337–47.
132. Nikolaou K, Sanz J, Poon M et al. Assessment of myocardial perfusion and viability from routine contrast-enhanced 16-detector-row computed tomography of the heart: Preliminary results. *Eur Radiol.* 2005;15:864–71.
133. Busch JL, Alessio AM, Caldwell JH et al. Myocardial hypo-enhancement on resting computed tomography angiography images accurately identifies myocardial hypoperfusion. *J Cardiovasc Comput Tomogr.* 2011;5:412–20.
134. Henneman MM, Schuijf JD, Dibbets-Schneider P et al. Comparison of multislice computed tomography to gated single-photon emission computed tomography for imaging of healed myocardial infarcts. *Am J Cardiol.* 2008;101:144–8.
135. Rubinshtein R, Miller TD, Williamson EE et al. Detection of myocardial infarction by dual-source coronary computed tomography angiography using quantitated myocardial scintigraphy as the reference standard. *Heart.* 2009;95:1419–22.
136. Bauer RW, Kerl JM, Fischer N et al. Dual-energy CT for the assessment of chronic myocardial infarction in patients with chronic coronary artery disease: Comparison with 3-T MRI. *AJR Am J Roentgenol.* 2010;195:639–46.
137. George RT, Jerosch-Herold M, Silva C et al. Quantification of myocardial perfusion using dynamic 64-detector computed tomography. *Invest Radiol.* 2007;42:815–22.
138. So A, Wisenberg G, Islam A et al. Non-invasive assessment of functionally relevant coronary artery stenoses with quantitative CT perfusion: Preliminary clinical experiences. *Eur Radiol.* 2012;22:39–50.
139. Meier P, Zierler KL. On the theory of the indicator-dilution method for measurement of blood flow and volume. *J Appl Physiol.* 1954;6:731–44.
140. Lee TY, Purdie TG, Stewart E. CT imaging of angiogenesis. *Q J Nucl Med.* 2003;47:171–87.
141. Axel L. Tissue mean transit time from dynamic computed tomography by a simple deconvolution technique. *Invest Radiol.* 1983;18:94–9.
142. Groothuis DR, Lapin GD, Vriesendorp FJ, Mikhael MA, Patlak CS. A method to quantitatively measure transcapillary transport of iodinated compounds in canine brain tumors with computed tomography. *J Cereb Blood Flow Metab.* 1991;11:939–48.
143. Patlak CS, Blasberg RG, Fenstermacher JD. Graphical evaluation of blood-to-brain transfer constants from multiple-time uptake data. *J Cereb Blood Flow Metab.* 1983;3:1–7.
144. Patlak CS, Blasberg RG. Graphical evaluation of blood-to-brain transfer constants from multiple-time uptake data. Generalizations. *J Cereb Blood Flow Metab.* 1985;5:584–90.
145. Bassingthwaighte JB, Wang CY, Chan IS. Blood-tissue exchange via transport and transformation by capillary endothelial cells. *Circ Res.* 1989;65:997–1020.
146. Ho KT, Chua KC, Klotz E, Panknin C. Stress and rest dynamic myocardial perfusion imaging by evaluation of complete time-attenuation curves with dual-source CT. *JACC Cardiovasc Imaging.* 2010;3:811–20.
147. So A, Hsieh J, Li JY, Hadway J, Kong HF, Lee TY. Quantitative myocardial perfusion measurement using CT perfusion: A validation study in a porcine model of reperfused acute myocardial infarction. *Int J Cardiovasc Imaging.* 2012;28:1237–48.
148. Brooks RA, Di Chiro G. Beam hardening in x-ray reconstructive tomography. *Phys Med Biol.* 1976;21:390–8.
149. So A, Hsieh J, Li JY, Lee TY. Beam hardening correction in CT myocardial perfusion measurement. *Phys Med Biol.* 2009;54:3031–50.

150. Alvarez RE, Macovski A. Energy-selective reconstructions in X-ray computerized tomography. *Phys Med Biol.* 1976;21:733–44.

151. So A, Lee TY, Imai Y et al. Quantitative myocardial perfusion imaging using rapid kVp switch dual-energy CT: Preliminary experience. *J Cardiovasc Comput Tomogr.* 2011;5:430–42.

152. Barrett JF, Keat N. Artifacts in CT: Recognition and avoidance. *Radiographics.* 2004;24:1679–91.

153. Lee TY, Chhem RK. Impact of new technologies on dose reduction in CT. *Eur J Radiol.* 2010;76:28–35.

154. Serafi AS, Evans SJ, Jones JV. Arrhythmogenic effect of ventriculography in patients with left ventricular dilation and/or hypertrophy. *Clin Sci* (Lond). 1998;95:453–8.

155. Choi SI, George RT, Schuleri KH, Chun EJ, Lima JA, Lardo AC. Recent developments in wide-detector cardiac computed tomography. *Int J Cardiovasc Imaging.* 2009;25(Suppl 1):23–9.

156. Johnson TR, Krauss B, Sedlmair M et al. Material differentiation by dual energy CT: Initial experience. *Eur Radiol.* 2007;17:1510–7.

157. Schwarz F, Ruzsics B, Schoepf UJ et al. Dual-energy CT of the heart—Principles and protocols. *Eur J Radiol.* 2008;68:423–33.

158. Walker PR, James MA, Wilde RP, Wood CH, Rees JR. Dipyridamole combined with exercise for thallium-201 myocardial imaging. *Br Heart J.* 1986;55:321–9.

159. Cury RC, Nieman K, Shapiro MD et al. Comprehensive assessment of myocardial perfusion defects, regional wall motion, and left ventricular function by using 64-section multidetector CT. *Radiology.* 2008;248:466–75.

160. Cerqueira MD, Weissman NJ, Dilsizian V et al. Standardized myocardial segmentation and nomenclature for tomographic imaging of the heart: A statement for healthcare professionals from the Cardiac Imaging Committee of the Council on Clinical Cardiology of the American Heart Association. *Circulation.* 2002;105:539–42.

161. Raff GL, Abidov A, Achenbach S et al. SCCT guidelines for the interpretation and reporting of coronary computed tomographic angiography. *J Cardiovasc Comput Tomogr.* 2009;3:122–36.

162. Chareonthaitawee P, Kaufmann PA, Rimoldi O, Camici PG. Heterogeneity of resting and hyperemic myocardial blood flow in healthy humans. *Cardiovasc Res.* 2001;50:151–61.

163. Hsu LY, Rhoads KL, Holly JE, Kellman P, Aletras AH, Arai AE. Quantitative myocardial perfusion analysis with a dual-bolus contrast-enhanced first-pass MRI technique in humans. *J Magn Reson Imaging.* 2006;23:315–22.

164. Muehling OM, Jerosch-Herold M, Panse P et al. Regional heterogeneity of myocardial perfusion in healthy human myocardium: Assessment with magnetic resonance perfusion imaging. *J Cardiovasc Magn Reson.* 2004;6:499–507.

165. Bergmann SR, Herrero P, Markham J, Weinheimer CJ, Walsh MN. Noninvasive quantitation of myocardial blood flow in human subjects with oxygen-15-labeled water and positron emission tomography. *J Am Coll Cardiol.* 1989;14:639–52.

166 Krivokapich J, Smith GT, Huang SC et al. ^{13}N ammonia myocardial imaging at rest and with exercise in normal volunteers. Quantification of absolute myocardial perfusion with dynamic positron emission tomography. *Circulation.* 1989;80:1328–37.

15

Pathologies of the Pericardium

Samuel Boynton and Philip A. Araoz

CONTENTS

15.1 Introduction

The pericardium is a very unassuming structure: thin and at the periphery of the heart, it can be easily overlooked. The effects of a diseased pericardium on cardiac function, however, can be significant and even fatal. It is important that a thorough evaluation of the heart includes the pericardium.

With the development and refinement of CT imaging, much information of the pericardium can be gained from one examination. The spacial resolution of computed tomography (CT) is high enough to delineate accurately the borders of the pericardium. The wide field of view (FOV) allows for the full extent of pericardial disease to be elucidated. Contrast-enhanced CT is useful for checking inflammation in pericarditis and neoplastic deposits. Because CT is extremely sensitive for the detection of calcium, pericardial calcification can reliably be seen. The temporal resolution of electrocardiography (ECG)-gated CT provides a valuable tool for reviewing the heart throughout the cardiac cycle with minimal blurring from motion. The effect of the diseased pericardium on cardiac hemodynamics can thus be studied dynamically.

15.2 Anatomy

The pericardium is a double-layered sac-like structure that envelopes most of the heart. It is composed of the inner visceral pericardium or epicardium and the outer parietal or fibrous pericardium. The visceral pericardium is a serosal membrane averaging between 0.05 and 1 mm thick, and is intimately associated with the epicardial fat. Under normal circumstances, it is not visible on imaging. The parietal pericardium consists of a thin inner surface of mesothelial cells responsible for producing the serous pericardial fluid. The bulk of the parietal pericardium, however, consists of a fibrous, somewhat elastic component that normally measures up to 2 mm in thickness. The fibrous pericardium is attached to the posterior sternum by the superior and inferior sternopericardial ligaments and to the central tendon of the diaphragm by the pericardiophrenic ligament. The pericardium is supplied by pericardiophrenic arterial and venous branches of the internal thoracic arteries and veins, respectively, and is innervated by the vagus and phrenic nerves and the sympathetic ganglion [1,2].

The visceral and parietal layers are continuous and can be thought of as a deflated balloon wrapped

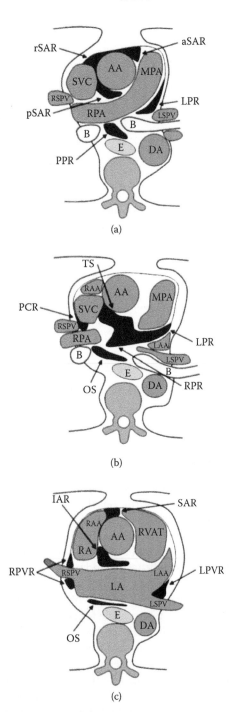

around the heart. There are several "extensions" of the pericardial space termed "pericardial recesses," which arise from two main "pericardial sinuses" that do not communicate with each other (Figure 15.1). Recognition of the location of the pericardial recesses is important as these structures may be prominent in normal individuals and can be mistaken for lymphadenopathy or mediastinal masses (Figure 15.2) [1]. Not all pericardial recesses will be visible in the same patient.

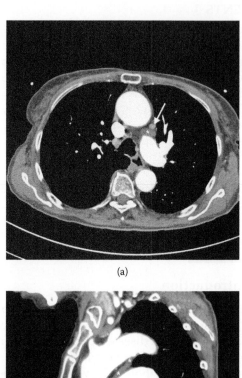

FIGURE 15.1
(a–c) Transverse drawings of the pericardial sinuses and recesses at three closely adjacent slice levels above the heart base. AA, ascending aorta; B, bronchus intermedius; DA, descending aorta; E, esophagus; IAR, inferior aortic recess; LA, left atrium; LAA, left atrial appendage; LPR, left pulmonic recess; LPVR, left pulmonic vein recess; LSPV, left superior pulmonary vein; MPA, main pulmonary artery; OS, oblique sinus; PCR, postcaval sinus; PRP, posterior pericardial recess; RA, right atrium; RAA, right atrial appendage; RPA, right pulmonary artery; RPR, right pulmonic recess; RPVR, right pulmonic vein recess; RSPV, right superior pulmonary vein; RVAT, right ventricular outflow tract; SAR, superior aortic recess; SVC, superior vena cava. (From Rienmuller R, Groll R, and Lipton MJ. *Radiol Clin North Am.*, 42(3): 587–601, 2004. With permission.)

FIGURE 15.2
Pericardial recess versus lymph node. (a) Single axial post contrast image showing a low-density structure anterior to the main pulmonary artery (asterisk). This could be mistaken for a mediastinal lymph node or mass. The white arrow points to an enhancing lymph node for comparison. (b) Oblique sagittal slice used for short-axis cardiac images is reconstructed from the axial raw data (inset). It also intersects the mystery structure: high extension of the posterior superior aortic pericardial recess (asterisks), which is continuous with the transverse sinus (white arrow), an extension of the pericardial space. There is also a pericardial effusion (black arrow).

The transverse sinus is located posterior to the ascending aorta and main pulmonary artery, and superior to the left atrium (Figure 15.3). It gives rise to the superior and inferior aortic recesses and the right and left pulmonary recesses. The superior aortic recess is composed of anterior, posterior, and right components (Figure 15.4). The anterior superior aortic recess is located anterior to the ascending aorta and the superior vena cava (SVC); the right superior aortic recess lies between the aorta and the SVC, and the posterior superior aortic recess lies posterior to the ascending aorta and SVC. The inferior aortic recess extends inferiorly from the transverse sinus and can be seen anterior to the left atrium. The right and left pulmonic recesses extend inferolaterally from the transverse sinus and are located caudal to the right and left pulmonary arteries (Figure 15.5) [2,3].

The oblique sinus lies posterior to the left atrium and is separated from the transverse sinus by the pericardial reflections. The posterior pericardial recess (also known as the pericardial sleeve recess) arises from the oblique sinus, and is located behind the right pulmonary artery and medial to the bronchus intermedius (Figure 15.6) [2].

A few pericardial recesses arise directly from the pericardium. The right and left pulmonary venous recesses are located between the right and left superior and inferior pulmonary veins, respectively. The postcaval recess is present along the posterolateral margin of the SVC.

Functionally, the pericardium fixes the position of the heart in the chest, provides some protection against the spread of disease, reduces friction via the pericardial fluid, and limits acute distension of the heart [3]. It is not an essential structure, however, and in some cases

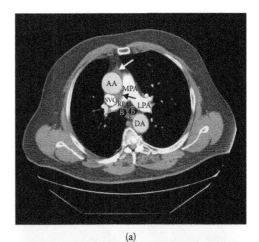

(a)

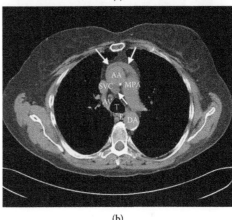

(b)

FIGURE 15.4
Figure showing superior aortic pericardial recess. (a) Anterior superior aortic recess (white arrow) and posterior superior aortic recess (black arrow). (b) Arrows show continuity of anterior, right, and posterior superior aortic recesses in a separate patient.

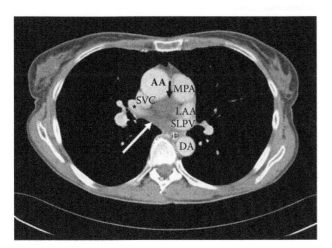

FIGURE 15.3
Figure showing oblique sinus (white arrow), transverse sinus (black arrow), and superior right pulmonary vein (asterisk). AA, ascending aorta; MPA, main pulmonary artery; SVC, superior vena cava; DA, descending aorta; SLPV, superior left pulmonary vein; LAA, left atrial appendage.

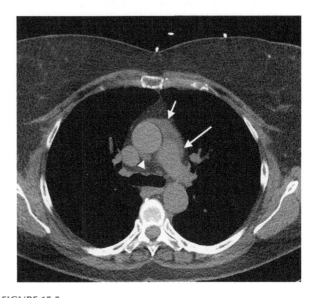

FIGURE 15.5
The left pulmonic recess (long arrow) merging with the anterior superior aortic recess (short arrow). The arrowhead points to the posterior superior aortic recess.

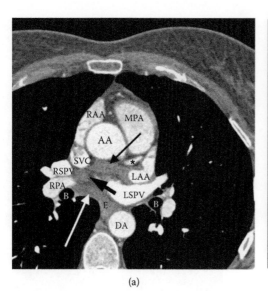

(a)

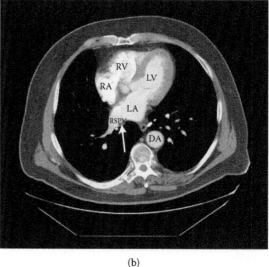

(b)

FIGURE 15.6
(a) Posterior pericardial recess (white arrow), postcaval recess (short black arrow), and transverse (long black arrow) sinuses. Asterisk, left main coronary artery. (b) Right pulmonary vein recess (arrow).

is incompletely developed or therapeutically excised without long-term complication.

15.3 Imaging the Pericardium on Computed Tomography

Improvements in gantry rotation times, detector size and number, and reconstruction algorithms over the last several years have allowed CT to obtain the spatial and temporal resolution necessary to image the pericardium [4]. ECG gating provides the necessary matching of acquired images to their respective phase of the cardiac cycle so the effect of the pericardium on cardiac function can be evaluated.

At our institution, the majority of pericardial CT scans are done on a dual-source 64- or 128-slice scanner. All images are obtained during an inspiratory breath-hold using retrospective ECG gating, a slice thickness of 0.6 mm, and dose modulation. Pitch is determined automatically and should not be more than 1. Scanning is done from the carina to the bottom of the heart, first without, and then with intravenous contrast. The noncontrast images are very important for showing pericardial calcium deposits, which may be difficult to distinguish from contrast the blood pool or nearby-enhancing structures on the contrast-enhanced images. Noncontrast images can also help identify subtle pericardial enhancement when compared side by side to matching postcontrast images.

Static pre- and postcontrast axial reconstructions are made with a thickness and increment of 3 mm each.

Multiphase images throughout the cardiac cycle are reconstructed in the axial and short-axis planes with a thickness and increment of 6 mm each. Lastly, a multiphase axial reconstruction using a 256 × 256 matrix is performed using a slice thickness of 1.5 mm and an increment of 0.7 mm. Beta blockers are typically not used with the dual-source scanners unless the patient's heart rate is above 90 beats/min, in which case 5 mL of metoprolol is administered intravenously.

15.4 Congenital Abnormalities of the Pericardium

15.4.1 Absence of the Pericardium

Congenital absence of the pericardium is a rare entity [5]. It is classified as either partial or complete and may involve the pericardium on the right, the left, or on both sides of the heart. Partial absence of the pericardium is the most common manifestation and occurs on the left 70% of the time and on the right 17% of the time. This is thought to be due to premature involution of the left common cardinal vein in utero; the microvasculature of which supplies nutrients to the pleuropericardium, the progenitor of the pericardium. Since the right superior common cardinal vein persists as the SVC, decreased blood supply and resultant hypogenesis or agenesis of the pericardium on the right is less common.

Most people with congenital pericardial defects are asymptomatic; it is usually discovered incidentally on imaging done for other reasons. However, a minority of patients have symptoms, the most common of which is precordial chest pain [5,6]. This is often a nonexertional paroxysmal chest pain from herniation of left ventricular myocardium with subsequent compression of coronary vessels [7]. Other signs and symptoms include dyspnea, murmurs, dysrhythmia, displaced apical impulse, syncope, and rarely sudden death. Thirty percent of patients with congenital absence of the pericardium will have a coexisting congenital cardiac abnormality such as an atrial septal defect, bicuspid aortic valve, mitral valve stenosis, patent ductus arteriosus, or tetralogy of Fallot. Congenital abnormalities with the lungs, chest wall, and diaphragm may also be seen. Prognostically, partial absence of the pericardium is more problematic than complete absence due to the risk of herniation through the defect. Herniation of the atrial appendage, myocardium, or a segment of a coronary artery may lead to myocardial ischemia [5,8,35]. Noncardiac structures and organs may also herniate into the pericardial space.

Although no treatment is required for complete bilateral absence of the pericardium, clinically concerning partial pericardial defects are treated with pericardiectomy or pericardioplasty. The location and extent of the lesion influences the surgical approach, thus precise description of imaging findings is important. CT is helpful for providing this information as well as any additional complications and overall assessment of the visible developed pericardium.

Direct discontinuity of the pericardium can often be seen on CT, primarily anteriorly along the right ventricle, the main pulmonary artery, and the aorta, as well as the cardiac apex (Figure 15.7) [9]. However, because a normal pericardium may not always be seen on CT, lack of visualization of the defect cannot provide the diagnosis. This is especially true along the left ventricular margin where the pericardium may not be seen due to a lack of substantial pericardial fat between it and the adjacent lung. In general, secondary signs are a more reliable indicator of pericardial defects.

Interposition of the lung between the aorta and the main pulmonary artery is the most common secondary finding and is almost pathognomonic when seen [5,9]. The anterior mediastinal margin of the left lung can be seen invaginated between and maintaining direct continuity with the ascending aorta and main pulmonary artery due to the absence of the pericardium. This may be seen on standard nongated axial images, however, ECG gating is recommended when possible so normal pericardium may also be evaluated with minimal motion artifact. Lung windows may improve conspicuity for subtle lesions (Figure 15.8).

A leftward shift of the heart in the thoracic cavity may be seen with complete absence of the pericardium. This results from a loss of the normal anchoring support of the heart by the pericardium [8]. The amount of rotation of the heart can vary from beat to beat and with the positioning of the patient during scanning (Figure 15.9). Although a direct complication from complete absence of the pericardium is rare, a thorough evaluation of the heart is warranted as it may coexist with other congenital malformations.

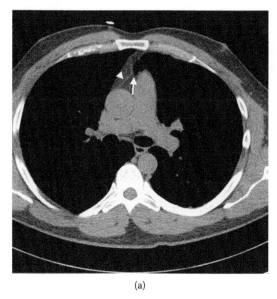
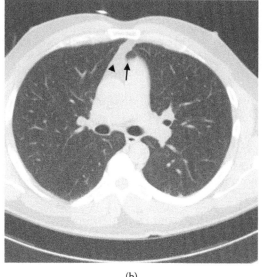

(a)   (b)

FIGURE 15.7
(a) Soft tissue and (b) lung windowing of a noncontrast CT done for calcium scoring shows the anteromedial left upper lobe in direct contact and wrapping around the main pulmonary artery (arrow) because of a partial pericardial defect. Some normally developed pericardium is visible (arrowhead).

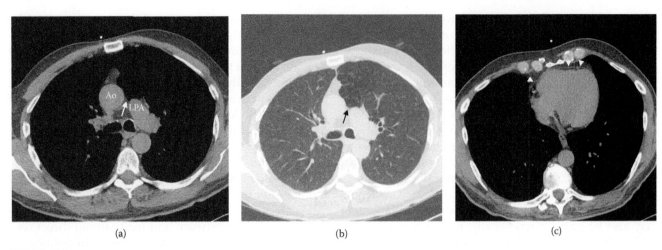

(a)   (b)   (c)

FIGURE 15.8

Partial pericardial defect. (a) Axial noncontrast CT with soft tissue windowing at the level of the carina shows part of the medial left upper lobe interposed between and directly in contact with the aorta and left pulmonary artery (arrow) because of the absence of the pericardium at this location. Ao, ascending aorta; LPA, left pulmonary artery. (b) Lung windows make the interposition (arrow) more conspicuous. (c) More inferiorly normally developed pericardium is seen along the right atrioventricular groove and right ventricular free wall (arrowheads).

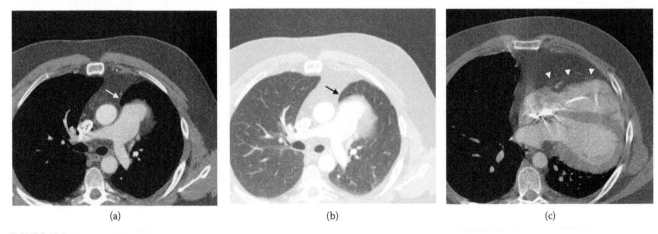

(a)   (b)   (c)

FIGURE 15.9

Complete absence of the left-sided pericardium. (a) Soft tissue and (b) lung windows of a contrast-enhanced computed tomography at the level of the mid ascending aorta. The anteromedial left lung is in direct contact with the main pulmonary artery and wraps around it (arrow). The ascending aorta and main pulmonary artery appear shifted to the left. (c) The heart has shifted to the left and is almost entirely within the left hemithorax. The pericardium on the right is faintly visible (arrowheads).

Herniations through partial defects, often initially seen as contour abnormalities, on chest x-rays, can be directly assessed on CT. Left atrial appendage herniation is rare but may appear as a congenital left atrial aneurysm; the latter of which is extremely rare but often associated with mural thrombus [10].

15.4.2 Pericardial Cysts and Diverticulum

Pericardial cysts are anomalous extensions of the pericardium, which maintain continuity with the pericardium proper but do not communicate with the pericardial space. They develop from a pinching off of redundant embryonic pericardium in utero. They are benign and are usually an incidental finding in an asymptomatic

patient, however, occasionally they can cause symptoms of tamponade through mass effect or present as chest pain. Pericardial cysts may show interval growth between examinations, and may appear like other thoracic masses both benign and malignant, such as esophageal and bronchial duplication cysts; pericardial, mediastinal, and pulmonary cystic neoplasms; loculated pleural effusions; hematomas; thoracic duct cysts; lymphangitic cysts; and lymphadenopathy (Figure 15.10).

While pericardial cysts can be located anywhere where there is pericardium, on imaging, 80% of pericardial cysts are located on the right cardiophrenic angle. Typically they are smooth, well-circumscribed, noncalcified ovoid masses with thin, sometimes imperceptible walls (Figure 15.11) [11]. They do not enhance,

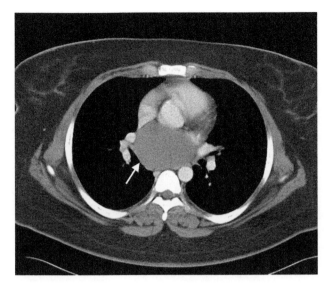

FIGURE 15.10
Bronchogenic duplication cyst. Well-circumscribed homogeneous mass located superior to the left atrium (arrow). The density is the same as muscle, not typical for a pericardial cyst. Histology confirmed it was a bronchogenic cyst with mucoid components accounting for the high density.

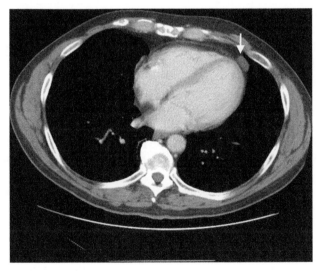

FIGURE 15.11
Pericardial cyst. A small ovoid, smoothly marginated homogeneous mass is seen at the cardiac apex (arrow). Comparison with multiple previous scans over several years showed this to be a stable pericardial cyst.

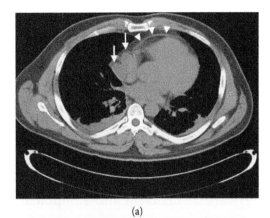

(a)

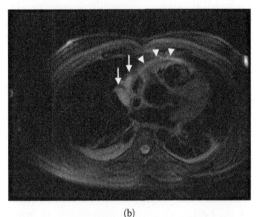

(b)

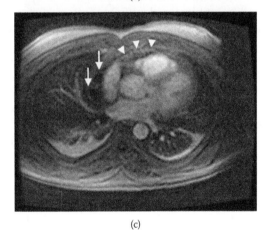

(c)

FIGURE 15.12
Pericardial cysts and pericarditis. (a) Noncontrast CT done for other purposes incidentally shows two homogeneous pericardial masses adjacent to the right atrium (arrows). The pericardium along the right ventricle is also thickened (arrowheads). (b) A triple inversion recovery magnetic resonance imaging showing homogeneous high signal within the mass, consistent with simple fluid (arrows). The internal signal of the masses followed that of cerebrospinal fluid on all sequences, showing these to be simple pericardial cysts. Note the high signal and thickening of the right-sided edematous pericardium (arrowheads), and small bilateral pleural effusions. (c) Early enhancement sequence after intravenous gadolinium injection. There is no internal enhancement of the cysts (arrows), however, faint enhancement of the walls is noted, as well as enhancement of the visible inflamed pericardium (arrowheads).

however, like the pericardium; thickening and faint early enhancement of the cyst walls may be seen in the setting of inflammation (Figure 15.12) [11]. They range in size from 2 to 20 cm in diameter, and may change shape with respiration and body positioning [12]. Internally, they are homogeneous, and have an attenuation at or near that of simple fluid. There should not be any internal enhancement or heterogeneity. Septations are typically not seen since most pericardial cysts are unilocular; however, 20% may be multiloculated.

Pericardial diverticula are very similar to pericardial cysts with the exception that they maintain continuity with the pericardial space, which may be difficult to appreciate on imaging.

15.5 Pericardial Effusion and Tamponade

The pericardial space normally contains between 15 and 50 mL of fluid. Any excess is abnormal and is termed a pericardial effusion. Clinical importance can vary depending on the cause, amount, type, acuity of accumulation, and physiologic effects of the pericardial fluid. Although most pericardial effusions are initially evaluated with echocardiography, CT can provide additional information regarding the size, location, and composition of the effusion. The wide FOV of CT provides thorough evaluation of the extent of the effusion as well as identification of extracardiac etiologies. ECG-gated CT can show any alterations to cardiac function related to the effusion; this is important as intervention often depends on hemodynamic compromise as opposed to other radiographically identifiable factors such as effusion size [13]. The compressive syndromes due to filling of the pericardial space can be divided into one of the three types: pericardial tamponade; constrictive pericarditis due to scarring and inelasticity of the pericardium; and effusive–constrictive pericarditis, which is a combination of constrictive physiology with coexistent pericardial effusion [14].

Pericardial effusions result from a wide variety of causes, such as myocardial infarction, congestive heart failure, pericardial inflammation, pericardial infection, malignancy, radiation, connective tissue disorders, traumatic hemorrhage, metabolic disorders, and adverse drug effects, among others. Most commonly, however, no cause is found [15]. The effusion itself may be serous, suppurative, hemorrhagic, or serosanguineous [13]. The fluid composition can be more broadly classified as exudative or transudative. Exudative effusions have greater fibrin or protein components and can be seen with any effusion, such as infectious, inflammatory, or malignant pericarditis. Transudative fluid is more serous in makeup, and is usually associated with congestive heart failure [13]. Often the density difference of the fluid on CT can offer clues as to which category it belongs (Figure 15.13).

Pericardial thickening is usually the first finding of a pericardial effusion. Because the pericardium and normal pericardial fluid are similar in density on CT, it can

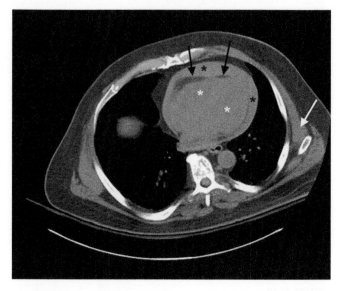

FIGURE 15.13
Hemorrhagic tamponade. Noncontrast CT shows the pericardial effusion (black asterisks) to be the same density as the blood pool (white asterisks) and muscle (white arrow). The epicardial fat along the right ventricle is displaced toward the septum (black arrows).

be difficult to separate the two, especially if the fluid is small in amount or localized. Review of suspected small effusions in cine mode can be helpful since pericardial thickening should remain constant throughout the cardiac cycle while an effusion may change in morphology [11]. In addition, pericardial thickening tends to occur anteriorly more than other locations [14].

Contrast administration is helpful for differentiating pericardium from underlying fluid, especially in the setting of pericarditis with small loculated effusions. Pericardial fluid should not enhance. Effusions with metastatic deposits or septations may show enhancement in these structures.

The density of pericardial fluid, along with the clinical history, can help limit the differential diagnosis [11]. If possible, density should be measured on a noncontrast scan to avoid the potential for volume averaging from adjacent enhancing structures, especially when evaluating small effusions [11]. Normal pericardial fluid has a Hounsfield unit (HU) density at or near that of water (0 HU). A density above 35 is suggestive of hemorrhage into the pericardial space (Figure 15.14). Aging blood coagulum will heterogeneously decrease in density as it evolves. A chylous effusion will have a median density of about −30 HU. Very high densities on a noncontrast scan should be suspected to have calcium components; narrowing the viewing window will help better define any pericardial calcium.

Filling of the pericardial space above 50 mL can cause alteration in the normal diastolic filling of the ventricles. This is termed pericardial tamponade and can be life threatening. The addition of fluid or mass into the

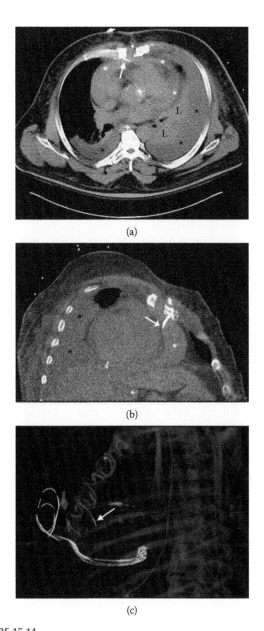

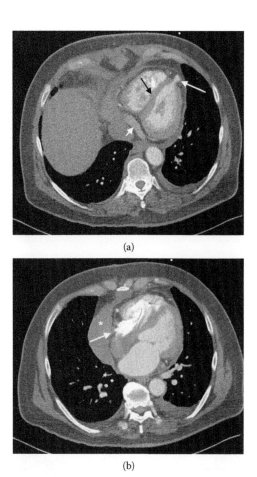

FIGURE 15.15
Tamponade. (a) Postoperative perforation of the apex shows high density contrast extravasating into the epicardial fat (white long arrow). Increased density is seen in the oblique sinus (short white arrow) from the hemorrhagic pericardial effusion. Note the sigmoid shape of the interventricular septum (black arrow). (b) The acute hemorrhagic pericardial effusion (asterisk) causes mass effect on the right atrium (arrow).

FIGURE 15.14
Hemorrhage effusion. (a) Fractured and displaced medial sternotomy wire (arrow) has perforated the right ventricle. A pericardial effusion (white asterisks) surrounds the heart. Compare the density of the pericardial effusion with the bilateral pleural effusion fluid (black asterisks). L, atelectatic lung. (b) Sagittal reformat showing the wire (arrow), the effusion (white asterisk), and pleural effusion (black asterisks). (c) Volume rendered reconstruction oblique sagittal projection shows the wire (arrow) projecting into the pericardial effusion, which is assigned a maroon color.

relatively rigid compartment defined by the pericardium increases the intrapericardial pressure, compresses the heart, and increases diastolic filling pressure, reducing stroke volume and cardiac output in the process [14,16]. Acute hemorrhagic pericardial tamponade will appear hyperdense and may be seen with trauma, recent surgery, myocardial rupture, coronary aneurysmal rupture, or rupture of the proximal great vessels (Figure 15.15).

Tamponade can also occur with gradual pericardial filling once the pericardium has reached its limit of accommodation, as seen with some neoplastic deposits and effusions [16,17]. The loss of intravascular volume from hemorrhage further the compressive effects of tamponade and reduction of ventricular filling, and cause rapid clinical deterioration from low cardiac output and hypotension [14]. Pneumopericardium, where air collects into the pericardial space from trauma to the tracheobronchial tree, may cause tamponade (tension pneumopericardium), as can herniation of adjacent organs into the pericardial space (Figure 15.16) [11,14].

Although pericardial tamponade is a clinical diagnosis, there are often accompanying signs that can be seen on CT. These include a pericardial effusion; a flattened or tubular appearance of the ventricles; dilatation of the inferior vena cava (IVC); reflux of contrast into the IVC, hepatic veins, and azygous vein; and periportal edema [14,18]. Increased transmural pressure

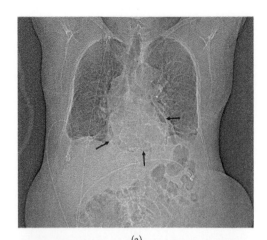

(a)

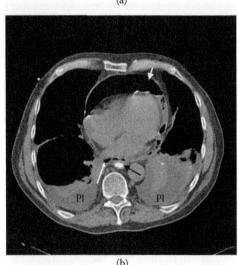

(b)

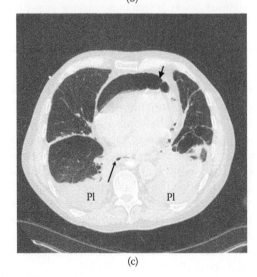

(c)

FIGURE 15.16
(a) Pneumopericardium. Topogram showing lucency surrounding the cardiac silhouette (arrows). (b) Air can be seen predominantly in the nondependent pericardial space (short arrow). Small amounts of air are also in the oblique sinus (long white arrow). Contrast is in the esophagus (black arrow), bilateral pleural effusions (Pl). (c) Lung windows make the pneumopericardial air more conspicuous (arrows).

caused by tamponade physiology can cause the anterior wall of the right ventricle to become compressed and convex to the ventricular lumen, a sign termed the flattened heart sign. Tamponade can also cause compression to intrapericardial vessels such as the main pulmonary trunk and the coronary sinus, as well as juxtapericardial vessels such as the intrathoracic IVC. Cine appreciation of abnormal diastolic septal motion, typically seen with constriction, can also be seen in tamponade.

15.6 Pericarditis

15.6.1 Nonconstrictive Pericarditis

When the pericardial sac surrounding the heart and origins of the great vessels becomes inflamed, it is termed pericarditis. The etiology of pericarditis is usually idiopathic or viral, but can be due to a variety of causes that can be split into infectious, and noninfectious categories [19,20]. Infectious causes include viruses such as mumps, HIV, varicella, and coxsackieviruses; gram-positive and gram-negative bacteria; tuberculosis; fungi such as candida; and parasites. In developed countries, infections causing a purulent pericarditis are often associated with an immunocompromised state [19]. Noninfectious causes include uremia from renal failure, hypothyroidism, acute myocardial infarction, neoplastic pericarditis, trauma, radiation therapy, iatrogenic causes such as pericardiotomy, sarcoidosis, connective tissue disorders such as scleroderma and lupus, and drugs such as procainamide, hydralazine and isoniazid [19]. Postmyocardial infarction pericarditis can occur 1–3 days after a transmural infarct due to interaction of the pericardium and myocardial necrosis, or weeks to months after the ischemic event (Dressler's syndrome) [20].

The chronicity of pericarditis is important to take into account as it can sometimes be elucidated on imaging. Pericarditis can be categorized as acute (<6 weeks), subacute (>6 weeks to 6 months), and chronic (>6 months). Depending on the underlying pathology, acute pericarditis can further be classified as effusive or fibrinous, and chronic pericarditis as effusive, adhesive, effusive–adhesive, and constrictive [19]. Specific imaging characteristics can favor acute versus chronic, but there is often overlap. Acute pericarditis is characterized by pericardial thickening, an effusion and fibrin deposition, whereas chronic pericarditis is associated with fibrosis and calcification (Figure 15.17) [3].

As in many areas of radiology, clinical history is helpful. Patients most often present with a pericardial

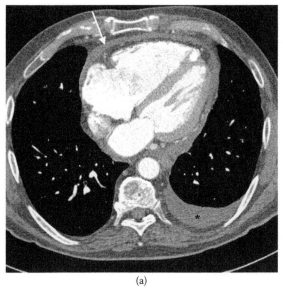 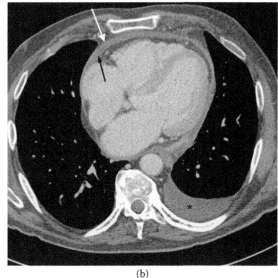

(a)   (b)

FIGURE 15.17
Pericardial thickening with effusion. (a) Arterial phase showing thickening of the pericardium (white arrow). Pericardial enhancement is subtle, making distinction of the underlying pericardial effusion difficult. Asterisk, pleural effusion. (b) Delayed images better differentiate the enhancing pericardium and the underlying pericardial effusion (black arrow).

friction rub, which is best heard when the patient is leaning forward. Retrosternal pain due to friction between the inflamed pericardium and cardiac and respiratory motion is relieved when sitting up and exacerbated when lying down. Other symptoms include palpitations, nonproductive cough, dyspnea, weakness, and fever. Alterations in hemodynamic physiology can be caused by tamponade and constrictive effects, and are reflected clinically by pulsus paradoxicus, Kussmaul sign, and ECG changes. Depending on the etiology, pericarditis may be accompanied with a pleural effusion and ascites [21,22].

Transthoracic or transesophageal echocardiography is usually the first line imaging modality when pericarditis is suspected. It offers real-time assessment of the pericardium and the pericardial space as well as wall motion abnormalities and certain other hemodynamic effects when combined with Doppler [23]. Optimal visualization of the pericardium with echocardiography relies heavily on a good acoustic window. Pericardial effusions in atypical locations may not be seen or underestimated in size due to shadowing from overlying bone or air in the lungs [23]. Echocardiography is also operator dependent. ECG-gated cardiac CT can provide additional valuable information in these situations. Characterizing features for pericarditis on CT include the thickness of the pericardium, pericardial enhancement, pericardial effusion, and associated constrictive findings.

The normal pericardial thickness is 2 mm or less; it is considered abnormally thickened if it is above 4 mm.

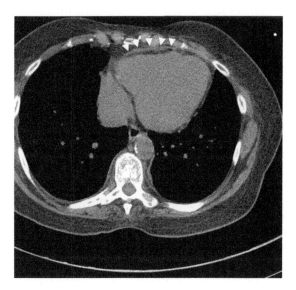

FIGURE 15.18
Thickened pericardium. Noncontrast CT done for coronary artery calcium scoring showing thickening of the right-sided pericardium (arrowheads).

This measurement can usually be made on the axial source images, but can also be made on any reformatted images. The measurement should be perpendicular to the plane of the pericardium in order not to overestimate the thickness. The pericardium adjacent to the right ventricle is the best place to look for thickening initially since the pericardium may normally not be seen on the left, and may blend with the pleura if the mediastinal fat in that area is sparse (Figure 15.18) [24].

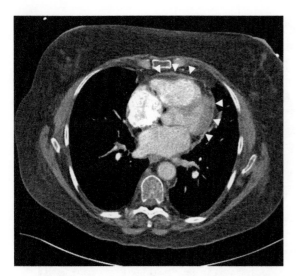

FIGURE 15.19
Thickened pericardium. Arrowheads point to thickened pericardium along the left and right ventricles.

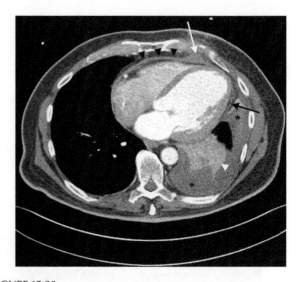

FIGURE 15.20
Pericardial thickening. White arrow points to focal thickening of the right pericardium at the site of previous right ventricle repair. The remainder of the right pericardium is mildly thickened (black arrowheads). Compare with the left ventricle pericardium (black arrow). Atelectatic lung (white arrowhead) and left pleural effusion (asterisks).

Pericardial thickening may be smooth or irregular and may involve the entire pericardium, or only focal portions (Figures 15.19 and 15.20). Pericardial thickness may be assessed on noncontrast images; however, differentiating pericardial thickening from a small or a dense effusion may be difficult [25]. Low-density effusions such as those seen with uremic or chylous usually provide enough of a natural contrast with the pericardium to make the distinction; however, purulent or hemorrhagic effusions with a higher density may obscure the pericardial border.

Unlike acute pericarditis, chronic pericarditis may not involve a thickened pericardium. The pericardium, in this instance, is often scarred down and has an irregular or nodular look, or it may not appear abnormal at all. Pericardial calcification is commonly seen with chronic pericarditis.

In the setting of acute pericarditis, the highly vascular inflamed pericardium may enhance following intravenous contrast administration [25]. Contrast enhancement helps differentiate the pericardium from an adjacent effusion as well as characterize associated masses such as metastatic deposits or developmental duplication cysts. The enhancement can be subtle, particularly with adjacent dense effusions. Window and level adjustments and side-by-side evaluation of pre- and postcontrast images can help make mild enhancement more conspicuous (Figure 15.21).

Pericarditis, particularly acute pericarditis, is usually accompanied with an effusion. The size of the effusion can vary greatly, and, as discussed earlier, the type of fluid will affect the density. The effusion may be serous, purulent, fibrinous, hemorrhagic, sanguineous, or chylous in composition and may appear loculated, heterogeneous, or septated. With metabolic etiologies, connective tissue diseases and congestive heart failure, an associated pleural effusion, may also be present.

As previously mentioned, CT can assess constrictive findings seen with tamponade or constrictive pericarditis that may occur in the setting of acute pericarditis. These findings include compression of one or both ventricles, a sigmoid shape of the interventricular septum, enlargement of the atria, coronary sinus and IVC, and pleural effusions and ascites [22]. The cine component of retrospective ECG-gated cardiac CT offers a unique ability to evaluate functional changes such as paradoxical motion of the septum throughout the cardiac cycle (the "septal bounce") and ventricular free wall motion abnormalities [22].

15.6.2 Constrictive Pericarditis

Constrictive pericarditis describes a subset of pericarditis, usually chronic, which results in diastolic dysfunction. Chronic or repetitive inflammation of the pericardium leads to reparative fibrosis, calcium deposits in the pericardium, and adhesions between the parietal and visceral pericardial layers. The pericardial layers become stiff and often thick, reducing compliance throughout the cardiac cycle [26]. This incompliance is transmitted to the ventricles, often compressing them,

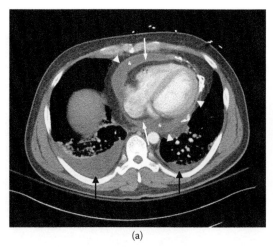 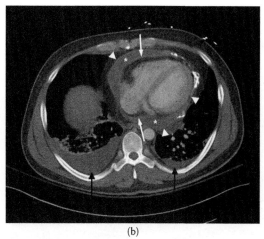

(a)   (b)

FIGURE 15.21
Pericarditis with pericardial effusion. (a) Post contrast images show enhancement of the parietal (arrowheads) and visceral (white arrows) pericardium with a pericardial effusion (asterisks). Bilateral pleural effusions (black arrows). (b) Narrowing the windows makes the pericardial enhancement more conspicuous and differentiates it better from the pericardial effusion.

and resulting in a decreased capacity for dilatation during diastole (preload), increased filling pressures, and a lowering of cardiac stroke volume. Systolic dysfunction may be seen in cases due to radiation and carry worse prognosis [27]. The physiologic changes can mimic those of the entirely separate disorder of restrictive cardiomyopathy. The distinction is an important one as it relates to prognosis: constrictive pericarditis, usually treated with pericardectomy, has a better prognosis than restrictive cardiomyopathy, which is treated medically [28].

The causes of constrictive pericarditis are similar to those of nonconstrictive pericarditis. Most cases are due to cardiac surgery, irradiation, or antecedent viral or idiopathic acute pericarditis [9,29]. Infectious causes such as bacterial, fungal, and tuberculous etiologies are more common in developing countries and with immunocompromised patients [28]. Metastatic tumor deposits are the most common neoplastic cause. Primary neoplastic causes include mesothelioma, leukemia, lymphoma, and sarcoma. Other etiologies include connective tissue diseases, uremia, previous myocardial infarction, and trauma.

Development of constrictive pericarditis usually ranges from 2–3 months to several years, although atypically an acute timeframe may occur after cardiac surgery [3,27]. Clinical presentation is variable and nonspecific. Frequently seen signs and symptoms of dyspnea, pleural effusions, ascites, and peripheral edema are similar to those of heart failure, reflecting the pathophysiologic changes of the diseased pericardium on cardiac function [28]. The natural history of constrictive pericarditis is progressive and irreversible. A rare exception to this is transient constrictive

pericarditis that most commonly occurs in patients with prior coronary artery bypass graft surgery and is treated medically [30].

Constrictive pericarditis can be divided into four subtypes: Chronic fibrous pericarditis is the most common presentation due to fibrosis and calcification of the pericardium. Acute inflammatory pericarditis describes constrictive physiology in the setting of acute pericarditis. Effusive–constrictive pericarditis combines constriction of the visceral pericardium with a chronic effusion, often discovered when symptoms persist after the effusion is drained [15,26]. Adhesive constrictive pericarditis is caused by adhesion of the two pericardial layers, usually due to a previous exudative pericardial effusion [31,34].

CT evaluation of constrictive pericarditis should include assessment of pericardial morphology and cardiac function. Morphological signs include pericardial thickening and calcification, changes in the appearance of the cardiac chambers, and extracardiac findings. Review of ECG-gated dynamic cine images in multiple planes allows for the evaluation of cardiac septal and ventricular wall motion. Volumetric assessment of the cardiac chambers can be done with the review of the cardiac cycle images for end systole and maximum diastole. The complete heart should be imaged with and without contrast to distinguish calcium deposits from enhancing structures [31].

The majority of constrictive pericarditis cases present with pericardial thickening, with a minority of about 5% having a fibrotic pericardium of normal thickness (Figure 15.22). The thickened pericardium will measure >4 mm and is often global in distribution, although focal

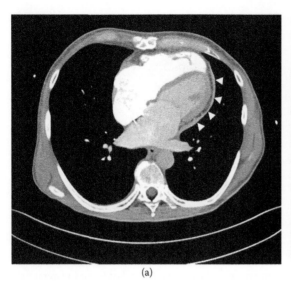
(a)

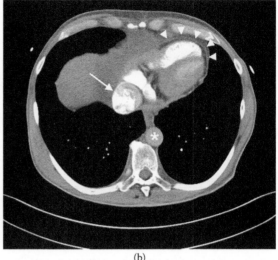
(b)

FIGURE 15.22
Constrictive pericarditis. (a) The left pericardium along the ventricle is thickened (arrowheads). There is straightening of the septum and the atria are enlarged bilaterally. (b) Lower down mild pericardial thickening is seen along the apex (is this artificial due to curvature of pericardium?). The inferior vena cava (arrow) is more than twice as large as the descending aorta (asterisk).

thickening may occur, usually over the right ventricle [9]. Thickening >6 mm with findings of congestive heart failure is highly supportive of constrictive pericarditis [26]. It may be difficult to distinguish the thickness from an adjacent focal pericardial effusion. Enhancement of the thickened pericardium is uncommon but may occur, indicating active inflammation [26].

Pericardial calcification is detected by CT better than any other imaging modality. The pattern of composition is variable and can be found bordering the right or left ventricle, the atrioventricular groove, the atria, and along the diaphragmatic margin (Figure 15.23). Calcification is not required for constrictive physiology, however, its presence excludes restrictive cardiomyopathy [2]. The association of calcification with constrictive pericarditis varies, ranging from 5% to over 50% depending on the population studied [29]. In the past, pericardial calcification was mostly seen with prior tuberculous pericarditis, however, it is now most commonly associated with idiopathic causes in developed countries [29].

The increased pericardial rigidity and calcification often deforms the normal contours of the right and left ventricles. They become compressed and assume a tubular configuration, decreasing in dimension along the ventricular longitudinal axis. The atrioventricular groove is frequently involved and can become narrowed and extend medially toward the septum (Figure 15.24). The septum often appears straightened or sigmoid in shape. One or both atria are often dilated due to altered filling pressures of the ventricles. Extracardiac findings reflect those seen in heart failure. There is a dilatation of the SVC and IVC when compared to the descending

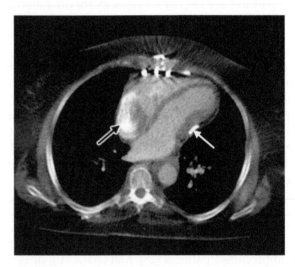

FIGURE 15.23
Left-sided morphology of constrictive pericarditis. There is focal calcification (white arrow) along the free wall of the lateral ventricle, causing the left ventricle to have a tubular appearance. The septum curves to the left (black arrow).

aorta (1 ≥ 1 and 2 ≥ 1, respectively), dilatation of the hepatic veins, pleural effusions, ascites, and peripheral edema [24,26,31].

The morphological findings of constrictive pericarditis can be combined into one of six recognizable patterns on cardiac CT as described by Rienmuller (Table 15.1) [31]. "Global" constrictive pericarditis involves bilateral thickening or calcification of the pericardium along both ventricles and enlargement of both atria, SVC, and IVC (Figure 15.25). "Annular" constrictive pericarditis consists of bilateral thickening or calcification, and

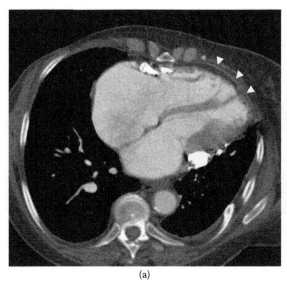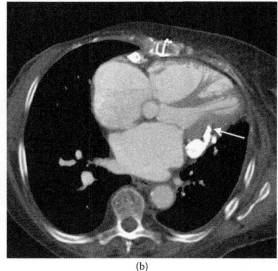

(a)   (b)

FIGURE 15.24
Annular morphology constrictive pericarditis. (a) Calcification is seen in the right and left atrioventricular (AV) grooves. The left ventricle is severely compressed and tubular in appearance, and both atria are enlarged. The septum has a sigmoid appearance. Mild pericardial thickening can be seen near the apex (arrows). (b) Slightly more superior slice shows left AV calcification indenting the lateral free wall of the left ventricle. Both atria are enlarged.

TABLE 15.1

Morphological Characteristics of Constrictive Pericarditis Subtypes

Constrictive Type	Distribution	Primary Pericardial Layer Thickened	Ventricle Compression	Atrial Enlargement	Other Findings
Global	Left and right pericardium, diffuse	Parietal	Variable	Biatrial	SVC/IVC enlargement
Annular	Bilateral AV grooves	Parietal	No	Biatrial	SVC/IVC enlargement
Left-sided	Left pericardium	Parietal	Left ventricle compressed	Right	Straightened or right-bending septum, SVC/IVC enlargement
Right-sided	Right pericardium	Parietal	Right ventricle compressed	Left	Straightened or left-bending septum, SVC/IVC enlargement
Epicardial	Variable	Epicardial	Variable	Varies	—
Effusive	Variable	Epicardial	Variable	Varies	Pericardial effusion, constriction remains after pericardiocentesis

narrowing of the atrioventricular (AV) grooves with normal-sized ventricles and enlargement of the atria, SVC and IVC (Figure 15.26). "Left-sided" constrictive pericarditis describes thickening or calcification along the compressed left ventricle with narrowing of the left AV groove, a straightened or leftward bending septum, and enlargement of both atria, SVC, and IVC. The right ventricle is normal size (see Figure 15.23). "Right-sided" constrictive pericarditis has thickening or calcification along the compressed right ventricle with narrowing of the right AV groove, a straightened or rightward bending septum, and enlargement of the right atrium, SVC, and IVC (Figure 15.27). "Epicardial" is when the global or focal form is predominantly caused by the epicardium. "Effusive" describes a general epicardial constriction and pericardial effusion. The epicardium does

not change regardless of the amount of pericardial fluid (Figure 15.28).

The physiologic changes that result from constriction on the cardiac chambers can be evaluated by reviewing dynamic images of the heart acquired through the entire cardiac cycle. Because matching cardiac images with the phase of the cardiac cycle is essential for correct interpretation, ECG gating is required for functional assessment.

The rigid pericardium causes increased pressure in the pericardial space, which is transmitted to the cardiac chambers, resulting in early filling of the ventricles and rapid normalization of pressure between the cardiac chambers. Diastolic volume accommodation for one ventricle is directly related to the other; a phenomenon termed "ventricular interdependence or

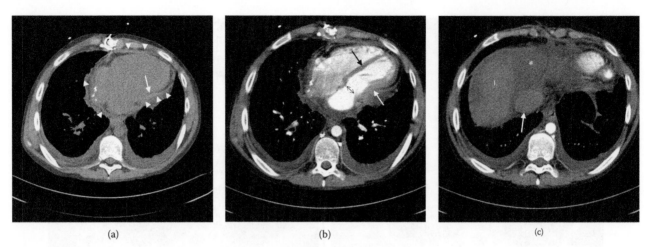

FIGURE 15.25

Global morphology of constrictive pericarditis. (a) Noncontrast CT showing a few foci of pericardial calcification limited to the right atrium. Noncalcified pericardial thickening can be seen along both atria and ventricles (arrowheads), however. The pericardial thickening and medially displaced epicardial fat suggests constriction of the left ventricle (arrow). Bilateral pleural effusions are also present. (b) Post contrast image shows narrowing of the left atrioventricular groove (double arrow) and left ventricle free wall near the base (white arrow) as well as straightening of the septum (black arrow). (c) Inferiorly the suprahepatic inferior vena cava is large (arrow) compared to the descending aorta. Low-density ascitic fluid (asterisk) is present next to the liver (L).

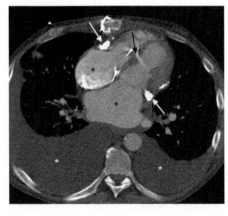

FIGURE 15.26

Annular morphology constrictive pericarditis. Calcification is present and causing narrowing predominantly in the right and left atrioventricular grooves (white arrows). There is narrowing of the ventricles, the septum has a slight sigmoid appearance (black arrow), both atria are enlarged (black asterisks), and there are bilateral pleural effusions (white asterisks).

ventricular coupling." Ventricular interdependence is reflected in the motion of the interventricular septum. Under normal conditions, the septum is concave to the left ventricle, and is displaced toward the right ventricle during most of diastole because of the lower filling pressures for the right ventricle. During inspiration, the negative thoracic pressure increases systemic flow to the right chambers of the heart. This, combined with the slightly earlier commencement of right ventricular filling, causes a transient mild deflection of the septum toward the left ventricle during early systole.

The constrictive effect of the abnormal pericardium accentuates the early diastolic transseptal pressure difference causing the septum to have an exaggerated displacement toward the left ventricle initially. As the ventricles quickly equalize in pressure because of the fixed pericardial volume, the septum will straighten. (The opposite scenario with exaggerated displacement of the septum toward the right ventricle during late diastole occurs during expiration because of increased flow to the left chambers of the heart; however, this may not be as easily appreciated on imaging since some diastolic septal motion to the right is normal). This abnormal septal movement is termed "septal bounce" and is a key diagnostic finding as it is typically seen with constrictive pericarditis but not with restrictive cardiomyopathy. Review of axial and short-axis reconstructions in dynamic cine mode will allow for assessment of septal bounce.

Cardiac function metrics such as end diastolic volume, stroke volume, and cardiac output can be calculated by measuring ventricular volumes at end systole and during diastole at the time of maximum diastolic distension (usually somewhere between 60% and 80% of the cardiac cycle). Depending on the reconstruction software, the optimal systolic and diastolic volumes may be determined automatically; however, review and editing of the ECG tracing for cardiac beats to be included or removed from the reconstruction algorithms may be necessary to help minimize artifacts because of arrhythmias. The endocardial surface is traced on sequential short-axis images, which, at our institution, are reconstructed

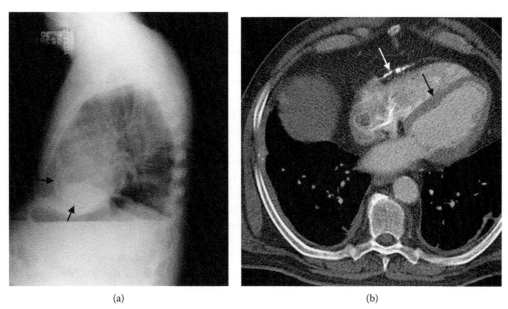

FIGURE 15.27
Right-sided morphology of constrictive pericarditis. (a) Lateral chest x-ray shows calcification of the anterior and inferior pericardium. The costophrenic angles are blunted due to pleural effusions. (b) Axial post contrast CT shows calcification along the right ventricle and right atrioventricular groove (white arrow). The right ventricle is narrowed and the septum is straightened (black arrow). The left ventricle is normal in size.

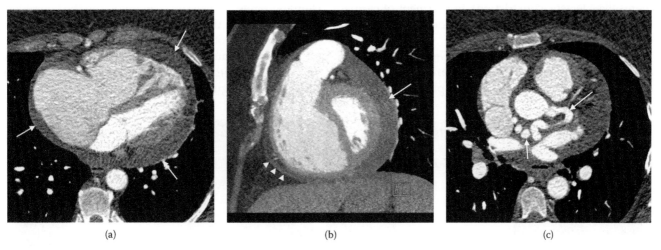

FIGURE 15.28
Effusive constrictive pericarditis. (a) There is a global low-density pericardial effusion (arrows). The septum is straightened. The left ventricle is compressed and has a tubular shape while the right atrium is dilated. (b) Short-axis reformatted image shows the pericardial effusion (arrow) and focal pericardial thickening (arrowheads). The septum bows toward the compressed left ventricle. (c) Arrows point to a coronary artery fistula to the superior vena cava, which was the cause of right ventricular overload and development of the pericardial effusion.

from the axial raw data in 6 mm increments with each slice having a thickness of 6 mm (in other words, no space between adjacent 6 mm slices). Tracing technique (e.g., including or excluding trabeculations and papillary muscles) is open to preference but should be consistent between systolic and diastolic images and done the same way for future examinations of a particular patient, if possible.

15.7 Pericardial Neoplasm

Pericardial neoplasms can be divided into "primary tumors," or those arising directly from the pericardium, and "secondary tumors" that result from metastatic spread. Of the two, metastases are a much more common source of pericardial masses. In patients with known cancer, 10%–20% have pericardial metastases on autopsy [12,32]. Distant primary tumor metastasis to the pericardium can occur through hematogenous seeding, lymphangitic spread, or direct extension. The most common sources of metastasis are breast and lung cancers (each of which account for about a third of cases), melanoma, lymphoma and leukemia, esophageal cancer, and renal cell carcinoma [32]. Sixty percent of metastatic melanoma involves the pericardium.

Primary pericardial lesions are rare and can be further classified as developmental, stromal, vascular, and miscellaneous. Common benign pericardial lesions include lipoma, hemangioma, teratoma, fibroma, lymphangioma, and neurofibroma. Of the malignant primary tumors, mesothelioma of the pericardium is the most common, accounting for 50% of cases. Other malignant primary tumors include sarcoma, liposarcoma, and lymphoma.

Patients with pericardial tumors are frequently asymptomatic; however, they may also present with pleuritic chest pain, dyspnea, edema, and effusions. Malignant pericardial effusions may result in tamponade [17]. Constrictive physiology can occur because of pericardial effusion (effusive constriction) or the tumors themselves (elastic constriction). Impairment of cardiac function can occur in up to 30% of patients with pericardial metastasis [32].

The high spatial resolution of ECG-gated cardiac CT allows for good evaluation of pericardial morphology and neoplastic invasion, as well as physiologic effects of constriction such as the septal bounce related to ventricular interdependence [33]. Evaluation should include assessment of pericardial thickness, irregularity and nodularity, the presence of a pericardial effusion, pericardial enhancement, extent of invasion, and constrictive physiology, if present. The wide FOV with CT also allows for potential identification and description of a distant source of pericardial metastases (Figure 15.29).

Attenuation and enhancement properties on CT can facilitate tissue characterization. Lipomas will have a low Hounsfield unit attenuation equal to that of fat. Teratomas may show gross fat as well as calcification. Fibromas often show poor or irregular enhancement. Hemangiomas are often low in attenuation and show slow enhancement.

The location and distribution of cardiac and extracardiac lesions directly extending into the pericardium may also suggest the diagnosis. For example, angiosarcoma, the most common primary malignant cardiac tumor in adulthood, typically arises from the right atrium, whereas the majority of leiomyosarcoma and undifferentiated sarcomas originate in the left atrium (Figure 15.30). These tumors can become quite large and necrotic, encasing large portions of the heart. Hemangiomas are usually seen involving the lateral left ventricular wall, the anterior right ventricular wall, or the septum. Mesothelioma may present as a focal nodule, plaques, or multiple coalescing masses, which often will obliterate the pericardial space while sparing the epicardial fat (Figure 15.31).

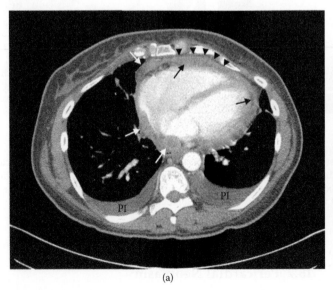
(a)

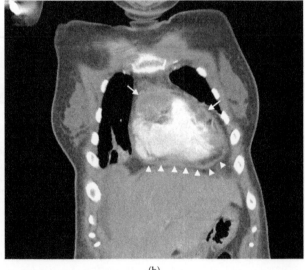
(b)

FIGURE 15.29
Metastatic adenocarcinoma. (a) Axial postcontrast image shows the pericardium to be diffusely thickened and irregular with discrete metastatic nodules (white arrows). Arrowheads point out pericardial enhancement, which contrasts with the small malignant pericardial effusion (black arrows). Pl, pleural effusion. (b) Coronal reconstructions through the right ventricle again show the pericardial metastases (arrows), as well as diffuse thickening and enhancement of the inferior pericardium (arrowheads).

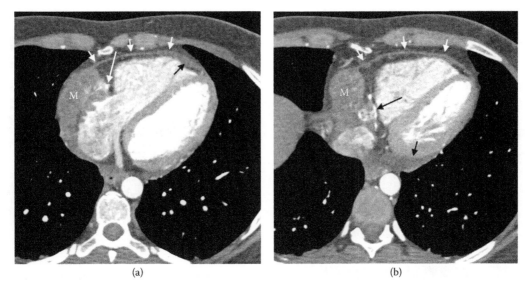

(a)   (b)

FIGURE 15.30
Angiosarcoma. (a) A lobulated heterogeneously enhancing mass (M), can be seen invading through the right atrial wall. It also involves right tricuspid annulus and encases the right coronary artery (white long arrow). The pericardium is mildly thickened and faintly enhances (short white arrows). A pericardial effusion is partially visible at the apex (black arrow). (b) There is partial encasement of the distal right coronary artery by the mass as it courses along the inferior right atrioventricular groove (long black arrow). Again noted is pericardial thickening, irregularity, and enhancement (white arrows), and a small pericardial effusion (short black arrow).

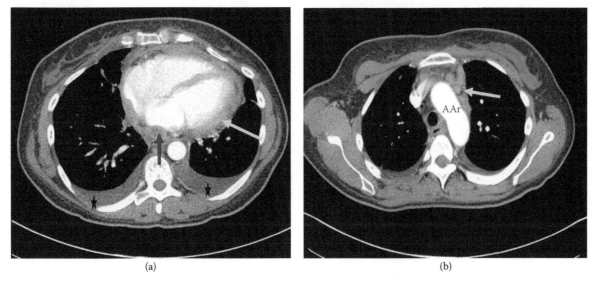

(a)   (b)

FIGURE 15.31
Mesothelioma. (a) There is diffuse pericardial thickening, irregularity and enhancement (yellow arrow), as well as discrete neoplastic masses (red arrow). Epicardial fat can be seen deep to the pericardial thickening. Stars, pleural effusions. (b) Prevascular lymphadenopathy (yellow arrow) can be seen more superiorly. AAr, aortic arch.

Unfortunately, many tumors are nonspecific in appearance (Figures 15.32 and 15.33). In addition, there are several mimics of pericardial neoplasms, including normal structures such as mediastinal or pericardiac lymph nodes and normal pericardial recesses, congenital duplication cysts, pericardial cysts, loculated pericardial effusions, and pericardial hematomas (Figures 15.34 and 15.35). While other imaging modalities such as magnetic resonance imaging may provide additional tissue character-ization, often a biopsy is necessary for a definitive diagnosis.

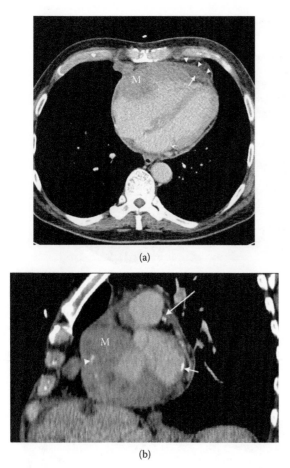

(a)

(b)

FIGURE 15.32
Lymphoma. (a) Delayed post contrast axial image at the mid level of the heart shows a mass (M), invading and causing mass effect on the right atrium and ventricle. A small pericardial effusion is visible near the apex (arrow), as well as enhancing pericardium (arrowheads). (b) Sagittal reformat shows the luminal calcifications of the right coronary artery (arrowhead), encased by the pericardial mass (M). The noninvolved left anterior descending (long arrow), and left circumflex (short arrow) arteries are also seen.

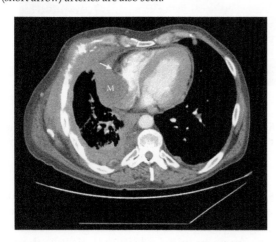

FIGURE 15.33
Metastatic colorectal carcinoma. A pericardial metastatic deposit (M), invades the right atrium resulting in an abrupt discontinuation of the epicardial fat (arrow). Involvement of the right pulmonary pleura and anterior right chest wall is also visible.

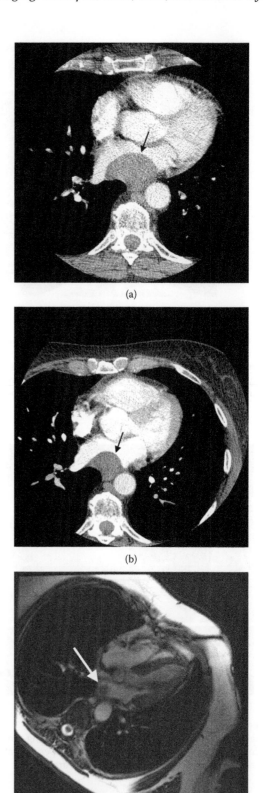

(a)

(b)

(c)

FIGURE 15.34
Hematoma. (a) A homogeneous, well-circumscribed, soft tissue density mass is present in the left atrium (arrow). (b) Follow up 1 month later showing the mass has decreased in size (arrow). (c) A magnetic resonance imaging exam performed a year later showing complete resolution of the mass (arrow).

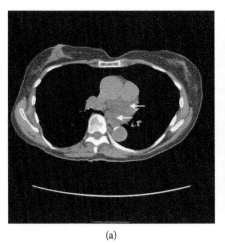
(a)

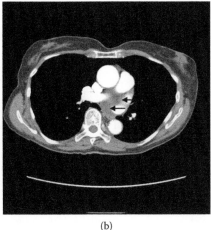
(b)

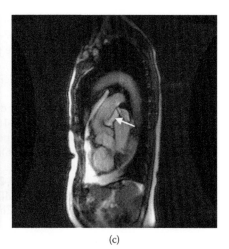
(c)

FIGURE 15.35

Pericardial recesses. (a) Nonenhanced and (b) enhanced images of the chest at the level of the carina showing two homogeneous low-density structures that do not enhance posterior to the aorta and main pulmonary artery (arrows). These were initially thought to be abnormal mediastinal masses. (c) A sagittal steady-state free-precession magnetic resonance imaging sequence shows that the questionable structures have the same characteristics as pericardial fluid (arrowheads). Careful review of the images showed them to be contiguous with the pericardial space.

References

1. Broderick LS, Brooks GN, and Kuhlman JE. Anatomic pitfalls of the heart and pericardium. *Radiographics*, 2005; 25(2): 441–453.
2. O'Leary SM et al. Imaging the pericardium: appearances on ECG-gated 64-detector row cardiac computed tomography. *Br J Radiol*, 2010; 83(987): 194–205.
3. Rajiah P and Kanne JP. Computed tomography of the pericardium and pericardial disease. *J Cardiovasc Comput Tomogr*, 2010; 4(1): 3–18.
4. Cody DD and Mahesh M. AAPM/RSNA physics tutorial for residents: technologic advances in multidetector CT with a focus on cardiac imaging. *Radiographics*, 2007; 27(6): 1829–1837.
5. Van Son JA et al. Congenital partial and complete absence of the pericardium. *Mayo Clin Proc*, 1993; 68(8): 743–747.
6. Garnier F et al. Congenital complete absence of the left pericardium: a rare cause of chest pain or pseudo-right heart overload. *Clin Cardiol*, 2010; 33(2): E52–E57.
7. Gatzoulis MA et al. Isolated congenital absence of the pericardium: clinical presentation, diagnosis, and management. *Ann Thorac Surg*, 2000; 69(4): 1209–1215.
8. Gassner I et al. Diagnosis of congenital pericardial defects, including a pathognomic sign for dangerous apical ventricular herniation, on magnetic resonance imaging. *Br Heart J*, 1995; 74(1): 60–66.
9. Grizzard JD and Ang GB. Magnetic resonance imaging of pericardial disease and cardiac masses. *Magn Reson Imaging Clin N Am*, 2007; 15(4): 579–607, vi.
10. Kunishima T et al. Congenital giant aneurysm of the left atrial appendage mimicking pericardial absence case report. *Jpn Circ J*, 2001; 65(1): 56–59.
11. Olson MC et al. Computed tomography and magnetic resonance imaging of the pericardium. *Radiographics*, 1989; 9(4): 633–649.
12. Oyama N et al. Computed tomography and magnetic resonance imaging of the pericardium: anatomy and pathology. *Magn Reson Med Sci*, 2004; 3(3): 145–152.
13. Palacios IF. Pericardial effusion and tamponade. *Curr Treat Options Cardiovasc Med*, 1999; 1(1): 79–89.
14. Restrepo CS et al. Imaging findings in cardiac tamponade with emphasis on CT. *Radiographics*, 2007; 27(6): 1595–1610.
15. Sagrista-Sauleda J et al. Effusive-constrictive pericarditis. *N Engl J Med*, 2004; 350(5): 469–475.
16. Goldstein JA. Cardiac tamponade, constrictive pericarditis, and restrictive cardiomyopathy. *Curr Probl Cardiol*, 2004; 29(9): 503–567.
17. Imazio M et al. Relation of acute pericardial disease to malignancy. *Am J Cardiol*, 2005; 95(11): 1393–1394.
18. Schairer JR et al. A systematic approach to evaluation of pericardial effusion and cardiac tamponade. *Cardiol Rev*, 2011; 19(5): 233–238.
19. Goyle KK and Walling AD. Diagnosing pericarditis. *Am Fam Physician*, 2002; 66(9): 1695–1702.
20. Little WC and Freeman GL. Pericardial disease. *Circulation*, 2006; 113(12): 1622–1632.
21. Kim EY et al. Multidetector CT and MR imaging of cardiac tumors. *Korean J Radiol*, 2009; 10(2): 164–175.
22. Lopez Costa I and Bhalla S. Computed tomography and magnetic resonance imaging of the pericardium. *Semin Roentgenol*, 2008; 43(3): 234–245.
23. Breen JF. Imaging of the pericardium. *J Thorac Imaging*, 2001; 16(1): 47–54.
24. Frank H and Globits S. Magnetic resonance imaging evaluation of myocardial and pericardial disease. *J Magn Reson Imaging*, 1999; 10(5): 617–626.

25. Wang ZJ et al. CT and MR imaging of pericardial disease. *Radiographics*, 2003; 23 Spec No: S167–S180.
26. Misselt AJ et al. MR imaging of the pericardium. *Magn Reson Imaging Clin N Am*, 2008; 16(2): 185–199, vii.
27. Troughton RW, Asher CR, and Klein AL. Pericarditis. *Lancet*, 2004; 363(9410): 717–727.
28. Glockner JF. Imaging of pericardial disease. *Magn Reson Imaging Clin N Am*, 2003; 11(1): 149–162, vii.
29. Ling LH et al. Calcific constrictive pericarditis: is it still with us? *Ann Intern Med*, 2000; 132(6): 444–50.
30. Haley JH et al. Transient constrictive pericarditis: causes and natural history. *J Am Coll Cardiol*, 2004; 43(2): 271–275.
31. Rienmuller R, Groll R, and Lipton MJ. CT and MR imaging of pericardial disease. *Radiol Clin North Am*, 2004; 42(3): 587–601, vi.
32. Chiles C et al. Metastatic involvement of the heart and pericardium: CT and MR imaging. *Radiographics*, 2001; 21(2): 439–449.
33. Jimenez-Juan L et al. Multimodality imaging in the evaluation of cardiovascular manifestations of malignancy. *Cardiol Res Pract*, 2011; 2011: 378041.
34. Higgins CB and de Roos A. *MRI and CT of the Cardiovascular System*, 2006. Philadelphia, Lippincot Williams & Wilkins.
35. Dadds V, Masters PL. Strangulation of the left ventricle following herniation through a congenital defect in the pericardial sac. *Aust Paediatr J*, 1972; 8(2):98–101.

16

Pulmonary Embolism and Pulmonary Hypertension

Tobias De Zordo, Karoline Netzer, Gudrun Feuchtner, and Werner Jaschke

CONTENTS

16.1 Introduction

Computed tomography (CT) is the standard of care for evaluation of patients with pulmonary vessel disease including both pulmonary embolism and pulmonary hypertension. In this chapter, we discuss CT protocols, diagnostic criteria, common pitfalls, and future developments in this field.

Pulmonary embolism is one of the most common indications for CT. CT angiography has become the method of choice for diagnosing pulmonary embolism. Clinical suspicion of pulmonary embolism can be confirmed or ruled out by CT angiography of the pulmonary arteries. Pulmonary embolism causes partial or complete intraluminal filling defects easily visualized by pulmonary CT angiography. Before the introduction

of multi-detector CT, radiological studies were of limited diagnostic value due to motion artifacts, and even today in noncompliant or unconscious patients, the quality of pulmonary CT angiography might be poor. Therefore, besides assessing pulmonary embolism, the radiologist should always address if the image quality was sufficient for diagnosing pulmonary embolism also on a subsegmental level.

Pulmonary hypertension can be caused by different etiologies. It may be idiopathic or may arise in association with various pathologies: chronic pulmonary thromboembolism, parenchymal lung disease, vasculitis, virus infection, or congenital or acquired heart disease. CT features of pulmonary hypertension are central pulmonary artery dilatation, right ventricular hypertrophy, right ventricular and atrial enlargement, dilated bronchial arteries, and a mosaic pattern of attenuation due to variable lung perfusion. Pulmonary CT is able to identify underlying disorders and to differentiate among the different etiologies of secondary pulmonary hypertension.

16.2 Pulmonary Embolism

16.2.1 Background

Pulmonary embolism is a blockage of a central or peripheral pulmonary artery. Most commonly, it is caused by a thrombus from the deep veins of the pelvis or leg. Pulmonary embolism is the third most common acute cardiovascular disease after myocardial infarction and stroke [1]. The incidence of pulmonary embolism in the Western countries is estimated to be approximately 1 case per 1000 persons per year [2]. Diagnosis of pulmonary embolism is challenging since pathognomic symptoms are not present in many cases [3]. Pulmonary embolism can present with subtle findings in otherwise healthy patients with cardiac reserve [3]. With increasing age, pulmonary embolism tends to masquerade as other illnesses such as acute coronary syndrome or exacerbation of chronic obstructive pulmonary disease (COPD) [3]. Accurate diagnosis of pulmonary embolism is particularly difficult when patients present with additional illnesses, such as pneumonia or congestive heart failure [3].

Wells et al. have developed a designated pulmonary embolism likelihood score including [4] the following:

- Clinical signs and symptoms of deep venous thrombosis (3 points)
- Alternative diagnosis less likely than pulmonary embolism (3 points)
- Heart rate higher than 100 beats/min (1.5 points)
- Immobilization or surgery in the previous 4 weeks (1.5 points)
- Previous deep venous thrombosis or pulmonary embolism (1.5 points)
- Hemoptysis (1 point)
- Cancer (1 point)

A Wells score of 4 points or less is unlikely to be associated with pulmonary embolism. They found pulmonary embolism in only about 5% in this low-risk group [4].

Clinical and laboratory tests, such as D-dimer assays, arterial blood gas analysis, and electrocardiography, are often indeterminate; hence, imaging studies play an important role in the diagnostic algorithm [5].

Ventilation-perfusion scintigraphy was recommended as a first-line procedure in patients with suspected pulmonary embolism [6], but examinations last relatively long and in most institutions availability is limited. Lower limb ultrasonography has high sensitivity and high specificity for diagnosing symptomatic deep vein thrombosis, but can only be used as indirect sign of pulmonary embolism [7]. Conventional pulmonary angiography is the diagnostic standard of reference for pulmonary embolism, but due to its invasiveness and high costs, it has not gained widespread acceptance. Furthermore, conventional angiography cannot provide diagnostic information that is suggestive of an alternative diagnosis [8].

Since the introduction of multi-detector CT with high spatial and temporal resolution, CT angiography has become the method of choice for imaging the pulmonary vasculature in routine clinical practice when pulmonary embolism is suspected. Sensitivity and specificity vary between 83% and 100%, and 89% and 97%, respectively [9–11]. The good diagnostic accuracy of multi-detector CT is linked to the improvement in image quality by substantial advances in CT technology over the past decades [12–14]. The improvements in spatial and temporal resolution, as well as the overall quality of arterial opacification, have allowed the routine analysis of pulmonary arteries down to the subsegmental level [15]. Therefore, multi-detector CT angiography has replaced conventional pulmonary angiography as the reference standard for the diagnosis of acute pulmonary embolism [8], since thrombi can be directly visualized and alternative diagnoses can be established accurately.

16.2.2 CT Examination Techniques

In general, CT data are acquired in a single breath-hold during inspiration in the caudocranial direction from the costophrenic angles to the lung apex. An intravenous access by an 18–20 gauge catheter into a right antecubital vein is preferred. An automated injector should be used to administer approximately 100 mL (depending on body mass index) of contrast material at a rate of 4–5 mL/s followed by a saline chaser bolus of 40 mL. A test bolus or automatic bolus tracking may be used, with a trigger attenuation threshold of 100 HU within the pulmonary trunk and a 5 s delay before the start of the acquisition. The chest field of view is the widest rib-to-rib distance acquired during breath-hold after inspiration. In our institution, a 64 slice scanner or higher is used for pulmonary CT angiography—higher slice scanners allow for faster image acquisition and reduce breathing artifacts. In patients with a body mass index of <30, tube voltage is set at 100 kV and in patients with a body mass index of >30 at 120 kV. Transverse images are reconstructed with a slice thickness of 1 and 0.8 mm increment using a medium smooth soft tissue kernel for optimal visualization of pulmonary vasculature. Additionally, maximum intensity projections are reformatted in a coronal plane to provide longitudinal views of the vessels. Multiplanar reformatted images can help differentiate between true pulmonary embolism and a variety of patient-related, technical, anatomic, and pathologic factors that can mimic pulmonary embolism.

CT venography of the iliac veins and lower extremities is performed with the same contrast material bolus that is used for chest CT. Images of the iliac, femoral, and popliteal veins are obtained 4 minutes after the onset of enhancement from the initial contrast material injection. Multisection CT venography is simple and accurate, and when combined with lung imaging, it allows fast and comprehensive evaluation for thromboembolic disease [16]. The Fleischner Society for Thoracic Imaging and Diagnosis recommends the use of CT venography when emphasis must be placed on a complete vascular examination that can be accomplished expeditiously [8]. When there are concerns about radiation exposure, they recommend substituting lower extremity ultrasound. When evaluation of the lower extremity veins is not clinically important, CT venography can be omitted.

16.2.3 Diagnostic Criteria

Pulmonary trunk, main, lobar, segmental, and subsegmental arteries are examined for signs of pulmonary embolism. Pulmonary embolism causes intraluminal filling defects that should have a sharp interface with the intravascular contrast material [17]. We shall differentiate between central and peripheral pulmonary embolism. Central pulmonary embolism involves the pulmonary trunk or main left and main right pulmonary arteries (Figure 16.1). This entity is more likely to lead to acute cardiac arrest. Pulmonary CT angiography is reported as either normal, containing acute and/or chronic pulmonary embolism, or indeterminate. The reason for indeterminacy depends on the quality of the study [17].

16.2.3.1 Acute Pulmonary Embolism

The diagnostic criteria for acute pulmonary embolism include direct and indirect signs of pulmonary embolism [17]:

- Direct signs include complete arterial occlusion leading to a filling defect of the affected pulmonary artery and forming an acute angle with the arterial wall (Figures 16.2 and 16.3). The pulmonary artery may be enlarged compared with adjacent patent vessels.

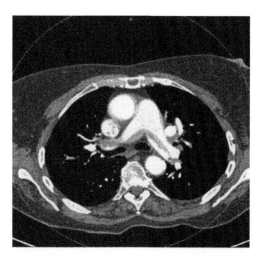

FIGURE 16.1
Central pulmonary embolism with a saddle thrombus in left and right main pulmonary arteries.

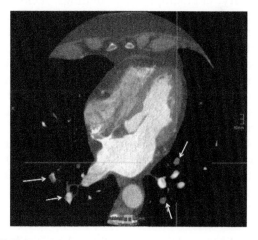

FIGURE 16.2
Multiple segmental and subsegmental emboli in the left and right lower lobes (arrows).

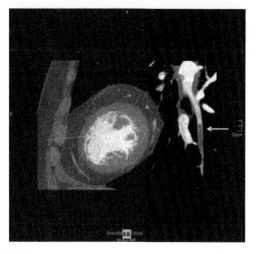

FIGURE 16.3
Longitudinal reconstruction of the left lower lobe artery showing an embolus with acute angles and consecutive tapering of the pulmonary artery toward the periphery.

- Another direct sign is a partial occlusion of a pulmonary artery. A partial filling defect surrounded by contrast material is named as "railway track sign" on images acquired longitudinally to the long axis of the vessels and as "polo mint sign" on axial views of a pulmonary artery (Figures 16.4 and 16.5).

- Indirect signs include peripheral wedge-shaped areas of hyperattenuation that may represent infarcts (Figure 16.6).

- Other indirect findings that are not specific for acute pulmonary embolism are linear bands or mosaic patterns with areas of hypoperfusion and/or hypoventilation.

Additional diagnostic analysis should address right ventricular failure that can be quantified by CT pulmonary angiography. CT findings include right ventricular dilatation (right ventricle > left ventricle) and/or deviation of the interventricular septum toward the left ventricle (Figure 16.7). A prognostic role of right ventricular enlargement in acute pulmonary embolism was reported for a ratio between right and left ventricular diameter. A ratio of 0.9 or higher was predictive for adverse events [18]. However, right ventricular function is better monitored by echocardiography.

Another predictive analysis for patients with acute pulmonary embolism is a CT obstruction index >60% [19]. To define a CT obstruction index, the arterial tree of each lung is regarded as having 10 segmental arteries. The presence of embolus in a segmental artery is scored 1 point and emboli in the most proximal arterial level are scored a value equal to the number of segmental arteries arising distally. A weighting factor is assigned to each value, depending on the degree of vascular obstruction. This factor is equal to 0, when no thrombus is observed; 1, when partially occlusive thrombus is observed; or 2, with total occlusion. Thus, the maximal CT obstruction index is 40 per patient and a percentage can be calculated [20].

16.2.3.2 Chronic Pulmonary Embolism

Chronic pulmonary embolism is mostly diagnosed on follow-up CT. The diagnostic criteria for chronic pulmonary embolism include a variety of patterns [17]:

- Mostly thrombi are adjacent to the wall with only partial filling defects of the pulmonary arteries (Figure 16.8).

- Complete occlusion of a vessel that is smaller than adjacent patent vessels.

- Peripheral, crescent-shaped intraluminal defect forming obtuse angles with the vessel wall (Figure 16.9).

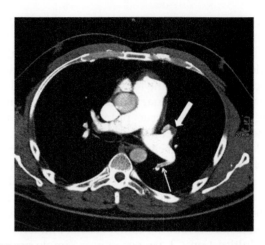

FIGURE 16.4
Peripheral pulmonary embolism with complete obliteration of the segment artery of the lingula (thick arrow) and subtotal occlusion of the posterobasal lower lobe artery (thin arrow) showing the "railway track sign."

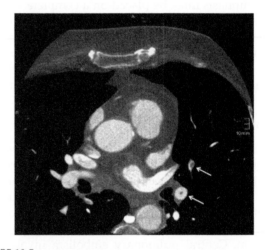

FIGURE 16.5
Peripheral pulmonary embolism showing the "polo mint sign."

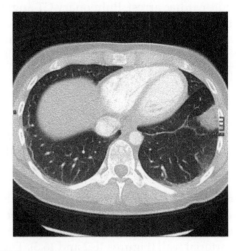

FIGURE 16.6
Pulmonary infarction secondary to pulmonary embolism of the laterobasal lobe of the left lung and bands in the left lower lobe.

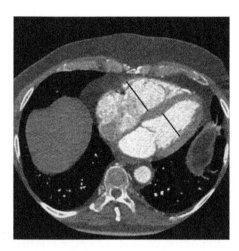

FIGURE 16.7
Moderately dilated right ventricle (right ventricle/left ventricle >1) in a patient with pulmonary embolism.

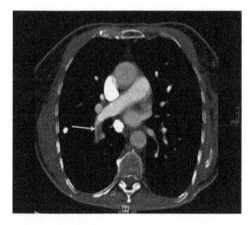

FIGURE 16.8
Chronic pulmonary embolism of the right lower lobe artery with wall adherent thrombus and subtotal occlusion of the pulmonary artery.

- Contrast enhancement in thickened, partially occluded arteries due to recanalization.
- Webs or flaps within pulmonary arteries.
- Secondary signs include extensive bronchial or other systemic collateral vessels, accompanying mosaic perfusion pattern, or calcification within eccentric vessel thickening.
- Fibrotic scars, bands, or atelectasis are more commonly found in chronic pulmonary embolism than in acute settings (Figure 16.10).

16.2.3.3 Differential Diagnosis

Pulmonary CT angiography is also able to identify thoracic diseases with symptoms similar to those of pulmonary embolism [17].

- Myocardial infarct: An occlusion of a coronary artery causing acute myocardial ischemia.
- Pericard: Pericardial thickening and pericardial effusion indicate pericarditis.
- Aorta: A "doubled" aorta can be seen in aortic dissection where a tear of the inner aortic wall creates a second aortic lumen. Penetrating aortic ulcera (contrast infiltrating the arteriosclerotic aortic wall) or intramural hematoma of the aorta (blood in the aortic wall) can often be identified.
- Lung and pleura: Other common differential diagnoses of pulmonary embolism include parenchymal lung disease, such as pneumonia or lung cancer, and pleural disease, such as pneumothorax and pleuritis.

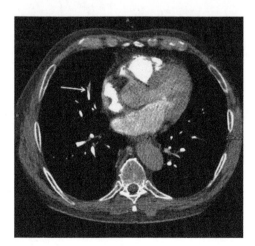

FIGURE 16.9
Subtle CT pulmonary angiography finding in a patient with chronic pulmonary embolism of the segmental artery of the medial middle lobe, note the obtuse angle with the vessel wall.

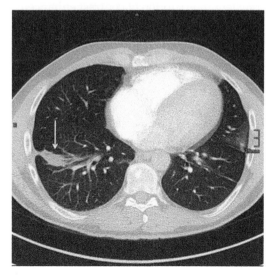

FIGURE 16.10
Scarring and hypoventilated areas are commonly found in patients with chronic pulmonary embolism.

- Skeletal: Bony alterations of the chest such as rib fractures, vertebra fracture, and metastatic bony lesions can also mimic pulmonary embolism symptoms.

- Esophagus: Less commonly esophagitis and esophageal rupture can be identified.

- Vascular tumor: Rare differentials are tumor emboli or primary pulmonary artery sarcoma, displayed as enhancing intraluminal masses.

16.2.3.4 Artifacts

We differentiate patient-related artifacts, such as motion artifacts, and technical-related artifacts [17]:

- Respiratory motion artifacts are the most common cause of indeterminate CT pulmonary angiography and can cause misdiagnosis of pulmonary embolism.

- Another patient-related artifact is image noise occurring especially in a large number of patients and making the evaluation of segmental and subsegmental vessels difficult.

- Technical artifacts leading to indeterminate pulmonary CT angiography include improper scanning technique. CT scans might be started early or late with insufficient opacification of pulmonary arteries. Also, atypical blood circulation time, for example, in critical care patients may cause such indeterminate exams.

- Bilateral lower lobe flow-related artifacts due to a too low amount of contrast agent leads to poor mixture of blood and contrast material causing transient interruption of contrast enhancement.

- Beam hardening streak artifacts from dense contrast material within the superior vena cava are commonly seen and can superimpose the right pulmonary and upper lobe arteries. Reducing the amount of injected contrast agent and adjusting contrast injection time to scan time can reduce such artifacts.

- Finally, the appropriate window width and level settings are important for identifying small emboli, webs, or flaps. Very bright vessel contrast can obscure small pulmonary emboli and window settings should be adjusted.

16.2.4 Recent Developments

Recent technical advances in CT angiography include high-pitch dual-source protocols and dual-energy protocols. Dual-source scanners are based on simultaneous data acquisition using two tubes and detectors of a dual-source CT system [21]. Using high-pitch dual-source CT, fast, nonoverlapping, but continuous volume coverage can be achieved by using a pitch factor of up to 3.4, allowing CT acquisitions of the entire thorax within less than 1 second [22]. Dual-energy CT uses two different tube energies (kV) and allows analyses of the chemical composition of tissues by means of dual-energy data acquisition according to the material decomposition theory [23]. A dual-energy CT dataset can be used to calculate iodine maps of the lungs, which represent blood volume in the lungs (Figure 16.11). A series of studies has already shown the potential of pulmonary blood volume maps obtained by dual-energy CT for showing perfusion impairment due to pulmonary embolism (Figure 16.12) [24–26]. High-pitch dual-source CT protocols allow a significant dose reduction compared to conventional multi-detector CT. The effective radiation doses of 16–64 slice CT units are estimated to be 3–5 mSv [27]. Dual-energy CT was reported to have a radiation dose similar to single-source CT (~2–3 mSv), whereas the radiation exposure of high-pitch dual-source CT is significantly lower with 1–2 mSv while maintaining diagnostic image quality [14].

Although advances in the multi-detector CT technique make it possible to evaluate peripheral subsegmental pulmonary arteries, physicians might oversee small emboli due to the high amount of images (>300 axial slices). Several studies have already reported that small peripheral embolisms may still be missed [28,29]. Therefore, several providers introduced computer-aided diagnosis (CAD) systems to assist the clinicians in the detection of pulmonary embolism. Studies comparing CAD systems with human readers reported that

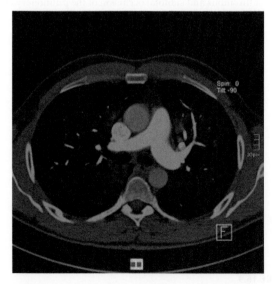

FIGURE 16.11
Regular pulmonary blood volume map acquired by dual-energy CT showing homogeneous "perfusion" of the right and left lungs.

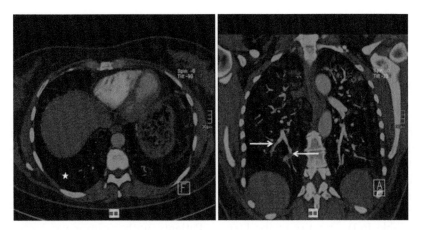

FIGURE 16.12
Peripheral pulmonary embolism of the right lower lobe (posterobasal and laterobasal segments, arrows) showing a "perfusion" defect on dual-energy CT pulmonary blood volume maps on axial and coronal projections (asterisk).

the sensitivity of CAD systems was superior for peripheral pulmonary embolism, while sensitivity of human readers was superior for proximal pulmonary embolism [30]. When CAD was utilized as a second reader, the diagnostic performance was improved [31] and the interobserver agreement was also improved, especially for inexperienced radiologists [32].

16.3 Pulmonary Hypertension

16.3.1 Background

Pulmonary hypertension is defined as a group of diseases characterized by a progressive increase in pulmonary vascular resistance leading to right ventricular failure and premature death [33]. Recently, the diagnostic approach has been more clearly defined according to a clinical classification established in Dana Point, California. Consensus was reached on algorithms of various investigative tests and procedures that exclude other causes and ensure an accurate diagnosis of pulmonary arterial hypertension [34,35].

The diagnostic procedures include clinical history and physical examination, electrocardiography, chest x-ray, transthoracic Doppler echocardiography, pulmonary function tests, arterial blood gas analysis, ventilation and perfusion lung scan, high-resolution CT of the lungs, contrast-enhanced spiral CT of the lungs and pulmonary angiography, blood tests and immunology, abdominal ultrasound scan, exercise capacity assessment, and hemodynamic evaluation [35].

CT is helpful to establish the diagnosis, to identify secondary causes of pulmonary hypertension, and to rule out other causes with similar symptoms [36]. Furthermore, CT is able to detect causes of pulmonary

hypertension that may be surgically treatable or where adverse reactions to vasodilator therapies during the course of treatment may occur [36].

16.3.2 Clinical Considerations

The estimated incidence of primary pulmonary hypertension is one to two cases per one million people in the general population. Pulmonary hypertension is more common in women than in men (ratio: 1.7:1) [37]. Pulmonary hypertension is most prevalent in persons 20–40 years of age [38]. In people over 50 years of age, cor pulmonale, the consequence of untreated pulmonary arterial hypertension, is the third most common cardiac disorder after coronary heart disease and hypertensive heart disease [37].

Pulmonary hypertension is defined as an elevation of pressure in the pulmonary circulation, with a mean pulmonary arterial pressure higher than 25 mm Hg or higher than 30 mm Hg with exercise [39]. Pulmonary arterial hypertension often presents with nonspecific symptoms and in the early stage it may be asymptomatic. The most common symptoms—dyspnea, chest pain, and syncope—reflect right-sided heart failure [40]. The clinical course of pulmonary hypertension is divided into three phases: asymptomatic compensated, symptomatic decompensating, and advanced decompensated [36].

The normal adult pulmonary vascular bed is a low-pressure, low-resistance system that is able to accommodate increases in blood flow with minimal elevation in pulmonary arterial pressure [36]. In patients with pulmonary hypertension, pulmonary arterial pressure and vascular resistance are chronically elevated, leading to right ventricular hypertrophy, followed by dilatation and right atrial enlargement [36,41]. Initially, these changes are compensatory mechanisms that allow the right ventricle to produce a larger stroke volume and maintain cardiac output [36]. In patients with severe pulmonary hypertension, the hypertrophied right ventricle has an impaired abnormal septal motion and consequently abnormal left ventricular function [36,37]. Eventually, the demand of the right ventricle for oxygen exceeds the available supply, causing chamber dilation that leads to tricuspid regurgitation, a result of tricuspid annular dilatation and incomplete valve closure [36,37]. These processes eventually result in decreased cardiac output and right heart failure [36,37].

The clinical classification system for pulmonary hypertension was updated in 2008 at the 4th World Symposium on Pulmonary Hypertension in Dana Point, California [42] (Table 16.1). The aim of the Dana Point classification system is to group together different manifestations of the disease that share similar pathophysiologic traits. A diagnosis of pulmonary arterial hypertension is made only in the absence of other causes of precapillary pulmonary hypertension such as that resulting from lung disease (group 3), chronic thromboembolic pulmonary hypertension (group 4), and disease resulting from multifactorial mechanisms (group 5). Pulmonary hypertension resulting from heart disease (group 2) implies an increase in pulmonary arterial pressure due to backward transmission of pressure elevation (postcapillary pulmonary hypertension) and is defined as a mean pulmonary arterial pressure of 20 mm Hg or more and a pulmonary wedge pressure greater than 15 mm Hg [42].

16.3.3 General Radiological Considerations

Patients with pulmonary hypertension usually complain of symptoms suspicious for cardiac or pulmonary disease. First diagnostic imaging steps for detecting pulmonary hypertension include plain films of the chest and echocardiography. If pulmonary hypertension is presumed, a systematic approach based on the Dana Point classification should be used to determine its origin. Treatment is based on the etiology of pulmonary hypertension; hence, accurate classification is mandatory with CT imaging playing a central role. CT is used to rule out the more common clinical groups of pulmonary hypertension such as left-sided heart disease, lung parenchyma disease, and chronic thromboembolic pulmonary hypertension. While typical CT findings of the central pulmonary arteries and right heart are present in advanced stages of pulmonary hypertension, morphologic and functional assessment of the right ventricle of the heart is more accurately assessed at cardiac magnetic resonance imaging (MRI). High-resolution CT of the lungs allows for assessing fibrotic lung parenchyma changes due to various causes such as COPD or interstitial lung disease. If untreated, pulmonary hypertension has a high mortality rate, typically from decompensated right-sided heart failure with an estimated median survival of approximately 2.8 years [40].

Catheterization of the right side of the heart is the gold standard for diagnosing pulmonary hypertension because it is the only test whose findings confirm the presence of pulmonary hypertension by enabling direct measurement of pulmonary pressures, resistance, and cardiac output [36]. However, it is invasive, it requires exposure to ionizing radiation, and it does not provide morphologic information [36].

16.3.4 CT Examination Technique

The classical CT findings in pulmonary hypertension may be divided into three categories: vascular, cardiac, and parenchymal. In patients with suspected pulmonary hypertension, visualization of the heart chambers and the pulmonary arteries is required. Therefore, a slightly modified CT protocol as used for pulmonary embolism and

TABLE 16.1

Clinical Classification of Pulmonary Hypertension

1.		Pulmonary arterial hypertension
	1.1.	Idiopathic pulmonary arterial hypertension
	1.2.	Heritable
	1.3.	Drug- and toxin-induced
	1.4.	Associated with connective tissue disorders, HIV infection, portal hypertension, congenital heart disease, schistosomiasis, chronic hemolytic anemia
	1.5.	Persistent pulmonary hypertension of the newborn
	1.6.	Pulmonary veno-occlusive disease, pulmonary capillary hemangiomatosis
2.		Pulmonary hypertension owing to left heart diseases (systolic or diastolic dysfunction, valvular disease)
3.		Pulmonary hypertension owing to lung disease and/or hypoxia
	3.1.	Chronic obstructive pulmonary disease
	3.2.	Interstitial lung disease
	3.3.	Other pulmonary diseases with mixed restrictive and obstructive pattern
	3.4.	Sleep-disordered breathing
	3.5.	Alveolar hypoventilation disorders
	3.6.	Chronic exposure to high altitude
	3.7.	Developmental abnormalities
4.		Chronic thromboembolic pulmonary hypertension
5.		Pulmonary hypertension with unclear multifactorial mechanisms
	5.1.	Hemtologic disorders
	5.2.	Systemic disorders: sarcoidosis, Langerhans cell histiocytosis, lymphangioleiomyomatosis, vasculitis
	5.3.	Metabolic disorders
	5.4.	Others: tumoral obstruction, fibrosing mediastinitis, chronic renal failure, dialysis

Source: Adapted from Castañer E. et al., *Radiographics.*, 29, 31–50, 2009.

described before can be used. The intravenous administration of the contrast material bolus is timed so that both the pulmonary circulation and the systemic circulation are opacified. The bronchial circulation, which usually originates from the descending aorta, is markedly increased in patients with chronic pulmonary thromboembolism, and the enhancement of bronchial vessels may aid in the differential diagnosis [43]. Bolus timing also allows assessment of all cardiac chambers. The desired opacification of the pulmonary and systemic circulation can be achieved by using a longer delay from contrast material injection to image acquisition; we use a higher trigger threshold, 200 HU, with a circular region of interest centered on the main pulmonary artery [43]. Obviously, a slightly higher amount of contrast agent is needed for such a protocol (>100 mL depending on body mass index) to allow best assessment of all cardiac chambers and the pulmonary vascular tree. When cardiac disease is suspected, cardiac CT with electrocardiographic triggering should be performed. Images are assessed by using three different gray scale settings for interpretation: a lung window (window width, 1500 HU; window level, −600 HU), a mediastinal window (window width, 350 HU; window level, 40 HU), and a pulmonary thromboembolism–specific window (window width, 700 HU; window level, 100 HU) [43]. In cases of unclear findings of lung parenchyma fibrosis, CT scan should be repeated in prone position.

16.3.5 Diagnostic Criteria

16.3.5.1 Pulmonary Arteries

The characteristic morphologic CT features of chronic pulmonary arterial hypertension are dilatation of the pulmonary artery trunk to 29 mm or more (Figure 16.13). The diameter of the pulmonary trunk often exceeds that of the ascending aorta and may be associated with dilatation of the right and left main pulmonary arteries (Figures 16.14 and 16.15) [39,44]. On transverse images, the main pulmonary artery is evaluated at the level of its bifurcation, orthogonal to its long axis. Furthermore, a high positive predictive value (>95%) for the presence of pulmonary hypertension was described when the pulmonary artery diameter exceeds that of the ascending aorta, or the segmental artery-to-bronchus ratio is greater than 1:1 in three of four pulmonary lobes [45,46]. However, it is important to emphasize that a diameter of less than 29 mm does not necessarily exclude pulmonary hypertension [47]. While central pulmonary arteries show dilatation, peripheral pulmonary vessels show abrupt narrowing and tapering [39,44].

Newer studies using electrocardiographically gated multi-detector CT show that functional parameters such as right pulmonary artery distensibility,

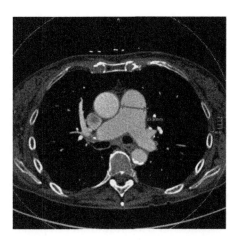

FIGURE 16.13
Dilated pulmonary trunk showing a diameter of 3.4 cm on axial CT angiography.

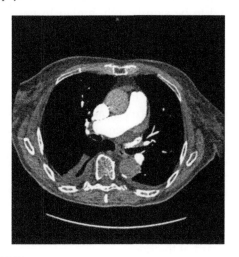

FIGURE 16.14
Minimal dilatation of the pulmonary trunk with 3 cm and a more obvious dilatation of the right pulmonary artery with 3.2 cm. Minimal pleural effusion is present on both sides.

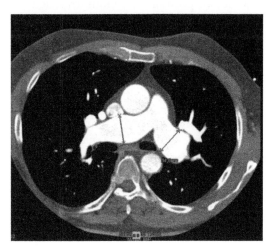

FIGURE 16.15
Distinct dilatation of the right and left pulmonary arteries of approximately 3.5 cm.

systolic-diastolic right ventricular outflow tract dimensions, and diastolic wall thickness can be measured with good interobserver agreement and used as reliable criteria for a diagnosis of pulmonary hypertension [48]. Decrease in right pulmonary artery distensibility—which is defined as the change in cross-sectional area between diastole and systole and is calculated by dividing the difference between the maximum cross-sectional area and the minimum cross-sectional area by the maximum cross-sectional area and multiplying the result by 100—is an accurate noninvasive marker of pulmonary hypertension, with the strongest correlation with mean pulmonary arterial pressure. The cutoff for distinguishing between patients with pulmonary hypertension and those without was a pulmonary artery distensibility of 16.5%. Furthermore, systolic right ventricular outflow tract diameter and cross-sectional area measurements were found to be significantly higher in patients with pulmonary hypertension [48].

16.3.5.2 Cardiac Assessment

In pulmonary arterial hypertension, the heart shows right ventricular hypertrophy and right ventricular and atrial enlargement with inversion of the interventricular septum. In severe pulmonary hypertension, dilatation of the tricuspid valve annulus may occur [39,44].

In suspected pulmonary arterial hypertension, a number of cardiac features should be looked for as follows:

- Cardiac chamber size
- Myocardial thickness
- Position and shape of the interventricular septum
- The presence of congenital cardiac abnormalities
- Anomalous pulmonary venous drainage
- Contrast reflux into the inferior vena cava and hepatic veins indicating the presence and severity of tricuspid regurgitation

Right ventricular dilatation is easy to assess by CT, even without electrocardiographic gating. Comparing right ventricular and left ventricular diameters at mid-ventricular level on axial images, a diameter ratio greater than 1:1 indicates right ventricular dilatation (Figures 16.16 and 16.17) [49]. Findings of adaptation and failure of the right side of the heart include right ventricular hypertrophy, which is defined as wall thickness of more than 4 mm, straightening or leftward bowing of the interventricular septum (Figures 16.18 and 16.19) [50]. Dilatation of the inferior vena cava and hepatic veins occurs in advanced disease when tricuspid regurgitation is present (Figure 16.20) [51]. Pericardial effusion is another common

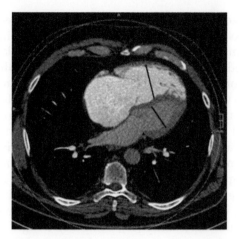

FIGURE 16.16
Dilated right ventricle and right atrium in a patient with pulmonary arterial hypertension. (right ventricle 4.9 cm, left ventricle 3.4 cm).

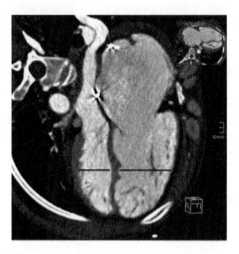

FIGURE 16.17
Massive pulmonary arterial hypertension: reformatted three-chamber view of the heart showing massive dilatation of the right ventricle and the right atrium.

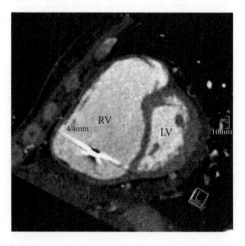

FIGURE 16.18
Enlarged right ventricle in a patient with pulmonary hypertension with moderate ventricle wall thickening of 4.4 mm. Note streaks artifacts due to an implanted heart pacemaker.

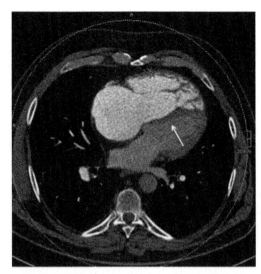

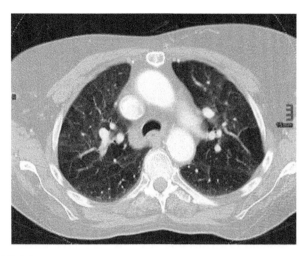

FIGURE 16.21
Axial CT images in lung window showing a mosaic pattern on the left and right sides caused by inhomogeneous lung perfusion.

FIGURE 16.19
Enlarged right atrium and right ventricle with ventricular wall thickening (6 mm) and bulging of the septal wall toward the left ventricle in advanced pulmonary hypertension.

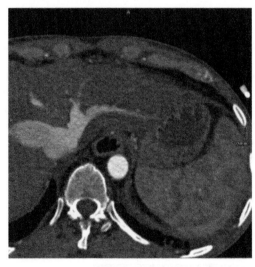

FIGURE 16.20
Advanced pulmonary hypertension with tricuspidal insufficiency showing contrast enhancement in the inferior vena cava and liver veins although an arterial phase scan was acquired.

finding in pulmonary hypertension [52]. Recently, also, low-dose CT techniques for functional analysis of the right heart were introduced especially by using advanced 64 slice or more CT scanners. Additionally, congenital abnormalities such as sinus venosus, atrial septal defect, patent ductus arteriosus, and anomalous pulmonary venous drainage can be assessed.

16.3.5.3 Lung Parenchyma

Alterations of lung parenchyma depend on the etiology of pulmonary hypertension. Centrilobular ground-glass nodules are a feature of pulmonary hypertension

and are especially common in patients with idiopathic pulmonary arterial hypertension caused by ingestion of red blood cells by pulmonary macrophages, a result of repeated episodes of pulmonary hemorrhage representing cholesterol granulomas [53,54]. Centrilobular ground-glass nodules are also seen in patients with pulmonary capillary hemangiomatosis; however, in these patients, the pathologic substrate is thought to result from profuse proliferation of capillaries [55]. Neovascularity, tiny serpiginous intrapulmonary vessels that often emerge from centrilobular arterioles but do not conform to usual pulmonary arterial anatomy, has also been seen as a manifestation of severe pulmonary hypertension [56]. A mosaic pattern of attenuation caused by regional variations in lung perfusion is another frequent finding in patients with pulmonary arterial hypertension (Figure 16.21).

16.3.5.4 Typical CT Findings in Pulmonary Hypertension Listed According to the Dana Classification

Idiopathic pulmonary arterial hypertension: Histopathologically, this subtype is known as plexogenic arteriopathy manifesting as proliferation of the intima with focal disruption in small and medium-sized arteries [39]. Generally, on CT, no specific findings other than central pulmonary artery dilatation can be detected. In some patients, small tortuous peripheral vessels representing plexogenic arteriopathy and an abrupt decrease in the caliber of segmental and subsegmental arteries might be detectable [44]. The mosaic pattern seen in idiopathic pulmonary arterial hypertension is characterized by small, scattered, well-defined areas of low attenuation corresponding to the anatomic unit of a secondary pulmonary lobule [44]. One of the most important diagnostic criteria for the diagnosis of idiopathic pulmonary arterial hypertension is to rule out chronic pulmonary embolism.

Congenital heart disease: Symptomatic cardiac shunts are typically diagnosed before or immediately after birth, but some left-to-right shunts such as sinus venosus defects, patent ductus arteriosus, and anomalous pulmonary venous are identified by CT [36]. Most common findings are interatrial septal defects (Figures 16.22 through 16.24).

Rare causes of pulmonary arterial hypertension include heritable, drug- and toxin-induced, association with connective tissue disorders (e.g., CREST syndrome, rheumatoid arthritis, and scleroderma), HIV infection,

portal hypertension with hepatopulmonary syndrome or portopulmonary hypertension, schistosomiasis, chronic hemolytic anemia, and persistent pulmonary hypertension of the newborn [42]. Clinical and/or laboratory findings mostly lead to the correct diagnosis in these etiologies.

Pulmonary veno-occlusive disease, pulmonary capillary hemangiomatosis: Both diseases are rare causes of pulmonary arterial hypertension characterized by the occlusion of postcapillary veins in children or young adults. At CT, the presence of the combination of features of pulmonary arterial hypertension and interstitial and alveolar edema leads to the diagnosis. Small central pulmonary veins, interlobular septal thickening, and patchy centrilobular ground-glass opacities representing interstitial and alveolar edema are characteristic for pulmonary veno-occlusive disease [44]. Detection of venous causes of pulmonary hypertension is critical since vasodilator agents are contraindicated in these patients [57].

Pulmonary hypertension owing to left heart disease: Systolic or diastolic dysfunction of the left heart and valvular disease are common causes of pulmonary hypertension (Figure 16.24). Echocardiography and MRI are generally used for assessment, but incidental detection by CT is possible [58].

Pulmonary hypertension owing to lung disease: In COPD, vascular remodeling leads to reduced distensibility of small pulmonary vessels and this may lead to increased pulmonary vascular resistance and elevated pulmonary vascular pressure (Figures 16.25 and 16.26) [59]. CT detects emphysema and fibrotic changes (Figures 16.27 and 16.28). Furthermore, total cross-sectional area of small pulmonary vessels (<5 mm^2) assessed on CT scans has shown to correlate with the degree of pulmonary hypertension estimated by right heart catheterization [60]. Interstitial lung diseases such as idiopathic

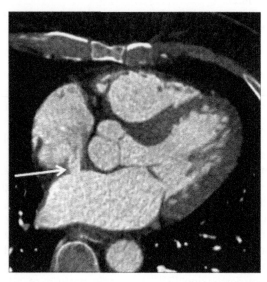

FIGURE 16.22
Atrial septum defect showing contrast enhancement in a patent foramen ovale.

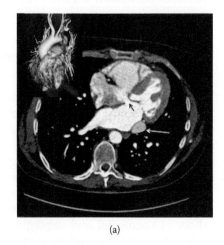

(a)

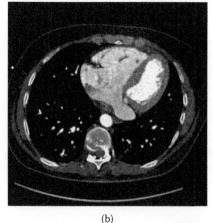

(b)

FIGURE 16.23
(a) Congenital heart disease showing a doubled superior vena cava (white arrow), whereas the left-sided superior vena cava (VCS) is connected to the coronary sinus. Additionally, an atrial septal defect was detected on CT (black arrow). (b) Both pathologies may be causative for the enlargement of the right ventricle.

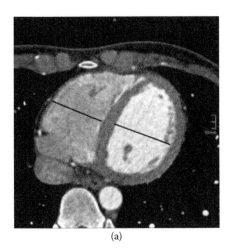
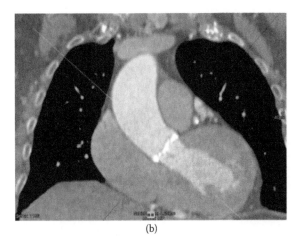

FIGURE 16.24
(a) Biventricular dilatation in a patient with (b) aortic valve stenosis and consecutive pulmonary arterial hypertension.

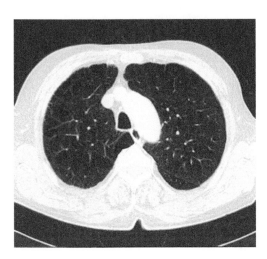

FIGURE 16.25
A patient with chronic obstructive pulmonary disease showing moderate emphysema.

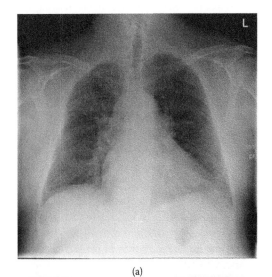

(a)

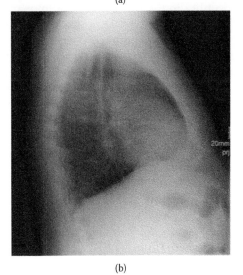

(b)

FIGURE 16.27
Posteroanterior (a) and lateral (b) chest x-ray showing biventricular dilatation of the heart, fibrotic lung changes, increased radiotransparency, and prominent central pulmonary vessels.

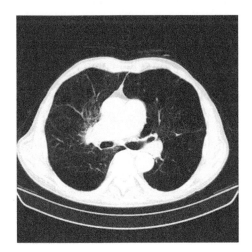

FIGURE 16.26
Panlobular emphysema with consecutive pulmonary hypertension.

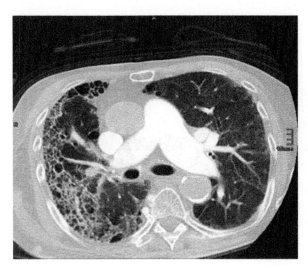

FIGURE 16.28
Corresponding axial CT image in lung window showing dilated central pulmonary arteries, retinacular fibrotic changes especially on the right side, and panlobular emphysema in a patient with COPD.

pulmonary fibrosis, nonspecific interstitial pneumonia, or chronic hypersensitivity pneumonitis lead to fibrosis in advanced stages and consequently to pulmonary hypertension. In early stages, no typical signs of pulmonary arterial hypertension can be detected, and only in advanced disease, dilatation of central pulmonary arteries and right heart involvement might be present (Figure 16.29). CT signs of fibrosis include reticulation often associated with traction bronchiectasis, ground-glass opacity, architectural distortion, and honeycombing. However, the pulmonary artery diameter does not always correlate with the presence or degree of pulmonary hypertension [61] and vascular measurements were shown to be of limited utility in the prediction of pulmonary hypertension [62]. The category of lung disease characterized by a mixed obstructive and restrictive pattern includes chronic bronchiectasis, cystic fibrosis, and a newly identified syndrome characterized by the combination of pulmonary fibrosis, mainly of the lower zones of the lung, and emphysema, mainly of the upper zones of the lung [42]. CT findings in sleep-disordered breathing, alveolar hypoventilation disorders, chronic exposure to high altitude and developmental abnormalities are unspecific.

Chronic thromboembolic pulmonary hypertension: Increased vascular resistance due to obstruction of the vascular bed caused by chronic pulmonary thromboembolism leads to pulmonary hypertension. It is mainly a consequence of incomplete resolution of pulmonary thromboembolism [43] and it occurs in up to 4% of patients after acute pulmonary embolism [63]. Patients with chronic thromboembolic pulmonary hypertension and central obstruction should consider pulmonary thromboendarterectomy, currently the only curative treatment [42]. CT is used for diagnosing chronic pulmonary thromboembolism,

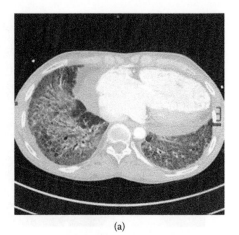

(a)

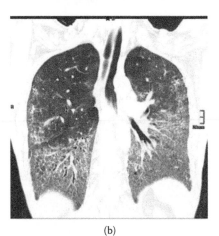

(b)

FIGURE 16.29
(a) Axial and coronal planes of lung window showing a patient with enlarged right ventricle and atrium. (b) Fibrotic changes and bronchiectasis of the lower lobes due to advanced scleroderma can be appreciated.

for determining treatment options, and postoperative follow-up [43]. Besides signs of pulmonary hypertension, CT shows findings as described for chronic pulmonary embolism including complete obstruction, partial obstruction, eccentric thrombus, calcified thrombus, bands, webs, and poststenotic dilatation, and systemic collateral supply with enlargement of bronchial and nonbronchial systemic arteries (Figure 16.30) [43]. Parenchymal signs include scars, a mosaic perfusion pattern, focal ground-glass opacities, and bronchial anomalies [43]. Dual-energy CT pulmonary angiography is a novel technique providing both functional and anatomical information with the potential to give further information of decreased lung perfusion (Figure 16.31) [64].

Pulmonary hypertension with unclear multifactorial mechanisms: CT findings in unclear mechanism are dependent on the origin. While in most etiologies only central pulmonary artery dilatation and right heart chamber enlargement can be found, additional typical findings of some underlying diseases might be found. Hematologic

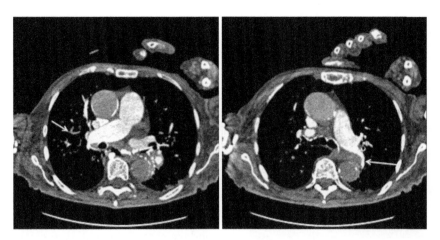

FIGURE 16.30
Patient with chronic thromboembolic pulmonary hypertension showing dilated central pulmonary arteries, multiple peripheral emboli, and tapering of the peripheral pulmonary arteries.

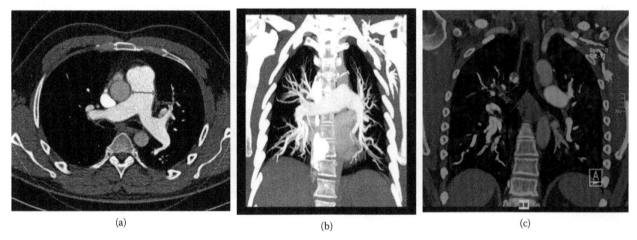

(a) (b) (c)

FIGURE 16.31
(a) Patient with chronic pulomary thromboembolic pulmonary hypertension showing a dilated pulmonary trunk, (b) serpinginous peripheral pulmonary arteries on maximal intensity projections, and (c) multiple small "perfusion" defects on dual-energy CT.

disorders include chronic myeloproliferative disorders such as polycythemia vera, essential thrombocythemia, chronic myeloid leukemia, and splenectomy [42]. Systemic disorders that are associated with an increased risk of developing pulmonary hypertension are sarcoidosis (bilateral hilar lymph node enlargement and/or interstitial lung disease, Figure 16.32) [65], pulmonary Langerhans cell histiocytosis (Figure 16.33) [66], neurofibromatosis type 1 (von Recklinghausen disease), vasculitis, and lymphangioleiomyomatosis (Figure 16.34) [67]. Metabolic disorders are rare causes of pulmonary hypertension and diagnosis is based on clinical and laboratory findings. Other rare causes of pulmonary hypertension include tumoral obstruction, fibrosing mediastinitis, and chronic renal failure. In tumor obstruction such as pulmonary artery sarcomas or metastasis, a tumor grows into the central pulmonary arteries, which is usually rapidly fatal (Figure 16.35) [42].

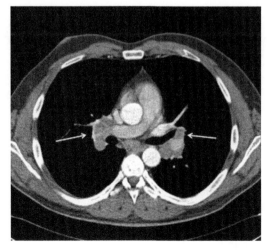

FIGURE 16.32
In patients with sarcoidosis, pulmonary interstitial disease or hilar lymphadenopathy may lead to pulmonary hypertension.

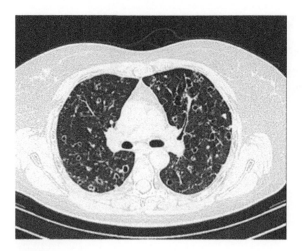

FIGURE 16.33
Typical pattern of pulmonary histiocytosis showing multiple relatively thick-walled cysts in a young, smoking female patient.

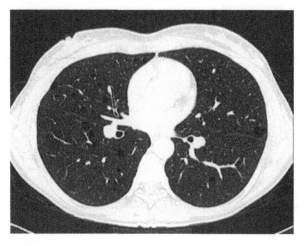

FIGURE 16.34
A 30-year-old woman with initial findings of lymphangioleiomyomatosis. Multiple cystic areas are shown in upper and lower lobes of both lungs.

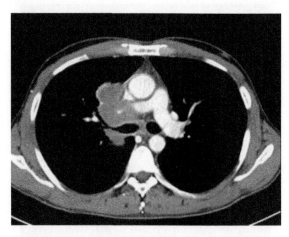

FIGURE 16.35
Central bronchial carcinoma infiltrating the mediastinum. Stenosis or occlusion of the pulmonary arteries may lead to pulmonary hypertension.

On CT, the tumor appears as an enhancing intraluminal soft-tissue mass, unlike apposition thrombi, which are nonenhancing [44]. Fibrosing mediastinitis is a rare condition after granulomatous infection resulting in a fibrotic reaction causing narrowing of the pulmonary arteries or veins [36].

16.4 Summary

CT is the method of choice for detecting pulmonary embolism. Knowledge of the typical primary and secondary signs is essential to establish the correct diagnosis in an acute setting. CT findings in pulmonary hypertension typically show pulmonary artery dilatation and right heart chamber enlargement. Often underlying causes such as chronic pulmonary thromboembolism or lung parenchyma fibrosis can be detected or ruled out by CT.

References

1. Giuntini C, Ricco GD, Marini C, Mellilo E, Palla A. Pulmonary embolism: Epidemiology. *Chest* 1995; 107: 3–9.
2. Ozsu S, Oztuna F, Bulbul Y, Topbas M, Ozlu T, Kosucu P, Ozsu A. The role of risk factors in delayed diagnosis of pulmonary embolism. *Am J Emerg Med* 2011; 29: 26–32.
3. Goldhaber SZ. Pulmonary embolism. *Lancet* 2004; 363: 1295–1305.
4. Wells PS, Anderson DR, Rodger M, Ginsberg JS, Kearon C, Gent M, Turpie AG, Bormanis J, Weitz J, Chamberlain M et al. Derivation of a simple clinical model to categorize patients probability of pulmonary embolism: Increasing the models utility with the SimpliRED D-dimer. *Thromb Haemost* 2000; 83: 416–420.
5. Pistolesi M, Miniati M. Imaging techniques in treatment algorithms of pulmonary embolism. *Eur Respir J Suppl* 2002; 35: 28–39.
6. Bajc M, Neilly JB, Miniati M, Schuemichen C, Meignan M, Jonson B. EANM guidelines for ventilation/perfusion scintigraphy: Part 2. Algorithms and clinical considerations for diagnosis of pulmonary emboli with V/P(SPECT) and MDCT. *Eur J Nucl Med Mol Imaging* 2009; 36: 1528–1538.
7. Rose SC, Zwiebel WJ, Nelson BD, Priest DL, Knighton RA, Brown JW, Lawrence PF, Stults BM, Reading JC, Miller FJ. Symptomatic lower extremity deep venous thrombosis: accuracy, limitations, and role of color duplex flow imaging in diagnosis. *Radiology* 1990; 175: 639–644.
8. Remy-Jardin M, Pistolesi M, Goodman LR, Gefter WB, Gottschalk A, Mayo JR, Sostman HD. Management of suspected acute pulmonary embolism in the era of CT angiography: A statement from the Fleischner Society. *Radiology* 2007; 245: 315–329.

9. Qanadli SD, Hajjam ME, Mesurolle B, Barré O, Bruckert F, Joseph T, Mignon F, Vieillard-Baron A, Dubourg O, Lacombe P. Pulmonary embolism detection: Prospective evaluation of dual-section helical CT versus selective pulmonary arteriography in 157 patients. *Radiology* 2000; 217: 447–455.

10. Winer-Muram HT, Rydberg J, Johnson MS, Tarver RD, Williams MD, Shah H, Namyslowski J, Conces D, Jennings SG, Ying J et al. Suspected acute pulmonary embolism: Evaluation with multi-detector row CT versus digital subtraction pulmonary arteriography. 2004; *Radiology* 233: 806–815.

11. Stein PD, Fowler SE, Goodman LR, Gottschalk A, Hales CA, Hull RD, Leeper KV Jr, Popovich J Jr, Quinn DA, Sos TA et al. Multidetector computed tomography for acute pulmonary embolism. *N Engl J Med* 2006; 354: 2317–2327.

12. Schoepf UJ, Goldhaber SZ, Costello P. Spiral computed tomography for acute pulmonary embolism. *Circulation* 2004; 109: 2160–2167.

13. Patel S, Kazerooni EA, Cascade PN. Pulmonary embolism: Optimization of small pulmonary artery visualization at multidetector row CT. *Radiology* 2003; 227: 455–460.

14. De Zordo T, von Lutterotti K, Dejaco C, Soegner PF, Frank R, Aigner F, Klauser AS, Pechlaner C, Schoepf UJ, Jaschke WR et al. Comparison of image quality and radiation dose of different pulmonary CTA protocols on a 128-slice CT: High-pitch dual source CT, dual energy CT and conventional spiral CT. *Eur Radiol* 2011; 22: 279–286.

15. Brunot S, Corneloup O, Latrabe V, Montaudon M, Laurent F. Reproducibility of multidetector spiral computed tomography in detection of subsegmental acute pulmonary embolism. *Eur Radiol* 2005; 15: 2057–2063.

16. Loud PA, Katz DS, Bruce DA, Klippenstein DL, Grossman ZD. Deep venous thrombosis with suspected pulmonary embolism: Detection with combined CT venography and pulmonary angiography. *Radiology* 2001; 219: 498–502.

17. Wittram C, Maher MM, Yoo AJ, Kalra MK, Shepard JA, McLoud TC. CT angiography of pulmonary embolism: Diagnostic criteria and causes of misdiagnosis. *Radiographics* 2004; 24: 1219–1238.

18. Quiroz R, Kucher N, Schoepf UJ, Kipfmueller F, Solomon SD, Costello P, Goldhaber SZ. Right ventricular enlargement on chest computed tomography: Prognostic role in acute pulmonary embolism. *Circulation* 2004; 109: 2401–2404.

19. Wu AS, Pezzullo JA, Cronan JJ, Hou DD, Mayo-Smith WW. CT pulmonary angiography: Quantification of pulmonary embolus as a predictor of patient outcome-initial experience. *Radiology* 2004; 230: 831–835.

20. Qanadli SD, El Hajjam M, Vieillard-Baron A, Joseph T, Mesurolle B, Oliva VL, Barré O, Bruckert F, Dubourg O, Lacombe P. New CT index to quantify arterial obstruction in pulmonary embolism: Comparison with angiographic index and echocardiography. *AJR Am J Roentgenol* 2001; 176: 1415–1420.

21. Petersilka M, Bruder H, Krauss B, Stierstorfer K, Flohr TG. Technical principles of dual source CT. *Eur J Radiol* 2008; 68: 362–368.

22. Sommer WH, Schenzle JC, Becker CR, Nikolaou K, Graser A, Michalski G, Neumaier K, Reiser MF, Johnson TR. Saving dose in triple-rule-out computed tomography examination using a high-pitch dual spiral technique. *Invest Radiol* 2010; 45: 64–71.

23. Johnson TRC, Krauss B, Sedlmair M, Grasruck M, Bruder H, Morhard D, Fink C, Weckbach S, Lenhard M, Schmidt B et al. Material differentiation by dual energy CT: Initial experience. *Eur Radiol* 2007; 17: 1510–1517.

24. Fink C, Johnson TR, Michaely HJ, Morhard D, Becker C, Reiser M, Nikolaou K. Dual-energy CT angiography of the lung in patients with suspected pulmonary embolism: Initial results. *Rofo* 2008; 180: 879–883.

25. Pontana F, Faivre JB, Remy-Jardin M, Flohr T, Schmidt B, Tacelli N, Pansini V, Remy J. Lung perfusion with dual-energy multidetector-row CT (MDCT): Feasibility for the evaluation of acute pulmonary embolism in 117 consecutive patients. *Acad Radiol* 2008; 15: 1494–1504.

26. Thieme SF, Becker CR, Hacker M, Nikolaou K, Reiser MF, Johnson TR. Dual energy CT for the assessment of lung perfusion-correlation to scintigraphy. *Eur J Radiol* 2008; 68: 369–374.

27. International Commission on Radiological Protection and Measurements. *Radiological protection and safety.* International Commission on Radiological Protection Measurements publication no. 60. Oxford, England: Pergamon; 1991.

28. Ghanima W, Nielssen BE, Holmen LO, Witwit A, Al-Ashtari A, Sandset PM. Multidetector computed tomography (MDCT) in the diagnosis of pulmonary embolism: Interobserver agreement among radiologists with varied levels of experience. *Acta Radiol* 2007; 48: 165–170.

29. Brunot S, Corneloup O, Latrabe V, Montaudon M, Laurent F. Reproducibility of multi-detector spiral computed tomography in detection of sub-segmental acute pulmonary embolism. *Eur Radiol* 2005; 15: 2057–2063.

30. Buhmann S, Herzog P, Liang J, Wolf M, Salganicoff M, Kirchhoff C, Reiser M, Becker CH. Clinical evaluation of a computer-aided diagnosis (CAD) prototype for the detection of pulmonary embolism. *Acad Radiol* 2007; 14: 651–658.

31. Das M, Muhlenbruch G, Helm A, Bakai A, Salganicoff M, Stanzel S, Liang J, Wolf M, Günther RW, Wildberger JE. Computer-aided detection of pulmonary embolism: influence on radiologists' detection performance with respect to vessel segments. *Eur Radiol* 2008; 18: 1350–1355.

32. Engelke C, Schmidt S, Bakai A, Auer F, Marten K. Computer-assisted detection of pulmonary embolism: Performance evaluation in consensus with experienced and inexperienced chest radiologists. *Eur Radiol* 2008; 18: 298–307.

33. Simonneau G, Galiè N, Rubin L, Langleben D, Seeger W, Domenighetti G, Gibbs S, Lebrec D, Speich R, Beghetti M, Rich S, Fishman A. Clinical classification of pulmonary arterial hypertension. *J Am Coll Cardiol* 2004; 43: 5–12.

34. Barst R, McGoon M, Torbicki A, Sitbon O, Krowka MJ, Olschewski H, Gaine S Diagnosis and differential assessment of pulmonary arterial hypertension. *J Am Coll Cardiol* 2004; 43: 40–47.

35. Galiè N, Manes A, Branzi A. Evaluation of pulmonary arterial hypertension. *Curr Opin Cardiol* 2004; 19: 575–581.

36. Peña E, Dennie C, Veinot J, Muñiz SH. Pulmonary hypertension: How the radiologist can help. *Radiographics* 2012; 32: 9–32.

37. Nauser TD, Stites SW. Diagnosis and treatment of pulmonary hypertension. *Am Fam Physician* 2001; 63: 1789–1798.

38. Rubin LJ. Primary pulmonary hypertension. *N Engl J Med* 1997; 336: 111–117.

39. Frazier AA, Galvin JR, Franks TJ, Rosado-de-Christenson ML. Pulmonary vasculature: hypertension and infarction. *Radiographics* 2000; 20: 491–524.

40. Schannwell CM, Steiner S, Strauer BE. Diagnostics in pulmonary hypertension. *J Physiol Pharmacol* 2007; 58: 591–602.

41. Moraes D, Loscalzo J. Pulmonary hypertension: newer concepts in diagnosis and management. *Clin Cardiol* 1997; 20: 676–682.

42. Simonneau G, Robbins IM, Beghetti M, Channick RN, Delcroix M, Denton CP, Elliott CG, Gaine SP, Gladwin MT, Jing ZC et al. Updated clinical classification of pulmonary hypertension. *J Am Coll Cardiol* 2009; 54: 43–54.

43. Castañer E, Gallardo X, Ballesteros E, Andreu M, Pallardó Y, Mata M, Riera L CT diagnosis of chronic pulmonary thromboembolism. *Radiographics* 2009; 29: 31–50.

44. Grosse C, Grosse A. CT findings in diseases associated with pulmonary hypertension: A current review. *Radiographics* 2010; 30: 1753–1777.

45. Tan RT, Kuzo R, Goodman LR, Siegel R, Haasler GB, Presberg KW. Utility of CT scan evaluation for predicting pulmonary hypertension in patients with parenchymal lung disease. Medical College of Wisconsin Lung Transplant Group. *Chest* 1998; 113: 1250–1256.

46. Ng CS, Wells AU, Padley SP. A CT sign of chronic pulmonary arterial hypertension: The ratio of main pulmonary artery to aortic diameter. *J Thorac Imaging* 1999; 14: 270–278.

47. Devaraj A, Hansell DM. Computed tomography signs of pulmonary hypertension: Old and new observations. *Clin Radiol* 2009; 64: 751–760.

48. Revel MP, Faivre JB, Remy-Jardin M, Delannoy-Deken V, Duhamel A, Remy J. Pulmonary hypertension: ECG-gated 64-section CT angiographic evaluation of new functional parameters as diagnostic criteria. *Radiology* 2009; 250: 558–566.

49. Reid JH, Murchison JT. Acute right ventricular dilatation: A new helical CT sign of massive pulmonary embolism. *Clin Radiol* 1998; 53: 694–698.

50. van der Meer RW, Pattynama PM, van Strijen MJ, van den Berg-Huijsmans AA, Hartmann IJ, Putter H, de Roos A, Huisman MV. Right ventricular dysfunction and pulmonary obstruction index at helical CT: Prediction of clinical outcome during 3-month follow-up in patients with acute pulmonary embolism. *Radiology* 2005; 235: 798–803.

51. Groves AM, Win T, Charman SC, Wisbey C, Pepke-Zaba J, Coulden RA. Semi-quantitative assessment of tricuspid regurgitation on contrast-enhanced multidetector CT. *Clin Radiol* 2004; 59: 713–714.

52. Baque-Juston MC, Wells AU, Hansell DM. Pericardial thickening or effusion in patients with pulmonary artery hypertension: A CT study. *AJR Am J Roentgenol* 1999; 172: 361–364.

53. Horton MR, Tuder RM. Primary pulmonary arterial hypertension presenting as diffuse micronodules on CT. *Crit Rev Comput Tomogr* 2004; 45: 335–341.

54. Nolan RL, McAdams HP, Sporn TA, Roggli VL, Tapson VF, Goodman PC. Pulmonary cholesterol granulomas in patients with pulmonary artery hypertension: Chest radiographic and CT findings. *AJR Am J Roentgenol* 1999; 172: 1317–1319.

55. Hansell DM. Small-vessel diseases of the lung: CT-pathologic correlates. *Radiology* 2002; 225: 639–653.

56. Sheehan R, Perloff JK, Fishbein MC, Gjertson D, Aberle DR. Pulmonary neovascularity: A distinctive radiographic finding in Eisenmenger syndrome. *Circulation* 2005; 112: 2778–2785.

57. Resten A, Maître S, Humbert M, Sitbon O, Capron F, Simoneau G, Musset D. Pulmonary arterial hypertension: Thin-section CT predictors of epoprostenol therapy failure. *Radiology* 2002; 222: 782–788.

58. Rosenkranz S, Bonderman D, Buerke M, Felgendreher R, ten Freyhaus H, Grünig E, de Haan F, Hammerstingl C, Harreuter A, Hohenforst-Schmidt W et al. Pulmonary hypertension due to left heart disease: Updated Recommendations of the Cologne Consensus Conference 2011. *Int J Cardiol* 2011; 154: 34–44.

59. Kubo K, Ge RL, Koizumi T, Fujimoto K, Yamanda T, Haniuda M, Honda T. Pulmonary artery remodeling modifies pulmonary hypertension during exercise in severe emphysema. *Respir Physiol* 2000; 120: 71–79.

60. Matsuoka S, Washko GR, Yamashiro T, Estepar RS, Diaz A, Silverman EK, Hoffman E, Fessler HE, Criner GJ, Marchetti N et al. Pulmonary hypertension and computed tomography measurement of small pulmonary vessels in severe emphysema. *Am J Respir Crit Care Med* 2010; 181: 218–225.

61. Zisman DA, Karlamangla AS, Ross DJ, Keane MP, Belperio JA, Saggar R, Lynch JP III, Ardehali A, Goldin J. High-resolution chest CT findings do not predict the presence of pulmonary hypertension in advanced idiopathic pulmonary fibrosis. *Chest* 2007; 132: 773–779.

62. Alhamad EH, Al-Boukai AA, Al-Kassimi FA, Alfaleh HF, Alshamiri MQ, Alzeer AH, Al-Qtair HA, Ibrahim GF, Shaik SA. Prediction of pulmonary hypertension in patients with or without interstitial lung disease: Reliability of CT findings. *Radiology* 2011; 260: 875–883.

63. Pengo V, Lensing AW, Prins MH, Marchiori A, Davidson BL, Tiozzo F, Albanese P, Biasiolo A, Pegoraro C, Iliceto S et al. Incidence of chronic thromboembolic pulmonary hypertension after pulmonary embolism. *N Engl J Med* 2004; 350: 2257–2264.

64. Hoey ET, Agrawal SK, Ganesh V, Gopalan D, Screaton NJ. Dual energy CT pulmonary angiography: Findings in a patient with chronic thromboembolic pulmonary hypertension. *Thorax* 2009; 64: 1012.

65. Criado E, Sánchez M, Ramírez J, Arquis P, de Caralt TM, Perea RJ, Xaubet A. Pulmonary sarcoidosis: typical and atypical manifestations at high-resolution CT with pathologic correlation. *Radiographics* 2011; 30: 1567–1586.

66. Chaowalit N, Pellikka PA, Decker PA, Aubry MC, Krowka MJ, Ryu JH, Vassallo R. Echocardiographic and clinical characteristics of pulmonary hypertension complicating pulmonary Langerhans cell histiocytosis. *Mayo Clin Proc* 2004; 79: 1269–1275.

67. Taveira-DaSilva AM, Hathaway OM, Sachdev V, Shizukuda Y, Birdsall CW, Moss J. Pulmonary artery pressure in lymphangioleiomyomatosis: An echocardiographic study. *Chest* 2007; 132: 1573–1578.

17

Computed Tomography of Carotid and Vertebral Arteries

Luca Saba

CONTENTS

Everything must be made as simple as possible.
But not simpler

Albert Einstein—Nobel Prize 1921

17.1 Introduction

Computed tomography (CT) can provide exquisite, rapid, high-resolution imaging of the body and, in particular, the vascular system. In the early 1990s, spiral CT was introduced, which enabled volumetric data acquisition through continuous x-ray source rotation and simultaneous continuous table movement so that the vascular enhancement following intravenous injection could be captured during one scan by allowing the development of so-called computed tomography angiography (CTA). Using this technique, noninvasive imaging of blood vessels became widely available. The steady increase in longitudinal coverage of x-ray detectors, that is, the number of slices, further improved the feasibility of CTA. The introduction of multi-detector-row technology gave a tremendous boost to CTA, which is now considered by several authors as a reference standard in advanced vascular imaging. CT technology has seen more rapid improvements than other radiological techniques: over the past decade, the performance of scanners doubled approximately every 2 years and the number of slices in CT doubled approximately every 2.5 years. Advances in spatial and temporal resolution and image reconstruction software have helped in the evaluation of vascular artery pathology and, in particular, in coronary artery anatomy (and vessel patency) and carotid artery plaque detection and characterization.

Over the years, CTA—together with ecocolor Doppler and magnetic resonance angiography (MRA)—has taken over most diagnostic vascular procedures from invasive catheter angiography. In fact, CTA has several advantages and is highly standardized, which makes it a very fast and robust procedure and the technique of choice in many vascular diseases. In particular, in the study of carotid arteries the use of CTA instead of catheter angiography allows one to analyze the luminal narrowing of the carotid plaque, the carotid wall, as well as the surrounding structures. Moreover, by using CTA it is possible to have three-dimensional (3D) information with high spatial resolution.

This chapter details the role of CTA for the assessment of cardiovascular pathology with an emphasis on detection, analysis, and characterization of carotid atherosclerosis.

17.1.1 Anatomy of Carotid Arteries

Carotid arteries are the principal arteries of supply to the head and neck. In human beings, the most common aortic branch pattern consists of three great vessels originating from the arch of the aorta: innominate artery, left "common carotid artery" (CCA), and left subclavian artery.

CCAs originate from the innominate artery on the right and form the highest part of the arch of aorta on the left; they ascend in the neck, and each one divides into two branches (Figure 17.1): (1) external carotid, supplying to the exterior of the head, the face, and the greater part of the neck; and (2) internal carotid, supplying to a great extent parts within the cranial and orbital cavities. For this reason, the length of the left CCA is bigger than that of the right CCA; moreover, the left

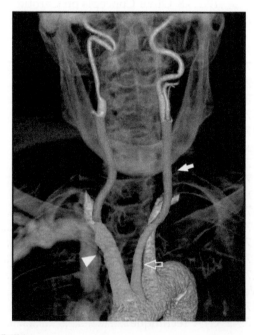

FIGURE 17.1

Anatomy of the common carotid artery (CCA): the innominate artery in green (white arrowhead), the cervical portion of CCA in red (white arrow), and the thoracic portion of the left CCA in blue (open white arrow).

CCA consists of a thoracic portion and a cervical portion, whereas the right CCA consists of only a cervical portion. The thoracic portion of the left CCA ascends from the arch of aorta through the superior mediastinum to the level of the left sternoclavicular joint, where it is continuous with the cervical portion. The CCA is contained in a sheath, which is derived from the deep cervical fascia and encloses also the internal jugular vein and vagus nerve. Behind the angle of bifurcation of the CCA is a reddish-brown oval body, which is known as glomus caroticum. Sometimes, anatomical variations can occur and one of the most common ones is the so-called "bovine arch" that occurs when the left CCA has a common origin with the innominate artery. Other common variants are the right CCA that arises as a separate branch from the arch of aorta, or in conjunction with the left carotid. The left common carotid varies in its origin more than the right. In the majority of abnormal cases, it arises with the innominate artery; if that artery is absent, the two carotids can originate as a single trunk. It is rarely joined with the left subclavian, except in cases of transposition of the aortic arch.

The internal carotid artery (ICA) originates at the bifurcation of the common carotid, opposite the upper border of the thyroid cartilage, and runs perpendicularly upward, in front of the transverse processes of the upper three cervical vertebrae, to the carotid canal in the petrous portion of the temporal bone reaching at the end the circle of Willis where it gives off its terminal or cerebral arteries. In the past years, as reported by the *Gray's Anatomy of the Human Body*, the anatomical division of ICA subdivided the artery into four parts: "cervical," "petrous," "cavernous," and "cerebral" (or supraclinoid). The cervical portion of ICA extends from the carotid bifurcation until it enters the carotid canal in the skull anterior to the jugular foramen. The petrous portion of ICA begins when the ICA enters the canal in the petrous portion of the temporal bone; it first ascends a short distance, then curves forward and medialward, and again ascends as it leaves the canal to enter the cavity of the skull between the lingula and petrosal process of the sphenoid. The cavernous portion of ICA identifies the section of the artery situated between the layers of dura mater forming the cavernous sinus. In the cerebral portion, the ICA having perforated the dura mater on the medial side of the anterior clinoid process passes between the optic and oculomotor nerves to the anterior perforated substance at the medial extremity of the lateral cerebral fissure, where it gives off its terminal or cerebral branches in the circle of Willis.

In 1996, Bouthillier [1] published a seminal paper describing seven segments of ICA that were designated C1 through C7 (Figures 17.2 and 17.3). The author's classification has the following seven segments: C1, "cervical"; C2, "petrous"; C3, "lacerum"; C4, "cavernous"; C5, "clinoid"; C6, "ophthalmic"; and C7, "communicating." The Bouthillier system is often used clinically by neurosurgeons, neuroradiologists, and neurologists (Table 17.1). The C1-C3-C5 segments of ICA do not branch.

The external carotid artery (ECA) originates at the level of the upper border of thyroid cartilage, and at the level of the neck of the mandible, where it divides

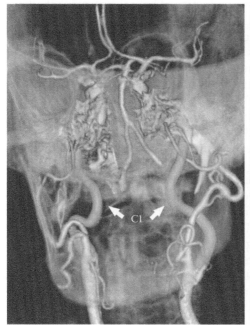 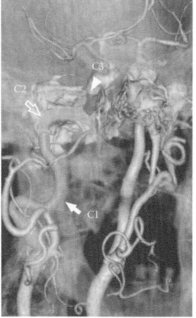

FIGURE 17.2
Anatomy of the internal carotid artery (ICA): C1 (white arrows), C2 (white open arrow), and C3 (white arrowhead) portions.

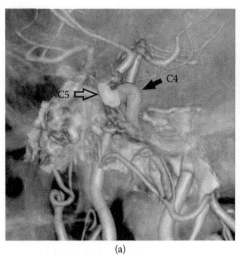
(a)
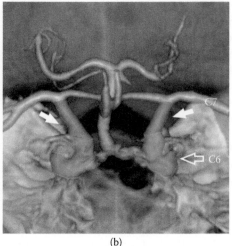
(b)

FIGURE 17.3
Anatomy of ICA: C4 (black arrow), C5 (black open arrow), C6 (white open arrow), and C7 (white arrows) portions.

TABLE 17.1

Intracranial ICA Classification

Gray's Anatomy	Bouthillier's Classification
G1: cervical portion	C1: cervical
G2: petrous portion	C2: petrous
	C3: lacerum
G3: cavernous portion	C4: cavernous
NC	C5: clinoid
G4: cerebral portion	C6: ophthalmic
	C7: communicating

into the superficial temporal and maxillary artery within the parotid gland (terminal branches). ECA rapidly diminishes in size in its course up the neck, owing to the number and size of the branches it gives off. In children, it is somewhat smaller than the internal carotid; but in adults, the two vessels are of nearly equal size. The branches of ECA are the following: superior thyroid artery, ascending pharyngeal artery, lingual artery, facial artery, occipital artery, posterior auricular artery, maxillary artery, and superficial temporal artery (terminal branches).

Moreover, it is important to note that it is not uncommon for carotid arteries to show tortuosity in their course. Usually, there are three tortuosity configurations: elongation, coiling, and kinking (Figure 17.4). "Elongation" identifies the simple increase in length of the carotid that shows some curve along its course. "Coiling" is considered as the elongation of the carotid artery in a restricted space, causing tortuosity and resulting in a C-, S-, or U-shaped curvature or a circular (or double circular) configuration, and "kinking" is a variant of coiling (less than or Z shape), that is, an angulation of one or more segments of ICA (an acute angle

with 60° or less). Vessel tortuosity is generically considered as the presence of kinking or coiling.

17.1.2 CTA: General Concepts

CTA, in particular multi-detector-row CTA (MDCTA), is a powerful noninvasive imaging tool that has experienced tremendous technological developments since its introduction more than 35 years ago. The first generation of CT scanners was developed in the 1970s [2], and since then numerous innovations have improved the utility and application field of CT such as the introduction of helical systems that allowed the development of the "volumetric CT" concept. In the first generation of CT scanners the acquisition of a single image took several minutes, whereas nowadays large volumes are covered in a few seconds.

A major improvement in CT technology was the incorporation of continuously rotating x-ray tubes with a single detector row longitudinally positioned in the gantry. This was the introduction of "third-generation geometry" (spiral CT), resulting in fundamental and far-reaching improvements of CT imaging and opening up a spectrum of entirely new applications including CTA with new visualization techniques such as maximum intensity projection (MIP), multiplanar reconstruction (MPR), curved-planar reconstruction (CPR), and volume rendering technique (VRT). With these scanners, an x-ray tube and a detector array rotate synchronously and continuously around the patient and it is possible to acquire a data volume in a continuous fashion. This technique became the basis of CTA because it allowed rapid and continuous imaging of large volumes so that the vascular enhancement following intravenous injection could be captured within one scan. Single-detector-row

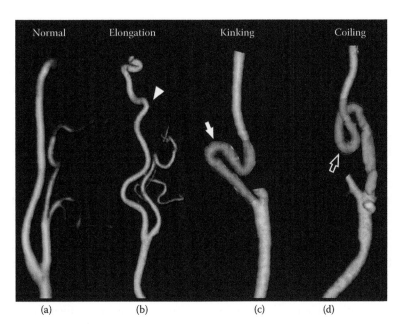

FIGURE 17.4
Vessel tortuosity: (a) normal morphology, (b) elongation, (c) kinking, and (d) coiling.

scanners used a single detector arc or detector ring that consists of parallel detector elements that are much smaller in the direction of the arc (*xy* plane) than in the *z* direction. In multi-detector technology, each element on a detector array is subdivided along the *z* axis and the parallel detector rows can be electronically combined to yield between 4 and 256 separate sections per rotation depending on the type of the scanner.

However, by using spiral CT technology the goal of isotropic imaging within one breath-hold could not be reached because a compromise among scan range, longitudinal resolution, and scan time should be accepted. In 1998, the first four-detector-row scanner with a rotation time of 0.5 second was proposed. This scanner allowed an increase in scanning performance by a factor of 6 compared with the previous single-slice scanners rotating at 0.75 second. The most important clinical benefit was the possibility of scanning a given scan range in a given time at a substantially improved spatial resolution. The introduction of 16-slice CT scanners in 2001 finally allowed true isotropic CT scanning with the potential to produce 1000 images in less than 15 seconds. Compared to 4-detector-row scanners, the performance of 32- to 64-detector-row scanners has been increased more than 20 times owing to more detector rows and faster rotation speeds.

A major recent improvement in CT technology is the introduction of dual-source CT [3–6]. Isotropic voxels, high spatial and temporal resolutions, use of fast contrast material injection rates, and postprocessing tools improved the sensitivity and specificity of MDCTA [7,8]. MDCTA allows full vascular imaging in a few seconds from the aorta to the circle of Willis. By providing this large coverage, MDCTA can now evaluate, besides carotid bifurcation, important atherosclerotic sites like the aortic arch, the origin of supra-aortic vessels, the carotid siphon, vertebrobasilar arteries, and the circle of Willis in one single exam [7,8]. Faster acquisitions provide better image quality, reducing artifacts (respiration, swallowing, pulsation of the aorta, short arteriovenous circulation). MDCT can provide lesser artifacts than single-row helical CT with faster table speeds. Another advantage of MDCTA for atherosclerotic plaque evaluation is its increased in-plane resolution, decreased slice thickness, and subsequent ability to obtain isotropic voxels so that more detailed analysis of atherosclerotic plaque morphology and luminal plaque surface may now be possible.

17.1.3 CTA Scanning Parameter

Scanning parameters are extremely important in CTA for the study of carotid arteries and the circle of Willis. It is possible to group scanning parameters into three major categories: (1) "acquisition" parameters, (2) "derivative" parameters, and (3) "reconstruction" parameters.

The acquisition parameters are number of active detector rows, section collimation, rotation time, table feed per rotation, pitch factor, scan length, tube voltage, and tube load. The number of active detector rows is one for single-detector-row CT, four for 4-MDCT detector row, and so on. Table feed indicates how much the table moves during the rotation time. The pitch provides the relation between table feed and total width of the acquired volume according to the formula, pitch = table feed/(number of active detector rows × section collimation). Section collimation is determined by the total width of the acquired volume in the center of the scan field divided by the number of sections. Rotation time is the time it takes for the tub-detector unit to rotate one time around the patient. The scan length may vary according to clinical indications.

The derivative parameters are table speed (that is determined by the ratio of table feed and rotation time) and scan duration (measured in seconds; it is determined by scan length divided by table speed).

The reconstruction parameters include field of view (FOV), matrix size, reconstruction filter, section thickness, and reconstruction interval. FOV determines which part of data will end up in images. The matrix size of a reconstructed image usually is a 512 × 512 matrix, but it is possible to use other matrices like 256 × 256, 768 × 768, or even 1024 × 1024 for modern scanners. The matrix size works as a limiting factor for spatial resolution. A too small matrix can reduce spatial resolution; however, a very large matrix size cannot increase resolution beyond the system resolution. A reconstruction filter is necessary to reconstruct usable images from projectional raw data.

17.1.4 CTA Principles of PostProcessing Techniques

The introduction of extremely fast scanners in the last 10 years has markedly changed the modality of view of the vascular system and, in particular, in those arteries where small alterations may produce significant damage (like a plaque in the carotid artery bifurcation or a small aneurysm in the circle of Willis). The impact has especially been felt with the ability to visualize isotropic datasets as true volume in a 3D world.

The latest generation of CT systems allows for truly isotropic imaging in virtually any application. As a consequence, the distinction between transverse and in-plane resolution is gradually becoming a historical remnant and the traditional axial slice is losing its clinical predominance because nowadays it is possible to observe images according to multiple planes in real time thanks to the interactive viewing manipulation of isotropic volume images. The routine availability of high-quality volume datasets opens the way for new visualization paradigms and novel evaluation techniques; the corresponding large number of images also poses a challenge to the viewing and reading environment of the radiologist. Image processing and 3D reconstruction of diagnostic images represents a necessary tool for depicting complex anatomical structures and understanding pathological changes in terms of both morphology and function.

To study carotid arteries and the circle of Willis using MDCTA, it is possible to use different techniques of postprocessing in addition to axial scan (Figure 17.5). First introduced in the late 1980s, postprocessing methods currently show an impressive visual capacity of representing anatomic structures, but they are not always adequate in detecting and visualizing all pathologic conditions. Therefore, they have to be used critically to obtain the best diagnostic efficacy. Several types of image reconstructions are available, and authors believe that the simultaneous use of all of these tools is time consuming and incorrect.

It is possible to classify the technique that displays 3D models into projectional and perspective methods. Projectional methods are those in which a 3D volume

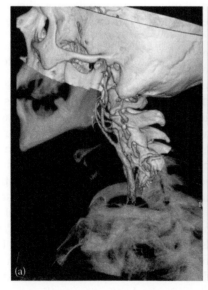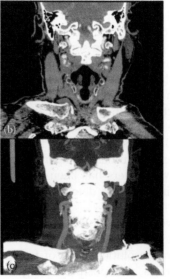

FIGURE 17.5
A 65-year-old male patient with minor stroke; example of different postprocessing methods: (a) volume rendering, (b) multiplanar reconstruction, and (c) maximum intensity projection (MIP) images.

is projected into a bidimensional plane; in perspective methods, a 3D virtual world is displayed by means of techniques that aim at reproducing the perspective of the human eye looking at the physical world.

Projectional methods include CT image-reformatting approaches such as multiplanar reconstructions in different spatial planes. More specific projection techniques include MIP and minimum intensity projection (MinIP). The reformatting process does not modify CT data but uses them in off-axis views and displays the images in an orientation different from native acquisition. Surface rendering and volume rendering (VR) use algorithms that generate 3D views of sectional two-dimensional (2D) data. VR displays the entire volume and preserves the whole dynamic range of an image, whereas surface rendering is based on the extraction of an intermediate surface description of relevant objects from the volume data.

Several reformatting techniques were introduced in the last 20 years, but nowadays the most frequently used in the assessment of circle of Willis and carotid arteries are the following four: MPR, CPR, MIP, and VR. All of these techniques show strengths and pitfalls since they are based on postprocessing procedures of CT data.

MPR is a simple reformatting method in which the images result from retrospectively reconstructed axial data and an obtained image may be oriented in every spatial direction. Two-dimensional MPR is a widely used postprocessing technique, and with arbitrarily chosen views it is very useful in CTA. With the use of 16-detector-row (or higher) scanners, it is possible to generate isotropic images. Oblique sectioning, particularly when interactive, requires a visualization method for plane placement and orientation verification. One method uses selected orthogonal images with a line indicating the intersection of the oblique image with the orthogonal images. MPR images show great utility in the quantitative lumen analysis of carotid arteries and in axial image plane definition because they depict lumen shape. This technique shows suboptimal results in studying the circle of Willis because of its tortuosity.

CPR is a bidimensional postprocessing method that shows the cross-sectional profile of a vessel along its length [9–11]. Often, structures of interest may have a curvilinear morphology that orthogonal and oblique reformations cannot capture in a single 2D image. This restriction of planar sections can be overcome using curvilinear reformatting techniques. A trace along an arbitrary path on any orthogonal plane identifies a set of pixels in the orthogonal image that has a corresponding row of voxels through the volumetric dataset. Each row of voxels for each pixel on the trace can be displayed as a line of a new image, which corresponds to the curved planar structure lying along the trace. It is possible to consider curved planar reformatting as a variation of

MPR. However, in using MPR, there are some limitations. An important issue concerning the use of CPR is that vascular images depend on the course of the selected curved plane; in fact, if the operator selects an inexact plane it will generate an erroneous stenosis morphology and degree. In general, CPR is operator dependent and not suitable for measurement of diameters while the operator may not accurately point the center of the vessel, leading to distortions of anatomic structures. However, there is commercially available software with automatic assessment of the vessel using CPR, where automatic assessment of the center of the lumen facilitates automatic measurements of vessel cross-sectional dimensions in diameters and area value.

MIP is a technique in which only the voxel with the highest CT number is displayed depending on the voxel position along the projecting ray [12]; therefore, MIP enables the evaluation of each voxel along a line from the viewer's eye through the volume of data and selects the maximum voxel value, which is used as the displayed value. When the dataset is obtained with a good quality, MIP may generate digital subtraction angiography (DSA)-like images providing an overview of the target vessel. Often, it is relevant to use thin- or thick-slab MIP [13] to limit the overprojection phenomenon, to avoid time-consuming editing to exclude ebony structures (Figure 17.6). MIP has a number of related artifacts that must be considered to properly interpret a rendered image. The displayed pixel intensity represents only the structure with the highest intensity along the projected ray. A high-density structure such as calcifications will obscure information from intravascular contrast material. Therefore, the use of MIP in the intrapetrous course of ICA is not possible because the high-density bones exclude the opacified lumen from the analysis. This limitation can be partially overcome with the use of a nonlinear transfer function or through volume editing to eliminate undesired data. Another limitation of MIP is that this technique misses the visualization of depth, and this may determine some errors, in particular, at the level of the circle of Willis. In MIPs, differences in attenuation can be detected; thus plaque mural calcifications are distinguishable, but an especially extensive mural calcification hampers the demonstration of vessel lumen. Intraluminal pathology may be obscured if it is surrounded by enhanced blood flow; hence, the detection of intravascular trombi, emboli, or dissection is limited in MIPs.

VR is an extremely useful system to visualize carotid arteries and the circle of Willis [10,14]. This technique incorporates all CT raw data into a resulting image, producing high-quality 3D images. The rendering technique is the computer algorithm used to transform conventional serial transaxial CT imaging data into simulated 3D images. The VR technique uses data from all

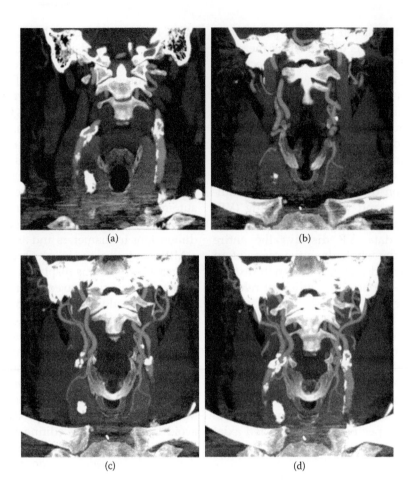

FIGURE 17.6
Thick-slab MIPs: the thickness of the slab determines a different visualization of the carotid artery: (a) 5 mm, (b) 10 mm, (c) 20 mm, and (d) 30 mm.

imaged voxels through volume data management, and the voxels are assigned with an "opacity" value and this value can be chosen between total transparency and opacity. The key to high-quality 3D imaging is the use of thin sections reconstructed at close interslice spacing. To optimally display anatomical structures, VR enables the modulation of window width and level, opacity, and percentage classification and also enables the interactive change of perspective of 3D rendering in real time.

Manual or semiautomatic editing is typically performed to "eliminate" an object such as an organ from surrounding structures; in particular, in the analysis of carotid arteries it is frequently used by the bone removal function that allows the deletion of bones that are superimposing with carotid arteries. Rendering parameters are applied to the full-volume datasets, and they affect the appearance of the image to be displayed. VR typically segments data on the basis of voxel attenuation. The window can be adjusted to standard settings; however, real-time rendering also permits the user to interactively alter the window setting and instantly see the changes. Opacity refers to the degree with which structures that appear close to the user obscure structures

that are farther away. Low opacity values allow the user to "see through" structures. The use of percentage classification is a more advanced feature of VR, which distinguishes between different groups of voxels pertaining to different tissues in an optimal way. Each group is approximated by a trapezoid in the software that can be interactively manipulated to alter the visibility of the tissue, and multiple trapezoidal distributions can be displayed simultaneously.

Image display is the final step of image processing and relates to the process by which a virtual 3D representation of a volume dataset is "flattened" onto one or more 2D planes; this process is required because a 3D model must be represented with a computer monitor, which is a bidimensional device. The most commonly used display method is ray casting, which is a basic technique for displaying a volume of data in two dimensions. In this technique, an array of parallel lines (rays) is mathematically projected through the volume in alignment with each pixel within a desired 2D plane. A weighted sum of the voxel values encountered by a ray is calculated for each pixel and then scaled to the particular range of grayscale values in the display. By using advanced

VR algorithms, it is possible to distinguish mural calcifications from the residual lumen and detect ulcerated carotid plaques [15].

17.1.5 Imaging of Extracranial Arteries

The choice of a specific imaging modality to assess the carotid artery depends on several parameters and depends largely on the clinical indication for imaging and the skills available in individual centers. Recently, Jaff and colleagues [16] proposed a diagnostic algorithm for the correct use of imaging modalities according to the different clinical indications of patients. They proposed that for patients with a high likelihood of vascular disease, CTA may represent an appropriate first exam. On the other hand, for screening patients with a lower likelihood of neurovascular pathology US-ECD (ultrasound) should be selected. If significant stenotic disease of the ICA is detected, CTA can be used to confirm the diagnosis and to accurately determine the precise degree of stenosis. For those asymptomatic patients scheduled for surgery for coronary artery bypass graft, abdominal aortic aneurysm, and lower limb ischemia,

US-ECD represents an accurate and cost-effective, noninvasive screening tool. DSA is infrequently necessary and is needed only in cases of severe multiple vessel disease, for which assessment of flow direction and collateral patterns may be important or when the image quality of noninvasive procedures is of limited value. In the pathology of carotid arteries atherosclerosis plays a major role, but there other pathological conditions for which it is necessary to correctly image carotid artery dissections (CADs), aneurysms, and neoplasms.

17.1.6 CT General Technique for the Study of Extracranial Arteries

The technique for the study of extracranial arteries is quite simple and should be tailored to the diagnostic suspect. The examination should cover the whole length of the carotid and vertebral arteries (VAs), and it requires a scanning range from the aortic arch to the circle of Willis (Figure 17.7). Usually unenhanced and enhanced phases are acquired, but for the characterization of atherosclerotic disease some authors use only the enhanced phase (Figure 17.8). The use of

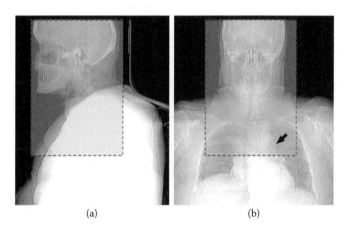

(a)   (b)

FIGURE 17.7
Scout images in (a) laterolateral view and (b) anteroposterior view: the red dotted rectangles indicate the volume of interest.

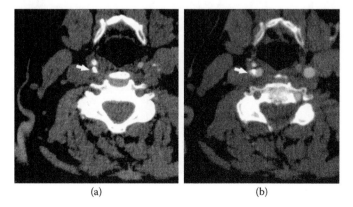

(a)   (b)

FIGURE 17.8
A 61-year-old female patient with minor transient ischemic attack (TIA): (a) image without the administration of contrast material and (b) image after the administration of contrast material.

only the enhanced phase can be important because it reduces the dose delivered to the patient by about 50%. On the other hand, some recent investigations (see Section 17.2.3.6) have demonstrated that contrast-plaque enhancement may play a role in stroke risk stratification. Therefore, whether to use the unenhanced phase or not is still being debated. In other diagnostic suspects like CAD, the use of the unenhanced phase (other than the enhanced phase) is mandatory because some findings (crescent-shaped sign) can be identified only without the administration of contrast material.

Correct timing of contrast material administration is fundamental to reach optimal arterial opacification and CTA image quality. With multi-detector scanners of up to 16 sections, a "fixed delay" (20 seconds) between contrast material injection and the start of scanning has been suggested, but, given the physiologic variability of blood flow among patients (suboptimal cardiac output) and the very fast imaging times of 64-section CT, accurately timing the delay between contrast material administration and scanning initiation with either a "bolus-tracking" technique or a preprocedure timing bolus becomes important.

With bolus tracking, the main contrast material bolus is injected and then a designated vessel of interest is monitored in real time with low-dose dynamic scanning. When a certain enhancement threshold is reached in the monitored vessel, the table moves to the start position and scanning begins. Some authors suggest that the test bolus is superior because CTA can be performed in the pure arterial phase, with optimal enhancement of the carotid and VAs and minimal enhancement in cervical veins. Also, there is no intrinsic delay with the timing-bolus approach; the volume of contrast material given for CTA can be kept as low as possible.

The amount of contrast material should be the minimum amount necessary to obtain optimal intravessel opacification. At the University of Cagliari, we administer a bolus of 50–60 mL of nonionic contrast medium (iodine, 350–400 mg/mL) with a flow rate of 4–6 mL/s. The injection of contrast material should be followed by a 25 mL saline bolus chaser. Flushing of the veins with a saline bolus should be used to remove the contrast material from the vein and reach better image quality. For contrast material infusion, an 18-gauge intravenous catheter is typically used. We suggest administering intravenous contrast material from a right-sided injection for two reasons: first, the left brachiocephalic vein takes a more transverse course into the superior vena cava, which produces a higher likelihood of undiluted contrast material obscuring the origins of the great vessels. Second, compression of the brachiocephalic vein by an ectatic aorta, which is especially common in elderly patients, can lead to contrast material pooling and subsequent reflux into neck veins. The rapid acquisition of CTA images with modern CT scanners can generate a variety of flow artifacts, which are very important for radiologists to recognize so that they are not misled by pseudodissection, pseudo-occlusion, and pseudo venous thrombosis appearances.

The acquisition direction can be caudocranial or craniocaudal. Some authors found that craniocaudal acquisition reduces streak artifacts due to beam hardening, especially at the thoracic inlet. Before the exam, it is important to ask the patient to remove (when it is possible) dental hardware to avoid artifacts (Figure 17.9).

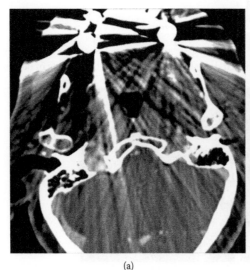 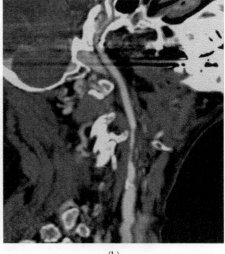

(a)   (b)

FIGURE 17.9
Streak artifacts due to dental hardware: (a) axial view and (b) sagittal view.

17.2 Carotid Atherosclerosis

17.2.1 Carotid Artery Atherosclerosis and Risk of Stroke

Nowadays, atherosclerosis is a very common problem, and several investigations have demonstrated that some degree of carotid artery narrowing is reported in up to 75% of men and 62% of women aged 65 years [17]. The first study that correlated the presence of carotid artery lesions with an increased incidence of stroke is attributed to Savory [18] who reported in 1856 the case of a woman affected by right hemiplegy, dysesthesia, and left monocular symptoms. The autoptic examination of this patient revealed an occlusion of the distal tract of left ICA associated with a bilateral obstruction of the subclavian artery. In the end of 1800s and the first years of 1900s, many other investigations (Gowers in 1875 [19], Chiari in 1905 [20], and Gulthrie and Mayou in 1908 [21]) showed that there is a deep correlation between carotid pathology and cerebral symptoms.

Currently, stroke is the third leading cause of severe disability in the Western world, causing 4.5 million deaths every year [22–24], and this pathology represents a severe health problem and the identification of its risk factors is extremely important [25]. The pathogenesis of stroke is still debated and not completely understood, even if it may be shortly ascribed to two major process: (1) hypoperfusion from high stenosis/occlusion of the vessel [26,27] and (2) distal embolization [28,29]. However, although it is likely that some strokes, associated with carotid artery disease, result from hypoperfusion, the majority of such events appear to be consequence of embolization of an atherosclerotic plaque or acute occlusion of the carotid artery with distal propagation of the thrombus.

17.2.2 Quantification of the Degree of Stenosis

Studies have demonstrated that the risk of stroke in patients with carotid atherosclerosis is closely associated with the severity of luminal stenosis: for asymptomatic patients with less than 75% stenosis the yearly risk of stroke is less than 1%, but this risk increases to 5% for patients with stenosis greater than 75% and is much higher in symptomatic patients with 10% in the first year and rising to 35% over the next 5 years [30–32].

Three fundamental prospective multicentric randomized studies, North American Symptomatic Carotid Endarterectomy Trial (NASCET), European Carotid Surgery Trial (ECST), and Asymptomatic Carotid Atherosclerosis (ACAS) group, provided cutoff values for stenosis degree, indicating possible benefits of carotid endarterectomy (CEA) [33–36]. In particular, the pooled analysis of these three trials proved

the benefits (70%–99% NASCET stenosis with a risk reduction of 16%, $p < .001$) of undergoing an endarterectomy for patients with symptomatic high-grade stenosis (70%–99%) after 5 years of follow-up. For symptomatic patients with mild stenosis (50% or less in NASCET) the risks during surgical procedure outweighed the benefits, whereas in patients with moderate stenosis (50%–70% in NASCET) there was moderate benefit with an absolute risk reduction of 4.6% after 5 years of follow-up. These results came almost four decades after the discovery of relationship of atherosclerotic carotid stenosis to stroke disease and surgical endarterectomy as a treatment. Previous randomized trials presumably failed to produce a positive result because of the high complication rates of the surgery and anesthesia. NASCET, ECTS, and ACAS evaluated the degree of carotid artery stenosis by using DSA, and for this reason these methods evaluated the degree of stenosis as the percentage reduction in linear diameter of the artery. Differences exist in the evaluation of stenosis degree between NASCET, ECST, and the carotid stenosis Index (CSI) (Figures 17.10 and 17.11), and values derived from these three classification methods are not equal if we consider the same carotid stenosis; so it is always important to specify the classification used to avoid errors in the interpretation of the degree of stenosis [37–40].

With NASCET criteria, the ratio between the lumen diameter at stenosis and the normal lumen diameter distal where there is no stenosis is calculated [33,40–43]. With ECST criteria, the ratio between the lumen diameter at stenosis and the total carotid diameter (including the plaque) is calculated [34,44,45]. With CSI-index criteria [35,46,47], the ratio between the lumen diameter at stenosis and the normal lumen of proximal CCA, first multiplied by 1.2, is calculated. In fact, the CSI method uses a fixed conversion factor of 1.2 to estimate the carotid bulb

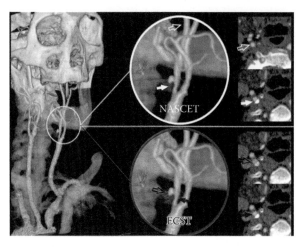

FIGURE 17.10
North American Symptomatic Carotid Endarterectomy Trial (NASCET) and European Carotid Surgery Trial (ECST) methods for the quantification of carotid artery degree of stenosis.

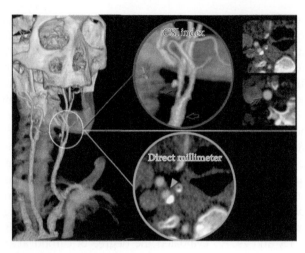

FIGURE 17.11
CSI-index method and direct millimeter method for the quantification of carotid artery degree of stenosis.

size based on a "fixed anatomic relationship" between the CCA and the carotid bulb.

To correctly quantify the degree of stenosis with NASCET criteria (this is the most used technique worldwide) to measure the stenosis of the carotid artery, it is important to follow some rules:

1. To measure the carotid diameter not in the bulb but usually 4–5 cm up to the bifurcation. In fact, the carotid bulb may be considered as an anatomic aberration, being an unusually dilated part of an artery [48] and if we consider this anatomic level as the "normal level" we obtain a more severe degree of stenosis because the carotid bulb can have nearly twice the diameter of the carotid artery beyond the bulb. However, the carotid bulb may determine another problem when it is the area where the plaque is present: if the carotid bulb was reduced to a parallel lumen by atherosclerosis, the NASCET percentage may be 0% even if anatomic purism suggests that this is a 50% reduction in diameter [48].

2. To not calculate the percentage of stenosis when a "near occlusion condition" is present (Figure 17.12). This condition will be further analyzed in this chapter, but at this point it is important to note that a near occlusion makes the calculation incorrect because the diameter of the ICA is diffusely reduced.

3. To quantify the degree of stenosis, measurements have to be performed on a plane strictly perpendicular to the carotid axis and these should be performed for both NASCET and ECST methods.

Moreover, the NASCET method (as well the ECST method and the CSI index) is a ratio between diameters and not between areas (because these studies were performed with angiography).

It was demonstrated by Saba et al. [53] that NASCET and ECST methods show a strength correlation and that interobserver and intra-observer agreement values are high for both NASCET and ECST.

The methodology of carotid stenosis quantification is widely debated because NASCET, ECTS, and CSI index are indirect ratio–percentage methods. These trials imaged carotid arteries by using conventional angiography, and methods of deriving percentage stenosis ratios were adopted because standardized stenosis measurements were not consistent with film in conventional angiography and because when they were used in digital angiography there were different degrees of magnification and lack of millimeter calibration. With the introduction of MDCTA, thanks to its high spatial resolution (with an isotropic voxel of 3 mm), a new direct millimeter method was proposed by Bartlett and colleagues [50–52] (Figure 17.11) to overcome the limitations of classical percentage methods. It was demonstrated well that there is a linear relationship between millimeter carotid bulb stenosis diameter and NASCET. Threshold values of 1.4–2.2 mm can be used to evaluate moderate stenosis (50%–69% according to NASCET) with a sensitivity of 75% and a specificity of 93.8%. A carotid diameter of 1.3 mm corresponds to 70% stenosis, and this value was proposed by Bartlett as a threshold for severe carotid stenosis with a sensitivity of 88% and a specificity of 92%. Saba and colleagues [53] demonstrated that the simple millimeter measurement of stenosis can reliably predict NASCET-type, ECST-type, and CSI-type percentage stenosis. Similar correlations are present between ECST and millimeter method and CSI index and millimeter method. The use of a direct millimeter method for the quantification of carotid arteries is an excellent option because it is possible to avoid cumbersome calculus and because the direct millimeter method overcomes the use of three different methods of measurement. The simple millimeter measurement of stenosis can reliably predict NASCET-type, ECST-type, and CSI-type percentage stenosis.

In the analysis of carotid arteries, sometimes it is possible to find complete occlusion of vessels. This condition is easily detected using CTA because there is the complete absence of contrast material into the lumen (Figure 17.13).

Another extremely important point in the CTA study of carotid arteries is the correct selection of the window parameter. CTA shows high sensitivity in detecting calcified plaques; but sometimes a bias in the exact quantification of stenosis degree occurs, mainly caused by the high linear attenuation coefficient of the calcified

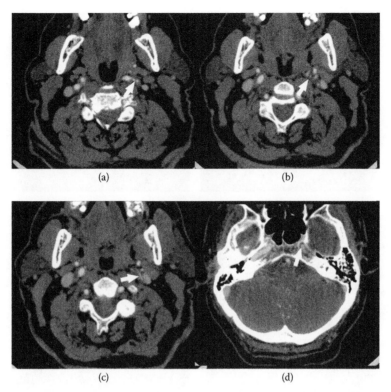

FIGURE 17.12
A 54-year-old male patient: (a–d) the near-occlusion condition of the left ICA with the small diameter from its origin to the C4 level is visible.

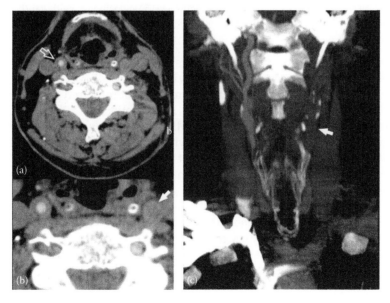

FIGURE 17.13
Complete occlusion of the left CCA (white arrows) with the absence of contrast material in the lumen of the carotid. In panels (a) and (b) axial views are given, whereas in panel (c) a coronal MIP is given. The contralateral carotid artery shows regular opacification (white open arrow).

plaques. Some authors found that a window width pre-set at 850 Hounsfield unit (HU), level of 300 HU, shows the best values (Figure 17.14).

Nowadays, MDCTA probably represents the best imaging method to quantify carotid artery stenosis with a sensitivity in the evaluation of stenosis degree

that may be compared with angiography but with fewer risks [54–56].

In the evaluation of carotid artery stenosis, US-ECD and MRA are widely used. US-ECD has come into widespread use for the classification of carotid stenosis since 1975 when a quantitative examination protocol

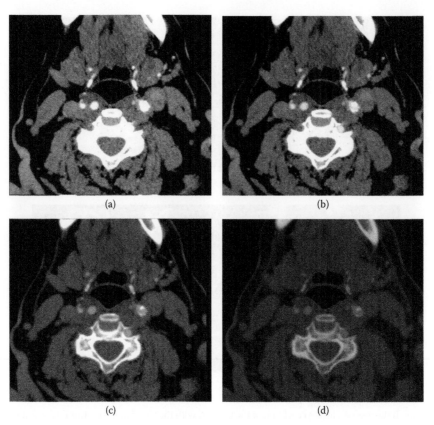

FIGURE 17.14
Effect of different window levels in carotid artery visualization: (a) window level 50 and window width 200, (b) window level 150 and window width 400, (c) window level 300 and window width 850, and (d) window level 450 and window width 1200.

that is now nearly universal was developed, and currently this technique is performed to screen patients with possible carotid artery disease. However, the accuracy of US-ECD in the quantification of the degree of stenosis is moderate and US-ECD should not be used as the only imaging diagnostic test for patients' selection for CEA [56–58]. MRA has come to be widely used as a noninvasive diagnostic imaging modality for carotid artery stenosis quantification. It avoids the radiation and iodinated contrast exposure associated with CTA. MRA sensitivity is quite good in determining stenosis degree. In a wide series of studies that assumed carotid angiography as the gold standard, the median sensitivity for a high-grade lesion was 93% and the median specificity was 88% [59]. A recent meta-analysis of Debrey and colleagues [60], published in 2008, indicated that MRA is highly accurate for the diagnosis of high-grade ICA stenosis and occlusion with both time of flight (TOF) and contrast enhanced (CE) techniques, with CE MRA having the edge over TOF MRA; that MRA has a high accuracy for distinguishing occlusions from high-grade stenosis, particularly CE MRA; and that both CE MRA and TOF MRA appear to be poor diagnostic tools for moderate ICA stenoses. 3D TOF provides a superior resolution, but

its sensitivity in measuring the flow is lower compared with 2D TOF. CE MRA is a very promising technique, and it is not impaired by slow-flow situations.

Investigations [61,62] showed that both US-ECD and MRA have the tendency to overestimate stenosis degree, whereas CTA underestimates it. In a recent study, Saba et al. [63] demonstrated that NASCET stenosis measured in MDCTA and PSV values measured by US-ECD have a good correlation: the use of a threshold of 283 cm/s obtains good values of sensitivity and specificity (75% and 88.6%, respectively).

17.2.3 Carotid Vulnerable Plaque

Nowadays, the degree of luminal stenosis is considered the most important element to grade atherosclerotic disease severity. However, several investigations have shown that plaque structure and composition represents a key element in the development of cerebrovascular ischemic events. From a conceptual point of view, this is easy to understand: in fact, the majority of ischemic infarcts occur because some emboli occlude an arterial vessel of the brain and not because there is a reduction in blood flow (hypoperfusion) that is usually well compensated thanks to the circle of

Willis collateralization. In the late 1980s the first angiographic studies on coronary arteries showed that also coronary with plaques that determine a moderate degree of stenosis can lead to an acute myocardial infarction [64–66]; histopathological studies showed that in these plaque there were also erosions and ulcers by confirming that the "luminal narrowing" was only one of the cause of the myocardial infarction. In the following year, similar conclusions were found for carotid arteries also because studies found that cerebrovascular events can occur in low-grade stenosis also by demonstrating that it is fundamental to look beyond the degree of stenosis and to characterize plaque morphology [67–69]. These findings have created tremendous interest in the development of noninvasive methods that can quantify the total plaque volume of a plaque and reliably identify the morphologic features of the "vulnerable plaque" [70–72]. Following these observations, the concept of vulnerable plaque, which refers to an atherosclerotic plaque that contains a large necrotic lipid core covered by a thin or disrupted fibrous cap (FC), was introduced and it is characterized by a higher tendency to rupture, resulting in embolization or thrombosis. In the analysis of a vulnerable plaque, at least three main classes of plaque determinants should be analyzed: (1) plaque luminal morphology (normal, irregular, and ulcerated), (2) plaque components (FC, intraplaque hemorrhage, thrombus, calcification), and (3) plaque eccentricity/remodeling. Before analyzing these plaque characteristics, it is fundamental to explain some other basic concepts of a carotid artery vulnerable plaque, in particular the fact that carotid artery plaques change during the time: in fact, the composition of a carotid plaque changes during the progression of atherosclerotic disease and some phases seem to be more prone to the vulnerability [73].

The American Heart Association (AHA) proposed a classical plaque classification based on plaque composition, which is considered to reflect the temporal natural history of the disease. AHA distinguishes six stages (Table 17.2).

This classification was modified by Virmani [74], suggesting seven categories of lesions, and more recently by a new classification system describing five phases of plaque development by introducing the acute phase [75]:

Phase 1: comprising the AHA histological stages I–III; constitutes early plaque development and is clinically silent.

Phase 2: advanced lesions can histologically be either stage IV (atheroma) or stage Va (thick cap) and carry the risk of rupture but may not be stenosing the vessel.

TABLE 17.2

AHA Classification

Stage	Definition
I	Incorporation of scattered macrophages and foam cells within the arterial wall triggered by intralesional atherogenic lipoprotein.
II	Development of fatty streaks.
III	Extracellular fats that break up cell–cell connections in smooth-muscle layers.
IV	The classic atheroma that contains a fatty necrotic core. The presence of atheroma may not narrow the vascular lumen since the affected vessels can compensate for the increase in plaque volume through a widening of their external circumference rather than protrusion of plaque into the vascular lumen.
V	Stage V is further classified into three different class, where stage Va indicates those plaques having a fatty core as well as a multilayered thick FC (fibroatheroma), stage Vb lesions are largely calcified, and in stage Vc lesions are predominantly fibrous.
VI	Complex plaque: there are areas of internal hemorrhage or focal apposition thrombosis. These lesions may undergo repeated cycles of rupture, thrombosis, and remodeling.

Phase 3: defines acute phases with plaque rupture and subsequent thrombosis. Phase 3 may still be clinically silent.

Phase 4: defines acute phases with plaque rupture and repeated thrombosis; phase 4 through its increasing hemodynamic effect is always symptomatic.

Phase 5: the plaque is a hemodynamically symptomatic lesion, which actively remodels through the in-sprouting of vasa vasorum, dense dystrophic calcification (stage Vb), or fibrous scarring (stage Vc).

17.2.3.1 Luminal Morphology of the Carotid Artery Plaque

Luminal plaque morphology represents an important element of plaque vulnerability because previous investigations have shown that there are different risks of embolic events according to the different types of luminal morphology. In particular, CTA allows the analysis of plaque surface by distinguishing between plaque irregularities and plaque ulceration [7,15]. De Weert and colleagues [76] showed that one can assess atherosclerotic carotid plaque surface morphology with differentiation between smooth, irregular, and ulcerated surfaces (Figures 17.15 and 17.16):

Smooth surface: this term refers to a regular luminal morphology at the level of the plaque without any sign of ulceration or irregularity.

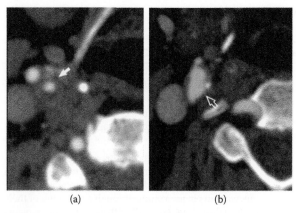

FIGURE 17.15
Different types of lumen surfaces: in panel (a) an example of a smooth surface (white arrow) is given, whereas in panel (b) an irregular plaque surface (white open arrow) is shown.

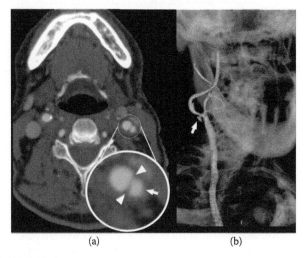

FIGURE 17.16
A 78-year-old male patient with an ulcerated carotid plaque in the left carotid artery bifurcation: in (a) the axial image the ulceration is clearly visible (white arrow) and also the pseudoflap (white arrowheads). In (b) the volume-rendered image, the ulcer is also clearly visible and its morphology is the "button-of-shirt" one.

Usually, the lumen profile should be plain (Figure 17.15). This type of morphology configuration indicates plaque stability (Figure 17.15).

Plaque irregularities: irregularities in the surface of a plaque are frequently associated with stroke/transient ischemic attack (TIA). Rothwell and colleagues [116] demonstrated with DSA that irregularities of a plaque's surface are an independent predictor of ischemic stroke; these observations were later confirmed using MDCTA. The presence of plaque irregularities should always be verified because they represent a risk factor (Figure 17.16).

Plaque ulceration: when a carotid artery plaque is ulcerated, there is an increased risk of stroke.

Pathologists define an ulceration of the plaque as "an intimal defect larger than 1000 micrometers in width, exposing the necrotic core of the atheromatous plaque"(p. 1232) [77]. Plaque ulceration has more frequently been observed proximal to the point of maximum luminal stenosis, which is exposed to a higher wall shear stress.

The association between carotid artery plaque and ischemic events was already demonstrated in the NASCET study that showed that in a group of patients who received medical therapy 30% of patients who had severe carotid stenosis associated with an ulcerated plaque suffered an ischemic cerebral event within 2 years, whereas only 17% of patients with severe stenosis but no ulcerated plaques had an ischemic cerebral event within 2 years [78–80]. Recently, some authors showed that the presence of ulceration alone represents an important risk for neurological symptoms and the presence of an ulceration associated with high-grade stenosis determines an increased risk of stroke. The presence of ulcerations in the plaque is very common; in fact, Redgrave et al. published a study based on the analysis of CEA specimens from 526 consecutive symptomatic patients with a stenosis degree of 75%–90% and found ulceration in 58% of cases. This is an extremely high value compared with the findings of MDCTA, MRA, US, and DSA, but it can be explained by three reasons: (1) a higher resolution of histology that enables the detection of even small ulcerations; (2) the presence of thrombus formation on the location of a rupture that may fill the ruptured site, which may lead to a nonvisualization with MDCTA; and (3) a higher volume of calcifications in severe stenosis, which may hamper the accurate detection of small ulcerations by MDCTA.

For the detection of ulceration, it is well demonstrated that DSA is not sufficiently reliable with a sensitivity of only 46% [81–84]. Also, US-ECD does not offer optimal results. A recent study compared MDCTA and US-ECD in the detection of plaque ulceration, and it was observed that MDCTA had markedly higher results compared to US-ECD (93% vs. 37.5%) [15,85–87].

Nowadays, the best imaging modality for the identification of carotid artery plaque is probably MDCTA. With this technique, it is quite easy to identify even small ulcers thanks to its extremely good spatial resolution. In MDCTA analysis, the most common criterion used to identify the presence of an atherosclerotic carotid plaque is the presence of extension of contrast material beyond the vascular lumen into the surrounding plaque. In identifying the ulcer, the plane (axial, sagittal, and coronal) of analysis of the dataset is important because ulcers may show some different morphologies (Figures 17.16 through 17.18). It is

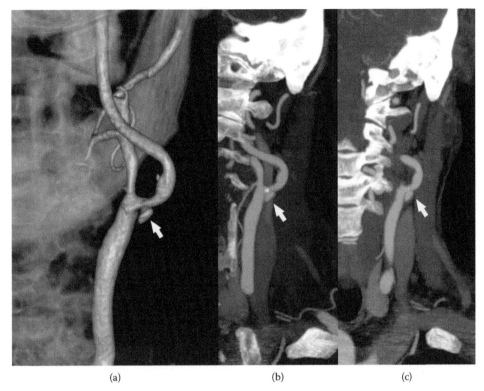

(a)   (b)   (c)

FIGURE 17.17
A 78-year-old male patient with an ulcerated carotid plaque in the left carotid artery bifurcation: in (a) the volume-rendered images and (b, c) the thick-slab MIP, the ulceration is clearly visible (white arrows).

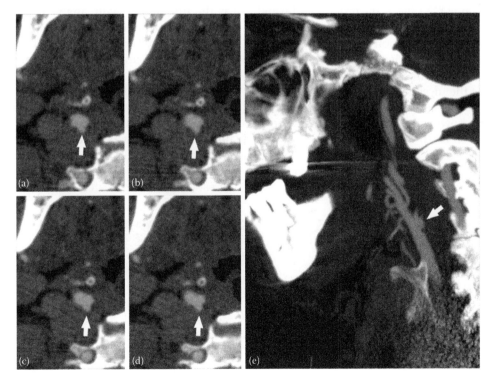

FIGURE 17.18
A 72-year-old male patient with an ulcerated carotid plaque in the right carotid artery bifurcation: in the (a, b, c, d) contiguous axial images, the ulceration is clearly visible (white arrows). Also in the (e) sagittal MIP, the ulcer is easily detectable (white arrow).

important to remember that ulcers may show at least four different morphologies:

1. Hook pointing upward
2. Hook pointing down
3. Shirt button
4. Rift of the plaque

In the axial view, types 1 and 2 (hook pointing upward and hook pointing down) may show an aspect similar to dissection; in this case, the use of sagittal or coronal image may help to clearly define the exact morphology by identifying the ulcer.

Lovett et al. [69] proposed a classification of carotid artery plaques into four categories, where type 1 is an ulcer that points out perpendicular to the lumen, type 2 has a narrow neck and points out proximally and distally, type 3 has an ulcer neck proximally and points out distally, and type 4 has an ulcer neck distally and points out proximally. Type 1 and type 3 are the most frequent types of rupture, but, at present, there is no evidence that a specific type of plaque is associated with a specific clinical behavior.

The localization of an ulcer can be proximal or distal according to the point of maximum stenosis, and it is extremely interesting to observe that ulcerated plaques are more frequently encountered with a higher degree of stenosis. This data was first demonstrated in the ECST study by using DSA (71% at the proximal site) and then by Saba and de Weert. It is interesting to note that the higher frequency of ulceration in the proximal site observed in the carotid artery is similar to that in coronary arteries; in fact, an intracoronary ultrasound study found that 69% of the ulcerated, ruptured plaques were proximal to the narrowest luminal point. The fact that the proximal site shows a predilection for ulceration is in concordance with shear stress theories; in fact, it is thought that a high shear stress on the plaque surface, determined by luminal narrowing, weakens the FC and determines the development of ulceration.

The use of postprocessing techniques may further help in the detection/characterization of carotid plaque ulcers. In particular, Saba et al. [15] showed that VR algorithms are the best postprocessing techniques to visualize the ulcerations of plaque. One of the limitations in identifying ulcerations by using MDCTA is the presence of a heavy calcified plaque. In this case, it can be very difficult to detect the plaque (in particular, the small plaques) because of the halo and edge blur that may mask it [88,89]. However, this is a problem that MDCTA shares with other imaging modalities and, in particular, with ultrasound where the acoustic shadowing from calcifications obscures the presence of ulcerations.

17.2.3.2 Different Types of Plaque

Atherosclerosis can show different pathways, and during this time carotid artery plaques may change their composition [73]. In the field of CT the first studies were performed by Porsche et al., [90,91] in which 55 patients undergoing CEA were imaged preoperatively using single-slice spiral CTA. Identifying the type of plaque is important because previous investigations have shown that a specific type of plaque (and therefore a consequent specific plaque histological composition) is associated with an increased or a reduced risk of developing cerebrovascular events. In fact, even in the presence of a plaque that determines a low-grade stenosis it is possible to observe a cerebrovascular event. Schroder et al. was the first author who, analyzing coronary arteries, observed the association between presence of symptoms and plaque type. Schroder categorized plaques as "fatty," "mixed," and "calcified" (Figure 17.19). In this classification, fatty (soft) plaques were considered to be those with a density value <50 HU, mixed plaques those with a density value between 50 and 119 HU, and calcified plaques, those with a density value >120 HU. This classification was used by other groups also. In particular, Saba et al.[15] proposed for the measure of HU attenuation the use of a circular or elliptical region-of-interest (ROI) cursor located in the predominant area of

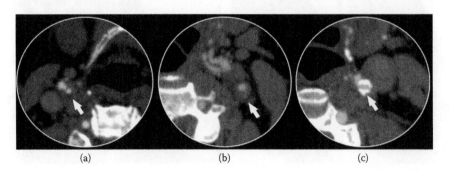

(a)   (b)   (c)

FIGURE 17.19
Examples of different types of carotid artery plaque: in panel (a) a fatty plaque (white arrow) is visible, in panel (b) a mixed plaque (white arrow), and in panel (c) a calcified plaque.

a plaque of at least 1 mm²; those areas showing contamination by contrast medium or calcification that is noncontributory to stenosis should be avoided. One possible bias in this analysis is the presence of beam hardening.

However, simply identifying the type of plaque is an important limitation because usually in the plaque several components are present at the same time and their different percentages may represent an important element. For this reason, the classification of Schroder et al. was modified by de Weert et al. [92] who changed the HU threshold to consider a plaque as fatty, mixed, or calcified by using automated computer software that can measure volume and percentages of the plaque's components. In this classification, fatty plaques were considered those with a density value <60 HU, mixed plaques those with a density value between 60 and 129 HU, and calcified plaques those with a density >130 HU. This method is time consuming because it is necessary to manually draw the ROI for the opacified lumen and the ROI for the plaque in each slice of the visible plaque (Figure 17.20). Moreover, there are some limitations in the use of this system that should be fully understood. First, it can be difficult to differentiate normal vessel wall and a slightly thickened vessel. Second, in some cases it can be difficult to distinguish the limit of carotid artery plaque from the paravertebral and sternocleidomastoid muscles, which are frequently positioned along the artery even if in most cases the vessel wall can be differentiated from the surrounding tissue by the low density of periarterial fat or the presence of calcifications at the outer border of the plaque [92]. Third, the erroneous manual inclusion of periarterial fat in the ROI leads to the classification of this fat as lipid in

the plaque. Fourth, contrast-enhanced lumen is differentiated from atherosclerotic plaque. Another investigation demonstrated that very low HU values in plaques (<0 HU) are associated with the presence of intraplaque hemorrhage [93,94].

17.2.3.3 Carotid Plaque Volume

Investigations have demonstrated that, more than luminal narrowing, atherosclerotic plaque rupture plays an important role in the development of cerebrovascular events like TIA and stroke. It is possible to observe very big plaques that do not determine significant stenosis degree because of the presence of a positive remodeling in which the artery enlarges to preserve the luminal area. Consequently, plaque volume is usually underestimated by the degree of stenosis.

There are many reasons for this because severity of stenosis is not a good reflection of the severity of atherosclerotic disease. First, extensive atherosclerotic disease can be present without stenosis of the lumen, and vice versa; stenosis can be caused by the focal accumulation of a small amount of atherosclerotic plaque. Second, vessel remodeling plays an additional role since the discrepancy between atherosclerotic plaque load and angiographic appearance of the lumen is also present in other vessel beds. Third, the configuration of a normal carotid bulbus and bifurcation allows the accumulation of extensive atherosclerotic plaque before luminal stenosis becomes visible on angiography.

Recent studies hypothesize that plaque volume may be a better descriptor of the severity of atherosclerotic disease than the degree of stenosis [95]. The

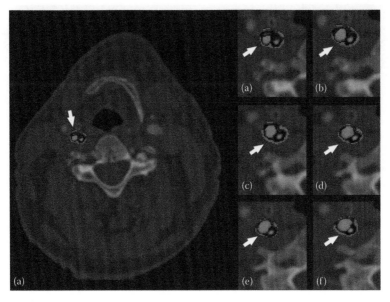

FIGURE 17.20
A 65-year-old male patient: an example of the automated analysis of carotid artery plaques. The different colors represent the different types of plaques (yellow = fatty, red = mixed, and blue = calcified), whereas the green color represents opacified lumen.

noninvasive in vivo assessment of atherosclerotic plaque volume and the relative contribution of different plaque components have important clinical implications; in particular, they provide optimal parameters, together with the severity of stenosis, for cardiovascular risk assessment. In particular, lipid component volume is associated with the presence of plaque ulceration, which represents a significant risk factor for the development of cerebrovascular events [96]. De Weert et al. [93] found a good association between severity of luminal stenosis and plaque volume, but it is interesting to observe that a relatively large proportion of patients with cerebrovascular symptoms had atherosclerotic plaque with no luminal narrowing measured according to the NASCET criteria. Other investigations found that there is excellent interobserver agreement in the quantification of plaque volume by using CT [97]. It is interesting to note that plaque composition changes with increasing plaque volume, and there is an increase in the proportions of lipid and calcification with increasing plaque volume.

17.2.3.4 Plaque Eccentricity and Remodeling

In coronary arteries, it is well demonstrated that plaque eccentricity is associated with the development of acute coronary syndrome; recent investigations have shown that also in carotid arteries plaque eccentricity is associated with the presence of ischemic cerebrovascular events. Plaques change over time, and it is possible that some determinants of instability are transitory and the concept of remodeling indicates the morphological and ultrastructural variation of a plaque in time.

In coronary plaques, histological analysis performed within 1 week after infarction showed morphological features of instability, whereas plaques taken later were histologically similar to those in patients with stable angina.

The computational simulation of carotid bifurcation models showed an important difference in the severity and distribution of wall shear stress, as well as the size of the post-stenotic recirculation zone between concentric and eccentric stenoses [98]. These data were confirmed using CTA [99], showing that the presence of eccentric plaques is associated with a significantly increased incidence of ipsilateral events compared with patients with concentric stenosis. Hardie and colleagues [100] studied the eccentricity index and the remodeling ratio of atherosclerotic carotid plaques by using CTA, and they found that in patients with cerebral ischemic symptoms expansive carotid remodeling was significantly greater than in asymptomatic patients. This finding indicated that the extent of expansive remodeling quantified by CTA may indicate underlying atherosclerotic plaque vulnerability (Figures 17.21 and 17.22).

17.2.3.5 Plaque Components

17.2.3.5.1 FC

An FC is a thin layer of fibrous connective tissue, derived from the migration and proliferation of vascular smooth muscle cells, that contains macrophages and smooth muscle cells. In the case of atherosclerosis, the histological composition of the FC changes and smooth muscle cells, macrophages, foam cells, lymphocytes,

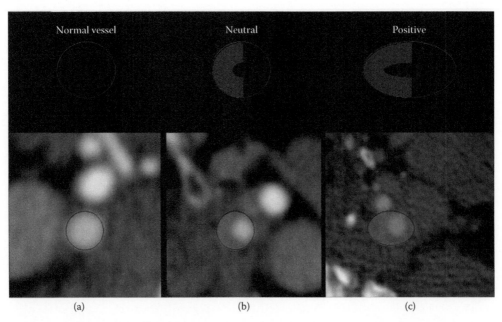

(a)   (b)   (c)

FIGURE 17.21
Plaque remodeling: (a) normal vessel without plaque, (b) carotid with plaque and neutral remodeling, and (c) positive remodeling.

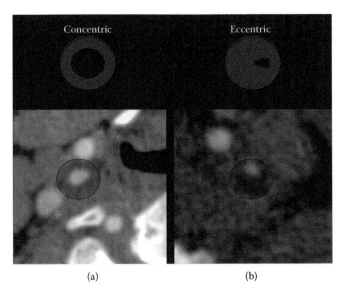

FIGURE 17.22
Plaque localization: (a) concentric plaque and (b) eccentric plaque.

elastin, and collagen can be found. The thickness of FC is an important element for entire carotid plaque stability, and Loree and colleagues [101] found that circumferential stress on a plaque was exquisitely linked to the thickness of the FC and the degree of arterial remodeling. Therefore, the thinner the cap, the greater the stress even at relatively low levels of stenosis. The rupture of the FC is considered a trigger for the development of coronary and carotid ischemic events [102,103].

The thickness of the FC can be extremely variable with values obtained ranging from 10 to 1750 μm. However, the main problem is to identify the FC with a high risk of rupture and therefore to identify the thin or ruptured FC. The modified AHA classification defines a coronary thin FC as one that is below 65 μm in thickness because this is the ninety-fifth percentile cap thickness at the point of rupture, but the degree of cap thickness that renders a carotid plaque prone to rupture is still being debated. Studies show that the risk of plaque rupture increases exponentially as FC thickness decreases. In 1997, Bassiouny et al. found that the mean distance between the necrotic core and the lumen was 500 μm in asymptomatic subjects and 270 μm in symptomatic subjects.

Nowadays, MRA is considered the best imaging technique to identify ruptured FCs, as well as to distinguish thick FCs from thin ones in carotid plaques [104–107]. Some authors also propose CT for the study and identification of ruptured FCs, but the value of this technique remains uncertain [108,109]. Saba et al. [109] suggested the study of FCs in CT by using the following four criteria: [1] the presence of a contrast material in a cleft located at the inner carotid surface, [2] whose dimension was less than 1 mm in depth, [3] with an angle of 230° or more with the lumen, and [4] the presence of an atherosclerotic plaque into which the contrast material in a cleft projects. With these four criteria, the interobserver agreement obtained was good (0.781) and, moreover, it was observed that the presence of a ruptured FC is significantly associated with cerebrovascular symptoms (or 3.86; $p = .0032$). In another recently published study, Wintermark et al. [6] demonstrated that it is possible to measure FC thickness using an automatic computer classifier algorithm for the detection of plaque components.

17.2.3.5.2 Intraplaque Hemorrhage

In the vulnerable plaque the presence of intraplaque hemorrhage is quite common, and several investigations have shown that the extravasation of red blood cells is associated with instability [110]; moreover, it is demonstrated that hemorrhage occurs in those plaques with stenosis > 70%. The mechanism that determines the hemorrhage is still debated and several authors have proposed different theories [111,112] : rupture of the vasa vasorum and cracks of the luminal surface. Like fissured fibrous cap (FFC) imaging, for the detection of intraplaque hemorrhage the best imaging modality is nowadays considered to be MR. Moody et al. [113] demonstrated that T1-weighted images can identify histologically confirmed complicated plaque with hemorrhage. Moreover, with MR it is possible to distinguish the temporal phase of the hemorrhage according to different signal sequences.

In CTA the identification of intraplaque hemorrhage is complex, and it is still debated whether it is possible to correctly detect intraplaque hemorrhage with CT without the use of automated software classification analysis [114,115]. In a paper published in 2009, Ajduk et al. [94] showed that the presence of HU values <31 HU is statistically associated with hemorrhage (a sensitivity of 100% and a specificity of 64%). However, these data should be further confirmed because of the limited number of patients analyzed (31 subjects). Moreover, Wintermark et al. [6] showed that there is an overlap in CT Hounsfield densities between connective tissue and hemorrhage.

17.2.3.5.3 Thrombus

The presence of thrombus in a plaque represents an important risk factor for the development of cerebrovascular events because it may determine distal embolization with ischemic events. Rothwell et al. [116] in the NASCET trial found that surface thrombus was visible in nearly 30% of cases of ulcerated plaque. The identification of thrombus using CT is quite difficult, and the best imaging technique for this kind of analysis is considered to be MR. The detection of thrombus and the determination of its age on MR images are mainly related to the physical characteristics and visual appearance of thrombus [117,118].

17.2.3.5.4 Calcification

Investigations have demonstrated that in coronary arteries the amount of calcium is associated with an increase in mortality [119,120], but in carotid arteries it seems that the presence of calcium represents a protecting factor [121–124] because the calcium is associated with the more stable plaques. Moreover, it is likely that calcium confers stability to atheromatous carotid plaques, resulting in protection against biomechanical stress and disruption. The mechanism by which calcium confers stability to plaques has both a mechanical basis and a functional basis. In fact, it was demonstrated that calcification does not significantly impact the biomechanical stress on FC unlike lipid pools, which increase the stress.

The presence and amount of calcium in carotid artery plaques can be evaluated using CT, MR, or US-ECD, but the most sensitive technique is considered to be CT because calcification can be easily detected with CT due to the high attenuation of x-rays by calcium hydroxyapatite, which leads to a high-density structure in the plaques. Some authors propose to use a density of 130 HU in an ROI having an area > 1 mm. By using CT, the presence of calcium can be detected without the injection of luminal contrast media; however, even in the presence of contrast media the threshold value is allowed to easily differentiate calcium from contrast media.

17.2.3.6 Carotid Plaque Enhancement

The significance, analysis, and quantification of carotid plaque enhancement in a carotid plaque using CT form an extremely new topic. Histological studies have demonstrated the presence of neovascularization of adventitial vasa vasorum in symptomatic ICA walls and plaques. In a recent paper by Romero et al., [125] the enhancement in the carotid wall was analyzed and it was found that using a threshold of contrast enhancement of 10 HU there was a positive association with the presence of cerebrovascular ischemic symptoms. The authors suggest that the carotid wall enhancement found by CT may represent vasa vasorum neovascularization.

Saba et al. [126] found that the carotid artery plaque enhancement at CT is associated with microvessel density and that the degree of intraplaque neovascularization is statistically associated with carotid plaque enhancement. For this reason, the plaque enhancement at CT should be considered when assessing vulnerable plaques because it represents a strong marker of instability [127] It is interesting that carotid plaque enhancement shows a very good reproducibility between observers.

The authors also found that the type of plaque (fatty, mixed, or calcified) plays a role in the enhancement of plaque. In fact, fatty plaques show a bigger enhancement compared with mixed ones and fatty plaques show a more frequent enhancement compared with mixed ones. For this reason, plaque enhancement ipso facto cannot be considered a good marker of plaque instability (in fact, 50% of patients without symptoms showed contrast enhancement, whereas 84% of patients with cerebrovascular symptoms showed plaque instability); the measurement of degree of enhancement may represent a good solution. Using CT it is possible to reliably quantify HU variation in tissues, and it was suggested that 15 HU may represent a good threshold to consider a carotid plaque enhancement as symptomatic. The use of 15 HU as threshold allows a specificity of 83.33% and a sensitivity of 76.47%.

The analysis of contrast plaque enhancement in CT is important because it may be used for plaque risk stratification and identification of vulnerable plaques. Plaque neovascularization has been well established and confirmed in histological studies as a consistent feature of plaque in patients with cerebrovascular symptoms [128,129], and researchers have indicated neovascularization as an important factor contributing to the vulnerability of atherosclerotic plaques [129,130].

The demonstration that carotid plaques may have enhancement (Figure 17.23) has an implication in the classification of carotid arteries, and a recent study performed in 380 patients showed that carotid artery plaques significantly change according to whether the analysis is performed before or after the administration of contrast material; therefore, the classification of plaque type should be performed in the basal scans [131].

17.2.3.7 Multispectral Imaging

In the past years (see Chapter 1), a new type of CT scanner has been introduced: dual-energy CT. With this technique, it is possible to obtain the attenuation value of a tissue at multiple energy levels and to postprocess a dataset to evaluate the tissue attenuation determined by only one specific keV value [132,133]. In a recently published study [134], the effect of multispectral imaging in carotid artery plaque classification was explored and it was found that the HU values of carotid artery plaques can change according to the selected keV (Figure 17.24); therefore, the HU-based plaque type (fatty and mixed) should be classified according to the energy level applied. With the use of multienergy imaging, the exact definition of the energy level is possible with a consequently improved and reliable classification of the carotid artery plaque type according to the level of energy applied.

17.2.3.8 Other Concepts on Carotid Artery Imaging

17.2.3.8.1 Carotid Artery Wall Thickness

The so-called intima-media thickness (IMT) nowadays represents a powerful parameter for stoke risk

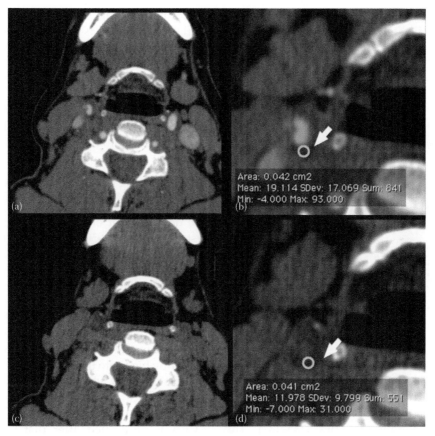

FIGURE 17.23

A 58-year-old male patient with right stroke: the analysis of carotid artery plaques clearly shows that there is contrast plaque enhancement (a, b) after and (c, d) before the administration of contrast material (white arrows). The region-of-interest analysis shows that the contrast plaque enhancement (CPE) is 7 HU.

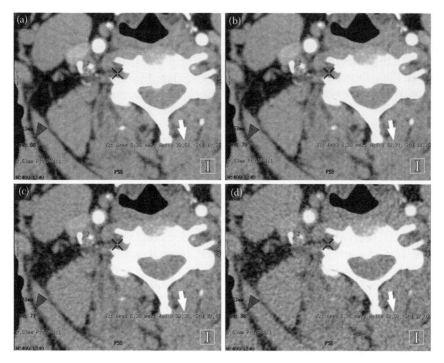

FIGURE 17.24

Effects of different energy levels in carotid artery plaque Hounsfield unit analysis at (a) 66 keV, (b) 70 keV, (c) 77 keV, and (d) 86 keV.

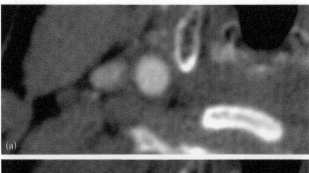

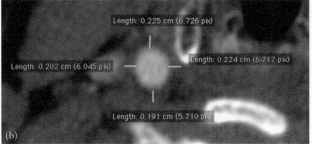

FIGURE 17.25
(a, b) Carotid artery wall thickness analysis.

prediction; several investigations have demonstrated by using ultrasound that an increase in thickness of the wall of carotid arteries is present in several pathologies that are associated with stroke risk [135–137]. The average value of IMT in healthy people ranges from 0.25 to 1 mm [138]. When IMT > 1 mm, the risk of stroke increases. However, it is important to note that the IMT increases by 0.01-0.02 mm per year. One of the limits in IMT analysis by using ultrasound is the low inter-\ intra-observer reproducibility [139]. In the past years, CT has been indicated as the imaging technique for the study of carotid artery wall thickness (CAWT) [140–145]. Using CAWT, Saba et al. [140] showed that a threshold of 1 mm is associated with the presence of stroke with a *p* value of .0001 (Figure 17.25).

17.2.3.8.2 Automated Plaque Volume Analysis

In previous sections, it was explained that a commonly used classification for carotid artery plaques categorizes them into three different groups: fatty plaques, mixed plaques, and calcified plaques. However, in a carotid plaque these three components are usually present all together in different percentages according to the type of the plaque. In fact, carotid artery plaques are extremely complex and multiple elements are visible in them. Some recent studies demonstrated that the volume and percentage of subplaque components may represent a marker of plaque vulnerability. For a reader, it is impossible to calculate the volume in cubic millimeter of the fatty-mixed-calcified components, but recently developed algorithms allow the (semi)automatic measurement of the volume of plaque and the

different percentages of the plaque's components. This kind of information is important because it is now demonstrated that the total volume of a plaque is a better descriptor of the atherosclerotic process and stroke risk than stenosis degree [35]. The use of automated software analysis can further help in the classification of tissue components of plaque, and Wintermark et al. [6] found a κ value of 0.712 between CTA and histology by using specific automatic software.

17.2.4 Imaging of Carotid Arteries after CEA and Interventional Therapy

The development of carotid surgery dates back to the first years of the 1950s (the first terminoterminal anastomosis between CCA and distal ICA was performed in 1954 by Eastcott, Pickering, and Rob and the first CEA in 1953 by Debakey and colleagues). In the CEA after incision, a surgeon has to expose the carotid sheath by dissecting and retracting posteriorly the medial and inner borders of the sternocleidomastoid muscle. A major difficulty is encountered in achieving exposure for lesions extending high into the ICA of patients with high carotid bifurcations, and when exposure is required above the second cervical vertebra it can be necessary to subluxate the mandible.

CEA is performed after that CCA, ECA, and ICA are clamped. Afterward, a procedure of isolation of the internal carotid is performed and with a scalpel blade the surgeon begins an arteriotomy that begins in the CCA and extends into the ICA. Then the surgeon searches for the dissection plane between the internal elastic lamina and the intima to start plaque excision. When normal intima is reached in the CCA, the intima is sharply dissected and transacted so as to allow no loose flap. In some cases, the entire CCA has eccentric thickening, necessitating leaving a small shelf of plaque. Particular attention must be paid in the presence of unstable plaques showing intraplaque hemorrhages or fatty and ulcerated plaques. Then the suture is placed, usually vertically rather than horizontally to avoid constricting the lumen. During the procedure, surgeons can use electroencephalography to determine the need for shunting. Arterial flow is then reactivated, first at the external maxillary artery level to direct a possible microembolization toward the ECA area and finally at the internal carotid level.

Usually after CEA there is no need to perform an image analysis, but it is important to remember that when a CEA is performed the carotid artery intimal layer is removed together with the atherosclerotic plaque. In follow-ups with CTA of patients who underwent a CEA, an increase in vasal lumen with the absence of a visible plaque and the formation of a small pseudoaneurysm is a common finding.

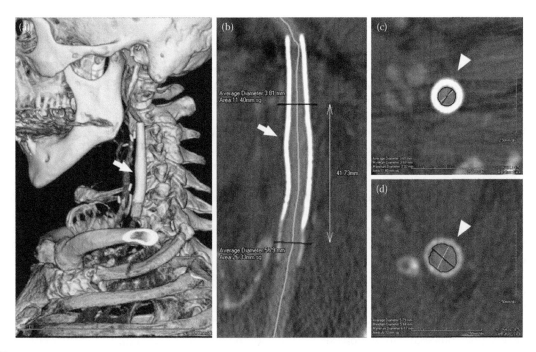

FIGURE 17.26
A 63-year-old male patient who underwent PTA and stent procedure: (a) the volume-rendered postprocessed image shows the position of the stent, whereas the (b) curved-planar reconstruction (CPR) and (c, d) computed tomography angiography (CTA) axial images show the patency of the stent (white arrows). (Courtesy of Michele Anzidei MD, Sapienza University of Rome, Rome, Italy.)

Another approach to treat carotid artery plaques that determine significant stenosis is the interventional approach and, in particular, carotid artery stenting (CAS). Over the past three decades, CAS has evolved to become a promising alternative to CEA, especially for patients deemed to have high surgical risks.

After the placement of a stent, it is important to check the normal patency of the treated vessel (Figure 17.26) and promptly identify the occlusion or res-stenosis of the vessel. CTA can be very helpful in the analysis of carotid artery patency, in particular, by using the new generation of CT scanners that have very high spatial resolutions. Moreover, multispectral imaging is extremely useful because the application of different keV values allows the optimization of visualization of the patent lumen.

17.3 CAD

17.3.1 General

CAD identifies a tear in the wall of the carotid artery, leading to the intrusion of blood within the layers of the arterial wall (intramural hematoma). This pathology is a significant cause of ischemic stroke in all age groups [146]. CAD accounts for a much larger percentage of strokes in young patients, but it occurs most frequently

in the fifth to sixth decade of life [146,147]. Dissection of ICA can occur intracranially or extracranially, with the latter being more frequent [148]. Dissections tend to affect extracranial segments of arteries much more commonly than intracranial segments. The site predilection for CAD is different from that for atherosclerosis: CAD usually involves the pharyngeal and distal parts of ICA, whereas atherosclerosis usually affects the origin and the carotid bulb. Intracranial dissections are usually more severe and carry a poorer prognosis than extracranial dissections: a mortality of 75% has been reported in these dissections. CAD can be caused by major or minor trauma, or it can be spontaneous, in which case genetic, familial, or heritable disorders are likely etiologies. The causes of CAD can be broadly categorized into two classes: "spontaneous" or "traumatic" [149,150].

Spontaneous CAD in the past years was considered uncommon, but nowadays it is an increasingly recognized cause of stroke that preferentially affects middle-age. Its incidence is 2.6–2.9 per 100,000 people [151]. Previous investigations showed that patients with spontaneous CAD may also have a history of stroke in their family and/or hereditary connective tissue disorders, such as autosomal dominant polycystic kidney disease, Marfan syndrome, Ehlers–Danlos syndrome, and fibromuscular dysplasia (FMD); but although an association with connective tissue disorders does exist, most people with spontaneous arterial dissections do not have associated connective tissue disorders [152–154].

Traumatic CAD is commonly determined by severe trauma to the head and/or neck. Up to 0.5% of patients admitted to hospitals after major motor vehicle accidents were found to have CAD [151,155]. Some authors [156] hypothesized that the mechanism of injury for most CAD cases is rapid deceleration, with resultant hyperextension and rotation of the neck, which stretches the carotid artery over the upper cervical vertebrae, producing an intimal tear.

After the CAD, patients can present in a variety of settings, which depends on if the CAD determines an occlusion. It was demonstrated that in patients with CAD, 60% had infarcts documented on neuroimaging [157]. CAD can cause neurological deficits either because of hemodynamic failure (caused by stenosis of the carotid lumen) or by artery-to-artery thromboembolism. When complete occlusion occurs after CAD, it may lead to ischemia; however, even a complete occlusion is totally asymptomatic because bilateral circulation keeps the brain well perfused.

Typical clinical features of CAD can be categorized as local and ischemic. "Local clinical features" include unilateral neck pain, headache, and ipsilateral Horner's syndrome followed by manifestations of cerebral or ocular ischemia and cranial nerve palsies [158–161]. In particular, neck pain and headache usually are the most prominent features of extracranial internal CAD and may be the only manifestations. The pain is usually sharp and may affect the jaw or face, and the headache is usually constant and nonthrobbing. Nearly 50% of people with CAD present with the Horner's syndrome that can occur because the sympathetic fibers that travel along the ICA can be affected in CAD. It is important to note that the syndrome is usually partial and is characterized by ptosis and miosis. Anhidrosis does not occur as fibers for sweat function in the face travel along the ECA. Other symptoms that may occur are pulsatile tinnitus (in about one third of patient) and ipsilateral cranial nerve palsies. In particular, isolated palsies of the hypoglossal nerve and sixth nerve have been reported and taste disturbance and tongue weakness are the most common manifestations, which are the result of compression and ischemia of the seventh nerve because of its proximity to the carotid sheath.

"Ischemic clinical features" (ipsilateral cerebral or retinal ischemia) can be found in 40%–90% of cases [162]. The ischemia may cause TIAs or infarctions, or both. Usually, ischemic signs tend to follow local symptoms by hours to a few days.

Extracranial CADs generally carry a good prognosis with 50% of cases with no neurological deficits,

21% mild deficits, 25% moderate to severe deficits, and the remaining 4% died [163]. The prognosis depends on the severity of the neurological deficit but is generally good in extracranial dissections. The treatment of symptomatic CAD is essentially medical, and neurosurgical interventions are rarely required. Asymptomatic CAD does not require any intervention. The treatment of symptomatic extracranial dissections is essentially medical. As thromboembolism is the most probable mechanism behind a neurological deficit, anticoagulants (heparin and warfarin) and antiplatelets are commonly used, although there have not been any randomized studies to evaluate their effectiveness. Sometimes in the site of CAD an aneurysm may follow, and in this case surgical treatment may be necessary, in particular if the aneurysm is symptomatic.

17.3.2 CTA of CAD

In the past years, DSA had been the method of choice to diagnose CAD; but with the advent of US-ECD, MRA, and CTA, most types of CAD can now be diagnosed noninvasively. Using DSA, the most common finding is the so-called "string sign," a long segment of narrowed lumen. The pathognomonic features of dissection, such as an intimal flap or a double lumen, are found in less than 10% of cases [164,165]. Sometimes, the artery may show sudden tapering because of occlusion of the lumen; aneurysmal dilatations are also found in some cases, but these are usually findings of the chronic phase.

Nowadays, CTA represents a frequently used technique for CAD detection and characterization; in a review by Provenzale and Sarikaya [166], CTA was compared with DSA and the sensitivities for retrospective CTA studies ranged from 64% to 100%, whereas those for prospective studies ranged from 51% to 98%. Specificities for retrospective CTA studies ranged from 82% to 95%, whereas those for prospective studies ranged from 67% to 100% (Figures 17.27 and 17.28). Some authors suggested that the variability in test performance can be explained with the different levels of CT technology used in the different studies. In the past 10 years, significant advances have been made in CT technology from hardware and software points of view. In the study of CT detection of CAD, 2D and 3D visualization methods are routinely used to create images comparable to those acquired with conventional angiography [167].

In CTA studies, unenhanced and enhanced CT of the whole length of carotid and VAs should be performed. In the scan obtained before the administration of contrast material, CAD is visible as a hyperdense

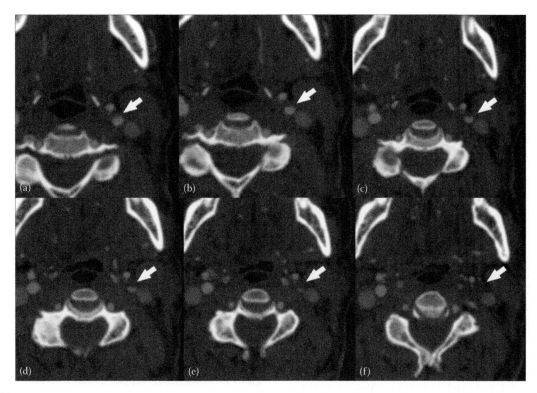

FIGURE 17.27
Carotid artery dissection (CAD) in a 37-year-old female patient: The (a–f) CTA axial images show the progressive dissection of ICA (white arrows).

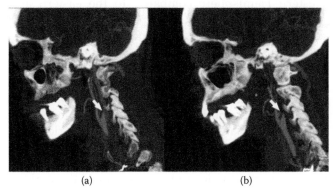

(a)   (b)

FIGURE 17.28
CAD in a 37-year-old female patient: The (a, b) MIP postprocessed images show the typical morphology of the dissection of the carotid artery.

area within the carotid artery, the so-called crescent-shaped sign [168], whereas in other cases in the basal scan there are no findings that can be due to CAD. The crescent-shaped hyperattenuating area corresponds to a wall hematoma. It is important to note that the window parameters are fundamental to identify the crescent-shaped sign because when incorrect window settings are applied intramural hematoma appears isoattenuating to the surrounding muscles and cannot

be distinguished. After the administration of contrast material, CAD is characterized by a narrow eccentric lumen with an increase in external diameter of the carotid. Sometimes, it is possible to find the typical "target" [168] picture when there is a narrow eccentric lumen surrounded by crescent-shaped mural thickening and thin annular enhancement. Some authors hypothesize that the peripheral enhancement occurring after the administration of contrast material is due to the contrast medium that enters the vasa vasorum at the adventitial layer. The presence of an intimal flap and the identification of true and false lumen are rare. Sometimes CTA can identify an aneurysm with dissection, but this condition usually occurs in the chronic stages.

In CTA analysis, some errors can occur in the diagnosis. A typical interpretation error is atherosclerotic luminal narrowing and arterial wall thickening, which are relatively commonly noted as causes of a false-positive interpretation of CTA studies. Moreover, the presence of ulcers sometimes may determine confusion in the radiologists because the presence of a collection of contrast material within the plaque (and outside of the expected location of the arterial lumen) and apparently separated from the arterial contrast enhancement by an intimal flap can closely simulate an arterial dissection. Streak artifacts caused by dental amalgam can also be a cause of a false-positive CTA examination for dissection, as well as beam hardening from dense contrast material within the venous phase causing obscuration of arteries.

17.3.3 Differential Diagnosis

Other pathological conditions may mimic CAD, and this condition should be differentiated from FMD, Takayasu arteritis (TA), dysgenesis of the ICA, Behcet's disease (BD), and other causes of arterial wall thickening (atherosclerosis, radiation treatment, and vasculitis).

Dysgenesis of the ICA: the prevalence of hypoplasia and congenital absence of the ICA is 0.13% [169]. Dysgenesis of the ICA may mimic occlusion or long stenosis of the ICA. The diagnosis is suggested when the carotid canal is absent or hypoplastic.

FMD: FMD is a vascular disease affecting small- to medium-sized vessels with a prevalence of 0.6%–1.1%. Usually, FMD occurs in young women. It is most frequently found in renal arteries (60%–75%) and craniocervical arteries (25%–30%). Most lesions occur adjacent to the C1-C2 space [170]. Bilateral involvement of cervical ICA is reported in 65% of cases. VA involvement is less common (10%) and frequently coexists with carotid disease. The classic hallmark of this pathology is the presence of tubular, multifocal stenosis with adjacent dilatations, the so-called "string-of-beads" sign [171,172].

TA: this is a pathology that affects large vessels, usually the aorta (and its main branches) and the pulmonary arteries. It is a chronic inflammatory disease that primarily involves the media and adventitia of vessel walls and thus results in luminal abnormalities [173,174]. It is considered a rare condition with a prevalence of 2.6 per million and most of the affected patients are young women. Of the extracranial arteries, the CCA and the subclavian artery are often affected over long segments on both sides.

Giant cell arteritis: the incidence of this pathology, which usually affects patients older than 50 years of age, is 20 per 100,000. It is an inflammatory disease that primarily involves internal elastic lamina [228], and its most typical manifestation is headache [175]. Any portion of the extradural arterial circulation within the head and neck may be involved because carotid arteries and VAs contain an internal elastic

lamina from the aortic arch up to 5 mm after their point of entry into the dura mater [176,177]. In the differential diagnosis with the CAD can be helpful to remember that the carotid siphon is most severely affected and the cervical segment is only rarely involved.

BD: this is an inflammatory disease that affects patients in the third and fourth decades of life, and it is characterized by uveitis and oral and genital ulcerations [178–180]. Behçet usually affects large vessels and histologically is characterized by a vasculitis of the vasa vasorum.

17.4 Glomus Tumor

17.4.1 General Introduction

The glomus tumor (GT) (also known as "solitary glomus tumor," "solid glomus tumor," or "glomangioma") is a rare benign neoplasm arising from the glomus body [181,182]. In 1742, von Haller described the carotid body as a glomus body–like structure situated just inferior to the carotid bifurcation. GTs were first described by Hoyer in 1877 and later by Masson in 1924. Incidence of GTs is higher in the Western Hemisphere compared to the eastern and more in female patients. GTs are associated with both von Hippel–Lindau disease and multiple endocrine neoplasia II. GTs are true neoplasms that arise from paraganglionic chemoreceptor cells. These paraganglia are distributed symmetrically and segmentally in the para-axial regions of the trunk. On the basis of anatomical distribution, innervation, and microscopic structure, they are grouped into branchiomeric, intravagal, aortosympathetic, and visceral-autonomic paraganglia. Paragangliomas can be subdivided into two groups: sympathetic and parasympathetic derived tumors. Virtually all GTs arise from the parasympathetic nervous system.

Paragangliomas can be familial or nonfamilial. Investigations found that germ line mutations in mitochondrial complex II genes, *SDHB*, *SDHC*, and *SDHD*, cause hereditary paragangliomas [183]. Mutations in *SDHD* and *SDHB* accounted for 70% of familial cases and approximately 8% of nonfamilial cases. *SDHD* mutations predispose to PGL-1, mutations in an unidentified gene on chromosome 11 to PGL-2, *SDHC* mutations to PGL-3, and *SDHB* mutations to PGL-4.

Hypoxia determined by high altitudes induces hyperplasia of the chemoreceptor tissue. This is reflected in the difference in volume of the carotid body at sea level, which is about 20 mg, and at high altitude, which is about 60 mg [184]. Authors [185] found that at high altitudes carotid body tumors are about 10 times more frequent than in the same population living at sea level.

In 80% of cases the most common presenting symptom of GT is pulsatile tinnitus, followed by hearing loss in 60% of cases [186]. Other symptoms can Browne's sign (up to 30% of cases) and cranial nerve deficit (deficits of ninth and tenth nerves are most commonly seen, but seventh, eighth, eleventh, and twelfth nerves can also be affected). Only a small percentage of these patients will suffer symptoms due to vasoactivity such as palpitation, hypertension, and flushing. Usually, GTs are benign neoplasms; malignant forms of paraganglioma are more frequent in the case of functioning GTs, more particularly in cases of tumors that secrete dopamine. Some authors [187,188] found that GTs arising in the vicinity of the organ of Zuckerkandl have the highest malignant potential. This neoplasm is highly vascular, and these characteristics are reflected in the enlargement of the feeding arteries, the intense staining of the tumor, and a rapid venous drainage.

GTs can present as a cervical mass, and these tumors cause splaying of the carotid bifurcation. The ICA usually becomes displaced posterolaterally and the ECA anterolaterally or anteromedially [189]. Sometimes, GTs can cause the encasement of ICA. The "Shamblin classification" graded GTs according to their position in type I tumors that are defined as localized in between internal and external carotid arteries and can be easily resected. Type II tumors are adherent to or partially surround the vessels, and type III tumors completely encase the carotids. This classification is important because it is associated with the degree of difficulty of resection of GTs. The morbidity related to surgical resection for Shamblin types I and II carotid body tumors is lower than that for type III tumors, the incidence of cerebrovascular complications is less than 5%, and permanent cranial nerve impairment occurs in approximately 20% for type III tumors [190,191].

17.4.2 CTA

Among the different imaging techniques US-ECD is usually performed to explore patients with cervical masses, but the role of color Doppler ultrasound in the diagnostic work-up of paragangliomas is limited because only a limited area of the neck can be investigated. After US-ECD, MR and CT are performed to better characterize the lesions. Some authors hypothesize that MR can provide more diagnostic information than CT because of the former's better soft-tissue contrasts compared with the latter. However, nowadays CT (especially CTA) also offers excellent diagnostic potentiality in the detection/characterization of GTs.

GTs are hypervascular, and CT appearance reflects this condition (Figures 17.29 and 17.30). In fact, after the administration of contrast material a GT shows homogeneous and intense enhancement. In the arterial phase, it is possible to identify a big ascending pharyngeal artery that is considered "the artery of the paraganglioma." However, occipital artery, posterior auricular artery, muscular branches of the VA and deep cervical artery, and thyrocervical trunk can also contribute to vascularization. As previously described, this neoplasm can cause the splaying of carotid bifurcation. Sometimes, when the diagnosis is not yet clear a DSA can confirm the diagnosis. The differential diagnosis for GTs should include lymph nodes, salivary gland tumors, schwannomas, or an aneurysm of the cervical ICA.

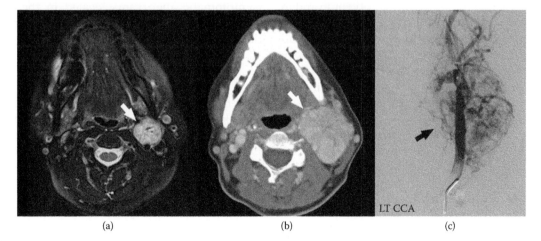

(a) (b) (c)

FIGURE 17.29
A 61-year-old male patient: (a) a magnetic resonance (MR) axial image obtained in 2008 that shows the glomic neoplasm (white arrow), and (b) CTA axial images obtained in 2012 indicating the dimensional increase of the glomic tumor (white arrow). The diagnosis is confirmed with (c) diagnostic angiography (black arrow). (Courtesy of Eytan Raz MD, Lanngone University, New York.)

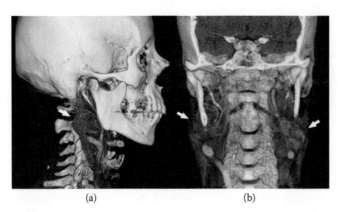

(a)   (b)

FIGURE 17.30
A 58-year-old male patient with bilateral glomic tumor clearly visible (white arrows) in (a, b) volume-rendered postprocessed images. (Courtesy of Michele Anzidei MD, Sapienza University of Rome, Rome, Italy.)

17.5 Extracranial Carotid Artery Aneurysm

17.5.1 General Introduction

Extracranial carotid artery aneurysm (ECAA) is a rare pathology with a prevalence of 0.2%–0.4% among aneurysms in general [192]. Some authors consider ECAA as localized increases of the caliber of more than 50% compared with the reference values of ICA (0.55 ± 0.06 cm in men; 0.49 ± 0.07 in women) [193]. This condition is extremely rare, and the largest, single-center study to date was carried out by the Texas Heart Institute (THI), Houston, Texas, between 1960 and 1995 with only 67 cases.

Sometimes, in the physical examination it is possible to find an increased left carotid artery pulse. Its most common location is at the level of the carotid bulb and in the proximal internal carotid [194], and the treatment of choice is open surgery with exclusion of aneurysm and restoration of circulation through a graft. They can be classified according to their different physiopathologies into "true" or "false" aneurysms. False aneurysms are less frequent, and they are responsible for only 14% of ECAA. Usually, false aneurysms are secondary to previous CEA with the onset of symptoms ranging from 1 month to 15 years after the original carotid procedure [193]. False aneurysms can also be determined by infections (recurrent tonsillitis or pharyngitis reaching the carotid artery wall, following peritonsillar abscess with subsequent ischemia of the wall leading to acute rupture) and trauma (stab wounds, car accidents, iatrogenic like the central venous cannulation). Sometimes, false aneurysms can be determined by Eagle syndrome (see Section 17.6.5), which is abnormal elongation of the styloid process associated with calcification of the

stylohyoid ligament [243]. True aneurysms are most commonly due to atherosclerosis or FMD.

ECAA can be classified according to its etiology into atherosclerotic (the most common, up to 40% of all cases), dysplastic, infective, post-traumatic, and iatrogenic [195]. Other rare contributing factors to ECAA formation include neck irradiation, neurofibromatosis, Marfan syndrome, Behcet's syndrome, and TA.

Atherosclerotic degeneration is assumed to be the most frequent cause of ECAA, and usually patients aged 50–70 years old are more frequently affected (with a male–female ratio of 1.9:1) [196,197]. Usually, atherosclerotic aneurysms affect the common artery bifurcation and the proximal ICA with a size ranging from 1.5 to 5.0 cm.

Infective cause, first described by Liston in 1843, used to be the main cause of ECAA, but nowadays it is quite uncommon because of the introduction of antibiotics. *Staphylococcus aureus* and *Streptococcus pyogenes* are the most common infection agents [198–200].

Many cases remain asymptomatic until ischemic neurological symptoms appear (about 35% of ECAA appears with neurological deficit), so their early detection and treatment are important [201,202] and the natural history of ECAA is associated with spontaneous progression of the aneurysm, most commonly associated with a high risk of neurological thromboembolic events and cranial nerve compression and, more rarely, rupture [203]. Most of the neurological symptoms are secondary to TIA, stroke, or ischemic retinopathy by embolisms. However, other compressions of the aneurysm on surrounding structures may determine other symptoms. With respect to treatment, surgery (resection or endovascular treatment) is indicated in most cases because the risk of vascular events in patients managed conservatively is over 50%. Conservative treatment is considered only in cases of very small or asymptomatic aneurysms located in the most distal section, near the base of the skull, due to the high surgical risk involved.

17.5.2 CTA

The first diagnosis of ECAA is usually performed with ultrasound, which is then confirmed by CTA or MRA. The purpose of CTA is to delineate extension, detect stenosis, and help during surgical planning. The morphology of the aneurysm, saccular or fusiform, should be described to offer further information to plan the therapeutic approach (Figure 17.31). To correctly characterize ECAA, it is useful to postprocess axial source images by selecting MPR planes oriented perpendicular to the long axis of the aneurysm. Sometimes, thrombotic components can be found. It is important to know the clinical history of patients and to verify a previous CEA because usually a dilatation is visible [204].

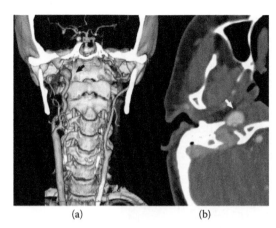

(a) (b)

FIGURE 17.31
A 68-year-old female patient: the (a) volume-rendered postprocessed image shows an aneurysm of the distal portion of the extracranial ICA (black arrow). The aneurysm (white arrow) is also visible in the (b) CTA axial image. (Courtesy of Michele Anzidei MD, Sapienza University of Rome, Rome, Italy.)

17.6 Other Pathologies of the Carotid Artery

17.6.1 FMD

FMD is an idiopathic, segmental, noninflammatory, and nonatherosclerotic vascular disease of small- to medium-sized arteries that most commonly affects the renal and carotid arteries but has been described in almost every arterial bed in the body [205,206]. The first histologically proved case of FMD of the carotid artery was reported by Connett and Lansche in 1965. Little is known about the epidemiology of cervical and intracranial FMD. The exact frequency of the disease is difficult to assess because many cases are asymptomatic. According to different authors, the prevalence of FMD ranges from 0.2% to 3% [207,208]. Investigations have demonstrated that extracervical FMD is less common that renal FMD. Stanley et al. [209,210] found a prevalence of 9% of extracranial carotid or VA dysplasia among 196 patients with renal FMD and in a study of 92 patients it was found that 28% of the subjects had FMD involving two or more arterial sites, corresponding most commonly to combined carotid and renal lesions. Intracranial aneurysms are usually considered a frequent finding in patients with carotid or vertebral FMD, with prevalence ranging from 20% to 50%.

Macroscopically FMD is characterized by alternating areas of thickening and thinning of the arterial wall, with mural aneurysms, and histologically FMD lesions are heterogeneous, with various degrees of collagen hyperplasia, internal elastic lamina rupture, and disorganization of the media layer. Pathologists classify FMD into three types (intimal-medial-adventitial FMD) according to the dominant arterial wall layer involved.

"Intimal FMD" accounts for 10% of all FMD lesions. It corresponds to the circumferential or eccentric deposition of collagen in the intima. Intimal FMD occurs primarily in children and adolescents. "Medial FMD" accounts for 80% of all FMD lesions. In this type, histological analysis reveals alternating areas of thinned media and thickened fibromuscular ridges containing collagen, resulting in multiple stenoses alternating with aneurysmal outpouchings. This subtype offers the characteristic aspect of a string of beads. "Adventitial FMD" is uncommon (<1%); histologically, the fibrous tissue of the adventitia is replaced by dense collagen, whereas the other arterial layers and elastic lamina remain intact.

FMD is associated with focal ischemic symptoms due to either a thromboembolic mechanism or a hemodynamic compromise of distal circulation. Moreover, some patients can develop complications of this disorder, including aneurysms, spontaneous CAD, carotid-cavernous fistulas, or vertebral arteriovenous fistulas [211–215].

CTA can exquisitely identify FMD, and there is no more need to use DSA to perform this type of diagnosis [216,217]. FMD involves ICA (95%), often bilaterally (60%–85%), and affects the middle and distal portions of ICA at the levels of the C1 and C2 vertebrae: this is an important element for differential diagnosis because these levels are not usually affected by atherosclerotic disease.

By using CTA, it is possible to distinguish four main FMD subtypes: the "multifocal-type FMD," with multiple stenoses and a string-of-beads appearance (Figure 17.32) is the most common angiographic subtype, and it is generally associated with medial FMD on histology. "Unifocal-type FMD" includes the "tubular" subtype, corresponding to a long concentric stenosis, and the "focal" type, corresponding to a short isolated stenosis of 1 cm in length. These unifocal subtypes cannot be related to specific histological lesions, although intimal FMD seems to be more common. Finally, up to 20% of patients have "mixed-type FMD" stenoses.

Some authors attribute to FMD unilateral involvement of the arterial wall ranging from a corrugated diverticulum-like outpouching with noncircumferential narrowing to a true aneurysm. However, this subtype has not been proved to correspond with FMD histologically and is likely to correspond with acute dissecting aneurysm or the aftermath of a dissection.

17.6.2 TA

TA was first described in 1908 and named in 1942 [218]. TA is considered a rare condition with a prevalence of 2.6 per million; it has a much higher incidence in women than in men and is most frequently found

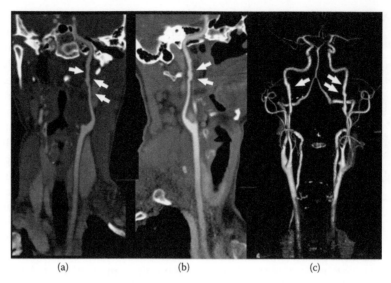

(a)   (b)   (c)

FIGURE 17.32
A 48-year-old female patient with fibromuscular dysplasia (FMD): panels (a) and (b) give CPR postprocessed images that show the string-of-beads appearance (white arrows). The volume-rendered postprocessed images confirm the bilateral involvement of ICAs. (Courtesy of Eytan Raz MD, Lanngone University, New York.)

in Asian patients, although the condition may occur in North American, European, African, and Middle Eastern patients also [219]. TA is a rare, idiopathic chronic inflammatory disease of unknown etiology, which determines a granulomatous panarteritis that mainly affects large vessels (aorta, pulmonary arteries, and carotids). In patients with TA, 95% had aortic involvement with or without aortic branch involvement, whereas 5% had only aortic branch involvement. TA determines the destruction of arterial media, with secondary aneurysm formation. Histopathologically, early TA changes are characterized by the presence of adventitial mononuclear infiltrates with perivascular cuffing of the vasa vasorum, followed by medullary mononuclear inflammation [220–222]. Intimal hyperplasia, the result of myofibroblast proliferation, is followed by fibrosis of the tunica media and intima, leading to stenosis and, on occasion, thrombosis. Some authors found that in 15%–20% of lesions, local destruction of the medial layer predominates and this, combined with an inadequate fibrotic response, results in dilatation and aneurysm formation.

TA typically presents with nonspecific systemic signs and symptoms such as arthralgia, fever, fatigue, headaches, rashes (including erythema nodosum), and weight loss. Chronic inflammation of the aorta and its major branches, including subclavian, common carotid, coronary, pulmonary, and renal arteries, may result in localized stenoses, vascular occlusion, dilatation, and aneurysm formation. In TA of carotid arteries, vessel wall thickening and stenosis are the most common findings, but aneurysmal dilatations occur less frequently [223,224]. Cerebral ischemia may occur

in up to 16% of patients with TA and can be due to several mechanisms such as subclavian steal in the arm, vessel stenosis/occlusion, and embolism from the aorta or the heart.

However, only a small percentage of patients experience a self-limiting monophasic inflammatory episode, which does not require chronic immunosuppressive therapy and does not progress to the occlusive stage.

The gold standard for the diagnosis of TA is considered to be histology, but histopathologic specimens are seldom available and therefore the diagnosis of TA is largely based on the combination of laboratory evaluation clinical information and diagnostic imaging. Therefore, a knowledge of the radiologic features of TA is essential for accurate diagnosis and early treatment.

In the past years angiography was widely used for the diagnosis of TA, but nowadays CTA and magnetic resonance imaging (MRI) are commonly used as the diagnostic techniques of choice. In particular, CTA can evaluate both the vessel wall and the lumen and may thus show vessel wall alterations when the lumen is still unaffected on angiography (Figure 17.33). In early TA some authors demonstrated that CTA may show arterial wall thickening with mural enhancement and low-attenuation rings on delayed images, whereas advanced-stage CTA shows the typical late-stage complications, including vessel stenosis, occlusion, and aneurysm.

Some authors hypothesize that CTA may have a role in monitoring the disease course. Aortic wall enhancement was shown to resolve after immunosuppressive therapy in 50% of patients with TA.

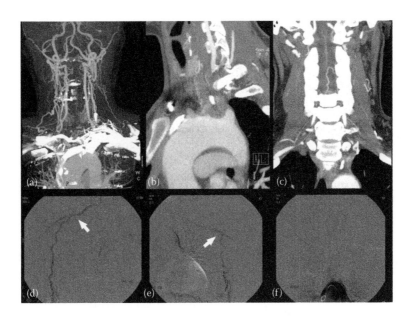

FIGURE 17.33
A 45-year-old female patient with Takayasu arteritis: in panels (a) and (b), complete occlusion of supra-aortic vessels is visible with the head flow given by filling of carotids and vertebral through collaterals. In panel (c), anterior spinal artery and deep cervical quite enlarged. In panels (d) and (e), the right and left T8 intercostal arteries to mammary to subclavian to vertebral is shown (white arrows). The aortic arch is visible in panel (f). (Courtesy of Eytan Raz MD, Lanngone University, New York.)

17.6.3 BD

BD is defined as a chronic, relapsing, multisystemic disorder characterized by mucocutaneous, ocular, vascular, and central nervous system manifestations. This pathology was first described by the Greek ophthalmologist Benediktos Adamantiades during the annual meeting of the Medical Association of Athens on November 15, 1930 [225,226]. The prevalence of BD is higher in the Mediterranean area and eastern Asia with 80–370 cases per 100,000 population in Turkey, 10 per 100,000 in Japan, and 0.6 per 100,000 in Yorkshire, United Kingdom. In common with ankylosing spondylitis and psoriatic arthropathy, BD has major histocompatibility complex class I associations. HLA-B51 is the most strongly associated known genetic factor of BD. It has a much higher incidence in men than in women (male–female ratio is 7:1). BD usually affects subjects between 18 and 40 years.

The pathogenesis of BD remains poorly understood, and some authors hypothesize that autoimmune or auto-inflammatory syndromes and infectious (in particular *Streptococcus sanguis*) and/or environmental factors are able to trigger BD in individuals with particular genetic variants. Investigations have demonstrated that streptococcal antigens increase interleukin-6 and interferon-γ production by peripheral blood T cells from BD patients and cross-react with a 65 kD heat shock protein sharing antigenicity with oral mucosal antigens.

Some main clinical features occur in BD: mucocutaneous lesions, eye lesions, vascular lesions, neurological manifestation, and articular manifestation. In vascular involvement, three types of manifestation are described: venous thrombosis, arterial wall involvement, and cardiac involvement. In BD, arterial involvement is seen in 3%–5% of cases [227].

The incidence is probably underestimated because an autopsy survey showed that 33% of patients had arterial lesions most of which had been asymptomatic. Thrombosis and/or aneurysms are observed, mainly false aneurysms. These arterial aphthae are localized on carotid arteries, pulmonary arteries, the aorta, and renal and peripheral arteries. They can rupture suddenly. Vascular surgery is mandatory, but thrombosis of the graft and relapses of aneurysms at the site of bypass are frequent.

17.6.4 Giant Cell Arteritis

Giant cell arteritis (GCA), first described by Horton in 1932, is a systemic vasculitis usually affecting the superficial temporal artery (STA) and the extraocular parts of the central retinal, posterior ciliary, and ophthalmic arteries. Less common is the involvement of other branches of ECA, axillary artery, internal carotid, vertebral and coronary arteries, and the aorta [228]. GCA is considered a large-vessel vasculitis (according to the Chapel Hill Consensus Conference, Chapel Hill, NC, large-vessel vasculitis syndromes include GCA and TA).

This pathology usually affects patients older than 50 years of age (women:men = 2:1), and the incidence increases with age and peaks in groups of patients older than 70 years. The prevalence is 20 per 100,000. It is an inflammatory disease that primarily involves internal elastic lamina [228], and the most typical manifestation is headache [175]. Any portion of the extradural arterial circulation within the head and neck may be involved because carotid arteries and VAs contain an internal elastic lamina from the aortic arch up to 5 mm after their point of entry into the dura mater [176,177]. Prompt diagnosis and treatment are preconditions for the prevention of serious vascular complications, particularly visual loss. Up to now, temporal artery biopsy is the gold standard for the diagnosis of GCA.

In its best known form, GCA affects ECA and its major extracranial branches, leading to the classical symptoms of temporal headache, scalp tenderness, jaw claudication, and tender temporal arteries. It is noted that 20% of patients can suffer ocular ischemia with ensuing anterior ischemic optic neuropathy, leading to irreversible vision loss in 10%–15% of cases. Stroke, albeit rare, is a grave and sometimes fatal complication of GCA. Collazos et al. [229] described a case of a patient with a GCA that had a bilateral infarction in the distribution of posterior cerebral arteries.

In patients with GCA, a systemic inflammatory response can be found; it is usually reflected by fever, malaise, anorexia, weight loss, anemia, and thrombocytosis. In laboratory examinations, high erythrocyte sedimentation rates and C-reactive protein levels are typically seen in patients with GCA.

Modern imaging has taken center stage over the last years in the search for broadly applicable tools to establish or exclude the diagnosis of GCA. Some authors suggest that the use of ultrasound can be important because the presence of a hypoechogenic wall thickening around the temporal artery (the so-called "halo-sign") is usually present in patients affected by GCA [230]. Another frequently used imaging technique is MRA because, thanks to the use of TOF sequences, it can easily detect the presence of stenosis in the ICA [231]. In the past years, CTA did not play a significant role in the diagnosis because of the difficulties in detecting the small stenoses that are usually visible in distal ICA. When the carotid artery is affected, CTA may show small stenoses, which are easily visible with CTA MIP postprocessing techniques. It is important to remember that GCA usually affects the carotid siphon, and this is important for differential diagnosis with other pathologies. However, this position represents also the most severe limit of CTA diagnosis in the case of GCA because the bones may obscure ICA at this level and hide the stenosis that allows one to reach the diagnosis of GCA [232]. Dual-energy CT systems with automated bone removal function can solve this kind of problems and show distal ICA without the superimposition of bones.

17.6.5 Eagle Syndrome

Eagle syndrome refers to a clinical syndrome determined by the abnormal elongation of the styloid process associated with the calcification of the stylohyoid ligament [233,237]. The styloid process is an elongated conical projection of the temporal bone that lies anteriorly to the mastoid process that arises embryonically from the second brachial arch, also known as "Reichert cartilage." The Reichert cartilage is divided into four levels based on the subsequent development of the stylohyoid complex (tympanohyal-stylohyal-ceratohyal). The styloid process serves as a point of attachment for the stylohyoid ligament and the stylomandibular ligament, as well as the styloglossus, stylohyoid, and stylopharyngeus muscles. In the general population, the distribution of styloid process length falls into a bimodal distribution, with approximately one quarter of the surveyed processes measuring <20 mm and three quarters measuring >20 mm. Usually, when the length of an elongated styloid process is more than 3.0 cm, it is considered to be elongated.

The prevalence of abnormal elongation of the styloid process is quite variable according to different publications, but it has been estimated to be 4% of the general population. However, only a small subset of patients with an elongated styloid process ever experiences any symptoms. The abnormal elongation of the styloid process is usually bilateral, but symptoms generally appear on only one side. Stylocarotid compression, typically involving ICA, results in various symptomatic presentations. Usually asymptomatic, it occurs in adult patients ranging from 30 to 50 years. Females are affected more often than males.

Symptoms range from pain or sensation of a foreign body in the throat to stroke and possibly even sudden death [234,236]. Sometimes, Eagle syndrome may determine the development of a pseudoaneurysm [235]. In the original publication of 1937, Eagle described two forms of the syndrome: the "classic form" and the "stylocarotid form." The classic form is commonly found in patients after tonsillectomy, although it can occur in patients without a history of pharyngeal surgery, where it is easier for the development of compression of cranial nerves V, VII, IX, and X by the elongated styloid process. Patients usually describe cervicofacial pain, dysphagia, vertigo, tinnitus, and sensation of a foreign body in the throat. The stylocarotid form, which is also described by Eagle, is attributed to the impingement of ICA or ECA by a laterally or medially deviated styloid process caused by the stimulation of the sympathetic nerve plexus associated with the artery. In the case of impingement of ICA, pain is referred along the course of the ICA and includes parietal headache as well as eye pain.

Patients may also suffer cluster headache or migraine. Impingement and stimulation of the ECA plexus causes pain in the face below the eyes. However, sometimes neurological symptoms (phasia, visual disturbances, weakness, and syncope) can also occur when there is compression of ICA/ECA with the consequent interruption of blood flow. In particular, TIAs can occur in patients with an elongated styloid process on turning their head, and the TIA usually resolves once their head is returned to the neutral position [235,236]. A rare event that can occur in Eagle syndrome is the direct mechanical damage of the carotid artery wall cased by the impingement of the elongated styloid process with consequent CAD.

The pathogenesis of Eagle syndrome is still being debated. Some authors hypothesize that surgical trauma or local chronic irritation can cause osteitis and periostitis of the stylohyoid complex with consequent reactive ossifying hyperplasia [237,238], whereas others suggest that the anatomic anomaly of the styloid process can be genetically transmitted as a recessive autosomal character. Ossification of the stylohyoid ligament should also be related to endocrine disorders in postmenopausal women [240]. Abnormal development of the styloid process is also associated with malformation of the atlanto-occipital hinge [239].

Eagle syndrome should be suspected in individuals with symptoms of stylocarotid compression and can be suggested by characteristic CT findings (Figures 17.34

and 17.35), most pertinently a heavily ossified and calcified styloid process. In Eagle syndrome, CTA is considered the gold standard because it offers the opportunity to study the styloid process and its relationship with the carotid artery. CTA should be used to determine the length of the styloid process (in particular using

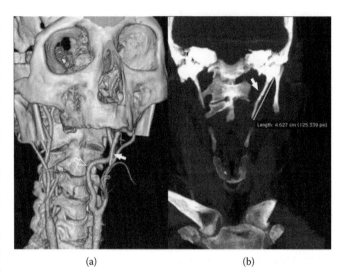

(a)   (b)

FIGURE 17.34
Eagle syndrome in a 49-year-old female patient: the (a) volume-rendered image shows the abnormal length of the styloid process (white arrow) and its relationship with the carotid artery (white open arrow). With (b) curved MIP, the entire length of the styloid process is measurable (46 mm).

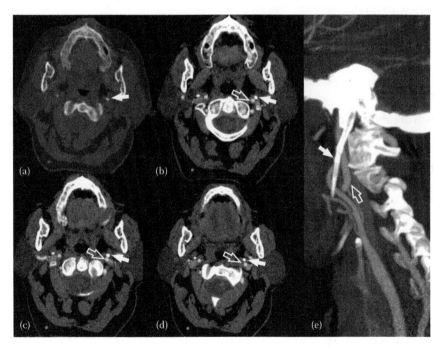

FIGURE 17.35
Eagle syndrome in a 49-year-old female patient (same as in Figure 17.26): in computed tomography, un-enhanced scan (a) is visible the styloid process (white open arrow) at the level of the ramus of the mandible. In (b–d) CTA axial scans, the styloid process and its relationship with the carotid artery is visible (styloid process = white arrow, ICA = white open arrow). The (e) MIP postprocessed image shows the abnormal length of the styloid process (white arrow) and the relationship with the carotid artery (white open arrow).

3D postprocessing techniques). The normal length of the styloid process is about 2.5 cm, and a length greater than 3 cm is considered to be elongated. Moreover, CTA should be explored regarding the relationship of the styloid process with the carotid wall by determining its compression. Chuang et al. [236] in a case of a patient with reversible left TIA caused by the elongation of the styloid process performed a CTA of the neck with the patient's head in the neutral position and a second CTA with the head oriented to the left and downward, in a position that was previously seen to elicit the patient's symptoms by showing that the left styloid process was compressing the carotid artery and no definite contrast material was found in the ICA. With the head in the neutral position, both internal carotids were widely patent. Therefore, in the case of symptomatic patients with an elongated styloid process a further acquisition with their heads in the non-neutral position is suggested.

17.7 Vertebral Arteries

The pathology of VAs is not uncommon, and therefore it is extremely important to correctly explore these arteries and characterize their alterations. In particular, imaging analysis of VAs is performed for dissection that usually occurs after trauma. However, other conditions can occur like aneurysm, pseudoaneurysm, and hypoplasia. In the study of VAs, CTA is an optimal technique because it allows the detection and characterization of their alterations.

17.7.1 Anatomy and Variants

VAs are the first branch of subclavian arteries and merge to form the single midline basilar artery in a complex called the vertebrobasilar system, which supplies blood to the posterior part of the circle of Willis. VAs, after originating from the subclavian arteries, one on each side of the body, enter the transverse process of the level of the sixth cervical vertebrae (in less than 10% of cases in C7). Then VAs proceed superiorly in the transverse foramen of each cervical vertebra until C1 when the VAs travel across the posterior arch of the atlas through the suboccipital triangle before entering the foramen magnum. Inside the skull, the two VAs join to form the basilar artery at the base of the medulla oblongata.

In up to 12% of the population, one VA is atretic (<2 mm in diameter) and makes little contribution to basilar artery flow. Lesser degrees of asymmetry are also frequent. In about 50% of the population, the left VA is larger than the right one; the right is larger in 25%, and only in the remaining quarter of cases are the two VAs of similar caliber. In 6% of cases, the left VA arises directly from the aortic arch. Unlike ICA, which is almost a direct extension of its parent vessel CCA, the VA branches almost at right angles to its feeding vessel. The normal diameter of the VA is between 3 and 5 mm.

The VA may be divided into four segments: "V1" (preforaminal), "V2" (foraminal), "V3" (from the second cervical vertebra to dura), and "V4" (intradural). In its intradural section, the VA pierces the dura and arachnoid mater at the base of the skull and ends as it meets its opposite VA to form the midline basilar artery at the level of the medullopontine junction.

The branches of VA may be divided into two sets: cervical branches (spinal arteries and muscular arteries) and cranial braches (meningeal arteries, posterior spinal arteries, anterior spinal arteries, posterior inferior cerebellar arteries, and medullary arteries).

Some anatomical variants can occur in the VA, and the most frequent are duplication and fenestration. The term duplication indicates an artery with two origins and a variable level of fusion in the neck, whereas fenestration represents a vessel with a single origin and two parallel segments anywhere along its course. Fenestration of VAs is identified in 0.23%–1.95% of angiographies, and duplication of the extracranial segments of VAs is rare. Both duplication and fenestration arise as a result of failed involution of fetal vessels.

17.7.2 CTA Technique

Techniques for the study of VAs are similar to those used for the study of carotid arteries. In the case of dedicated VA study, the unenhanced phase can be avoided (the unenhanced phase is important only for the analysis of carotid artery intraplaque vascularization. The examination should cover the whole length of the carotid and VAs, and it requires a scanning range from the aortic arch to the circle of Willis. For the other parameter, see Sections 17.1.3 and 17.1.4.

17.7.3 VA Dissections

17.7.3.1 General Information

VA dissection (VAD) indicates a tear in the wall of VAs with the development of intramural hematoma and secondary stenosis of the lumen when blood collects between the intima and the media or an aneurysmal dilatation of the artery when the hematoma predominantly involves the media and the adventitia. The overall incidence of VAD is approximately 1–1.5 per 100,000. Spontaneous VAD accounts for only about 2% of all ischemic strokes, but VAD is an important cause of ischemic stroke in young and middle-aged patients accounting for 10%–25% of such cases. Spontaneous dissections of VAs affect all age groups, including children, but there is a distinct peak in the fifth decade of life. Although there is no overall sex-based predilection, women are on average about 5 years younger than men at the time of dissection.

The pathophysiology of VAD is poorly understood. Possible constitutional factors include connective tissue disorders and genetic predisposition. Environmental factors include major and minor trauma and also recent infection. Extracranial VAD can be spontaneous or traumatic, and most of the traumatic dissections involve the atlantooccipital (V3) segment. Patients with spontaneous VAD are thought to have an underlying structural defect of the arterial wall (Ehlers–Danlos syndrome type IV, Marfan syndrome, autosomal dominant polycystic kidney disease, and osteogenesis imperfecta type I). However, these heritable disorders have been identified in only 1%–5% of patients with spontaneous dissection of VA. Frequently, VAD is associated with minor precipitating events associated with hyperextension or rotation of the neck including practicing yoga, painting a ceiling, coughing, vomiting, sneezing, the receipt of anesthesia, and the act of resuscitation. These neck movements, particularly when they are sudden, may injure the artery as a result of mechanical stretching.

Clinically [240–246], 70% of patients with VAD may present with occipital headache and neck pain, whereas 60% of patients have symptoms of vertebrobasilar circulation ischemia. It is also possible to divide VAD into two types: [1] the ischemic type, which is manifest by ischemic symptoms and/or infarction of vertebrobasilar circulation due to arterial narrowing and thromboembolism; and [2] the hemorrhagic type, which presents as a subarachnoid hemorrhage (SAH) caused by the rupture of an intradural VA dissecting aneurysm.

17.7.3.2 CTA of VAD

In the past years, DSA was considered the gold standard for imaging VAD. A number of terms are used to describe the various radiological appearances of dissections. The typical findings that are possible to find in VAD are the following: the string sign (arising as a result of a dissection that extends circumferentially around the lumen over a long segment), the double lumen sign, pseudoaneurysm formation, or complete occlusion. Stenosis is by far the most common finding resulting in luminal narrowing by subintimal hematoma formation [247–249]. Nowadays, MRI and CTA have become the new reference standards for the study of VAD because of their potentiality to evaluate extraluminal abnormalities and ability to further evaluate patients for a variety of clinical conditions associated with VAD, including stroke, SAH, and cervical spine abnormalities [250]. Although the DSA appearance of VAD is often characteristic, it does not assess the vessel wall for intramural hematoma; because of this feature, dissections in unusual locations or with atypical morphology may be misclassified or attributed to other processes.

In the CTA analysis of suspected VAD, it is possible to recognize some typical DSA findings like string sign and complete VA occlusion (Figure 17.36). Usually, stenosis is the most common finding that is caused by the intrawall hematoma. The identification of VAD should

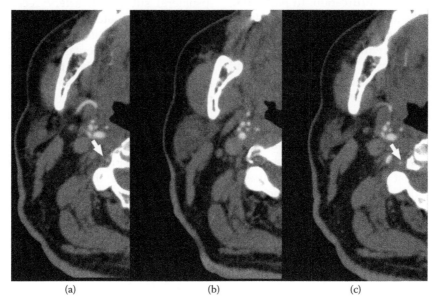

(a)   (b)   (c)

FIGURE 17.36
A 47-year-old female patient with right vertebral artery dissection (shown at different levels, (a), (b), and (c).

be performed when there is evidence of normal caliber of VA that suddenly becomes small or completely
occluded. Sometimes it is possible to find inside the VA
a hyperdense spot in the unenhanced scans that represent fresh hemorrhage (like the dissection of the carotid
artery). Some further findings have been described in
the CTA analysis of VAD. In particular, Lum et al. [250]
described cases of VAD in the segment between C2 foramen transversaria and foramen magnum (V3 segment)
in which lumen diameter was normal in caliber and the
only visible abnormality was a dorsal thickening of the
arterial wall against the adjacent fat; they called this the
"suboccipital rind" sign. The authors suggested that this
sign is a highly characteristic CTA finding of vessel wall
hematoma in the V3 portion. However, caution must be
exercised when abnormalities are detected in the V3
portion of the artery because the course of the obliquus
capitis inferioris muscle passes directly posterior to the
artery at the posterolateral aspect of the C1 arch and
the proximity of the anterior aspect of the muscle to the
posterior arterial wall could potentially lead to inaccu-
racies regarding arterial wall diameter in this location.
Moreover, in differential diagnosis in patients with wall
thickening at CTA, a diffuse vasculitis should also be
considered.

17.7.4 Atherosclerosis

TIA and stroke of the posterior circulation account for
20% of all TIA and stroke cases [251], and a number of
cases are determined by the atherosclerotic pathology
of VAs. Stenosis of the VA can occur in either its extracranial or its intracranial portions, and some authors consider the VA as the second most common site of stenosis
after ICA stenosis at carotid bifurcation. In particular,
at the origin of the VAs atherosclerotic plaques determining stenosis are not uncommon. In an angiographic
study of about 5000 patients with ischemic stroke, some
degree of proximal extracranial VA stenosis was found
in 18% of cases on the right VAs and in 22.3% on the left
VAs [252]. VA is of much smaller relative caliber than
the subclavian with special flow dynamics between
the origins of the carotid and vertebrobasilar cerebral
circulations, with a consequent predilection to forming a different type of atherosclerotic plaque. Some
authors hypothesize that the atherosclerotic disease
that affects VA (in particular at its origin) is "smoother"
and less prone to ulcerate with secondary thrombus
formation [253]. Some investigations explored the
differences between carotid and VA plaque morphologies using angiography, but there are few published
pathological data to support this [254]. Intracranial VA
stenosis in V4 often also involves the basilar artery and
is more strongly associated with brain stem infarction
than extracranial VA stenosis.

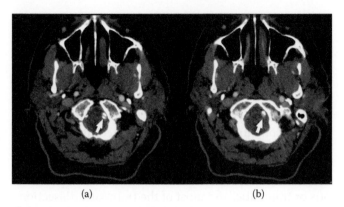

(a)   (b)

FIGURE 17.37
Calcification of the left vertebral artery (white arrows): in panels (a)
and (b), two contiguous levels are given.

Nowadays, with the advances in the techniques of
imaging it has become possible to image the posterior
circulation routinely at reasonable cost and negligible
risk and it is possible to determine the degree of stenosis of a VA. Usually most of the plaques that determine stenoses of VAs are calcified plaques (Figure 17.37),
but sometimes it is possible to find stenoses caused by
noncalcified plaques. It is important to remember that
the most affected segment is V4. Sometimes, it can be
necessary to distinguish between a stenosis and a VAD.
In this case, the length of the stenosis is important: the
stenosis determined by atherosclerosis usually is focal,
whereas the dissection usually shows the string sign
(or a nonfocal stenosis).

17.7.5 Subclavian Steal Syndrome

Subclavian steal describes any anomaly in which the
ipsilateral subclavian artery receives retrograde flow
from the contralateral circulation. Usually, ipsilateral
subclavian stenosis is caused by acquired atherosclerosis, which causes decreased upstream pressure to the
ipsilateral VA. Obviously, the stenosis must be proximal
to the origin of the VA and vascular flow travels in a
retrograde fashion from the contralateral VA to the basilar artery and finally to the ipsilateral VA, resulting in
the steal phenomenon. Subclavian steal syndrome (SSS)
should be a diagnostic consideration in any patient who
presents with a pulse deficit or a systolic blood pressure
difference greater than 15 mmHg [255,256]. However,
not only atherosclerotic disease but also other conditions like Takayasu, neoplasms, infiltration, and bone
anomalies may determine SSS [257,258].

In the early phase of SSS the patients usually are
asymptomatic as collateral flow from the opposite
VA and/or carotid circulation may compensate for
the steal, but when the collateral compensation is not
good (absence of the posterior communicating artery
or hypoplasia of the contralateral VA) and subclavian

stenosis becomes severe the high-resistance arterial supply may result in a characteristic syndrome that involves intermittent ipsilateral arm claudication, pain, and symptoms of vertebrobasilar insufficiency; typically, vertigo, diplopia, ataxia, dysarthria, or syncope may appear. SSS can often be provoked by rotating the head to the contralateral side and by arm exercises. Surgical therapy may solve this condition, and carotid–subclavian bypass has had a high technical success rate in patients with isolated atherosclerotic subclavian stenosis.

Imaging can help in the diagnosis and characterization of SSS, particularly MRA and ultrasound because these techniques have the potentiality of evaluating the direction of blood flow, which is the most important element in diagnosing the presence of this condition. In particular, using ultrasound the severity can be graded as "grade I," antegrade flow with diminished peak systolic velocity; "grade II," antegrade flow in the diastolic phase and retrograde flow in the systolic phase (the so-called "alternating flow"); and "grade III," completely retrograde flow.

References

1. Bouthillier A, van Loveren HR, Keller JT. Segments of the internal carotid artery: a new classification. *Neurosurgery* 1996 Mar;38(3):425–32.
2. Prokop M. General principles of MDCT. *Eur J Radiol* 2003;45:S4–10.
3. Fishman E. A brief overview of CT angiography. *Suppl Appl Radio* 2003;32:9–11.
4. Prokop M. Multislice CT: technical principles and future trends. *Eur Radiol* 2003;13:M3–13.
5. Das M, Braunschweig T, Muhlenbruch G et al. Carotid plaque analysis: comparison of dual source computed tomography (CT) findings and histopathological correlation. *Eur J Endovasc Surg* 2009;38:14–9.
6. Wintermark M, Jawadi SS, Rapp JH, Tihan T, Thong E, Glidden DV. High resolution CT imaging of carotid artery atherosclerotic plaques. *AJNR Am J Neuroradiol* 2008;29:875–82.
7. Saba L, Anzidei M, Sanfilippo R et al. Imaging of the carotid artery. *Atherosclerosis* 2012 Feb;220(2):294–309.
8. Saba L, Sanfilippo R, Montisci R, Mallarini G. Assessment of intracranial arterial stenosis with multidetector row CT angiography: a postprocessing techniques comparison. *AJNR Am J Neuroradiol* 2010 May;31(5):874–9.
9. Rankin SC. Spiral CT: vascular applications. *Eur J Radiol* 1998;28:18–29.
10. Rubin GD, Dake MD, Semba CP. Current status of three-dimensional spiral CT scanning for imaging the vasculature. *Radiol Clin North Am* 1995;33:51–70.
11. Rubin GD, Silverman SG. Helical (spiral) CT of the retroperitoneum. *Radiol Clin North Am* 1995;33:903–32.
12. Prokop M, Shin HO, Schanz A, Schaefer-Prokop C. Use of maximum intensity projections in CT angiography: a basic review. *RadioGraphics* 1997;17:433–51.
13. Ertl-Wagner BB, Bruening R, Blume J et al. Relative value of sliding-thin slab multiplanar reconstruction and sliding-thin-slab-maximum intensity projections as reformatting techniques in multisection CT angiography of the cervicocranial vessels. *Am J Neuroradiol* 2006;27:107–13.
14. Calhoun PS, Kuszyk BS, Heath DG, Carley JC, Fishman EK. Three-dimensional volume rendering of spiral CT data: theory and method. *RadioGraphics* 1999;19:745–64.
15. Saba L, Caddeo G, Sanfilippo R, Montisci R, Mallarini G. Efficacy and sensitivity of axial scans and different reconstruction methods in the study of the ulcerated carotid plaque by using multi-detector-row CT angiography. Comparison with surgical results. *Am J Neuroradiol AJNR* 2007;28:716–23.
16. Jaff MR, Goldmakher GV, Lev MH, Romero JM. Imaging of the carotid arteries: the role of duplex ultrasonography, magnetic resonance arteriography, and computerized tomographic arteriography. *Vascular Medicine* 2008;13:281–92.
17. O' Leary DH, Polak JF, Kronmal RA et al. Distribution and correlated of sonographically detected carotid artery disease in the cardiovascular health study. The CHS Collaborative research group. *Stroke* 1992;23:1752–60.
18. Savory WS. Case of a young woman in whom the main arteries of both upper extremities and of the left side of the neck were throughout completely obliterated. *Med Chir Trans Lond* 1856;39:205–19.
19. Gowers WR. On a case of simultaneous embolism of central retinal and middle cerebral arteries. *Lancet* 1875;2:794.
20. Chiari H. Uber des verhalten des teilungswinkels der carotis communis bei der endarteriitis chronica deformans (About the behavior of the distribution of the angle of carotid artery in chronic endarteritis deformans). *Verh Dtsch Ges Pathol* 1905;9:326–30.
21. Guthrie LG, Mayou S. Right hemiplegia and atrophy of left optic nerve. *Proc R Soc Med* 1908;1:180.
22. Adelman SM. Economic impact. In McDowell FM report on the National Survey of stroke. *Stroke* 1981;12:1.
23. Robins M, Baum H. National survey of stroke: incidence. *Stroke* 1981;12(1):45–57.
24. Gibbs RGJ, Todd JC, Irvine C et al. Relationship between the regional and national incidence of transient ischemic attack and stroke and performance of carotid endarterectomy. *Eur J Vasc Surg* 1998;16:47–52.
25. Holman RR, Paul SK, Bethel MA, Neil HA, Matthews DR. Long-term follow-up after tight control of blood pressure in type 2 diabetes. *N Engl J Med* 2008; 359:1565–76.
26. Grego F, Antonello M, Lepidi S. Is contralateral carotid artery occlusion a risk factor for carotid endarterectomy? *Ann Vasc Surg* 2005;19:882–9.
27. Fox AJ, Eliasziw M, Rothwell PM. Identification, prognosis, and management of patients with carotid artery near occlusion. *Am J Neuroradiol* 2005;26:2086–94.
28. Marcus HS, MacKinnon A. Asymptomatic embolization detected by Doppler ultrasound predicts stroke risk in symptomatic carotid artery stenosis. *Stroke* 2005; 36:971–5.
29. McCann RL. Surgical management of carotid artery atherosclerotic disease. *South Med J* 1994;86:S23–8.

30. Autret A, Pourcelot L, Saudeau D, Marchal C, Bertrand P, de Boisvilliers S. Stroke risk in patients with carotid stenosis. *Lancet* 1987;1:888–90.

31. Dennis MS, Bamford JM, Sandercock PA, Warlow CP. A comparison of risk factors and prognosis for transient ischemic attacks and minor ischemic strokes. The Oxfordshire Community Stroke Project. *Stroke* 1989;20:1494–9.

32. Meissner I, Wiebers DO, Whisnant JP, O' Fallon WM. The natural history of asymptomatic carotid artery occlusive lesions. *JAMA* 1987;258:2704–7.

33. North American Symptomatic Carotid Endarterectomy Trial Collaborators. Beneficial effect of carotid endarterectomy in symptomatic patients high with grade stenosis. *N Engl J Med* 1991;325:445–53.

34. European Carotid Surgery Trialists' Collaborative Group. Randomised trial of endarterectomy for recently symptomatic carotid stenosis: final results of the MRC European Carotid Surgery Trial (ECST). *Lancet* 1998;351:1379–87.

35. Asymptomatic Carotid Atherosclerosis Group. Endarterectomy for asymptomatic carotid artery stenosis. *JAMA* 1995;73:1421–8.

36. Rothwell PM, Eliasziw M, Gutnikov SA. Analysis of pooled data from the randomized controlled trials of endarterectomy for symptomatic carotid stenosis. *Lancet* 2003;361:107–16.

37. Fox AJ, Symons SP, Aviv RI et al. Falsely claiming use of NASCET percentage stenosis method. *Radiology* 2009 Nov;253(2):574–5; author reply 575.

38. Toole JF, Castaldo JE. Accurate measurement of carotid stenosis. Chaos in methodology. *J Neuroimaging* 1994 Oct;4(4):222–30.

39. Wardlaw JM, Lewis S. Carotid stenosis measurement on colour Doppler ultrasound: agreement of ECST, NASCET and CCA methods applied to ultrasound with intra-arterial angiographic stenosis measurement. *Eur J Radiol* 2005 Nov;56(2):205–11.

40. Bucek RA, Puchner S, Haumer M, Rand T, Minar E, Lammer J. Grading of internal carotid artery stenosis: can CTA overcome the confusion? *J Endovasc Ther* 2006 Aug;13(4):443–50.

41. Clinical alert: benefit of carotid endarterectomy for patients with high-grade stenosis of the internal carotid artery. National Institute of Neurological Disorders and Stroke Stroke and Trauma Division. North American Symptomatic Carotid Endarterectomy Trial (NASCET) investigators. *Stroke* 1991 Jun;22(6):816–7.

42. Eliasziw M, Smith RF, Singh N, Holdsworth DW, Fox AJ, Barnett HJ. Further comments on the measurement of carotid stenosis from angiograms. North American Symptomatic Carotid Endarterectomy Trial (NASCET) Group. *Stroke* 1994 Dec;25(12):2445–9.

43. Pelz DM, Fox AJ, Eliasziw M, Barnett HJ. Stenosis of the carotid bifurcation: subjective assessment compared with strict measurement guidelines. *Can Assoc Radiol J* 1993 Aug;44(4):247–52.

44. Warlow CP. Symptomatic patients: the European Carotid Surgery Trial (ECST). *J Mal Vasc* 1993;18(3):198–201. PubMed PMID: 8254241.

45. Alexandrov AV, Bladin CF, Maggisano R, Norris JW. Measuring carotid stenosis. Time for a reappraisal. *Stroke* 1993 Sep;24(9):1292–6.

46. Easton JD, Wilterdink JL. Carotid endarterectomy: trials and tribulations. *Ann Neurol* 1994 Jan;35(1):5–17.

47. Bladin CF, Alexandrov AV, Murphy J, Maggisano R, Norris JW. Carotid Stenosis Index. A new method of measuring internal carotid artery stenosis. *Stroke* 1995 Feb;26(2):230–4.

48. Fox AJ. How to measure carotid stenosis. *Radiology* 1993 Feb;186(2):316–8.

49. Hirai T, Korogi Y, Ono K et al. Maximum stenosis of extracranial internal carotid artery: effect of luminal morphology on stenosis measurement by using CT angiography and conventional DSA. *Radiology* 2001; 221:802–9.

50. Bartlett ES, Walters TD, Symons SP, Fox AJ. Quantification of carotid stenosis on CT Angiography. *AJNR Am J Neuroradiol* 2006;27:13–9.

51. Bartlett ES, Symons SP, Fox AJ. Correlation of carotid stenosis diameter and cross-sectional areas with CT angiography. *AJNR Am J Neuroradiol* 2006;27:638–42.

52. Bartlett ES, Walters TD, Symons SP, Fox AJ. Carotid stenosis index revised with direct CT angiography measurement of carotid arteries to quantify carotid stenosis. *Stroke* 2007;38:286–91.

53. Saba L, Mallarini G. Comparison between quantification methods of carotid artery stenosis and computed tomographic angiography. *J Comput Assist Tomogr* 2010 May–Jun;34(3):421–30.

54. Sameshima T, Futami S, Morita Y et al. Clinical usefulness and problems with three-dimensional CT angiography for the evaluation of atherosclerotic stenosis of the carotid artery: comparison with conventional angiography, MRA and ultrasound sonography. *Surg Neurol* 1999;51:300–9.

55. Seemann MD, Englmeier K, Schuhmann DR et al. Evaluation of the carotid and vertebral arteries: comparison of 3D SCTA and IA-DSA - work in progress. *Eur Radiol* 1999;9:105–12.

56. Goodson SF, Flanigan P, Bishara RA. Can carotid duplex scanning supplant arteriography in patients with focal carotid territory symptoms? *J Vasc Surg* 1987;5:551–7.

57. Polak JF, Kalina P, Donaldson MC. Carotid endarterectomy: preoperative evaluation of candidates with combined Doppler sonography and MR angiography: work in progress. *Radiology* 1993;186:333–8.

58. Dawson DL, Zierler RE, Strandness DE. The role of duplex scanning and arteriography before carotid endarterectomy: a prospective study. *J Vasc Surg* 1993;18:673–80.

59. Yucel EK, Anderson CM, Edelman RR et al. Magnetic resonance angiography. update on applications for extracranial arteries. *Circulation* 1999;100:2284–301.

60. Debrey SM, Yu H, Lynch JK et al. Diagnostic accuracy of magnetic resonance angiography for internal carotid artery disease: a systematic review and meta-analysis. *Stroke* 2008;39:2237–48.

61. Nederkoorn PJ, Mali WPT, Eikelboom BC et al. Preoperative diagnosis of carotid artery stenosis. Accuracy of non-invasive testing. *Stroke* 2002;33:2003–8.

62. Magarelli N, Scarabino T, Simeone AL et al. Carotid stenosis: a comparison between MR, and spiral CT angiography. *Neuroradiology* 1998;40:367–73.

63. Saba L, Sanfilippo R, Montisci R, Mallarini G. Correlation between US-PSV and MDCTA in the quantification of carotid artery stenosis. *Eur J Radiol* In press.

64. Little WC, Constantinescu M, Applegate RJ. Can coronary angiography predict the site of a subsequent myocardial infarction in patients with mild-to-moderate coronary artery disease? *Circulation* 1988;78:1157–66.

65. Ambrose JA, Tannenbaum MA, Alexopoulos D. Angiographic progression of coronary artery disease and the development of myocardial infarction. *J Am Coll Cardiol* 1988;12:56–62.

66. Libby P. The interface of atherosclerosis and thrombosis: basic mechanisms. *Vasc Med* 1998;3:225–9.

67. Lovett JK, Gallagher PJ, Rothwell PM. Reproducibility of histological assessment of carotid plaque: implications for studies of carotid imaging. *Cerebrovasc Dis* 2004;18:117–23.

68. Wasserman BA, Wityk RJ, Trout HH, Virmani R. Looking beyond the lumen with MRI. *Stroke* 2005;36:2504–13.

69. Lovett JK, Gallagher PJ, Hands LJ, Walton J, Rothwell PM. Histological correlates of carotid plaque surface morphology on lumen contrast imaging. *Circulation* 2004;110:2190–7.

70. Kullo IJ, Edwards WD, Schwartz RS. Vulnerable plaque: pathobiology and clinical implications. *Ann Intern Med* 1998;129:1050–60.

71. Budinger T, Berson A, McVeigh E et al. Magnetic resonance imaging of the cardiovascular system. *J Cardiovasc Magn Res* 1999;1:53–8.

72. Falk E, Fernandez-Ortiz A. Role of thrombosis in atherosclerosis and its complications. *Am J Cardiol* 1995;75:3B–11B.

73. van Gils MJ, Vukadinovic D, van Dijk AC, Dippel DW, Niessen WJ, van der Lugt A. Carotid atherosclerotic plaque progression and change in plaque composition over time: a 5-year follow-up study using serial CT angiography. *AJNR Am J Neuroradiol* 2012 Feb 16. [Epub ahead of print] PubMed PMID: 22345501.

74. Virmani R, Kolodgie FD, Burke AP, Farb A, Schwartz SM. Lessons from sudden coronary death: a comprehensive morphological classification scheme for atherosclerotic lesions. *Arterioscler Thromb Vasc Biol* 2000;20:1262–75.

75. Fuster V, Moreno PR, Fayad ZA, Corti R, Badimon JJ. Atherothrombosis and high-risk plaque. Part I: evolving concepts. *J Am Coll Cardiol* 2005;46:937–54.

76. de Weert TT, Cretier S, Groen HC et al. Atherosclerotic carotid plaque surface morphology in the carotid bifurcation assessed with multi-detector computed tomography. *Stroke* 2009 Apr;40(4):1334-40.

77. Sitzer M, Muller W, Siebler M et al. Plaque ulceration and lumen thrombus are the main sources of cerebral microemboli in high-grade internal carotid artery stenosis. *Stroke* 1995;26:1231–3.

78. Morgenstern LB, Fox AJ, Sharpe BL, Eliasziw HJ, Grotta JC. The risks and benefits of carotid endarterectomy in patients with near occlusion of the carotid artery. North American Symptomatic Carotid Endarterectomy Trial (NASCET) group. *Neurology* 1997;48:911–5.

79. Eliasziw M, Streifler JY, Fox AJ. Significance of plaque ulceration in symptomatic patients with high grade carotid stenosis: North American Symptomatic Carotid Endarterectomy Trial. *Stroke* 1994;25:304–8.

80. Barnett HJ, Taylor DW, Eliasziw M et al. Benefit of carotid endarterectomy in patients with symptomatic moderate or severe stenosis. North American Symptomatic carotid Endarterectomy Trial Collaborators. *N Engl J Med* 1998;339;1415–25.

81. Walker LJ, Ismail Á, McMeekin W, Lambert D, Mendelow AD, Birchall D. Computed tomography angiography for the evaluation of carotid atherosclerotic plaque: correlation with histopathology of endarterectomy specimens. *Stroke* 2002;33:977–81.

82. Randoux B, Marro B, Koskas F. Carotid artery stenosis: prospective comparison of CT, three-dimensional gadolinium-enhanced MR, and conventional angiography. *Radiology* 2001;220:179–85.

83. Streifler JY, Eliaziw M, Fox AJ et al. Angiographic detection of carotid plaque ulceration: comparison with surgical observations in to multicenter study. *Stroke* 1994;25:1130–2.

84. Runge VM, Kirsch JE, Lee C. Contrast-enhanced MR angiography. *J Magn Reson Imaging* 1993;3:233–9.

85. Debernardi S, Martincich L, Lazzaro D. CT angiography in the assessment of carotid atherosclerotic disease: results of more than two years' experience. *Radiol Med* 2004;108:116–27.

86. Lammie GA, Wardlaw J, Allan P, Ruckley CV, Peek R, Signorini DF. What pathological components indicate carotid atheroma activity and can these be identified reliably using ultrasound? *Eur J Ultrasound* 2000;11:77–86.

87. Bluth EI, McVay LV, Merritt CR, Sullivan A. The identification of ulcerative plaque with high resolution duplex carotid scanning. *J Ultrasound Med* 1998;7:73–6.

88. Cumming MJ, Morrow IA. Carotid artery stenosis: a prospective comparison of CT angiography and conventional angiography. *AJR Am J Roentgenol* 1994;163:517–23.

89. Schwartz RB, Jones KM, Chernoff DM et al. Common carotid artery bifurcation: evaluation with spiral CT. *Radiology* 1992;185:513–9.

90. Porsche C, Walker L, Mendelow AD, Birchall D. Assessment of vessel wall thickness in carotid atherosclerosis using spiral CT angiography. *Eur J Vasc Endovasc Surg* 2002;23:437–40.

91. Porsche C, Walker L, Mendelow D, Birchall D. Evaluation of cross-sectional luminal morphology in carotid atherosclerotic disease by use of spiral CT angiography. *Stroke* 2001;32:2511–5.

92. de Weert TT, de Moynè C, Meijering E et al. Assessment of atherosclerotic carotid plaque volume with multidetector-row CT Angiography. *Int J Cardiovasc Imaging* 2008;24:751–9.

93. de Weert TT, Ouholus M, Meijring E et al. In cico characterization and quantification of atherosclerotic plaque components with multidetector computer tomography and histopathological correlation. *Arteriosler Thromb Vasc Biol* 2006;26:2366–72.

94. Ajduk M, Pavić L, Bulimbasić S et al. Multidetector-row computed tomography in evaluation of atherosclerotic carotid plaques complicated with intraplaque hemorrhage. *Ann Vasc Surg* 2009;23:186–93.

95. Ouhlous M, Flach HZ, de Weert TT. Carotid plaque composition and cerebral infarction: MR imaging study. *Am J Neuroradiol* 2005;26:1044–9.

96. Saba L, Sanfilippo R, Sannia S et al. Association between carotid artery plaque volume, composition, and ulceration: a retrospective assessment with MDCT. *AJR Am J Roentgenol* 2012;199:151–6.

97. Nandalur KR, Hardie HD, Raghavan P, Schipper MJ, Baskurt E, Kramer CM. Composition of the stable carotid plaque: insights from a multi-detector computed tomography study of plaque volume. *Stroke* 2007;38:935–40.

98. Tambasco M, Steinman DA. Path-dependent hemodynamics of the stenosed carotid bifurcation. *Ann Biomed Eng* 2003;31:1054–65.

99. Ohara T, Toyoda K, Otsubo R et al. Eccentric stenosis of the carotid artery associated with ipsilateral cerebrovascular events. *Am J Neuroradio* 2008;29:1200–3.

100. Hardie AD, Kramer CM, Raghavan P. The impact of expansive arterial remodelling on clinical presentation in carotid artery disease: a multi-detector-row CT angiography study. *Am J Neuroradiol* 2007;28:1067–70.

101. Loree HM, Kamm RD, Stringfellow RG, Lee RT. Effects of fibrous cap thickness on peak circumferential stress in model atherosclerotic vessels. *Circ Res* 1992;71:850–8.

102. Virmani R, Burke AP, Kolodgie FD, Farb A. Vulnerable plaque: the pathology of unstable coronary lesions. *J Interv Cardiol* 2002;15:439–46.

103. Falk E. Coronary thrombosis: pathogenesis and clinical manifestation. *Am J Cardiol* 1991;68:28B–35B.

104. Wasserman BA, Smith WI, Trout HH III, Cannon RO 3rd, Balaban RS, Arai AE. Carotid artery atherosclerosis: in vivo morphologic characterization with gadolinium enhanced double-oblique MR imaging-initial results. *Radiology* 2002;223:566–73.

105. Kramer CM, Cerilli LA, Hagspiel K, DiMaria JM, Epstein FH, Kern JA. Magnetic resonance imaging identifies the fibrous cap in atherosclerotic abdominal aortic aneurysm. *Circulation* 2004;109:1016–21.

106. Yuan C, Zhang SX, Polissar NL et al. Identification of fibrous cap rupture with magnetic resonance imaging is highly associated with recent transient ischemic attack or stroke. *Circulation* 2002;105:181–5.

107. Mitsumori LM, Hatsukami TS, Ferguson MS, Kerwin WS, Cai J, Yuan C. In vivo accuracy of multisequence MR imaging for identifying unstable fibrous caps in advanced human carotid plaques. *J Magn Reson Imaging* 2003;17:410–20.

108. Saba L, Mallarini G. Fissured fibrous cap of vulnerable carotid plaques and symptomaticity: are they correlated? Preliminary results by using MDCTA. *Cerebrovasc Dis* 2009;27:322–7.

109. Saba L, Potters F, van der Lugt A, Mallarini G. Imaging of the fibrous cap in atherosclerotic carotid plaque. *Cardiovasc Intervent Radiol* 2010 Aug;33(4):681–9.

110. Kolodgie FD, Gold HK, Burke AP et al. Intraplaque hemorrhage and progression of coronary atheroma. *N Engl J Med* 2003;349:2316–25.

111. Constantinides P. Plaque fissuring in human coronary thrombosis. *J Atheroscler Res* 1966;6:1–17.

112. Davies MJ, Thomas AC. Plaque fissuring: the cause of acute myocardial infarction, sudden ischaemic death, and crescendo angina. *Br Heart J* 1985;53:363–73.

113. Moody AR, Murphy RE, Morgan PS. Characterization of complicated carotid plaque with magnetic resonance direct thrombus imaging in patients with cerebral ischemia. *Circulation* 2003;107:3047–52.

114. Oliver TB, Lammie GA, Wright AR. Atherosclerotic plaque at the carotid bifurcation: CT angiographic appearance with histopathologic correlation. *AJNR* 1999;20:897–901.

115. Saba L, Sanfilippo R, Pirisi R, Pascalis L, Montisci R, Mallarini G. Multi-detector Row CT Angiography in the study of atherosclerotic carotid artery. *Neuroradiology* 2007;49:623–37.

116. Rothwell PM, Gibson R, Warlow CP. Interrelation between plaque surface morphology and degree of stenosis on carotid angiograms and the risk of ischemic stroke in patients with symptomatic carotid stenosis. *Stroke* 2000;31:615–21.

117. Toussaint JF, Southern JF, Fuster V, Kantor HL. Water diffusion properties of human atherosclerosis and thrombosis measured by pulse field gradient nuclear magnetic resonance. *Arterioscler Thromb Vasc Biol* 1997;17:542–6.

118. Wentzel JJ, Aguiar SH, Fayad ZA. Vascular MRI in the diagnosis and therapy of the high risk atherosclerotic plaque. *J Interv Cardiol* 2003;16:129–42.

119. Kondos GT, Hoff JA, Sevrukov A. Electron beam tomography coronary artery calcium and cardiac events: a 37-month follow-up of 5635 initially asymptomatic low- to intermediate-risk adults. *Circulation* 2003;107:2571–6.

120. Sangiorgi G, Rumberger JA, Severson A. Arterial calcification and not lumen stenosis is highly correlated with atherosclerotic plaque burden in humans: a histologic study of 723 coronary artery segments using nondecalcifying methodology. *J Am Coll Cardiol* 1998;31:126–33.

121. Nandalur KR, Baskurt E, Hagspiel KD, Phillips CD, Kramer CM. Calcified carotid atherosclerotic plaque is associated less with ischemic symptoms than is noncalcified plaque on MDCT. *AJR* 2005;184:295–8.

122. Nandalur KR, Hardie AD, Raghavan P, Schipper MJ, Baskurt E, Kramer CM. Composition of the stable carotid plaque. Insights from a multidetector computed tomography study of plaque volume. *Stroke* 2007;38:935–40.

123. Saba L, Montisci R, Sanfilippo R; Mallarini G. Multidetector row CT of the brain and carotid artery: a correlative analysis. *Clin Radiol* 2009;64:767–78.

124. Fanning NF, Walters TD, Fox AJ, Symons SP. Association between calcification on the cervical carotid artery bifurcation and white matter ischemia. *AJNR Am J Neuroradiol* 2006;27:378–83.

125. Romero JM, Babiarz LS, Forero NP, Murphy EK, Schaefer PW, Gonzalez RG, Lev MH. Arterial wall enhancement overlying carotid plaque on CT angiography correlates with symptoms in patients with high grade stenosis. *Stroke* 2009;40:1894–6.

126. Saba L, Lai ML, Montisci R et al. Association between carotid plaque enhancement shown by multidetector CT angiography and histologically validated microvessel density. *Eur Radiol* 2012 May 10. [Epub ahead of print] PubMed PMID: 22572988.

127. Saba L, Mallarini G. Carotid plaque enhancement and symptom correlations: an evaluation by using multidetector row CT angiography. *AJNR Am J Neuroradiol* 2011 Nov–Dec;32(10):1919–25.

128. Moreno PR, Purushothaman KR, Fuster V et al. Plaque neovascularization is increased in ruptured atherosclerotic lesions of human aorta: implications for plaque vulnerability. *Circulation* 2004;110:2032–8.

129. McCarthy MJ, Loftus IM, Thompson MM et al. Angiogenesis and the atherosclerotic carotid plaque: an association between symptomatology and plaque morphology. *J Vasc Surg* 1999;30:261–8.

130. Dunmore BJ, McCarthy MJ, Naylor AR, Brindle NP. Carotid plaque instability and ischemic symptoms are linked to immaturity of microvessels within plaques. *J Vasc Surg* 2007;45:155–9.

131. Saba L, Piga M, Raz E, Farina D, Montisci R. Carotid artery plaque classification: does contrast enhancement play a significant role? *AJNR Am J Neuroradiol* 2012 May 3. [Epub ahead of print] PubMed PMID: 22555579.

132. Fleischmann D, Boas FE. Computed tomography—old ideas and new technology. *Eur Radiol* 2011;21:510–7.

133. Petersilka M, Bruder H, Krauss B, Stierstorfer K, Flohr TG. Technical principles of dual source CT. *Eur J Radiol* 2008 Dec;68:362–8.

134. Saba L, Argiolas GM, Siotto P, Piga M. Carotid artery plaque characterization using CT multi-energy imaging. *AJNR Am J Neuroradiol* In press.

135. Heliopoulos I, Papaoiakim M, Tsivgoulis G et al. Common carotid intima media thickness as a marker of clinical severity in patients with symptomatic extracranial carotid artery stenosis. *Clin Neurol Neurosurg* 2009;111(3):246–50.

136. Lorenz MW, von Kegler S, Steinmetz H, Markus HS, Sitzer M. Carotid intima-media thickening indicates a higher vascular risk across a wide age range: prospective data from the Carotid Atherosclerosis Progression Study (CAPS). *Stroke* 2006;37(1):87–92.

137. O'Leary DH, Polak JF, Kronmal RA, Manolio TA, Burke GL, Wolfson SK. Carotid-artery intima and media thickness as a risk factor for myocardial infarction and stroke in older adults. Cardiovascular Health Study Collaborative Research Group. *N Engl J Med* 1999;340(1):14–22.

138. Veller MG, Fisher CM, Nicolaides AN. Measurement of the ultrasonic intima-media complex thickness in normal subjects. *J Vasc Surg* 1993;17:719–25.

139. Dwyer JH, Sun P, Kwong-Fu H, Dwyer KM, Selzer RH. Automated intima-media thickness: the Los Angeles Atherosclerosis Study. *Ultrasound Med Biol* 1998 Sep;24(7):981–7.

140. Saba L, Sanfilippo R, Pascalis L, Montisci R, Caddeo G, Mallarini G. Carotid artery wall thickness and ischemic symptoms: evaluation using multi-detector-row CT angiography. *Eur Radiol* 2008 Sep;18(9):1962–71. Epub 2008 Apr 11. PubMed.

141. Saba L, Sanfilippo R, Montisci R, Suri JS, Mallarini G. Carotid artery wall thickness measured using CT: inter- and intraobserver agreement analysis. *AJNR Am J Neuroradiol* 2013 Feb;34(2):E13-8.

142. Saba L, Montisci R, Molinari F et al. Comparison between manual and automated analysis for the quantification of carotid wall by using sonography. A validation study with CT. *Eur J Radiol* 2012 May;81(5):911–8.

143. Saba L, Pascalis L, Sanfilippo R et al. Carotid artery wall thickness and leukoaraiosis: preliminary results using multidetector row CT angiography. *AJNR Am J Neuroradiol* 2011 May;32(5):955–61.

144. Saba L, Sanfilippo R, Montisci R, Mallarini G. Associations between carotid artery wall thickness and cardiovascular risk factors using multidetector CT. *AJNR Am J Neuroradiol* 2010 Oct;31(9):1758–63.

145. Saba L, Sanfilippo R, Montisci R, Mallarini G. Carotid artery wall thickness: comparison between sonography and multi-detector row CT angiography. *Neuroradiology* 2010 Feb;52(2):75–82.

146. Rao AS, Makaroun MS, Marone LK, Cho JS, Rhee R, Chaer RA. Long-term outcomes of internal carotid artery dissection. *J Vasc Surg* 2011 Aug;54(2):370–4.

147. Divjak I, Slankamenac P, Jovićević M, Zikić TR, Popović N. Factors predisposing to cervical artery dissection. *Med Pregl* 2011 Mar–Apr;64(3–4):198–201.

148. Shea K, Stahmer S. Carotid and vertebral arterial dissections in the emergency department. *Emerg Med Pract* 2012 Apr;14(4):1–23.

149. Sato S, Toyoda K, Matsuoka H et al. Isolated anterior cerebral artery territory infarction: dissection as an etiological mechanism. *Cerebrovasc Dis* 2010 Jan;29(2):170–7.

150. Suzuki I, Nishino A, Nishimura S et al. [Nontraumatic arterial dissection of the anterior cerebral artery: six cases report]. *No To Shinkei* 2005 Jun;57(6):509–15.

151. Lleva P, Ahluwalia BS, Marks S et al. Traumatic and spontaneous carotid and vertebral artery dissection in a level 1 trauma center. *J Clin Neurosci* 2012 Aug;19(8):1112–4.

152. Dohle C, Baehring JM. Multiple strokes and bilateral carotid dissections: a fulminant case of newly diagnosed Ehlers-Danlos Syndrome Type IV. *J Neurol Sci* 2012 Jul 15;318(1–2):168–70.

153. Willey JZ. The outer arterial wall layers are primarily affected in spontaneous cervical artery dissection. *Neurology* 2011 Nov 15;77(20):1859.

154. Ferruzzi J, Collins MJ, Yeh AT, Humphrey JD. Mechanical assessment of elastin integrity in fibrillin-1-deficient carotid arteries: implications for Marfan syndrome. *Cardiovasc Res* 2011 Nov 1;92(2):287–95.

155. Carprieaux M, Michotte A, Van Varenbergh D, Marichal MP. Spontaneous bilateral carotid artery dissection following cervical manipulation. *Leg Med (Tokyo)* 2012 Sep;14(5):249–51.

156. Huang YC, Chen CM, Lai SL et al. Spontaneous intrapetrous internal carotid artery dissection: a case report and literature review. *J Neurol Sci* 2007 Feb 15;253(1–2):90–3.

157. Lee VH, Brown RD Jr, Mandrekar JN, Mokri B. Incidence and outcome of cervical artery dissection: a population-based study. *Neurology* 2006;67:1809–12.

158. Bogousslavsky J, Despland PA, Regli F. Spontaneous carotid dissection with acute stroke. *Arch Neurol* 1987;44:137.

159. Silbert PL, Mokri B, Schievink WI. Headache and neck pain in spontaneous internal carotid and vertebral artery dissections. *Neurology* 1995;45:1517–22.

160. Sarikaya H. Hemifacial sweating after carotid artery dissection. *Lancet* 2011 Aug 13;378(9791):606.

161. Patel RR, Adam R, Maldjian C, Lincoln CM, Yuen A, Arneja A. Cervical carotid artery dissection: current review of diagnosis and treatment. *Cardiol Rev* 2012 May;20(3):145–52.

162. Guillon B, Levy C, Bousser MG. Internal carotid artery dissection: An update. *J Neurol Sci* 1998;153:146–58.

163. Saver JL, Easton JD. Dissection of cervicocerebral arteries. In: Barnett HJM, Mohr JP, Stein BM et al., eds. *Stroke: pathophysiology, diagnosis and management.* New York: Churchill Livingstone, 1998:769–86, 1459.

164. Houser OW, Mokri B, Sundt TM Jr, Baker HL Jr, Reese DF. Spontaneous cervical cephalic arterial dissection and its residuum: angiographic spectrum. *AJNR Am J Neuroradiol* 1984;5:27–34.

165. Djouhri H, Guillon B, Brunereau L et al. MR angiography for the long-term follow-up of dissecting aneurysms of the extracranial internal carotid artery. *AJR Am J Roentgenol* 2000;174:1137–40.

166. Provenzale JM, Sarikaya B. Comparison of test performance characteristics of MRI, MR angiography, and CT angiography in the diagnosis of carotid and vertebral artery dissection: a review of the medical literature. *AJR Am J Roentgenol* 2009 Oct;193(4):1167–74.

167. Lell MM, Anders K, Uder M et al. New techniques in CT angiography. *RadioGraphics* 2006;26(spec issue):S45–62.

168. Rodallec MH, Marteau V, Gerber S, Desmottes L, Zins L. Craniocervical arterial dissection: spectrum of imaging findings and diagnosis. *RadioGraphics* 2008;28:1711–28.

169. Tasar M, Yetiser S, Tasar A, Ugurel S, Gonul E, Saglam M. Congenital absence or hypoplasia of the carotid artery: radioclinical issues. *Am J Otolaryngol* 2004;25(5):339–49.

170. Osborn AG, Anderson RE. Angiographic spectrum of cervical and intracranial fibromuscular dysplasia. *Stroke* 1977;8(5):617–26.

171. Lassiter FD. The string-of-beads sign. *Radiology* 1998;206(2):437–8.

172. Herregods N, Beckers R, Van Rattinghe R, Verstraete K. Fibromuscular dysplasia of the carotid artery. *JBR-BTR* 2008 Sep–Oct;91(5):195–7.

173. Umekita K, Hashiba Y, Kariya-Kaneko Y, Matsuda M, Okayama A. Arteriosclerosis of whole aorta in takayasu arteritis. *J Rheumatol* 2012 Jun;39(6):1291.

174. Sadurska E, Jawniak R, Majewski M, Czekajska-Chehab E. Takayasu arteritis as a cause of arterial hypertension. Case report and literature review. *Eur J Pediatr* 2012 May;171(5):863–9.

175. Nahas SJ. Headache and temporal arteritis: when to suspect and how to manage. *Curr Pain Headache Rep* 2012 Aug;16(4):371–8.

176. Stacy RC, Rizzo JF, Cestari DM. Subtleties in the histopathology of giant cell arteritis. *Semin Ophthalmol* 2011 Jul–Sep;26(4–5):342–8.

177. Foss F, Brown L. An elastic Van Gieson stain is unnecessary for the histological diagnosis of giant cell temporal arteritis. *J Clin Pathol* 2010 Dec;63(12):1077–9.

178. Wakefield D, Cunningham ET Jr, Tugal-Tutkun I, Khairallah M, Ohno S, Zierhut M. Controversies in Behçet disease. *Ocul Immunol Inflamm* 2012 Feb;20(1):6–11.

179. Calamia KT, Schirmer M, Melikoglu M. Major vessel involvement in Behçet's disease: an update. *Curr Opin Rheumatol* 2011 Jan;23(1):24–31.

180. Geri G, Wechsler B, Thi Huong du L et al. Spectrum of cardiac lesions in Behçet disease: a series of 52 patients and review of the literature. *Medicine (Baltimore)* 2012 Jan;91(1):25–34.

181. Prasad SC, Thada N, Pallavi, Prasad KC. Paragangliomas of the head & neck: the KMC experience. *Indian J Otolaryngol Head Neck Surg* 2011 Jan;63(1):62–73.

182. Bozek P, Kluczewska E, Lisowska G, Namysłowski G. [Imaging and assessment of glomus jugulare in MRI and CT techniques]. *Otolaryngol Pol* 2011 May–Jun;65(3):218–27.

183. Baysal BE, Willett-Brozick JE, Lawrence EC et al. Prevalence of SDHB, SDHC, and SDHD germ line mutations in clinic patients with head and neck paragangliomas. *J Med Genet* 2002;39(3):178–83.

184. Heath D. The human carotid body in health and disease. *J Pathol* 1991;164(1):1–8.

185. Saldana MJ, Salem LE, Travezan R. High altitude hypoxia and chemodectomas. *Human Pathol* 1973;4(2):251–63.

186. Jackson CG. Glomus tympanicum and glomus jugulare tumors. *Otolaryngol Clin North Am* 2001;34(5):941–70.

187. Rinaldo A, Ferlito A, Myssiorek D, Devaney KO. Which paragangliomas of the head and neck have a higher rate of malignancy? *Oral Oncol* 2004;40:458–60.

188. Lee JH, Barich F, Karnell LH et al. National cancer data base report on malignant paragangliomas of the head and neck. *Cancer* 2002;94(3):730–7.

189. van den Berg R. Imaging and management of head and neck paragangliomas. *Eur Radiol* 2005 Jul;15(7):1310–8.

190. van der Mey AGL, Jansen JC, van Baalen JM. Management of carotid body tumors. *Otolaryngol Clin North Am* 2001;34(5):907–24.

191. Liapis C, Gougoulakis A, Karydakis V et al. Changing trends in management of carotid body tumors. *Am Surg* 1995;61(11):989–93.

192. Mattes NA, Hernández-Osma E, Fauria CB, Salvador VS. Extracranial internal carotid artery aneurysm: an uncommon disease of the supra-aortic arteries. *Neurologia* 2012 Jan;27(1):53–5.

193. Rittenhouse EA, Radke HM, Summer DS. Carotid artery aneurysm: review of the literature and report of a case with rupture into the oropharynx. *Arch Surg* 1972;105:786–9.

194. McCann RL. Basic data related to peripheral artery aneurysms. *Ann Vasc Surg* 1990;4:411–4.

195. Szopinski P, Clostek P, Kierlar M, Myrcha P, Pleban E, Noszcyzyk W. A series of 15 patients with extracranial carotid artery aneurysms: surgical and endovascular treatment. *Eur J Vasc Endovasc Surg* 2005;29:256–61.

196. Azzarone M, Cento M, Gobbi S, Tecchio T, Piazza P, Salcuni PF. Neuropathy as the only symptom of common carotid artery spontaneous rupture. *J Cardiovascular Surg* 2003;44:767–9.

197. Rosset E, Albertini JN, Magnan PE, Ede B, Thomassin JM, Branchereau A. Surgical treatment of extracranial internal carotid artery aneurysms. *J Vasc Surg* 2000;31(4):713–23.

198. Biasi L, Azzarone M, De Troia A, Salcuni P, Tecchio T. Extracranial internal carotid artery aneurysms: case report of a saccular wide-necked aneurysm and review of the literature. *Acta Biomed* 2008 Dec;79(3):217–22.

199. Liston R. On a variety of false aneurysms. *Br Foreign Med Rev* 1843;15:155–61.

200. Reisner A, Marshall GS, Bryant K, Postel GC, Eberly SM. Endovascular occlusion of a carotid pseudoaneurysm complication deep neck space infection in a child. Case report. *J Neurosurg* 1999;91:510–4.

201. Stevens HE. Vascular complication of neck space infection: case report and literature review. *J Otorinolaring* 1990;19:206–10.

202. Welling RE, Talisa A, Tarun G. Extracranial carotid artery aneurysms. *Surgery* 1983;93:319–23.

203. Mokri B, Piepgras DG, Sundt TM, Pearson BW. Extracranial internal carotid artery aneurysms. *Mayo Clin Proc* 1982;57:310–21.

204. Faggioli GL, Freyrie A, Stella A et al. Extracranial internal carotid artery aneurysms: results of a surgical series with long-term follow-up. *J Vasc Surg* 1996 Apr;23(4):587–94.

205. Slovut DP, Olin JW. Fibromuscular dysplasia. *N Engl J Med* 2004;350:1862–71.

206. Plouin PF, Perdu J, La Batide-Alanore A, Boutouyrie P, Gimenez-Roqueplo AP, Jeunemaitre X. Fibromuscular dysplasia. *Orphanet J Rare Dis* 2007;2:28.

207. So EL, Toole JF, Dalal P, Moody DM. Cephalic fibromuscular dysplasia in 32 patients: clinical findings and radiologic features. *Arch Neurol* 1981;38:619–22.

208. Houser OW, Baker HL Jr. Fibromuscular dysplasia and other uncommon diseases of the cervical carotid artery: angiographic aspects. *Am J Roentgenol Radium Ther Nucl Med* 1968;104:201–12.

209. Stanley JC, Gewertz BL, Bove EL, Sottiurai V, Fry WJ. Arterial fibrodysplasia. Histopathologic character and current etiologic concepts. *Arch Surg* 1975;110:561–6.

210. Lüscher TF, Keller HM, Imhof HG et al. Fibromuscular hyperplasia: extension of the disease and therapeutic outcome. *Nephron* 1986;44:109–14.

211. Cohen JE, Grigoriadis S, Gomori JM. Petrous carotid artery pseudoaneurysm in bilateral carotid fibromuscular dysplasia: treatment by means of self-expanding covered stent. *Surg Neurol* 2007 Aug;68(2):216–20.

212. Bellot J, Gherardi R, Poirier J, Lacour P, Debrun G, Barbizet J. Fibromuscular dysplasia of cervico-cephalic arteries with multiple dissections and a carotid-cavernous fistula. A pathological study. *Stroke* 1985;16:255–61.

213. Zimmerman R, Leeds NE, Naidich TP. Carotid-cavernous fistula associated with intracranial fibromuscular dysplasia. *Radiology* 1977;122:725–6.

214. Olin JW, Froehlich J, Gu X et al. The United States registry for fibromuscular dysplasia: results in the first 447 patients. *Circulation* 2012 Jun 26;125(25):3182–90.

215. Reddy SV, Karnes WE, Earnest F, Sundt TM Jr. Spontaneous extracranial vertebral arteriovenous fistula with fibromuscular dysplasia. Case report. *J Neurosurg* 1981;54:399–402.

216. Enterline DS, Kapoor G. A practical approach to CT angiography of the neck and brain. *Tech Vasc Interv Radiol* 2006 Dec;9(4):192–204.

217. Castillo M, Wilson JD. CT angiography of the common carotid artery bifurcation: comparison between two techniques and conventional angiography. *Neuroradiology* 1994 Nov;36(8):602–4.

218. Numano F. The story of Takayasu arteritis. *Rheumatology* 2002;41:103–6.

219. Matsunaga N, Hayashi K, Sakamoto I, Ogawa Y, Matsumoto T. Takayasu arteritis: protean radiologic manifestations and diagnosis. *RadioGraphics* 1997;17:579–94.

220. Matsunaga N, Hayashi K, Sakamoto I et al. Takayasu arteritis: MR manifestations and diagnosis of acute and chronic phase. *J Magn Reson Imaging* 1998;8:406–14.

221. Numano F. Vasa vasoritis, 1vasculitis and atherosclerosis. *Int J Cardiol* 2000;75:S1–8.

222. Cid MC, Cebrian M, Font C. Cell adhesion molecules in the development of inflammatory infiltrates in giant cell arteritis: inflammation-induced angiogenesis as the preferential site of leukocyte-endothelial cell interactions. *Arthritis Rheum* 2000;43:184–94.

223. Arnaud L, Haroche J, Toledano D et al. Cluster analysis of arterial involvement in Takayasu arteritis reveals symmetric extension of the lesions in paired arterial beds. *Arthritis Rheum* 2011;63:1136–40.

224. Maffei S, Di Renzo M, Bova G, Auteri A, Pasqui AL. Takayasu's arteritis: a review of the literature. *Intern Emerg Med* 2006;1:105–12.

225. Zouboulis CC, Keitel W. A historical review of early descriptions of Adamantiades-Behcet's disease. *J Invest Dermatol* 2002;119(1):201–5.

226. McGonagle D, McDermott MF. A proposed classification of the immunological diseases. *PLoS Med* 2006;3(8):e297.

227. Saadoun D, Asli B, Wechsler B et al. Long-term outcome of arterial lesions in Behcet disease: a series of 101 patients. *Medicine (Baltimore)* 2012;91(1):18–24.

228. Wilkinson IM, Russell RW. Arteries of the head and neck in giant cell arteritis. A pathological study to show the pattern of arterial involvement. *Arch Neurol* 1972 Nov;27(5):378–91.

229. Collazos J, García-Moncó C, Martín A, Rodriguez J, Gómez MA. Multiple strokes after initiation of steroid therapy in giant cell arteritis. *Postgrad Med J* 1994 Mar;70(821):228–30.

230. Schmidt WA, Kraft HE, Vorpahl K, Volker L, Gromnica-Ihle EJ. Color duplex ultrasonography in the diagnosis of temporal arteriitis. *N Engl J Med* 1997;337(19):1336–42.

231. Both M, Ahmadi-Simab K, Reuter M et al. MRI and FDG-PET in the assessment of inflammatory aortic arch syndrome in complicated courses of giant cell arteritis. *Ann Rheum Dis* 2008;67(7):1030–3.

232. Yahyavi-Firouz-Abadi N, Wynn BL, Rybicki FJ et al. Steroid-responsive large vessel vasculitis: application of whole-brain 320-detector row dynamic volume CT angiography and perfusion. *AJNR Am J Neuroradiol* 2009 Aug;30(7):1409–11.

233. Piagkou M, Anagnostopoulou S, Kouladouros K. Eagle's syndrome: a review of the literature. *Clin Anat* 2009; 22:545–58.

234. Farhat HI, Elhammady MS, Ziayee H. Eagle syndrome as a cause of transient ischemic attacks. *J Neurosurg* 2009;110(1):90–93.

235. Dao A, Karnezis S, Lane JS 3rd, Fujitani RM, Saremi F. Eagle syndrome presenting with external carotid artery pseudoaneurysm. *Emerg Radiol* 2011 Jun;18(3):263–5.

236. Chuang WC, Short JH, McKinney AM, Anker L, Knoll B, McKinney ZJ. Reversible left hemispheric ischemia secondary to carotid compression in Eagle syndrome: surgical and CT angiographic correlation. *AJNR Am J Neuroradiol* 2007 Jan;28(1):143–5.

237. Eagle WW. Elongated styloid process. Further observations and a new syndrome. *Archives of Otolaryngology* 1948;47:630–40.

238. Eagle WW. Symptomatic elongated styloid process; report of two cases of styloid process-carotid artery syndrome with operation. *Arch Otolaryngol* 1949 May;49(5):490–503.

239. Arnould G, Tridon P, Lazenaire M, Picard L, Weber M, Masingue M. [Stylohyoid apparatus and malformations of the occipito-vertebral joint. Apropos of 5 cases]. *Rev Otoneuroophtalmol* 1969 May–Jun;41(4):190–5.

240. Bogousslavsky J, Regli F. Ischemic stroke in adults younger than 30 years of age. Cause and prognosis. *Arch Neurol* 1987 May;44(5):479–82.

241. Arauz A, Márquez JM, Artigas C, Balderrama J, Orrego H. Recanalization of vertebral artery dissection. *Stroke* 2010 Apr;41(4):717–21.

242. Canadian Chiropractic Association, Canadian Federation of Chiropractic Regulatory Boards, Clinical Practice Guidelines Development Initiative et al. Chiropractic clinical practice guideline: evidence-based treatment of adult neck pain not due to whiplash. *J Can Chiropr Assoc* 2005 Sep;49(3):158–209.

243. Ahl B, Bokemeyer M, Ennen JC, Kohlmetz C, Becker H, Weissenborn K. Dissection of the brain supplying arteries over the life span. *J Neurol Neurosurg Psychiatry* 2004 Aug;75(8):1194–6.

244. Phan T, Huston J 3rd, Bernstein MA, Riederer SJ, Brown RD Jr. Contrast-enhanced magnetic resonance angiography of the cervical vessels: experience with 422 patients. *Stroke* 2001 Oct;32(10):2282–6.

245. Barinagarrementeria F, Amaya LE, Cantú C. Causes and mechanisms of cerebellar infarction in young patients. *Stroke* 1997 Dec;28(12):2400–4.

246. Schievink WI, Torres VE, Wiebers DO, Huston J 3rd. Intracranial arterial dolichoectasia in autosomal dominant polycystic kidney disease. *J Am Soc Nephrol* 1997 Aug;8(8):1298–303.

247. Provenzale JM, Morgenlander JC, Gress D. Spontaneous vertebral dissection: clinical, conventional angiographic, CT, and MR findings. *J Comput Assist Tomogr* 1996;20:185–93.

248. Mokri B, Houser OW, Sandok BA, Piepgras DG. Spontaneous dissections of the vertebral arteries. *Neurology* 1988;38:880–5.

249. Nakagawa K, Touho H, Morisako T et al. Long-term follow-up study of unruptured vertebral artery dissection: clinical outcomes and serial angiographic findings. *J Neurosurg* 2000;93:19–25.

250. Lum C, Chakraborty S, Schlossmacher M et al. Vertebral artery dissection with a normal-appearing lumen at multisection CT angiography: the importance of identifying wall hematoma. *AJNR Am J Neuroradiol* 2009 Apr;30(4):787–92.

251. Cloud GC, Markus HS. Diagnosis and management of vertebral artery stenosis. *QJM* 2003 Jan;96(1):27–54.

252. Hass WK, Fields WS, North RR, Kircheff II, Chase NE, Bauer RB. Joint study of extracranial arterial occlusion. II. Arteriography, techniques, sites, and complications. *JAMA* 1968 Mar 11;203(11):961–8.

253. Caplan LR. *Stroke: a clinical approach*, 3rd edition. New York: Butterworth-Heinemann, 2000.

254. Imparato AM, Riles TS, Kim GE. Cervical vertebral angioplasty for brain stem ischemia. *Surgery* 1981;90:842–52.

255. Dainton CJ, Iglar K, Prabhudesai V. A case of right-sided congenital subclavian steal. *Can J Cardiol* 2010 Jan;26(1):e15–6.

256. Aboyans V, Criqui MH, McDermott MM et al. The vital prognosis of subclavian stenosis. *J Am Coll Cardiol* 2007 Apr 10;49(14):1540–5.

257. Yamaguchi R, Kohga H, Kurosaki M et al. Acute basilar artery occlusion in a patient with left subclavian artery occlusion due to first rib anomaly: case report. *Neurol Med Chir (Tokyo)* 2008 Aug;48(8):355–8.

258. Yoneda S, Nukada T, Tada K, Imaizumi M, Takano T. Subclavian steal in Takayasu's arteritis. A hemodynamic study by means of ultrasonic Doppler flowmetry. *Stroke* 1977 Mar–Apr;8(2):264–8.

18

CT of the Aorta and Splanchnic Vessels

Jorge M. Fuentes-Orrego, Rocío Pérez-Johnston, and Dushyant V. Sahani

CONTENTS

18.1 Computed Tomography

Computed tomography (CT) has become an important imaging modality for assessing the vascular system, given its fast acquisition time and noninvasive approach. The introduction of multi-detector CT (MDCT) with hardware and software improvements and enhanced temporal and spatial resolution has enabled high-quality three-dimensional (3D) imaging of the aorta and its branches, aiding vascular surgeons as well as interventional radiologist to better plan therapeutic interventions. Another advantage provided by MDCT is its flexibility with the scanning protocols to target different vascular structures and anatomic regions specific to the clinical conditions [1]. The most common indications for CT angiography (CTA) are listed in Table 18.1.

18.2 Technique

As any other CT technique, CTA should be tailored to the region of interest and the clinical need. Every patient should be evaluated before the procedure for two principal risks directly related to intravenous (IV) contrast material: contrast-induced nephropathy and allergic reactions. If mild (nausea, vomiting, or itching)

to moderate (symptomatic urticaria, vasovagal reaction, bronchospasm, transient hypotension, or tachycardia) symptoms have been well documented in the past, premedication with antihistamines and steroids is indicated. Patients with mild and moderate symptoms are usually premedicated with diphenhydramine 25 or 50 mg intravenously or intramuscularly before the administration of contrast, whereas patients with moderate symptoms are premedicated with steroids (prednisone or methylprednisolone) beginning at least 12 hours before the scan.

Regarding contrast-induced nephropathy, particular attention should be drawn to patients with chronic renal disease or patients with predisposing clinical conditions such as diabetes mellitus, congestive heart failure, leukemia, and myeloma should be screened for risk of contrast material (CM)-induced nephropathy (CIN). Therefore, it is usually recommended that adequate hydration and renal function test should be assessed before reinstating metformin after IV contrast administration for at least 48 hours; if patients are already known for diabetic nephropathy, it is suggested that metformin be withheld 48 hours before the scan.

Patients are usually scanned in the supine position with their feet first. To avoid streak artifacts during the acquisition, it is recommended to scan patients with both arms above the head. Patients should be warned about the mild side effects of contrast injection such as warm feeling, burning sensation, and metallic taste.

Every patient should be advised to hydrate properly after the scan, and patients with a positive history of previous allergic reaction should be closely evaluated for at least 20–30 minutes after the scan.

Since the main interest of the protocol in these patients remains in vascular imaging, no oral contrast should be used since positive oral contrast can interfere with 3D reconstruction and identification of specific pathology such as aortointestinal fistulas, acute bleeding, and mesenteric ischemia. If necessary, to better delineate bowel, a negative oral contrast media can be administered, usually water ranging from 500 to 1000 mL for 20–30 minutes before the scan and additional 300–500 mL immediately before the scan.

In our institution, unenhanced images are acquired first, using 5–10 mm slice thickness and low mA (150–250) approach to cover the organ of interest. The role of unenhanced CT is controversial but usually helps with selecting the coverage for the CTA portion. It is agreed that it has a limited diagnostic role.

A good IV access with an 18–20 gauge catheter is recommended to sustain the faster injection for the CTA. Typically 100–120 mL of nonionic iodinated CM (300–370 mg iodine/mL) is bolus injected at a rate of 4–5 mL/sec. The initial arterial phase is acquired using slice thickness of 1.25–2.5 mm. The venous phase is acquired subsequently at a delay of 65–75 seconds

using 2.5–5 mm thick slices. Usually CTA involves only these two phases (arterial and venous), but recently some authors have found that important findings such as luminal and endoleak enhancement peaks are better shown at different acquisition times beyond the biphasic standard protocol [2]. The technical parameters are listed in Table 18.2. Given the advent of newer MDCT scanners from various vendors that offers 64 detector rows and more, the technical parameters vary and these are listed in Table 18.3.

High-quality MDCTA requires sufficient contrast enhancement, which depends on iodine administration rate, the injection duration, and the cardiac output and body weight of the patient [3]. It is preferable to adjust the CM volume based on its iodine concentration and body weight. For example, for CM of 300 mg I/mL, a total of 100–150 mL range can be used, whereas when higher concentration CM of 350–370 mg I/mL is being used, a CM dose of 80–120 mL is sufficient [4].

Generally, CM injections at 3–5 mL/sec have been shown to work effectively in obtaining a good quality CTA exam. However, with the faster MDCT scanners, a rate of 5 mL/sec is preferred because of its benefits for shortening the injection duration to match up with the scanning duration, thereby influencing CTA quality and optimal vascular enhancement [5–7]. Although injection rates as high as 8 mL/sec has been used in clinical studies to improve tumor-to-parenchyma contrast, but in general, their use is not supported in the outpatient clinical practice because of inherent increase in the CM extravasations risks [8].

The timing of CM delivery with respect to scan acquisition is crucial, and there are several methods to determine an appropriate scan delay. An empiric delay that is fixed based on the organ circulation time for the given CM injection rate is the most commonly used approach (as in our institution) (Table 18.4). Alternatively, a small bolus of CM can be injected first to get a handle on the peak enhancement time in the desired vessel and then adjust the scan delay accordingly.

Maintaining a fixed delay to match-up with each phase of CM enhancement is the most commonly employed technique because of its ease of use and practical application in the outpatient setting, despite the expertise of the operator. However, the rate of CM injection and patient cardiac output variability are not always factored into the equation by this approach,

TABLE 18.1

Indications for CT Angiography

	Indication
Abdominal aorta	• AAA (Diagnosis, treatment planning, posttreatment [EVAR] follow-up). • AAA rupture • AD • Inflammatory conditions
Renal arteries	• Renal artery dissection or aneurysm • Renal artery stenosis (diagnosis, follow-up) • Renal transplant planning or follow-up
Mesenteric arteries	• Acute or chronic mesenteric ischemia (emboli, thrombi, dissection, etc.) • Tumor invasion
Other indications	• Liver transplant • Pancreatic surgery

TABLE 18.2

Technical Parameters for CT Angiography

	Slice Thickness (mm)	Slice Interval (mm)	kV	mA	Pitch–Tube Rotation (s)	Delay (Seconds)	Retro Recon
Unenhanced	5	5	120	150–450	1.375–0.5	0	
MDCTA	0.625	0.625	140	150–715	1.375–0.5	40–50	2.5 mm
Venous phase	2.5	2.5	120	150–450	1.375–0.5	65–75	5.0 mm

TABLE 18.3

Proposed MDCT Scanning Parameters According to Different Vendors

	GE LightSpeed VCT	Philips Brilliance 64	Siemens Sensation 64	Toshiba Aquilion 64
Detector configuration (inner rows)	64×0.625 mm	64×0.625 mm	32×0.6 mm	64×0.5 mm
Detector configuration (outer rows)	NA	NA	8×1.2 mm	NA
Z-axis detector length (64-slice mode) (mm)	40	40	19.2	32
Fastest gantry rotation (second)	0.35	0.40	0.33	0.40
Scan field of view (mm)	25, 50	25–50	50 (option to 70)	18, 24, 32, 40, 50
Coverage in 1 second with pitch of one in 64-slice mode (mm)	114.3	100	58.2	80
X-ray generator power (kW)	100	60	80	60
Anode heat capacity (MHU)	8	8	Equivalent to 30	8
Maximum mA at 120 kV	800	500	665	500
Matrix	512	512, 768, 1028	512	512
Automatic dose reduction	3D dose modulation	Dose right	Care rose 4D	Sure exposure
Simultaneous ATCM in x-y and z-planes	Yes	Yes	Yes	Yes
Cone beam reconstruction algorithm	3D	3D	3D	3D
Automatic reformation in multiple planes	Source axial images	Source axial images	Raw data	Source axial images
Simultaneous functions	Yes	Yes	Yes	Yes
Speed of reconstruction (frame/sec)	22	14	2	2

NA, not applied; GE, General Electric Medical Systems, Milwaukee, WI; Philips, Philips Medical Systems, Best, the Netherlands; Siemens, Siemens Medical Solutions, Forchheim, Germany; Toshiba, Tokyo, Japan

TABLE 18.4

Fixed Scaning Delays According to the Vascular Phase

Injection Rate (mL/sec)	Arterial Phase Time (sec)	Portal Venous Phase (sec)
3	30	70
4	25	65
5	20	60

and in the select patients, this can impact the quality of vascular/organ enhancement. Especially, now with the faster MDCT scanners, most centers with high volume MDCTA practice a test bolus or automated scanning trigger technique that is available on all MDCT scanners.

Automated bolus tracking is more often used than the test-bolus technique, because it is simpler to perform and it reduces the total contrast medium dose. With bolus-tracking technique, the acquisition of the scan is performed during the plateau of attenuation, which offers a more homogenous enhancement in the main branches of the aorta [9].

Irrespective of the use of scan delay technique, it is generally agreed that a saline chaser/flush of 30–40 mL not only decreases the artifacts in the subclavian vein, but it also improves the iodine flux and provides more uniform vascular enhancement [10].

There are certain circumstances in which the defined protocols should be modified (Table 18.5).

TABLE 18.5

Adjustment of the Protocol Based on Patient's Weight, Venous Access, and Renal Function

Large patients > 300 pounds	kVP: 120–140
	Maximize mA
	Speed rotation: 0.8–1.0 second
	Slice thickness: 2.5 mm
	Rate of injection: 5.5–6 mL/sec
Patients < 200 pounds	kVP: 80–100 in arterial phase
Compromised renal function	Prescan: IV saline hydration
	Volume contrast: 60–75 ml
	Saline flush: 40 ml
	Rate of injection: 3.5–4.5 mL/sec
	Postscan: IV saline hydration
Poor venous access	Rate of injection: 3 mL/sec
	Delay: use automated trigger

Large Body Habitus: Patient body size and weight can affect the performance of CTA exam. Typically, the image quality degradation from excessive noise as a result of inadequate beam penetration and field of view restrictions is the main concern in these patients. In our practice, for patients weighing over 300 pounds, we increase the radiation delivery and beam penetration by using a kVP of 140 and increasing the effective milliampere to the maximum allowed on the scanner. Likewise, the rotation of the gantry is decreased to 0.8–1 second and the slice thickness is maintained over 2 mm to distribute the noise over more pixels. Also the CM injection rate is increased by 0.5–1 mL/sec faster than the existing rate of injection.

Compromised Renal Function: In patients with an estimated glomerular filtration rate (eGFR) under 45 mL/min/m², risk of CIN can be minimized by an adequate intravenous hydration before and after the IV CM injection. It is also recommended that the CM load be decreased by 20%–30% of the calculated dose. It has been shown that with the use of 60–75 mL of CM administered at 3.5–4.5 mL/sec combined with the use of a 50 mL saline flush can provide an adequate quality exam. In our practice, eGFR of ≤30 mL/min/m² is considered a contraindication for IV CM administration.

Venous Access Issues: In patients with poor IV access, the rate of CM injection should be adjusted not only to minimize the risks of extravasation but also to sustain a constant injection rate at 3 mL/sec, and the delay of arterial imaging acquisition should be increased from 45 to 55 seconds or established with the automated trigger approach.

Lately, efforts have been addressed to reduce the most important limitations related to CTA, which are CM and radiation dose. The use of low tube voltage results in higher CT attenuation, given that x-ray output energy at this level is closer to the iodine k edge of 33 keV [3]; therefore, recent studies [11,12] have investigated the possibility of lowering both contrast and scanning technique parameters with positive results, which in conjunction with latest denoising reconstruction algorithms will further aid in reducing both of these factors even further.

18.2.1 Postprocessing Techniques

Although a variety of postprocessing protocols have been advocated, the most frequently used approaches include multiplanar reconstruction (MPR), maximum intensity projections (MIP), volume rendering (VR), 3D and curved planar reformation (CPR). Each of these has a specific role for assessing regional anatomy and relationship of lesions in the vicinity. MPR generates views in arbitrary planes without losing information but limited to two-dimensional images; however, it is ideal to obtain precise measurements. MIP displays images with high attenuation values; therefore, enhanced vessels are depicted along with calcified plaques and bones, which can obscure areas of disease

and interfere when measuring strictures. Therefore, bone and plaque subtraction techniques need to be applied to overcome these obstacles. VR offers a good 3D impression of the vessel, better 3D visualization of the vasculature, and important adjacent structures (Figure 18.1). The postprocessing protocols used in our institution are listed in Table 18.6. In addition, advanced vessel and stent analysis can be achieved with applications such as automatic measurement of cross-sectional quantities along the vessel path as well as plaque and bone subtraction (Figures 18.2 and 18.3). One of the latest applications available is virtual angioscopy, which

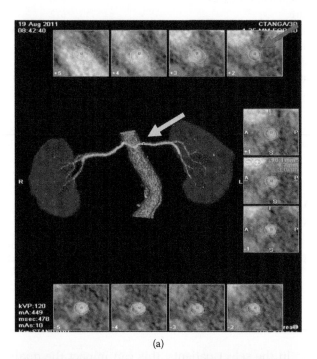

(a)

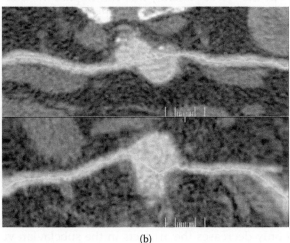

(b)

FIGURE 18.1

(a and b) Left artery stenosis identified at the origin showed by artery segmentation (solid red arrow), volume rendered (solid yellow arrow), and automatic centerline detection (solid blue arrow).

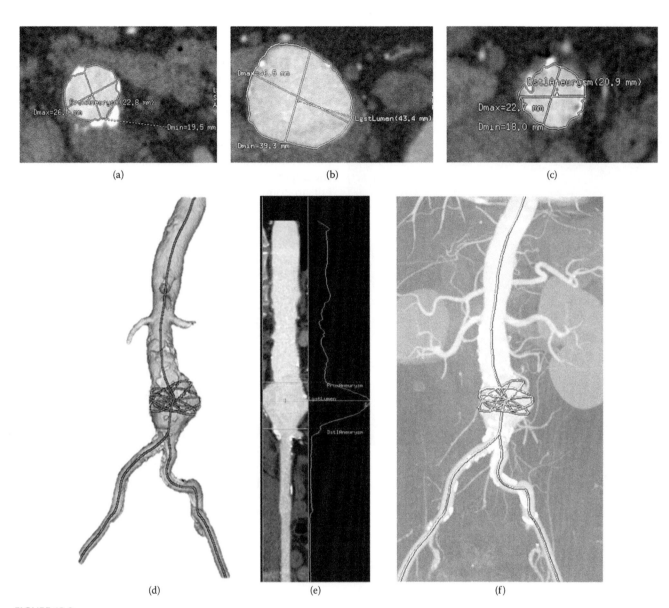

FIGURE 18.2
Automated analysis of a fusiform abdominal aortic aneurysm facilitates diameter measurements cross sectional images at the level of the (a) proximal, (b) middle, and (c) distal portions of abdominal aortic aneurysm. (d) Volume rendering and (e) stretched vessel image and diagram and (f) coronal maximum intensity projections.

TABLE 18.6

Postprocessed Views for CT Angiography

Hepatic artery	3D vascular maps
Celiac trunk and branches	Coronal and sagittal MPR, coronal VR
SMA	Curved CPR, MIP, VR
IMA	Curved CPR, MIP, VR

allows exploration of the inner surface of the vessels, providing information comparable to endovascular ultrasound (US), useful in the clinical context of aortic dissection (AD), atheroma plaques, poststent endothelial healing, and stent fractures (Figure 18.4).

18.2.2 Anatomy

The abdominal aorta has its origin below the diaphragm and extends distally up to the bifurcation of the common iliac arteries. The celiac trunk is the first major branch off the aorta arising approximately at the level of the first lumbar vertebrae along the anterior aspect of the aorta. In the majority of patients, the celiac artery gives rise to three vessels: common hepatic artery, splenic artery, and left gastric artery, which feed the liver, spleen, and lesser curvature of the stomach, respectively. The hepatic artery originates from the celiac trunk and divides into right and left branches; its branches classically follow the portal vein

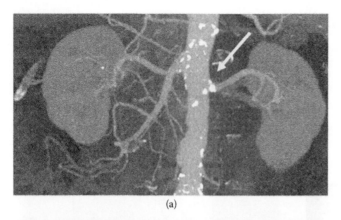

(a)

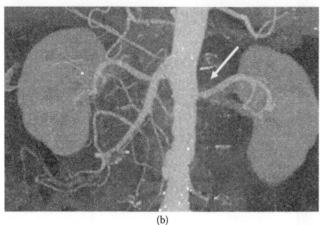

(b)

FIGURE 18.3
(a) Maximum intensity projections of computed tomography (CT) angiography show a calcified plaque at the origin of the left renal artery, impairing evaluation of the lumen. (b) After removal of bone and calcified plaques, the stenosis is better appreciated (arrow).

and bile duct distribution. In some patients, the right hepatic artery originates from the mesenteric artery, often called "right replaced hepatic artery," which is present in up to 18% of patients. Another important anatomical variation is an accessory left hepatic artery arising from the left gastric artery, usually seen in 12% of patients.

The renal arteries arise at the anterolateral and posterolateral aspect of the aorta, just below the level of the superior mesenteric artery (SMA). There are different anatomical variations that range from single renal artery to multiple and duplicated renal arteries.

The SMA is the next major branch of the aorta, followed by the inferior mesenteric artery (IMA). The SMA arises from the aorta just below the celiac trunk and posterior to the pancreatic neck; it courses inferiorly to become anterior to the uncinate process of the pancreas, alongside the SMV, and supplies most of the small bowel via the inferior pancreaticoduodenal, jejunal, and ileal arteries. The SMA also feeds the pancreas along with the celiac trunk and the ascending and the transverse colon by means of the ileocolic, right colic, and middle colic arteries, the former vessels branch off the appendiceal artery. An important pathway for blood flow is established between the SMA and IMA by means of the marginal artery of Drummond, which anastomoses these arteries by branching off vessels that ride along and parallel to the left side of the colon, which become clinically important in obstruction or stenosis of any of these vessels. The IMA arises at the level of L3 and feeds the rest of the colon by the left colic artery (descending colon); sigmoid artery (sigmoid colon); rectosigmoid

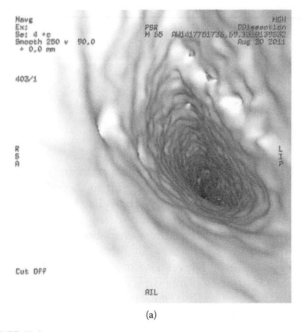

(a)

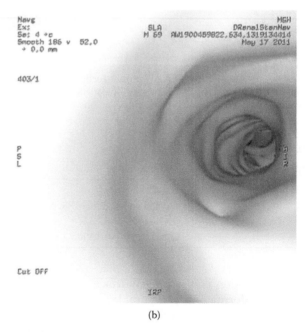

(b)

FIGURE 18.4
Virtual angioscopy in a patient with aortic dissection Type B showing the inner surface of (a) the false lumen and (b) the true lumen.

repair is indicated. These findings have been correlated at autopsies, where there is a 9.4% incidence of rupture for aneurismal diameters of 5.5 cm, which increases up to 32.5% in patients with diameters above 7 cm [14].

The symptoms can vary but patients often present with back pain, buttock, and groin pain, symptoms can also vary depending on if visceral arteries are involved.

Regarding the imaging evaluation of AAA, an unenhanced CT is useful. The unenhanced scan should be carefully searched for complications such as acute bleeding, which usually occurs at the periaortic area, retroperitoneum, either at the pararenal or perirenal space, given that a retroperitoneal hematoma is the most common imaging finding of rupture [15]. Concerning the enhanced phases, acute rupture can be easily shown during arterial phase by showing either leakage of contrast or the presence of a hematoma in the periaortic region, with mass effect on surrounding structures.

The AAA should be assessed for extension, involvement of visceral arteries (renal, superior mesenteric, and celiac arteries), morphology (fusiform, eccentric), and evaluation of true lumen and true vessel size, since the latter is important to assess the risk of rupture as previously described. It is also important to obtain the measurement of the transverse diameter, which is better assessed with the CPR images, since axial images are not as reliable especially if the AAA is tortuous. These features have to be included in the report, so the therapeutic approach can be planned accordingly (Figures 18.2 and 18.6).

Important imaging findings of AAA impending rupture include increased diameter of the aneurysm (0.6–1 cm per year), decreased thrombus-to-lumen ratio as the diameter increases, discontinuity of circumferential calcification in relation to previous studies, suggesting a contained rupture, and the increase in attenuating crescent sign in the periphery within the thrombus of AAA is a sign of acute or impending rupture [15–17].

A less common subtype of aneurysm include mycotic aneurysms, which are pseudoaneurysms, since they involve only the adventitia. Mycotic aneurysms are seen often in patients with septicemia and endocarditis, occurring secondary to hematogenous seeding, and as expected, they may show fat stranding, fluid, gas, and collections in the periaortic area. These aneurysms have a saccular morphology, and in contraposition to the AAA, they are found in the thoracic aorta and above the level of the renal arteries. These aneurysms can also be seen secondary to contiguous spread from vertebral osteomyelitis and abscesses originating in the psoas muscles or kidneys [18].

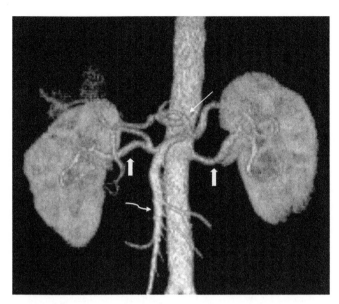

FIGURE 18.5
Three-dimensional volume rendering image depicting major arteries of abdominal aorta. Celiac axis (thin arrow), renal arteries (thick arrows), and superior mesenteric artery (curved arrow).

artery (terminal sigmoid colon) and the superior rectal arteries (superior rectum) (Figure 18.5).

18.2.3 Abdominal Aortic Aneurysm

Abdominal aortic aneurysm (AAA) is most commonly seen in patients with the following risk factors: male patients over 65-years old, smokers, family history of AAA, and patients with longstanding hypertension. AAA represents a focal dilation of the vessel wall, involving the three layers of the vessel (the intimae, media, and adventitia). The aortic dilatation has to have a transverse diameter above 3.0 cm, which often is found incidentally, and can be assessed using either US, magnetic resonance imaging (MRI), or CT, each of which has benefits and limitations. In clinical practice, patients usually are assessed in conjunction of these imaging modalities. The majority of AAA usually arise below the renal arteries which could extend to the iliac arteries in up to one-third of the patients; whereas dissection is not infrequent when aneurysms originates at the thoracic aorta usually extending to the abdomen (Figure 18.2).

Patients with known AAA are usually followed up with US [13]. If the sac diameter is between 3 and 4 cm, a yearly US scan is recommended; for patients with a diameter of 4–4.5 cm, every six month serial ultrasounds are suggested. If the diameter is above 4.5 cm, a vascular specialist should evaluate the patient, with a more dedicated exam, either a CTA or an MRA depending on the clinical context. If the estimated rate of AAA growth is about 0.6–1.0 cm yearly, or the diameter is above 5.5 cm,

18.2.4 Postendovascular Aortic Repair Surveillance

The main objective of therapy in patients with AAA is to exclude the weakened wall of the sac from the

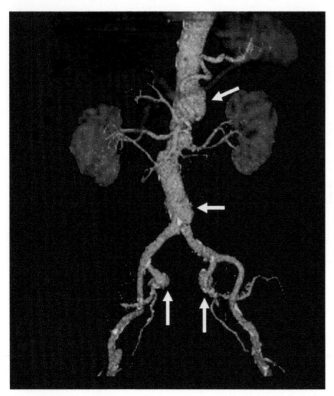

FIGURE 18.6
Volume rendering image of the abdominal aorta showing a supra and infra-renal abdominal aortic aneurysm in a 71-year-old male patient as well as aneurysms in both internal iliac arteries (arrows). Note extensive atherosclerotic disease involving the celiac axis, bifurcation of common iliac arteries, internal and external iliac arteries, and both femoral arteries.

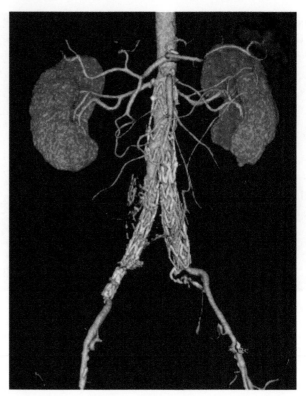

FIGURE 18.7
Volume rendering image of a 69-year-old patient with an abdominal aortic aneurysm status postendovascular aortic repair surveillance adequately positioned. Note that the stent shows no fracture or migration.

high-pressure system, because as the sac grows wider, the intravascular pressure becomes greater, which increases the chance of rupture, according to Laplace law. Therefore, AAA repair can be done with either open transabdominal or endovascular surgery, the latter is preferred because of reduced morbidity and mortality, since it is feasible in majority of patients [19]. All patients undergoing AAA repair need to have surveillance, especially in those who have had endovascular aortic repair surveillance (EVAR) given that endostents can either migrate or present with endoleaks, which are associated with a persistent increase in incidence of AAA and, as expected, result in an increase in diameter, which augments the risk of rupture. Endoleaks represent blood flow out of the endostent into the aneurismal sac and have been classified at least in five different types. Type I endoleaks, usually originate at the proximal or distal attachment site of the stent-graft and represent a failure to exclude the aneurismal sac. These leaks have been described after repair of thoracic aortic aneurysms and are usually seen in patients with tortuous and irregular vascular anatomy; as this prevents adequate sealing between the native arterial

wall and the endostent-graft, they are usually subclassified as type a or b, depending on if it involves [1] the proximal attachment site or [2] the distal attachment site. Type II, on the other hand, is the most common type of endoleak after EVAR and usually originates from retrograde blood flow through branch vessels of the aorta such as the lumbar arteries or IMA into the sac. Type III endoleaks are uncommon and occur when leaks originate within the stent, as a result of fabric holes, fracture, or any other structural problem. Type IV is described as graft porosity, and it is thought to arise secondary to full anticoagulation and is seen as "blush" after implantation, which requires no treatment. Finally, Type V has been described as aneurismal sac dilatation without the presence of an endoleak (Figures 18.7 and 18.8).

18.2.5 Aortic Dissection

AD is defined as the separation between the layers in the aortic wall, usually secondary to intimal disruption, which allows blood to enter the intima-media space, thus creating a less resistant pathway for blood to go

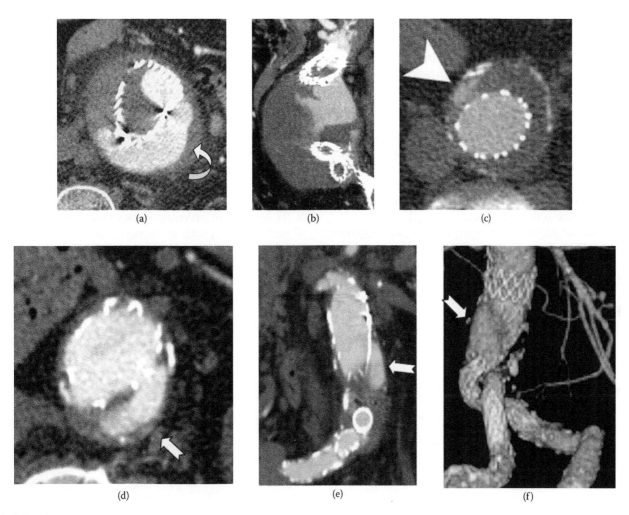

(a)　　(b)　　(c)

(d)　　(e)　　(f)

FIGURE 18.8
Axial image showing endoleak (arrow head) in follow up study postendovascular aortic repair surveillance.

through, which allows progression of dissection in a proximal-to-distal manner. Blood may reenter the true lumen (reentry tear) or not. AD has been classified according to the time frame as acute (>2 weeks) or chronic (more than 2 weeks) with a higher mortality rate in the former [20]. Even when different classifications have been created to characterize anatomically ADs, Stanford classification is still the most commonly used. Type A classification involves the ascending aorta, while Type B includes dissections occurring distal to the left subclavian artery [21]. By far, the most common type is A, which in acute clinical setting has the highest mortality rate [20] and requires emergently surgical procedure. Type B dissections are usually treated medically if no end organ damage has been established and represent about 40% of the cases, whereas type A is by far most common conforming 60%–70%.

The predisposing factors for AD include hypertension, aneurysm, trauma, surgery, infection, and inflammatory conditions as connective tissue disorders (Wegener's granulomatosis, systemic lupus erythematosus, etc.).

Regarding the clinical presentation, patients often complain of chest pain, located either anteriorly or posteriorly between the shoulders, resembling the clinical presentation of acute myocardial infarction. Up to 10% of patients with AD have no symptoms [22]; therefore, a high index of clinical suspicion is necessary to clinch the diagnosis.

Special attention should be paid to AD, since there are other entities that can mimic it, such as a mural thrombus in ectatic segments of the aorta or saccular aneurysm, periaortic soft tissue tumor or fibrosis, and even anemia given the low intraluminal attenuation compared to the aortic wall.

The classic imaging findings of AD include the intimal flap, dividing both the true and false lumen, which often becomes aneurismal given the high pressure system. Other signs habitually found in AD include delayed enhancement of the false lumen; widening of the aorta, mediastinal, pleural, or pericardial hematoma; and displacement of calcifications [23]. It is important to assess the intimal flap, the size of the aorta, patency of false lumen, and rupture of dissection. The false lumen is usually larger than the true lumen; the intimal flap adopts a linear configuration most of the times. If intimal calcifications are present, they are displaced as previously described and face the true lumen (Figure 18.9).

ADs have a higher rate of occurrence in the thoracic (70%), descending (20%), and aortic root (7%) and less commonly isolated in the abdominal aorta (2%) [24]. Several authors have reported isolated abdominal ADs since the wide availability of CT (25–27), which usually present with the dissection flap originating at or below the level of the renal arteries.

Abdominal AD is usually symptomatic, although none specific. Patients present with back pain, abdominal pain, pulsatile abdominal mass, peripheral ischemia, and distal embolization [27]. Dissection of the celiac axis (CA) can lead to splenic or hepatic infarction depending on the vessels involved [27].

The most common complications of dissection of the aorta are rupture of the dissection into the pericardium progressing to tamponade, occlusion of the coronary or supra aortic vessels, severe aortic insufficiency, and acute heart failure [28].

Intramural hematomas (IHs) have been described as an atypical variant of AD, but the underlying pathophysiology is different between both processes. IH results from rupture of the vasa vasorum with subsequent hemorrhage into the media, which has been associated with the formation of pseudoaneurysm, aneurysm, and dissections, given the resultant weakening of the wall [29]. IHs have shown a mortality rate of up to 21% and have been found in 20% of patients with symptoms of AD [30]. The imaging findings of IH include an eccentric hyperdense crescent, usually >7 mm diameter, with an average density of 60–70 HU in unenhanced scans [31]. The Stanford classification of AD is used to characterize IH, which have different implications, and has been shown by some authors who have found that Type A IHs have a higher rate to progress to classic AD, whereas Type B is usually treated medically [32].

IH, as do hematomas in other regions of the body, may become hypodense sometimes in periods as short as one

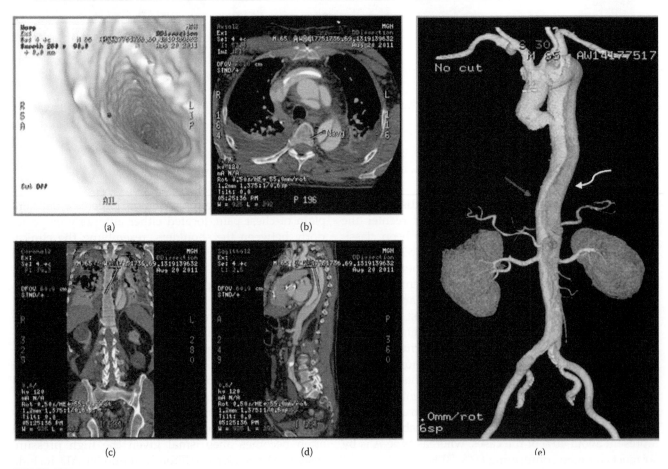

(a)   (b)   (c)   (d)   (e)

FIGURE 18.9
Aortic dissection in a thoraco–abdominal aneurysm in the same patient, as shown in Figure 18.4. (a) Virtual angioscopy of false lumen. (b–d) Axial, coronal, and sagittal images at the level of the thoracic descending aorta shows dissection flip (black arrow), bilateral pleural effusion, and mediastinal hemorrhage. (e) Volume rendering image showing the true (straight arrow) and false lumen (squiggly arrow), with the latter involving the celiac axis and superior mesenteric artery extending up to the common iliac arteries.

week long; therefore, IH may show a high or low density in acute and chronic stages, respectively. Another clue useful for the diagnosis of IH is the configuration of intimal calcifications, as previously described; calcifications in AD become linear, as opposed to the semicircular or ovoid configuration of intimal calcifications in IH. Secondary findings like pleural or pericardial effusions and mediastinal hematoma may be present.

It is fundamental to assess the diameter of the aorta at the level of the IH, given that weakening of the wall predisposes the vessel to rupture; therefore, it is recommended that patients be followed up to asses for new intimal tears, new dissections and rupture, with the former often seen as enhanced saccular out-pouchings along the wall of the vessel best seen in axial or CPR images. These intimal tears are more frequently seen in the thoracic aorta and aortic arch, which can progress to dissection and rupture. As in AD, IH may be confused with different conditions such as inflammation, soft tissue tumor (lymphoma, retroperitoneal, or mediastinal nodes), atheromatous plaques, but these entities usually involve longer segments of the aorta in an irregular manner and often in different clinical scenarios that set these conditions and IH apart.

18.2.6 Mesenteric Ischemia

Mesenteric arteries as well as celiac axis can become occluded both in acute and chronic conditions, leading to mesenteric ischemia presenting with nonspecific abdominal pain, bloody diarrhea, elevated liver, and/or pancreatic enzymes. In the acute setting, either one or both the celiac and SMA become obstructed by embolic or thrombotic events. In the embolic setting, other visceral end organ damage can be associated (renal and splenic infarcts), and these findings are an important clue for the diagnosis, which has most often a cardiac origin, whereas thrombosis is a superimposed condition that is usually found in the context of extensive atherosclerotic disease. Acute mesenteric ischemia can also be seen in patients with low cardiac output and/or low blood volume, which results in decreased blood flow to the mesentery, such as in patients with noncompensated congestive heart failure, bleeding, and septic shock. A less frequent cause of mesenteric ischemia is the median arcuate ligament syndrome, which consist of a fibrotic tissue that unites the diaphragmatic crura, arising from either side, and is often found superior to the celiac axis, but sometimes, it is located in a lower position in which compression of the celiac axis leads to epigastric abdominal pain, which can be depicted with either angiography or CTA. CTA is more useful to show its relationship to adjacent structures to better plan therapeutic approach and has the advantage of being noninvasive [33]. Other conditions associated with mesenteric ischemia include SMA dissection and/or aneurysm. Dissection of CA can lead to splenic or hepatic infarction depending on the vessels involved. The usual clinical setting of acute mesenteric ischemia is seen in elderly patients with abdominal pain out of proportion to the physical exam findings, which can deteriorate to abdominal distention, gastrointestinal bleeding, peritoneal irritation secondary to perforation, and bowel necrosis.

The imaging findings vary according to the etiology; therefore, when multiple filling defects as well as end organ damage is seen (renal, splenic, hepatic infarctions, etc.), an embolic event should be considered. On the other hand, whenever filling defects occur in the context of heavily calcified vessels, thrombotic events should be favored. Along with these findings, other frequently found image characteristics include lack of contrast enhancement in ischemic bowel loops, wall thickening, mural thumb printing because of edema or hemorrhage, pneumatosis intestinalis, and perforation. In low cardiac output/low blood volume conditions, findings that correlate with these clinical scenarios can be found such as pericardial and/or pleural effusion, ascitis, and pulmonary embolism. If none of these findings is present, one giveaway for the diagnosis of acute mesenteric ischemia is the decrease in diameter of the mesenteric arteries.

In the chronic setting, mesenteric ischemia has also been called abdominal angina, which is often seen in patients over 60 years old, with a prevalence of female to male ratio of about 3:1 [34]. It is usually associated with epigastric pain after meals, but can also present with diarrhea, constipation, flatulence, less often vomiting, and can involve the celiac, superior, and IMAs as well. It is commonly seen in patients with extensive atherosclerotic disease, which leads to obstruction or stenosis of these vessels. To become clinically symptomatic, the stenosis or obstruction should involve at least two out of three arteries. Weight loss can be seen, since patients can become "food fear," given the experienced postpandrial pain and also given the mucosal damage associated blood flow reduction.

Another important aspect of CTA concerns the evaluation of vessel encasement secondary to tumor spreading, which is usually seen in pancreatic neoplasm. A vessel is considered to be encased when tumor involves at least 180° of the vessel circumference, which precludes surgery as a primary treatment.

Concerning treatment, abdominal angina can be approached both surgically and percutaneously, with the latter being done preferentially given its low morbidity and mortality. Usually when the celiac axis and the SMA are involved, treatment should be directed to either one of them, unless a high grade stenosis is present (>70% luminal narrowing) in both arteries, then both of them should be treated accordingly (Figure 18.10).

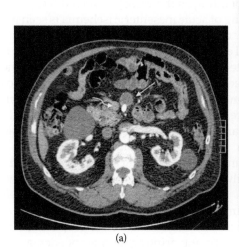
(a)

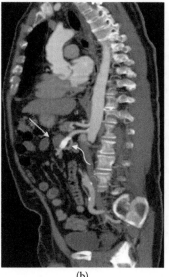
(b)

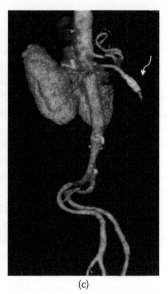
(c)

FIGURE 18.10

(A 69-year-old patient with a fusiform aneurysm (straight arrow) of the superior mesenteric artery with a patent stent (squiggly arrow) shown on (a) contrast enhanced axial, (b) sagittal, and (c) volume rendering images.

18.2.6.1 Patient Safety

Given that the two limitations of CTA are radiation and CM, we will describe a few strategies that can be used to reduce both.

CM can be reduced by different ways: first, by using a higher iodine concentration (>370 mg/mL) with a saline flush during the injection phase, second, by using low kVp (80–100) during CTA acquisition. Given that at low kVp, the energy in the x-ray beam moves closer to the k-edge of iodine, this approach can, therefore, enable contrast reduction by 20%–40%. This method not only offers the benefit of cutting down CM doses, but also provides the added value of lowering radiation dose to the patient. And third, CM can be reduced by using virtual monochromatic energies generated by dual energy CT (DECT, either single or double source) at low keV (50–70 keV), which provides a higher contrast than single energy CT scan at 120 kv.

Radiation dose reduction, on the other hand, can be achieved with different methods: first, by limiting the phases of the CTA scan, for example, by combining the arterial and venous phase (delaying arterial phase by 10–15 seconds). Second, by limiting the scanning region of interest to the AAA repair/stent area, instead of covering the entire abdominopelvic region. Utilization of DECT can further reduce dose, by using a virtual-non-contrast-enhanced image instead of true noncontrast images, limiting unnecessary exposition of patient to radiation. DECT can also be applied to obtain a late phase and reconstruct images for arterial-like-phase using low kVp/keV images (50–70 keV) and venous phase images from intermediate to high kVp/keV data (140 kVp or 70–80 keV). Finally, since the introduction of

TABLE 18.7

Different Approaches to Reduce CM and Radiation Doses

Reduce CM Utilization	Radiation Dose Reduction
Higher concentration of iodine (>370 mg/mL) during injection	
Acquisition of CTA	
Use of low kVp (80–100) during CTA acquisition	Use of low kVp (80 kVp, <180 lbs, 100 kVp, 181–300 lbs, 120 kVp, >300 lbs)
	Reduce phases of scan (combined arterial and venous phase) in conventional CT and use of late phase on DECT (50–70 keV)
	Limiting the scanning region (AAA repair/stent)
	Use of virtual-noncontrast image from DECT instead of true-noncontrast phase
Postprocessing (image reconstruction)	
Use of virtual monochromatic energies in DECT (50–70 keV) to increase contrast	Reconstruct images at low keV (50–70) for arterial phase and at intermediate-to-high keV (70–80) for venous phase
	Use of iterative reconstruction techniques to lower both kVp and mAs. Image quality is preserved.

improved iterative reconstruction techniques, low kVp and mAs protocols can be instituted more aggressively without image quality concerns (see Table 18.7).

18.3 Conclusion

CTA has become nowadays an important tool to evaluate vascular structures, especially in acute clinical settings where an early and noninvasive diagnosis can be obtained directing treatment and improve patient management and prognosis, especially with the latest and fast postprocessing techniques that allow for 3D visualization of the region of interest. Although other imaging methods such as US and magnetic resonance are already available, both of them have limitations that have allowed CTA to become the imaging method of choice in these scenarios. For example, US requires a high grade of expertise (user-dependent) and also visualization of vascular structures can be limited by bowel gas. Even when MRI has a high temporal and spatial resolution comparable to CTA, it is more expensive and the scanning times are greater, making it not suitable in urgent conditions. The ability to evaluate both vascular and extravascular disease in a single scan makes CTA a suitable exam when assessing patients with chronic conditions as well.

Nowadays, the two most important limitations for CTA are radiation dose and IV contrast media. Given the recent introduction of new technologies such as dual energy CT, higher row detector scanners, and new denoising software reconstruction techniques, both of these limitations can be addressed and patient safety can be increased.

References

1. Lawler LP, Fishman EK. Multi-detector row CT of thoracic disease with emphasis on 3D volume rendering and CT angiography. *RadioGraphics* 2001; 21: 1257–1273.
2. Lehmkuhl L, Andres C, Lücke C et al. Dynamic CT angiography after abdominal endovascular aneurysm repair: differences in contrast agent dynamics in the aorta and endoleaks-preliminary results. *J Vasc Interv Radiol* 2012; 23(6): 744–750.
3. Nakayama Y, Awai K, Funama Y et al. Abdominal CT with low tube voltage: preliminary observations about radiation dose, contrast enhancement, image quality, and noise. *Radiology* 2005; 237(3): 945–951.
4. Furuta A, Ito K, Fujita T et al. Hepatic enhancement in multiphasic contrast-enhancement MDCT: comparison of high and low-iodine-concentration contrast medium in same patients with chronic liver disease. *AJR Am J Roentgenol* 2004; 183: 157–162.
5. Pannu HK, Maley WR, Fishman EK. Liver transplantation: preoperative CT. *Radiographics* 2001; 21: S133–S146.
6. Horton KM, Fishman EK. 3D CT angiography of the celiac and superior mesenteric arteries with multidetector CT data sets: preliminary observations. *Abdom Imaging* 2000; 25: 523–525.
7. Tanikake M, Shimizu T, Narabayashi I et al. Three-dimensional angiography of the hepatic artery: use of multi-detector row helical CT and contrast agent. *Radiology* 2003; 227: 883–889.
8. Shueller G, Schima W, Schueller-Weidekamm C et al. Multidetector CT of the pancreas: effects of contrast material flow rate and individualized scan delay on enhancement of pancreas and tumor contrast. *Radiology* 2006; 241: 441–448.
9. Thomas A, Bernhard M. New trends in multidetector computed tomography angiography of peripheral arteries. *Advances in MDCT–an International Literature Review Service* 2005; 2(2): 1–6.
10. Tatsugami F, Matsuki M, Kani H et al. Effect of saline pushing after contrast material injection in abdominal multidetector computed tomography with the use of different iodine concentrations. *Acta Radiol* 2006; 47(2): 192–197.
11. Nakaura T, Awai K, Maruyama N et al. Abdominal dynamic CT in patients with renal dysfunction: contrast agent dose reduction with low tube voltage and high tube current-time product settings at 256-detector row CT. *Radiology* 2011; 261(2): 467–476.
12. Iezzi R, Cotroneo AR, Giammarino A et al. Low-dose-multidetector-row CT angiography of abdominal aortic aneurysm after endovascular repair. *Eur J Radiol* 2011; 79(1): 21–28.
13. Kent KC, Zwolak RM, Jaff MR, Hollenbeck ST, Thompson RW, Schermerhorn ML et al. Screening for abdominal aortic aneurysm. *J Vasc Surg* 2004; 39: 267–269.
14. Lederle FA, Johnson GR, Wilson SE et al. Rupture rate of large abdominal aortic aneurysms in patients refusing or unfit for elective repair. *JAMA* 2002; 287: 2968–2972.
15. Siegel CL, Cohan RH, Korobkin M et al. Abdominal aortic aneurysm morphology: CT features in patients with ruptured and non-ruptured aneurysms. *AJR Am J Roentgenol* 1994; 163: 1123–1129.
16. Mehard WB, Heiken JP, Sicard GA. High-attenuating crescent in abdominal aortic aneurysm wall at CT: a sign of acute or impending rupture. *Radiology* 1994; 192: 359–362.
17. Rakita D, Newatia A, Hines JJ et al. Spectrum of CT findings in rupture and impending rupture of abdominal aortic aneurysms. *Radiographics* 2007; 27: 497–507.
18. Macedo TA, Stanson AW, Oderich GS et al. Infected aortic aneurysms: imaging findings. *Radiology* 2004; 231: 250–257.
19. Moore WJ, Kashyap VS, Vescera CL et al. Abdominal aortic aneurysm: a 6-year comparison of endovascular vs. transabdominal repair. *Ann Surg* 1999; 230: 298–308.
20. Hagan PG, Nienaber CA, Isselbacher EM et al. The international registry of acute aortic dissection (IRAD): new insights into an old disease. *JAMA* 2000; 283(7): 897–903.
21. Daily PO, Truebold HW, Stinson EB et al. Management of acute aortic dissections. *Ann Thorac Surg* 1970; 10: 237–247.
22. Spittell PC, Spittell JA Jr, Joyce JW et al. Clinical features and differential diagnosis of aortic dissection: experience with 236 cases (1980 through 1990). *Mayo Clin Proc* Jul 1993; 68(7): 642.

23. Fisher ER, Stern EJ, Godwin JD et al. Acute aortic dissection: typical and atypical imaging features. *Radiographics* 1994; 14: 1263–1271.

24. Roberts CS, Roberts WC. Aortic dissection with the entrance tears in abdominal aorta. *Am Heart J* 1991; 121: 1834–1835.

25. Farber A, Wagner WH, Cossman DV, Cohen JL, Walsh DB, Fillinger MF et al. Isolated dissection of the abdominal aorta: clinical presentation and therapeutic options. *J Vasc Surg* 2002; 36: 205–210.

26. Baumgartner F, Omari B, Donayre C. Suprarenal abdominal aortic dissection with retrograde formation of a massive descending thoracic aneurysm. *J Vasc Surg* 1998; 27: 180–182.

27. Borioni R, Garofalo M, DePaulis R et al. Abdominal aortic dissections: anatomic and clinical features and therapeutic options. *Tex Heart Inst J* 2005; 32(1): 70–73.

28. Sebastia C, Pallisa E, Quiroga S et al. Aortic dissection: diagnosis and follow up with helical CT. *Radiographics* 1999; 19: 45–60.

29. Sawhney NS, DeMaria AN, Blanchard DG. Aortic intramural hematoma: an increasingly recognized and potentially fatal entity. *Chest* 2001; 120: 1340–1346.

30. Nienaber CA, Von Kodolitsch Y, Petersen B et al. Intramural hemorrhage of the thoracic aorta: diagnostic and therapeutic implications. *Circulation* 1995; 92: 1465–1472.

31. Chao CP, Walker TG, Kalva SP. Natural history and CT appearances of aortic intramural hematoma. *Radiographics* 2009; 29: 791–804.

32. Choi SH, Choi SJ, Kim JH et al. Useful CT findings for predicting the progression of aortic intramural hematoma to overt aortic dissection. *J Comput Assist Tomogr* 2001; 25: 295–299.

33. Horton KM, Talamini MA, Fishman EK. Median arcuate ligament syndrome: evaluation with CT angiography. *Radiographics* 2005; 25: 1177–1182.

34. Roobotom CA, Dubbins PA. Significant disease of the celiac and superior mesenteric arteries in asymptomatic patients: predictive value of Doppler sonography. *AJR Am J Roentgenol* 1993; 161: 985–988.

19

Peripheral CT Angiography of the Lower and Upper Limbs

Michele Anzidei, Eugenio Marotta, Luca Bertaccini, Alessandro Napoli, and Carlo Catalano

CONTENTS

19.1 Introduction

In the last few years, computed tomography angiograpy (CTA) has become the standard diagnostic method for lower and upper limbs vascular examination [1–3]. Steno-obstructive disease is the most frequent pathology requiring CTA studies, which recognizes atherosclerosis as the most frequent among causes of the disease, especially in older patients. One of the critical aspects in the study of peripheral arterial regions is represented by the examination technique, mostly with regard to the synchronization between contrast media administration and data acquisition [4]. While until a few years ago, peripheral CTA still required a compromise between temporal resolution and spatial resolution of the acquisition, with potential detrimental effects on diagnostic accuracy [5,6], the introduction of the latest (>16 slice) multi-detector computerized tomography (MDCT) scanners finally removed this kind of technical limitations, allowing at the same time to reduce iodine and radiation doses, enabling optimal image quality from the largest vessel to the small caliber branches. At the same time, the introduction of advanced postprocessing

systems produced an added value in image interpretation that, in combination with high resolution datasets examinations, largely increased the diagnostic value of CTA examinations. In this chapter, we will discuss the examination techniques for CTA of the lower and upper limbs as well as normal anatomy, anatomic variants, atherosclerotic disease, and post-treatment findings.

19.2 CTA of the Lower Limbs

19.2.1 Anatomy

For detailed anatomy or arterial circulation of the upper limbs, refer to Figures 19.1 through 19.5 and Tables 19.1 through 19.6

19.2.2 Examination Technique

The patient is placed supine on the CT scanner, with arms overhead to reduce beam hardening artifacts, the lower limbs are close together, facing the gantry, with feet slightly internally rotated (toes can

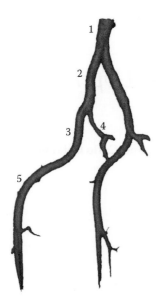

FIGURE 19.1
Abdominal aorta (1), common iliac artery (2), external iliac artery (3), internal iliac artery (4), and common femoral artery (5) (see also Table 19.1).

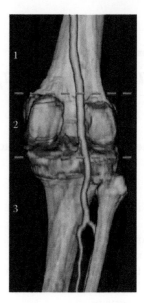

FIGURE 19.3
Popliteal artery (Table 19.3): sovra-articular (1), articular (2), and subarticular (3).

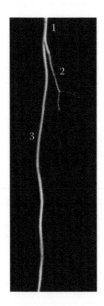

FIGURE 19.2
Femoral arteries: common (1), deep (2), and superficial (3) (see also Table 19.2).

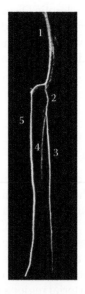

FIGURE 19.4
Leg and calf arteries: popliteal (1), tibio-peroneal trunk (2), anterior tibial artery (3), interosseous artery (4), and posterior tibial artery (5) (see also Tables 19.3 through 19.6).

be optionally fixed with tape to help maintain this position). Peripheral venous access should be placed on one arm, preferably on the elbow, and must be not less than 20 G. A positioning topogram (not less than 130 cm long) must be acquired on the coronal plane from the diaphragmatic dome to the tip of the feet (Figure 19.6a). In order to calculate the optimal delay between the contrast agent administration and the start of scans, a circular region of interest (ROI)

must be placed on the sovrarenal abdominal aorta, avoiding the inclusion of intimal calcifications, which could alter the diagram of density variation on both bolus tracking and bolus test techniques (Figure 19.6b and c). The aortic attenuation threshold must be set at 150–200 HU (Figure 19.6d) using the minimum delay allowed by the scanner for acquisition start. If abdominal aortic aneurysm have been previously diagnosed, it can be useful to place the ROI within the dilated

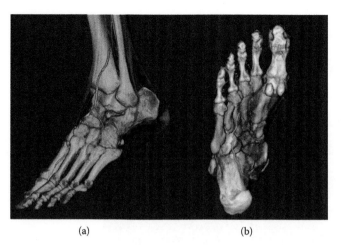

FIGURE 19.5
Foot arteries: (a) dorsal arteries and (b) plantar arteries (see also Tables 19.4 through 19.6).

TABLE 19.1

Iliac Arteries: Branches and Collaterals

Iliac Arteries		
Common iliac artery		
External iliac artery	Inferior epigastric artery	Cremasteric artery
	Deep circumflex iliac artery	
Internal iliac artery	Anterior branches	Vesical arteries
		Obturator artery
		Rectal arteries
		Uterine artery
		Vaginal artery
	Posterior branches	Ileo-lumbar artery
		Sacral artery
		Superior gluteal artery

TABLE 19.2

Femoral Arteries: Branches and Collaterals

Femoral Arteries	
Superficial femoral artery	Superficial epigastric artery
	Superficial iliac circumflex
	Superficial external pudendal
	Deep external pudendal
Deep femoral artery	Lateral femoral circumflex
	Medial femoral circumflex
	Perforating and muscular branches

TABLE 19.3

Popliteal Arteries: Branches and Collaterals

Popliteal Artery
Anterior tibial
Posterior tibial artery
Sural
Superior genicular (medial, lateral)
Middle genicular
Inferior genicular (medial, lateral)

TABLE 19.4

Anterior Tibial Arteries: Branches and Collaterals

Anterior Tibial
Posterior tibial recurrent
Anterior tibial recurrent
Muscular branches
Anterior medial malleolar
Anterior lateral malleolar
Dorsalis pedis

TABLE 19.5

Posterior Tibial Arteries: Branches and Collaterals

Posterior Tibial
Fibular artery
Medial plantar artery
Lateral plantar artery

TABLE 19.6

Peroneal Arteries: Branches and Collaterals

Peroneal (or Fibular) Artery
Communicating branch
Perforating branch

tract of the aorta since the turbulence of the blood flow will slow down the speed of blood, diluting the concentration of the contrast media, with the risk of inadequate opacification of the lower limbs arteries.

The use of high iodine concentration contrast media (350–400 mgI/mL) is recommended as well as high injection flows (at least 4 mL/s) in order to achieve a higher and more homogeneous arterial opacification (Tables 19.7 and 19.8). Using a monophasic contrast agent administration protocol, acquisition time should not be less than 35–40 seconds in patients with normal cardiac output and preserved peripheral circulation—faster scans could easily surpass the contrast agent bolus, mostly below the knee, with poor opacification in the distal segments. In these cases, it can be useful to set up a "rescue" scan for the calf with caudocranial acquisition direction; when needed, this

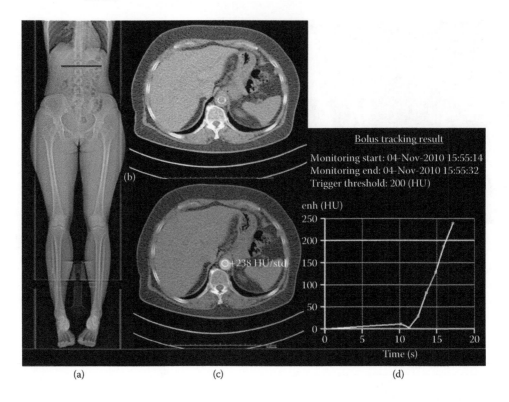

FIGURE 19.6
(a) Topogram acquisition in the coronal plane. (b) Red line represents the premonitoring, placed on the sovrarenal abdominal aorta. Density values variation on the area marked by region of interest, on the lumen of the sovrarenal abdominal aorta (c), until the achievement of threshold value (d).

TABLE 19.7

Contrast Agent Administration Parameters for Lower Limb Peripheral CTA

MDC	4 Slices	16 Slices	64 Slices	128 Slices	Dual Source
IV contrast iodine concentration (mgI/mL)	350–400	350–400	350–400	350–400	350–400
Volume (mL)	125	120	115	115	115
Saline flush volume (mL)	50	50	50	50	50
Flow rate (mL/s)	2.5	3	4–5	4–5	4–5

TABLE 19.8

Scan Parameters for Lower Limb Peripheral CTA

	4 Slices	16 Slices	64 Slices	128 Slices	Dual Source
kVp	120	120	120	120	120
mAs	140	160	190 (Dose Modulation)	190 (Dose Modulation)	190 (Dose Modulation)
Slice Collimation	4 × 2.5	16 × 1.5	64 × 0.6	128 × 0.6	64 × 0.6 × 2
Slice width (mm)	3	2	2	1	1
Recon increment (mm)	2	1	1	1	1

scan can be started immediately after the end of the first acquisition in order to avoid poor vessels opacification in patients with slow flow in the calf region. Similarly, setting up acquisition protocols lasting longer than 40 s must be avoided, since in this case, venous opacification may cause suboptimal image quality (Figure 19.7). It should be kept in mind that various pathological conditions, including advanced atherosclerotic disease, diabetic ulcers, and arterovenous fistulae, may asymmetrically alter the flow velocity, inevitably causing a reduction in image quality even with the above-mentioned tips.

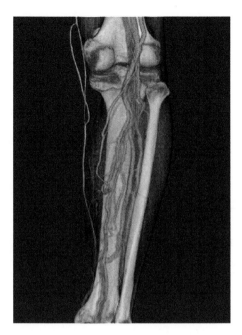

FIGURE 19.7
Venous contamination due to incorrect synchronization between the contrast media injection and the scan start.

19.2.3 Atherosclerotic Disease of the Lower Limbs

Atherosclerotic disease is the main cause of peripheral arterial disease, producing a reduction in arterial blood supply to the lower vascular district by major vessels stenosis or occlusion. It is actually impossible to provide a truly accurate assessment of the incidence of peripheral arterial obstructive disease (PAOD) since the early stages of the disease are asymptomatic or low-symptomatic and, in most cases, are misdiagnosed or diagnosed only in advanced stages. However, several epidemiological studies [7,8] calculated an overall prevalence of the disease between 3% and 10% in the Western population under 70 years of age, rising to 15%–20% after 70 years of age. The main risk factors are age, male sex, cigarette smoke, diabetes, and dyslipidemia (Table 19.9). The early stage of PAOD is clinically characterized by chronic cramping and soreness in the posterior compartment of the leg, mainly after exercise, while acute worsening of the symptoms occurs more commonly in the advanced stage of the disease. Critical limb ischemia (CLI) is the most severe evolution of advanced PAOD and develops when the blood flow does not meet the metabolic demands of tissue at rest. This condition, manifested by pain during rest and by nonhealing ulcers and gangrene that are usually located in the toes, forefoot, or heel of the affected limb, is the main nontraumatic indication for lower limb amputation. Diabetes is the most important risk factor for CLI, since in this case, atherosclerosis not only develops at a younger age, causing stenosis and obstruction of femoral arteries that can be compensated

TABLE 19.9

Risk Factors for PAOD

PAOD Risk Factors	
Sex	Dyslipidemia
Age	Hyperhomocysteinemia
Cigarette smoke	Chronic renal failure
Diabetes	
Arterial hypertension	

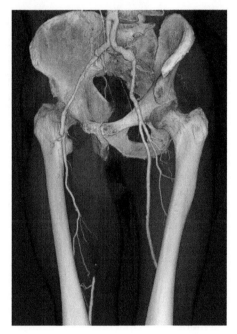

FIGURE 19.8
Patient with right superficial femoral artery obstruction.

(Figure 19.8) by collateral vessels, but more often, affects arteries below the knee and in the foot, which are more susceptible to occlude acutely (Figure 19.9). Symptoms can arise in a few days and patients present the five cardinal signs and symptoms—pain, pallor, pulselessness, paresthesia, and paralysis. With an occluding thrombosis, the patient will experience acute rest pain, the lower leg and foot will appear pale and have no pulse, and if the condition is left untreated, it can progress to paresthesia and paralysis and later, soft tissue necrosis. Acute embolism from other causes (atrial fibrillation, valvular disease, or vasculistis) can cause similar symptoms. The degree of limb ischemia dictates treatment planning—despite the benefits of pharmacologic therapy, surgical or interventional revascularization remains a mainstay in the management of CLI because the restoration of adequate blood flow to the foot is crucial to provide pain relief, promote wound healing, and avoid amputation.

From a clinical point of view, the two most commonly used classifications for PAOD staging are those of Rutherford and Fontaine, which allow an adequate

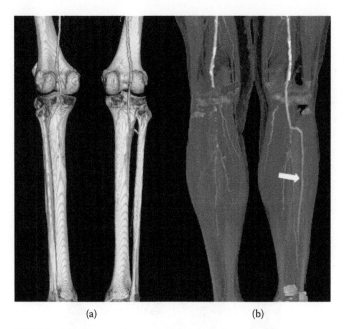

(a)   **(b)**

FIGURE 19.9
(a) Volume-rendered (VR) and (b) coronal plane maximum intensity projection (MIP) of a patient with peripheral arterial obstructive disease. Red arrow points to the obstruction of the right popliteal artery; left leg run off is sustained by the anterior tibial artery (white arrow).

clinical grading to address patients for imaging and treatment (Tables 19.10 and 19.11). From a radiological point of view, it is appropriate to refer to the current guidelines of the Transatlantic InterSociety Consensus (TASC) for the Management of Peripheral Arterial Disease [9,10], which classified the lesions according to their extension and possible surgical or endovascular approach. In particular, atherosclerotic lesions are divided into "inflow lesion" (those involving the aorta and the iliac arteries) and "run off lesions" (involving the femoral and popliteal arteries) (Figure 19.10). In these regions, atherosclerotic lesions are classified using a four-point scale:

1. Lesions that should be treated preferably with an endovascular approach.

2. Lesions that are treated with sufficiently good results using endovascular methods; surgical treatment should be limited to selected cases.

3. Lesions that are treated surgically with superior long-term results; endovascular treatment should be preferred only in patients with high surgical risk.

4. Lesions that should be treated preferably with a surgical approach.

In this scenario, it should also be noted that PAOD is almost always characterized by multifocal lesions in various anatomical regions; hence, the TASC

TABLE 19.10

Fontaine Classification of PAOD

	Fontaine Classification
Stage 1	No symptoms
Stage 2	Intermittent claudication subdivided into:
2a	without pain on resting, but with claudication at a distance of greater than 200 m
2b	without pain on resting, but with a claudication distance of less than 200 m
Stage 3	Nocturnal and/or resting pain
Stage 4	Necrosis (death of tissue) and/or gangrene in the limb

TABLE 19.11

Rutherford Classification of PAOD

	Rutherford Classification
Stage 0	Asymptomatic
Stage 1	Mild claudication
Stage 2	Moderate claudication
Stage 3	Severe claudication
Stage 4	Rest pain
Stage 5	Ischemic ulceration not exceeding ulcer of the digits of the foot
Stage 6	Severe ischemic ulcers or frank gangrene

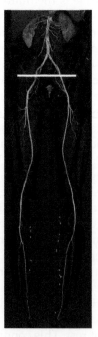

FIGURE 19.10
White line distinguishes inflow from outflow lesions.

classification is partly limited by the focus on single lesions (Figure 19.11). The role of imaging in PAOD is fundamental in the diagnostic–therapeutic process for the quantification and localization of the stenosis and in treatment planning, intended as analysis of the vascular anatomy and the choice of more effective therapeutic approach (Figure 19.12). Since digital subtraction angiography (DSA) is a procedure that needs hospitalization and is burdened by several complications, CTA represents the most cheap, fast, and readily available modality in the evaluation of clinically diagnosed PAOD; it should noted that this technique can be partly limited by the use of ionizing radiations and iodinated contrast and by the presence of artifacts caused by calcium and high density structures (Figures 19.13 and 19.14). However, with an expert use of reconstruction filters and advanced postprocessing techniques, this latter limitation could be easily overcome. A recent meta-analysis [11] of the diagnostic performance of CTA in patients with PAOD reported sensitivity and specificity values ranging from 73% to 100% for severe stenosis (>75%) and 92%–93% for moderate stenosis (≥50%, in the aorto-iliac, femoral-popliteal, and infra-popliteal regions (Figure 19.15). From a radiological point of view

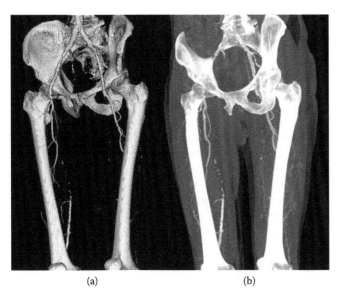

(a)   (b)

FIGURE 19.11
(a) VR and (b) MIP on the coronal plane of a patient with right femoral arterosclerotic obstruction.

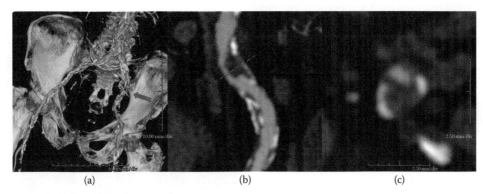

(a)   (b)   (c)

FIGURE 19.12
VR reconstruction of a CTA examination (a) in a patient with sever stenosis of the common iliac artery (red arrow). (b and c) Multiplanar reconstructions (MPRs) allow a correct analysis on the stenosis level with a precise quantification of the residual lumen.

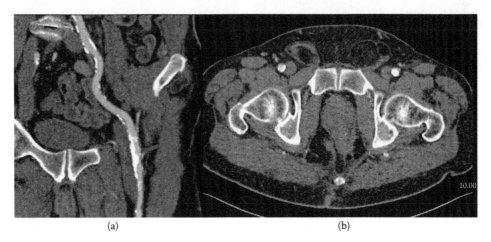

(a)   (b)

FIGURE 19.13
Patient with femoral calcified plaque: blooming artifacts due to the presence of calcium can be the cause of a stenosis overestimation on both (a) MPR and (b) axial reconstruction.

it is strictly necessary to follow a precise pattern in reporting peripheral CTA in PAOD patients, trying to cover all points that allow a correct patient classification from a clinical and surgical point of view:

1. Localize and characterize lesions, evaluating the degree of stenosis and plaque composition (calcified or noncalcified atheromas).
2. Describe collateral vessels in case of obstruction.
3. Describe anatomical abnormalities and vessel condition above and below the lesions (including caliber and wall status).
4. Evaluate leg circulation (including flow asymmetry) and the presence of additional parietal lesions, although of lesser magnitude, since

this can be necessary for accurate surgical planning.
5. Pay attention to nonvascular findings in the abdomen, soft tissues, and lung bases.

19.2.4 PAOD Treatment

Interventional and surgical therapy for PAOD commonly includes percutaneous transluminal angioplasty (PTA), thrombolytic infusion, bypass, and stent placement [12]. With the improvement of new angioplastic techniques, endovascular treatment is becoming a feasible and effective alternative to surgery, despite this latter option being preferred when symptoms cannot be controlled by changing the risk factors or by physical or pharmacological therapy; moreover, even if endovascular treatment allows immediate clinical success rates ranging from 85% (revascularization of occluded iliac arteries) to 100% (treatment of iliac stenosis), surgical bypass is still most durable even if various types of complications

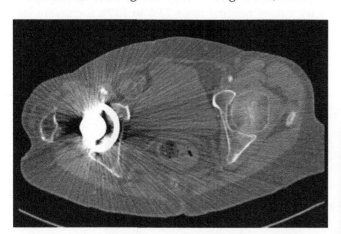

FIGURE 19.14
Beam hardening artifact by hip prosthesis on right femoral artery.

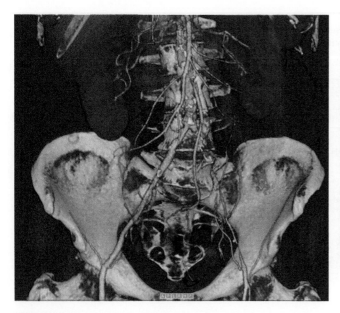

FIGURE 19.15
Patient with common left iliac artery obstruction.

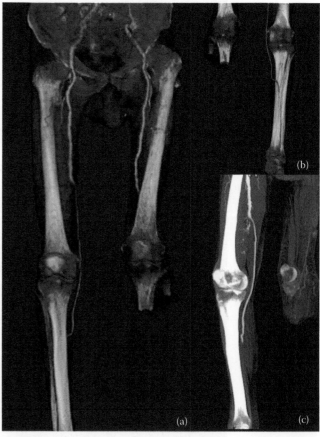

FIGURE 19.16
Diabetic patient with previous subarticular amputation of left leg and femoro-femoral right arterial bypass (a and b): vascular structures are completely occluded distally to the end of bypass (c).

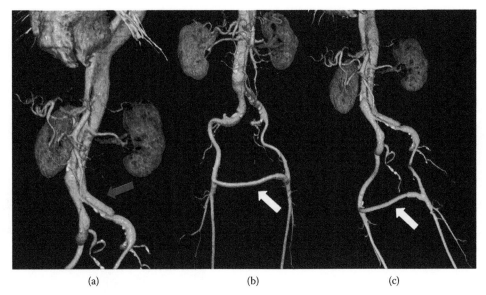

FIGURE 19.17
Patient with aorto-iliac dissection (a, red arrow) and femoro-femoral crossover bypass (b and c, white arrows).

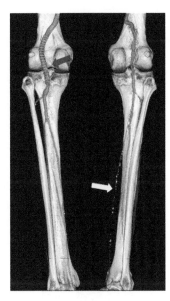

FIGURE 19.18
Patient with popliteal bypass (red arrow) an obstruction of posterior tibial artery.

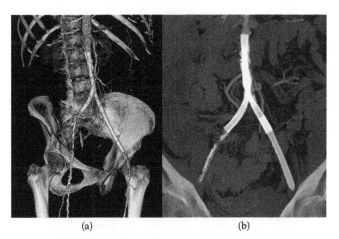

FIGURE 19.19
Patient with two aorto-iliac "kissing" stents (a) and complete obstruction of right branch (b).

19.2.5 Aneurysm

The cut off caliber ratio with contralateral vessels for the diagnosis of aneurysms is >0.7 for popliteal arteries and >1.5 for femoral arteries. Generally, aneurysms can be categorized as either true or false. True aneurysms occur when all layers of the arterial wall are abnormally dilated (Figure 19.22); these aneurysms occur mostly in the popliteal region and are mainly associated with atherosclerotic disease (Figure 19.23). False aneurysms (pseudoaneurysms) are due to a defect in the arterial wall related to trauma (most commonly, iatrogenic) or infection. About 45% of patients are asymptomatic at the time of diagnosis; in the remaining cases, symptoms

might occur (Figures 19.16 through 19.18). In the case of PTA coupled with stent placement, the success rate and duration of the procedure is strictly connected to the lesion's type and localization (87% at 1 year and 55% at 5 years from treatment) (Figures 19.19 through 19.21) [13]. Last, thrombo-endo-arterectomy (TEA), consisting in the removal of the atherosclerotic plaque along the intima, can be used in the presence of short lesions, but it is not widely adopted in PAOD patients due to the high chance of restenosis.

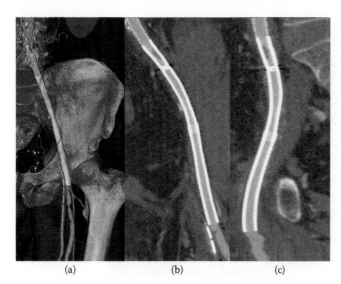

(a)   (b)   (c)

FIGURE 19.20
Patient with left iliac-femoral stent (a) with in-stent restenosis (b and c).

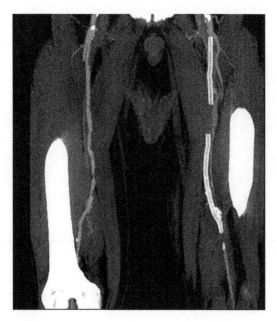

FIGURE 19.21
Patient with two left femoral stents, both occluded.

may include lower-extremity ischemia, thrombosis, and embolization. CTA technique should be adapted by increasing the delay between the contrast agent administration and the scan start by 3–4 seconds (the blood flow at the aneurysm level can be very turbulent, causing the dilution of contrast media); the above mentioned "rescue" technique should be adopted in case of bolus mistiming. Reporting must:

1. Describe the localization, size, and longitudinal extension of the aneurysm.
2. Describe the thrombotic apposition in the aneurysm (concentric/eccentric).

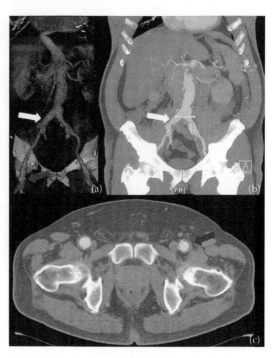

FIGURE 19.22
Patient with iliac (white arrow) and femoral aneurysms (red arrow): (a) VR, (b) MIP on coronal plane, and (c) axial reconstructions.

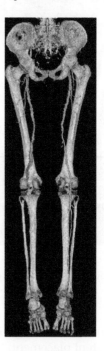

FIGURE 19.23
Asymmetry in calf blood flow due to aneurismatic left popliteal artery.

3. Provide the distance from the normal vessel above and below the aneurysm.
4. Identify the incipient rupture or occlusion signs.
5. Describe the relationship with the surrounding vascular and nonvascular structures.

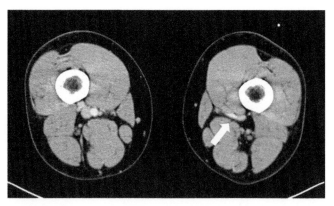

FIGURE 19.24
Axial computed tomography scan performed during feet plantar extension: left popliteal artery (white arrow) is compressed by the medial branch of gastrocnemius muscle.

19.2.6 Entrapment

Popliteal artery entrapment syndrome (PAES) is a developmental abnormality that results from an abnormal relationship of the popliteal artery with the gastrocnemius muscle or, rarely, an anomalous fibrous band or the popliteus muscle, causing a deviation and compression of the artery. There are essentially four anatomic variants of PAES. Type V is any of the four anatomic variants that include the popliteal vein. Stress CTA (scan performed in the neutral position as well as with the foot in either dorsiflexion or plantar flexion position to elicit vascular compression) is usually performed to confirm the diagnosis prior to surgery (Figure 19.24).

19.3 CTA of the Upper Limbs

19.3.1 Anatomy

For detailed anatomy of arterial circulation of the lower limbs refer to Figures 19.25 through 19.27 and Tables 19.12 through 19.17.

19.3.2 Examination Technique

The patient should be positioned prone or supine (prone position, if feasible, is preferred), with the hands as near as possible to the center of the gantry; bilateral examination should be preferred in order to provide comparative data. The arms should be extended to the maximum and pronated. Pillows or supports can be used to help the patient to maintain position and to extend the arms as much as possible. The venous access should be placed on one leg to avoid artifacts during the passage of highly concentrated contrast media in the arm veins

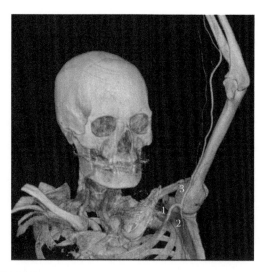

FIGURE 19.25
Subclavian artery (1), Axillary artery (2), and Brachial artery (3) (see also Table 19.2).

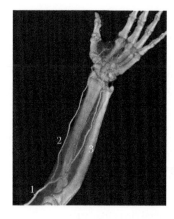

FIGURE 19.26
Brachial artery (1), Radial artery (2), and ulnar artery (3) (see also Table 19.2).

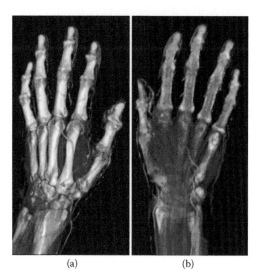

(a)   (b)

FIGURE 19.27
(a) Dorsal metacarpal arteries and (b) volar metacarpal arteries.

TABLE 19.12

Arteries of the Arm and Forearm

	Arm		Forearm
1	Subclavian artery	1	Brachial artery
2	Axillary artery	2	Radial artery
3	Brachial artery	3	Ulnar artery

TABLE 19.13

Subclavian Artery: Branches and Collaterals

Subclavian Artery	
Vertebral artery	
Internal mammary artery	
Thyrocervical trunk	Inferior thyroid artery
	Suprascapular artery
	Transverse cervical artery
Costocervical trunk	Deep cervical artery
	Supreme intercostal artery

TABLE 19.14

Axillary Artery: Branches and Collaterals

Axillary Artery	
Superior thoracic artery	
Thoracoacromial artery	Acromial branch
	Clavicular branch
	Deltoid branch
	Pectoral branch
Lateral thoracic artery	
Subscapular artery	Thoracodorsal artery
	Scapular circumflex artery
Anterior humeral circumflex artery	
Posterior humeral circumflex artery	

TABLE 19.15

Brachial Artery: Branches and Collaterals

Brachial Artery	
Deep brachial artery	Medial collateral artery
	Radial collateral artery
Superior ulnar collateral artery	
Inferior ulnar collateral artery	

TABLE 19.16

Radial Artery: Branches and Collaterals

Radial Artery	
Radial recurrent artery	
Palmar carpal branch of radial artery	
Superficial palmar branch of the radial artery	
Dorsal carpal branch of radial artery	Dorsal metacarpal arteries
Princeps pollicis artery	
Radialis indicis	
Deep palmar arch	Palmar metacarpal arteries

TABLE 19.17

Ulnar Artery: Branches and Collaterals

Ulnar Artery	
Anterior ulnar recurrent artery	
Posterior ulnar recurrent artery	
Common interosseous artery	Volar
	Dorsal
Dorsal carpal branch of radial artery	
Volar carpal	
Dorsal carpal	
Superficial volar arch	

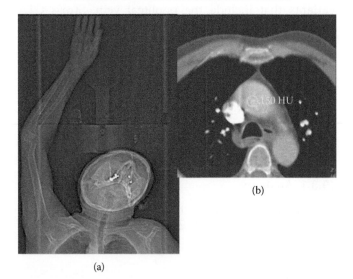

(b)

(a)

FIGURE 19.28

(a) Topogram acquisition on coronal plane; (b) premonitoring should be placed on the aortic arch.

immediately after the injection. A positioning topogram (not less than 130 cm long) must be acquired on the coronal plane from the aortic arch to the tip of the fingers (Figure 19.28a). In order to calculate the optimal delay between the contrast agent administration and the scan's start, a circular region of interest (ROI) must be placed on the aortic arch, avoiding the inclusion of intimal calcifications, which could alter the diagram of density variation on both the bolus tracking and bolus test techniques. The aortic attenuation threshold must be set at 150–200 HU (Figure 19.28b), using the minimum delay allowed by the scanner for the acquisition start. The other technical considerations are almost superimposable to those made for CTA of the lower limbs, apart from the suggested scan duration that should not exceed 25–30 seconds in normal patients since the arteries of the upper limbs lay more closely to the heart than those of the lower limbs, and their opacification occurs faster (Tables 19.18 and 19.19).

TABLE 19.18

Contrast Agent Administration Parameters for Upper Limb Peripheral CTA

	4 Slices	16 Slices	64 Slices	128 Slices	Dual Source
IV contrast iodine concentration (mgI/mL)	350–400	350–400	350–400	350–400	350–400
IV contrast iodine concentration (mgI/mL)	120	120	110	110	110
Saline flush-volume (mL)	50	50	50	50	50
Flow rate (mL/s)	4	4	4–5	4–5	4–5

TABLE 19.19

Scan Parameters for Upper Limb Peripheral CTA

	4 Slices	16 Slices	64 Slices	128 Slices	Dual Source
kVp	120	120	120	120	120
mAs	200–300	200–300	180–200	180	120–180
Slice collimation	4 × 2.5	16 × 0.75	64 × 0.625	128 × 0.6	64 × 0.6 × 2
Slice width (mm)	1–3	0.625–1	0.5–1	0.6	0.6

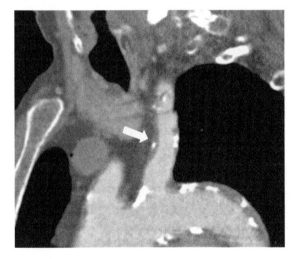

FIGURE 19.29
Atheromasic plaque localized at the basis of left subclavian artery (white arrow).

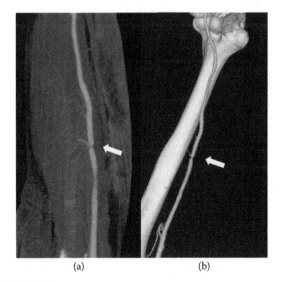

(a)   (b)

FIGURE 19.30
(a) Coronal MPR and (b) VR of a significant brachial artery stenosis (white arrows).

19.3.3 Atherosclerotic Disease of the Upper Limbs

In the upper limbs, atherosclerosis is far less common than in the lower limbs; when present, atherosclerotic lesions may involve the innominate artery and the origin of the subclavian artery [14]. Stenosis (Figure 19.29) or the occlusion of these arteries may be asymptomatic due to the development of collateral vessels, or lead to upper extremity claudication or ischemia. Symptomatic patients can undergo various procedures, such as carotid-subclavian bypass or subclavian transposition [15]. In these cases, CTA can be used to assess the graft location, anastomoses, lumen patency, and potential restenosis [16].

Acute arm ischemia is even more uncommon; this condition may be caused by thromboembolic disease, trauma, or iatrogenic injury (Figure 19.30), but it is the cardiac sources that account for the vast majority of cases (84%). Emboli derived from the heart that lodge in the upper limb are most likely to occlude the brachial and axillary arteries (in 95% of cases).

19.3.4 Thoracic Outlet Syndrome

Dynamically induced compression of the neural, arterial, or venous structures crossing the tunnels of the

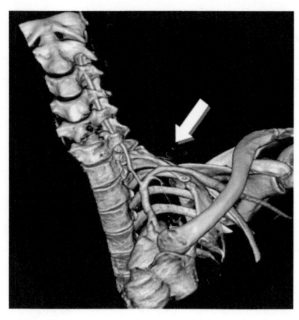

FIGURE 19.31
Patient with thoracic outlet syndrome caused by supranumerary cervical rib (white arrow).

TABLE 19.20

Causes of TOS

Principal Causes of TOS
Skeletal and bone abnormalities
Cervical rib elongated C7 transverse process
Exostosis or tumor of the first rib or clavicle
Excess callus of the first rib or clavicle
Soft tissue abnormalities
Fibrous band
Congenital muscle abnormalities (insertion variations, supranumerary muscles)
Acquired soft tissue abnormalities
Post-traumatic fibrous scarring
Postoperative scarring
Posture and predisposing morphotype
Poor posture and weak muscular support in thin women

thoracic outlet leads to thoracic outlet syndrome (TOS). The diagnosis is based on the results of clinical evaluation, particularly if the patient's symptoms can be reproduced when various dynamic maneuvers, including elevation of the arm, are undertaken. The thoracic outlet, or cervicothoracobrachial junction, includes three confined spaces, extending from the cervical spine and the mediastinum to the lower border of the pectoralis minor muscle, which are potential sites of neurovascular compression. These three compartments are the interscalene triangle, the costoclavicular space, and the retropectoralis minor space (Figure 19.31; Table 19.20). CTA can adequately depict vascular compressions related to TOS [17], but some technical adjustments are required—the examination must be performed first with the arms adducted alongside the body and during overhead arms abduction, in order to attempt to reproduce the neurovascular compression. Images should be then compared to assess vascular compression; a detailed analysis of the branches of the brachial plexus is more difficult and should performed with MRI.

19.3.5 Subclavian Steal Syndrome

Subclavian steal syndrome results from the occlusion or severe stenosis of the left subclavian artery or the brachiocephalic trunk proximal to the origin of the ipsilateral vertebral artery. As the demand for blood supply to the upper extremity increases (overhead activity, muscular stress), blood flow is diverted or "stolen" from the vertebrobasilar system and bypassed to the arm via retrograde flow in the ipsilateral vertebral artery. Stenosis or occlusion of the subclavian artery is most commonly caused by atherosclerotic disease, but the differential diagnosis includes trauma, vasculitis, dissection, and congenital anomaly. Subclavian steal affects the left subclavian artery three times more commonly than the right. In patients affected by this condition, CTA can confirm the stenosis or obstruction of the proximal subclavian artery (Figure 19.32), allowing at the same time, an evaluation of the ipsilateral reperfusion through the vertebral artery.

19.3.6 Hemodialysis Fistulae

Hemodialysis requires well-functioning vascular access to allow sufficient blood flow for adequate clearance and dialysis dosing. This is achieved temporarily by central vein catheterization and subsequently by surgical creation of an arteriovenous fistula or graft for more permanent and durable access. An upper extremity arterovenous fistula is commonly created by surgical end-to-side anastomosis of the radial or brachial artery to an adjacent basilic, cephalic, or medial antecubital vein. Complications of hemodialysis fistuale include venous stenosis, thrombosis, infection, aneurysms, and, rarely, arterial steal syndrome. CTA has proven to be a useful, safe, fast, and accurate imaging modality for the comprehensive evaluation of the anatomy (Figure 19.33) and function of hemodialysis fistulae [18], as well as for the diagnosis of related complications. It allows noninvasive monitoring and early detection of hemodynamically significant stenoses treatable with elective angioplasty, thereby substantially reducing the frequency of subsequent thrombosis and access failure.

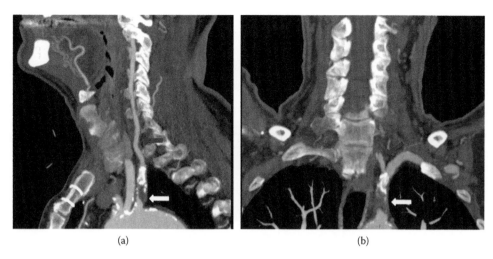

(a)   (b)

FIGURE 19.32
Subclavian steal syndrome. (a) Left subclavian artery is occluded at the origin by an atherosclerotic plaque (white arrow); (b) distal blood flow is sustained by retrograde perfusion from the Left vertebral artery (red arrow).

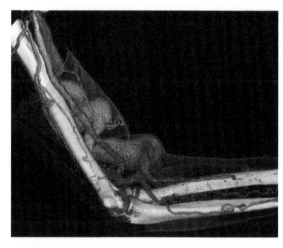

FIGURE 19.33
Latero-lateral hemodialytic fistula in the arm with ectasic drainage vein.

References

1. Fleischmann D. Present and future trends in multiple detector-row CT applications: CT angiography. *Eur Radiol* 2002; 12(Suppl 2): S11–S15.
2. Napoli A, Fleischmann D, Chan FP, Catalano C, Hellinger JC, Passariello R, Rubin GD. Computed tomography angiography: State-of-the-art imaging using multidetector-row technology. *J Comput Assist Tomogr* 2004; 28(Suppl 1):S32–S45.
3. Fleischmann D, Hallett RL, Rubin GD. CT angiography of peripheral arterial disease. *J Vasc Interv Radiol* 2006; 17(1): 3–26.
4. Fleischmann D, Rubin GD. Quantification of intravenously administered contrast medium transit through the peripheral arteries: Implications for CT angiography. *Radiology* 2005; 236(3): 1076–1082.
5. Catalano C, Fraioli F, Laghi A, Napoli A, Bezzi M, Pediconi F, Danti M, Nofroni I, Passariello R. Infrarenal aortic and lower extremity arterial disease: Diagnostic performance of multi-detector row CT angiography. *Radiology* 2004; 231: 555–563.
6. Rubin GD, Schmidt AJ, Logan LJ, Sofilos MC. Multidetector row CT angiography of lower extremity arterial inflow and runoff: Initial experience. *Radiology* 2003; 221: 146–158.
7. Ostchega Y, Paulose-Ram R, Dillon CF, Gu Q, Hughes JP. Prevalence of peripheral arterial disease and risk factors in persons aged 60 and older: Data from the National Health and Nutrition Examination Survey 1999–2004. *J Am Geriatr Soc* 2007; 55(4): 583–589.
8. US Department of Health and Human Service. *The Health Consequences of Tobacco Use: A Report to the Surgeon General.* Atlanta, GA: U.S Department of Health and Human Service, Public Health Service, Center for Disease and Control and Prevention, National Center for Chronic Disease Prevention and Health Promotion, Office on Smoking and Health, 2003.
9. Dormandy JA, Rutherford RB. Management of peripheral arterial disease (PAD). TASC Working Group. TransAtlantic Inter-Society Consensus (TASC). *J Vasc Surg* 2000; 31: S192–S274.
10. Norgren L, Hiatt WR, Dormandy JA, Nehler MR, Harris KA, Fowkes FG; TASC II Working Group, Bell K, Caporusso J, Durand-Zaleski I, Komori K et al. Inter-Society Consensus for the Management of Peripheral Arterial Disease (TASC II). *Eur J Vasc Endovasc Surg* 2007; 33(Suppl 1): S1–75.
11. Heijenbrok-Kal MH, Kock MC, Hunink MG. Lower extremity arterial disease: Multidetector CT angiography meta-analysis. *Radiology* 2007; 245: 433–439.
12. Zohu M, Liu CJ, Qiao T, Liu C, Huang D, Ran F, Wang W, Zhang M. Hybrid surgical and endovascular therapy in TASC type D atherosclerotic occlusive disease: A retrospective analysis of 48 cases. *Zhonghua Wai Ke Za Zhi* 2010; 48(22): 1735–1738.

13. Lopera JE, Trimmer CK, Josephs SG, Anderson ME, Schuber S, Li R, Dolmatch B, Toursarkissian B. Multidetector CT angiography of infrainguinal arterial bypass. *Radiographics* 2008; 28: 529–549.

14. Kaufman JA. Upper-extermity arteries. In: Kaufman JA, Lee MJ, eds. *Vascular and Interventional Radiology: The Requisites*. Philadelphia, PA: Mosby, 2004, p 142–162.

15. Johnston KW. Upper extremity ischemia. In: Rutherford RB, ed. *Vascular Surgery*. Philadelphia, PA: WB Saunders, 2000, p 1111–1115.

16. Anderson SW, Foster BR, Soto JA. Upper extremity CT angiography in penetrating trauma: Use of 64-section multidetector CT. *Radiology* 2008; 249(3): 1064–1073.

17. Demondion X, Herbinet P, Van Sint Jan S, Boutry N, Chantelot C, Cotten A. Imaging assessment of thoracic outlet syndrome. *Radiographics* 2006; 26: 1735–1750.

18. Cavagna E, D'Andrea P, Schiavon F, Tarroni G. Failing hemodialysis arteriovenous fistula and percutaneous treatment: Imaging with CT, MRI and digital subtraction angiography. *Cardiovasc Intervent Radiol* 2000; 23: 262–265.

20

CT Venography

Michele Anzidei, Goffredo Serra, Francesco Fraioli, and Carlo Catalano

CONTENTS

20.1 Introduction

Several imaging modalities allow the exploration of the anatomy and the evaluation of pathological conditions of the venous system.

Computed tomography (CT) venography is an easy and noninvasive imaging modality, which allows a wide anatomic coverage and short acquisition time. Compared to other imaging modalities (ultrasounds, conventional venography), CT venography offers several significant advantages: a wider field of view, three-dimensional reformations and the possibility to perform a CT-angiography evaluation in the same study, excellent anatomical detail and contrast resolution of surrounding structures, identification and characterization of pathological processes arising from inside and outside the vessel lumen, delineation of collateral circulation and evaluation of venous patency.

20.2 Highlights on the Anatomical Development of the Venous System

The cardinal veins represent the main vessels in the venous drainage of the embryo. The anterior and posterior cardinal veins run on the ventral and dorsal side of the common cardinal veins and empty into them before ending in the sinus venous.

At the eighth week, an oblique anastomosis connects the anterior cardinal veins; this anastomotic vessel will form the left brachiocephalic vein after the complete degeneration of the distal part of the anterior cardinal vein.

The superior vena cava (SVC) originates from the right anterior cardinal vein and the right common cardinal vein.

The posterior cardinal veins almost completely degenerate during development; their only residuals are represented by the origin of the azygos vein and the common iliac veins.

The posterior cardinal veins are gradually substituted by the subcardinal and supracardinal veins. The subcardinal veins, the first to appear, are interconnected by the subcardinal anastomosis; the mesophrenic sinusoids connect the subcardinal veins with the posterior cardinal veins; the subcardinal veins form the peduncle of the left renal vein, the suprarenal veins, gonadic veins (ovary and testis), and a part of the inferior vena cava (IVC).

The supracardinal veins appear later, ending in the region of the kidneys; in their upper part they get connected by an anastomosis, which will form the the azygos and hemiazygos veins.

Inferior to the kidneys, the left supracardinal vein disappears, whereas the right supracardinal vein will form a part of the IVC.

The SVC is formed by the right anterior cardinal vein and the right common cardinal vein.

20.2.1 Development of the Inferior Vena Cava

The IVC is formed by four main embryonal segments:

1. A hepatic segment derived from the hepatocardiac channel.
2. A suprarenal segment derived from the right subcardinal vein.
3. A renal segment derived from the subcardinal-supracardinal anastomosis.
4. A subrenal segment derived from the right supracardinal vein.

20.2.2 Anatomy of the Venous System

CT venography enables a detailed evaluation of the venous anatomy with a wide body coverage, allowing the identification of possible anatomical variants—often asymptomatic—and pathological conditions; a deep knowledge and familiarity with the ordinary venous anatomy and its most frequent variants is necessary in a correct and complete assessment of a venographic study.

20.2.3 Veins of the Neck

The jugular veins and their interconnections represent the principal vessels forming the venous circulation of the neck. The system of the jugular veins is given by three main veins: the internal jugular vein, the external jugular vein, and the anterior jugular vein (Figure 20.1).

The internal jugular vein begins in the posterior compartment of the jugular foramen, at the base of the skull. It runs down the side of the neck in a vertical direction, laterally to the internal carotid artery and then laterally to the common carotid artery; at the base of the neck, it unites with the subclavian vein to form the brachiocephalic vein, also called innominate vein, which ends in the right atrium through the SVC. The internal jugular vein presents two focal dilatations respectively localized at its origin (superior bulb) and its termination (the inferior bulb).

The internal jugular veins represent the main vessel draining the regions of the neck, part of the face and brain.

The external jugular vein is thinner and starts its path from the parotid gland running perpendicularly down the neck in a superficial position. In its way down it crosses the sternocleidomastoideus obliquely, and in the subclavian triangle it perforates the deep fascia ending

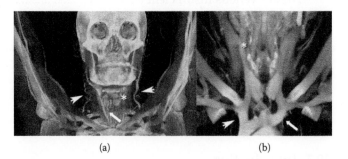

(a)   (b)

FIGURE 20.1
Computed tomographic (CT) venography of the (a) neck and (b) thoracic outlet. In subpart (a), the jugular system with the internal jugular veins (asterisk), anterior jugular veins (big arrow), and the external jugular veins (small arrows). In subpart (b), the right (small arrow) and left (big arrow) anonymous trunks and jugular veins (asterisk).

in the subclavian vein. The external jugular vein varies in size and it is sometimes double. It receives blood mainly from the exterior of the cranium and the deep parts of the face.

The anterior jugular drains the submandibular region, originating from the confluence of several superficial veins of the submaxillary region near the hyoid bone. It descends between the median line and the anterior border of the sternohyoideus, ending in the external jugular or the subclavian vein. It varies considerably in size and also in number (most frequently there are two anterior jugulars but sometimes only one).

Just above the sternum, the two anterior jugular veins communicate by a transverse trunk, the venous jugular arch.

20.2.4 Veins of the Thorax

The main vessels of the thorax are represented by the SVC, formed by the union of the two innominate veins and the azygos system (azygos and hemiazygos veins) (Figure 20.1). Other thoracic veins are the intercostal veins, the internal mammary veins, and the bronchial veins.

The SVC drains the blood from the upper half of the body and is formed by the junction of the two innominate veins. It begins immediately below the cartilage of the right first rib close to the sternum, and, descending vertically behind the first and second intercostal spaces, ends in the right atrium; the lower half of the vessel is within the pericardium.

The innominate veins are two large trunks, placed one on either side of the root of the neck, and formed by the union of the internal jugular and subclavian veins of the corresponding side.

The right innominate is a short vessel, which begins behind the sternal end of the clavicle and joins with the left innominate vein just below the cartilage of the first rib to form the SVC. The left innominate begins behind the sternal end of the clavicle and runs obliquely downward to the sternal end of the first right costal cartilage, where it unites with the right innominate vein to form the SVC.

The azygos vein begins opposite the first or second lumbar vertebra from the ascending lumbar vein; it enters the thorax through the aortic hiatus of the diaphragm, and passes along the right side of the vertebral column ending in the SVC.

The hemiazygos vein begins in the left ascending lumbar or renal vein. It enters the thorax, through the left crus of the diaphragm, and, ascending on the left side of the vertebral column, passes across the column, behind the aorta, esophagus, and thoracic duct, to end in the azygos vein.

20.2.5 Veins of the Upper Arms

As with the lower limbs, the venous system of the upper limbs is formed by two independent systems, richly interconnected: the superficial and deep veins.

The deep veins accompany the homonymous arteries.

The main vessels of the superficial system are the cephalic vein and the basilic vein (Figure 20.2).

The cephalic vein origins from the medial side of the forearm, crosses the elbow anteriorly, and runs up along the anterolateral surface of the biceps and brachioradialis muscle; after passing between the pectoralis major muscles and through the deltopectoral triangle, it ends into the axillary vein.

The basilic vein originates on the medial side of the forearm, it runs up on the posteromedial side of the forearm, and after crossing anteriorly the elbow, it travels between the muscles round pronator and biceps, crossing the brachial artery. It ends into the axillary vein at the inferior edge of the muscle teres major.

20.2.6 Veins of the Abdomen

The IVC is formed by the junction of the two common iliac veins on the right side of the fifth lumbar vertebra. It ascends along the front of the vertebral column, on the right side of the aorta; in its upper tract it runs on the posterior surface of the liver. It then passes through the diaphragm to open into the lower and back part of the right atrium.

The thoracic portion is only about 2.5 cm in length and is situated partly inside and partly outside the pericardial sac.

The renal veins are placed in front of the renal arteries. The left passes in front of the aorta, just below the origin of the superior mesenteric artery and receives the left spermatic; it opens into the IVC.

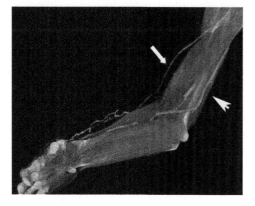

FIGURE 20.2
CT venography of the upper extremity showing the two main vessels of the superficial system: the cephalic vein (small arrow) and the basilic vein (big arrow).

The suprarenal veins are two in number: the right ends in the IVC and the left ends in the left renal or left inferior phrenic vein.

The spermatic veins emerge from the back of the testis; they unite to form a plexus, called the pampiniform plexus, which constitutes the greater mass of the spermatic cord; below the subcutaneous inguinal ring they unite to form three or four veins, which pass along the inguinal canal, and, entering the abdomen through the abdominal inguinal ring, coalesce to form two veins, which ascend on the psoas major, behind the peritoneum, along the internal spermatic artery. These unite to form a single vein, which opens on the right side into the IVC and on the left side into the left renal vein.

The ovarian veins correspond with the spermatic in the male; they form a plexus in the broad ligament near the ovary and uterine tube. They end in the same way as the spermatic veins in the male.

The hepatic veins arise from the liver, in the terminations of the portal vein and hepatic artery, and are arranged in two groups, upper and lower. The upper group usually consists of three large veins, which converge toward the posterior surface of the liver, and open into the IVC. The veins of the lower group vary in number, and are of small size; they come from the right and caudate lobes.

20.2.7 Veins of the Lower Limbs

The venous system of the inferior limbs is formed by two systems, largely interconnected: the deep and superficial veins. The blood drained by the superficial veins flows into the deep system through the perforating veins, reaching up the IVC and the heart. The veins of the deep system are accompanied by the homonymous arteries.

The posterior tibial veins accompany the posterior tibial artery and are joined by the peroneal veins.

The anterior tibial veins are the upward continuation of the venae comitantes of the dorsalis pedis artery. They unite with the posterior tibial to form the popliteal vein (Figure 20.3).

The popliteal vein is formed by the junction of the anterior and posterior tibial veins at the lower border of the popliteus; it ascends through the popliteal fossa ending in the aperture in the adductor magnus, where it continues into the femoral vein (Figure 20.4).

The femoral vein accompanies the femoral artery through the upper two-thirds of the thigh; below the inguinal ligament is joined by the deep femoral vein; near its termination it is joined by the great saphenous vein (GSV), from the superficial system.

The two main vessels of the superficial system are the GSV and the small saphenous vein (SSV) (Figure 20.5).

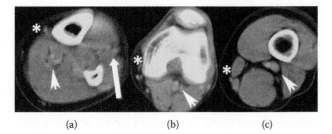

(a)   (b)   (c)

FIGURE 20.3
CT venography of the lower limbs showing: the deep vessels of the calf (small arrow), the great saphenous vein (asterisk), and the small saphenous vein (big arrow) in subpart (a); the popliteus vein after the sapheno–popliteal junction (small arrow) and the great saphenous vein (asterisk), running up on the medial side of the knee in subpart (b); deep and superficial veins of the thigh: great saphenous vein (asterisk) and femoral vein (small arrow) in subpart (c).

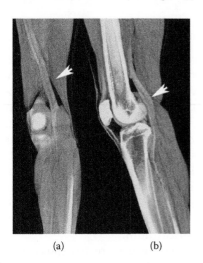

(a)   (b)

FIGURE 20.4
CT venography of the deep venous system of the lower limbs showing the popliteal vein (a - arrow) running up posteriorily to the omonymous artery after the sapheno–popliteal junction (b - arrow).

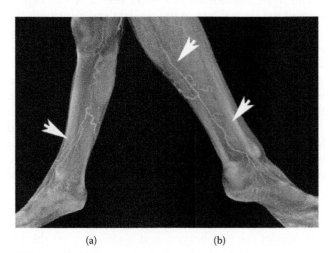

(a)   (b)

FIGURE 20.5
(a) Origin of the great saphenous vein from the medial marginal vein of the dorsum of the foot (arrow) and (b) origin of the small saphenous vein (arrows) behind the lateral malleolus as a continuation of the lateral marginal vein.

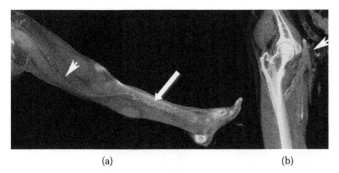

(a)   (b)

FIGURE 20.6
The entire path of the great saphenous vein (a) from its origin from the medial marginal vein to its termination in the sapheno–femoral junction (small arrow) (b); in subpart (a), signs of venous insufficiency with tortuous and dilatated vessel walls (big arrow).

The SSV originates from the lateral side of the foot and runs up on the posterolateral edge of the Achilles tendon; after reaching the popliteal fossa, between the two heads of the gastrocnemius muscle, it ends into the popliteal vein.

The GSV originates from the medial side of the foot, it travels anteriorly to the medial malleolus and runs up to the medial side of the knee; in the thigh it keeps running up in an antero–medial position, it passes through the foramen ovale and ends into the common femoral vein (saphenofemoral junction) (Figure 20.6).

20.3 Technique for CT Venography

CT venography can be performed with two different techniques, both after the administration of contrast media: the direct method and the indirect method, with recirculation of the contrast media.

20.3.1 Direct CT Venography

With the direct method, the contrast media is administered directly in a peripheral vessel draining the venous system of interest through a peripheral vein of the hand (for the evaluation of the upper limbs or chest) or of the foot (for the evaluation of the lower limbs) [1]. The scan starts toward the end of the injection, obtaining a first-pass phase of the contrast media in the vascular lumen: the result is a selective opacification of the venous vessels in evaluation. For better imaging results, it is mandatory to dilute the contrast media with saline solution (1:5); the dose of contrast media administered should be then customed for a selective opacification (usually not more of 55 cc) and the administration rate should be slow (1–2 cc/s).

20.3.2 Indirect CT Venography

With the indirect method (the most frequently used), the scan starts when the contrast media has already passed an arterial phase and the venous system starts to be opacified [2]. The dose of contrast media is about 2 cc/kg (100–150 cc); with this dose, a sufficient opacification even of the most distal vessels of the upper and lower limbs can be obtained. In the evaluation of the venous vessels, the rate of administration is slow, ranging between 2 and 3 cc/s. The optimal imaging delay is empiric, as it can significantly change from patient to patient depending on the cardiovascular status. A scan delay of 60 seconds is usually sufficient for a good evaluation of the upper extremities, thorax, abdomen, and pelvis; for the lower limbs, the scan should start with a delay of at least 3–3.5 minutes. The peak of enhancement after contrast administration in the peripheric veins can change from patient to patient, primarily reflecting the presence of wall alterations of the arterial vessels and possible obstacles to the blood flow directed to the right atrium (caval thrombosis, external compressions); once the peak is achieved (in some patients just 120 seconds after the administration of contrast media), it remains stable in a prolonged plateau, which allows a certain flexibility in the choice of the exact scan delay. Both techniques offer some advantages and disadvantages. Indirect venography allows the visualization at the same time of all vascular structures (pulmonary and arterial vessels included) and the injection from a peripheric vein of the hand of foot, sometimes difficult, can be avoided; its pitfalls are represented by the empiric, variable optimal scan delay and an unpredictable degree of opacification (depending on patients' cardiovascular status and the dilution of the contrast media when the contrast reaches the venous system). The direct venography offers a better and selective opacification of the vessel in study (no dilution of the contrast media in the venous phase) with a lower dose of ionizing radiations (unique acquisition with no recirculation of the contrast media).

20.4 CT Venography of the Neck and Thorax

20.4.1 Neck

Venous thrombosis represents the main pathological condition of the jugular veins system (Figure 20.7).

Thrombosis can result from an alteration of one or more mechanisms in Virchow's classic triad: endothelial damage, stasis, and hypercoagulable state. Even hyatrogenic factors (neck surgery, drugs inducing a condition of hypercoagulability) can play a significant role in the genesis of thrombosis.

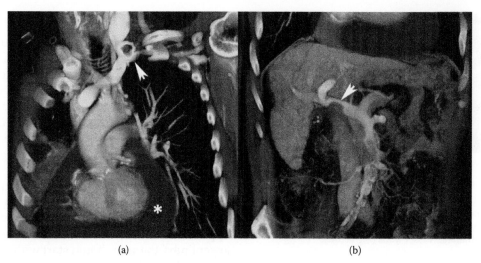

(a)   (b)

FIGURE 20.7
Venous thrombosis of the (a) left internal jugular vein (small arrow) and (b) portal vein (small arrow) in a patient with pulmonary carcinoma and pericardial effusion (asterisk).

The most common malformative alterations of the neck venous system are internal jugular vein aneurysms and phlebectasias [3]. Although these terms are frequently used as synonyms, they represent two conditions with different etiology and pathophysiology. Macroscopically, aneurysms are described as saccular and phlebectasias as fusiform. Although phlebectasia in the neck region is considered to be congenital in origin or to arise from a primary congenital weakness within the muscular layer of the venous wall, venous aneurysm and pseudoaneurysm often occurs secondary to trauma (i.e. before catheterization) or in association with other diseases involving the venous system. Fusiform jugular phlebectasia is most commonly seen in childhood, whereas secondary or acquired venous dilatations are usually saccular in form; these often thrombosed venous aneurysms, which are typically seen in adults, can be associated to a large spectrum of etiological factors.

20.4.2 Thorax

Complexity of the venous system development leads to the possible presence of multiple anomalous variants in its definitive structure, not frequently observed [4]. In most of the cases, these anomalies are asymptomatic and have no clinical significance; nevertheless, it is necessary to be aware of all the main anatomic venous anomalies to be able to recognize them in imaging studies made for other reasons (above all, in patients evaluated for thoracic surgery), in complex malformative syndromes, or when an anomalous venous vessel represents the cause of the clinical symptomatology for its interactions with surrounding normal structures.

20.4.3 Superior Vena Cava

The evaluation of the anomalies of the vessels forming the superior caval district is crucial in patients awaiting the placement of endovascular devices with subclavian or jugular access, such us central venous catheter or port-a-cath.

The persistent left SVC is a rare condition, occurring in the 0.3%–0.5% of the population. A unique left SVC occurs when the persistence of the left SVC is associated with the degeneration of the right common and anterior cardinal veins (normally forming the right SVC). Blood transported by the left SVC most commonly reaches the right atrium through the coronary sinus. This anomaly is usually asymptomatic and does not require treatment when it is not accompanied by other cardiac anomalies.

The most frequent anomaly is represented by the double SVC, which is seen in 0.3% of the general population and 11% of patients with congenital heart disease. This abnormality derives from the persistence of the left anterior cardinal vein. The anastomosis that usually forms the left brachiocephalic vein is small or absent.

Total absence of the SVC is extremely rare and is associated with undeveloped right anterior cardinal vein; in this condition, named SVC agenesis and drainage into the IVC through azygous vein, the blood from the upper extremities and the head reaches the right atrium through a venous plexus formed by the azygous vein, which appears dilatated, and blood flow is directed toward the IVC.

20.4.4 Thoracic Outlet Syndrome

This syndrome is caused by the compression of the superior thoracic outlet, which may occur because of the positional or even a static cause, involving one or more nerves of the brachial plexus, the subclavian artery, and—less frequently—the subclavian vein. When the compression principally involves the vein, the main symptoms are given by swelling and cyanosis of the extremity, with pain, a feeling of heaviness in the upper limb, and venous distention of the upper arm and shoulder region; the obstacled blood flow can lead, in prone patients, to subclavian axillary vein thrombosis.

The diagnosis of thoracic outlet syndrome is mainly based on the results of clinical evaluation; however, the use of imaging is required to show the location and extent of the neurovascular compression, to determine the nature of the structures undergoing compression (arteries, veins, nerves) and the structure producing the compression [5].

The principal causes of thoracic outlet syndrome are represented by skeletal and soft-tissue abnormalities: cervical ribs, elongated transverse process of C7, exostosis of the first rib or clavicle, and excessive callus of the clavicle or first rib, hypertrophy of the anterior or middle scalene muscles, congenital fibrous bands and ligaments connecting skeletal elements.

20.5 CT Venography of the Abdomen

CT venography of the abdomen is indicated in the evaluation of anatomical variants, which can be relevant in abdominal surgery planning or when associated to other systemic malformative conditions and in the assessment of venous thrombosis in patients with hypercoagulability or oncological diseases.

20.5.1 Inferior Vena Cava

The IVC can show several anomalies in its abdominal tract, which can be sometimes interrupted at different levels [6]; in such cases, the blood coming up from the lower limbs, abdomen and pelvis is drained by the azygos system through collateral circles. The clinical symptoms essentially depend from the obstructed and delayed blood flow on its way to the heart; this can lead, in prone patients, to the occurrence of deep venous thrombosis (DVT) in the iliac veins and in the deep veins of the lower limbs.

- *Left IVC*: a left IVC results from regression of the right supracardinal vein with persistence of the left supracardinal vein. Typically, the left IVC joins the left renal vein uniting with the right renal vein to form a normal right-sided IVC in its prerenal path (Figure 20.8).

- *Azygos continuation of the IVC (absence of the hepatic segment of the IVC)*: this anomaly derives from the failure to form the right subcardinal–hepatic anastomosis, with resulting atrophy of the right

subcardinal vein. As a consequence, the blood drained from the lower limbs is shunted to the azygos system; the hepatic veins end independently in the right atrium. It can be associated with severe congenital heart disease and asplenia or polysplenia syndromes (Figure 20.9).

- *Double IVC*: this anomaly originates from persistence of the lower tract of the left supracardinal vein and it results in the presence of two venous vessels constituting the inferior caval system inferiorly to the renal veins; the left vessel is generally smaller (Figure 20.10).

- *Absence of the entire posthepatic IVC*: this condition suggests that all three paired venous systems failed to develop properly and leads to the constitution of multiple collateral circles in the lombar, sacral, and inferior epigastric systems.

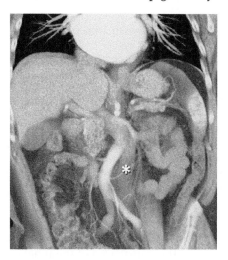

FIGURE 20.8
CT venography showing a left inferior vena cava (asterisk).

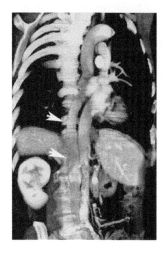

FIGURE 20.9
Azygos continuation of the inferior vena cava: absence of the intrahepatic tract of the inferior vena cava; blood from the lower abdomen and limbs reaches the right atrium through an enlarged azygos vein (arrows).

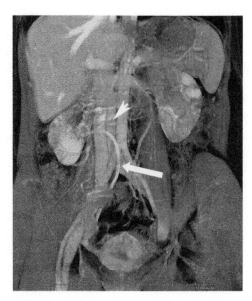

FIGURE 20.10
Double inferior vena cava (small arrow) with compression of the right urether treated with a double J stent placement (arrow) in a patient with recurrent episodes of pyelonephritis.

20.5.2 Renal Veins

The renal veins can show several abnormalities in number and path, with direct consequences in their anatomical relations with other anatomical structures, first of all the aorta. The identification of such abnormalities is fundamental in the kidney surgical planning (nefrectomy, tumorectomy, transplantation).

- *Retroaortic left renal vein*: it results from the persistence of the dorsal arch of the renal collar; in this variation the ventral arch (intersubcardinal anastomosis) regresses so that a single renal vein passes posterior to the aorta.
- *Circumaortic left renal vein*: one left renal vein crosses anterior to the aorta and drains the surrenalica vein; another crosses posterior to the aorta and drains the gonadic vein.

20.5.3 "Nutcracker" Phenomenon

"Nutcracker" phenomenon, also known as left renal vein entrapment, is characterized by impeded flow from the left renal vein into the IVC due to its extrinsic compression, often accompanied by lateral (hilar) dilatation and medial (mesoaortic) narrowing. In most of the cases, the compression of the left renal vein occurs between the aorta posteriorly and the superior mesenteric artery anteriorly [7]. The frequence and clinical significance of the syndrome are unpredictable, varying from asymptomatic microematuria to severe pelvic congestion.

20.5.4 Venous Thrombosis

Thrombosis of the abdominal venous vessels can be differentiated in benign and malign thrombosis and it can occur in any vessel of the upper abdomen and the pelvis; benign thrombosis is related to the presence of a bland thrombus in the vessel lumen, occurring in prone patients with alteration of the classic Virchow's triad in patients with congenital or acquired conditions associated with a hypercoagulability; malign thrombosis is given by a clot of neoplastic cells invading the vessels lumen. Venous thrombosis can be diagnosed by CT when a filling defect (with partial or complete occlusion of the lumen) is detected in a venous vessel after contrast media administration. Imbibition and edema of the surrounding soft tissue and wall enhancement represent indirect signs of thrombosis. The differentiation between a bland (benign) thrombus and a malignant (neoplastic) thrombus is crucial in clinical management: benign thrombosis can be treated with anticoagulants and fibrinolytic therapy or—in selected cases—with the placement of intravenous filters to prevent secondary distant embolization; the treatment of malignant thrombosis is based and customized on the tumor of origin.

20.5.4.1 Bland Thrombosis

The definition of bland thrombosis includes all kinds of intraluminal filling defect not determined by neoplastic cells. The main imaging feature of bland thrombosis is thrombus the absence of enhancement after contrast media administration (Figures 20.11 and 20.12) [8]. Nevertheless, the distinction between bland thrombosis and neoplastic thrombosis can be challenging in patients affected by tumoral diseases, which can lead to a condition of plasmatic hypercoagulability, related to the treatment or to the tumor itself.

20.5.4.2 Neoplastic Thrombosis

Neoplastic thrombosis is given by a group of neoplastic cells invading the vessel lumen. Its identification and characterization is crucial in the formulation of patient's prognosis and in the surgical or medical therapeutical planning.

The tumors most frequently associated with neoplastic thrombosis are renal cell carcinoma (Figure 20.13) and hepatocarcinoma (Figure 20.14). Thrombus enhancement after contrast administration, explained by the necessary blood flow feeding the neoplastic cells forming the thrombus, represents a highly suggestive imaging sign of neoplastic thrombosis [8]; however, even some chronic bland thrombi in an advanced phase of organization can show a significant contrast enhancement.

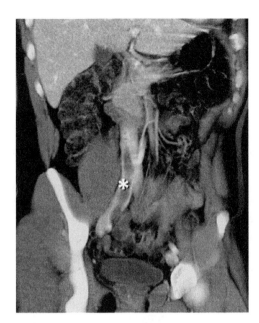

FIGURE 20.11
Venous thrombosis of the inferior vena cava (asterisk) with extension to the right common iliac vein in a patient with congenital hypercoagulability assuming oral anabolic steroids for bodybuilding.

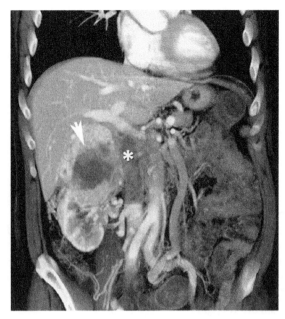

FIGURE 20.13
Neoplastic thrombosis of the inferior vena cava in a patient with renal cell carcinoma (arrow) with venous invasion (asterisk).

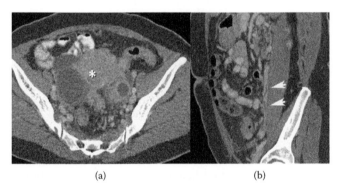

(a)   (b)

FIGURE 20.12
A 25-year-old patient with (a) pelvic inflammatory disease (asterisk) and (b) thrombosis of the left ovarian vein (small arrows).

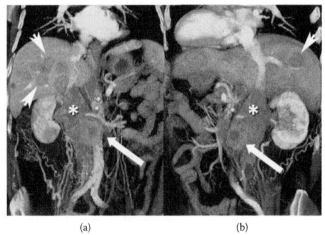

(a)   (b)

FIGURE 20.14
Patient with multifocal hepatocellular carcinoma (small arrows) (a), with neoplastic thrombosis of the inferior vena cava (asterisk) showing enhancement after contrast media administration (big arrow) (b).

Neoplastic thrombosis not only occurs in presence of malignant tumoral lesions: some intravascular benign lesions (lipomas endothelial papillary hyperplasia) can appear as filling defect within the vessel lumen showing a mild enhancement after contrast media administration.

20.5.5 CT Venography of the Lower Limbs

The main pathological conditions occurring in the venous system of the lower extremities are represented by venous insufficiency, with the presence of varicose veins, DVT, and venous compressions due to anatomical variants.

An exhaustive knowledge of the venous system of the lower limbs and the exact discrimination between the vessels of the superficial and deep districts is not only crucial in an anatomical and functional analysis, but, more importantly, it can also have direct clinical implications: venous thrombosis principally occurs in the vessels of the deep system (DVT) being a possible cause of distant embolism.

The superficial system is more frequently affected by other pathological conditions, such as varicosis and phlebitis; thrombosis of the superficial vessels is rare and with less relevant possible consequences.

20.5.6 Venous Insufficiency

Varicose veins are enlarged and tortuous veins caused by a prolonged high intraluminal pressure and loss of the physiological resistance of the vessels walls. Varicose veins are most common in the superficial veins of the legs, which are subject to high pressure when standing. This condition more frequently affects patients older than 50 years, women, and obese subjects. Varicose veins are cause of blood stasis, edema, congestion, and can predispose to intravascular thrombus formation. In spite of the frequency of thrombosis occurring in varicose veins, distal embolism is infrequent; distal embolism is much more common in the deep veins, for the mobilization of the thrombi caused by the surrounding muscular compression.

In the evaluation of venous insufficiency, CT venography allows the assessment of presence and extent of varicose veins and it allows the identification of possible complications [9].

20.5.7 Venous Thrombosis

Direct CT venography allows the visualization of the thrombus after the administration of intravenous contrast into a foot vein. Compared to standard venography, its sensitivity is 100% and its specificity is 96% for both femoropopliteal and calf vein thromboses [10].

Indirect CT venography with the administration of contrast media from a venous vessel of the arm allows a CT pulmonary angiography and the evaluation of DVT in the same study. Indirect CT venography is as accurate as ultrasonography in detecting DVT, and accurately images the veins of the abdomen, pelvis, and calves.

Venous thrombosis can be differentiated in acute and chronic, which are characterized by peculiar clinical manifestations and different CT patterns.

Venous thrombosis (also known as phlebothrombosis) occurs in the 90% of cases in the veins of the lower extremities, both in the superficial and in the deep venous systems. The vessels forming the systems of the GSV and the SSV represent the main sites of thrombus formation in the superficial system, especially occurring in varicose vessels; the thrombi of the superficial system rarely cause distant embolism.

Deep thrombosis can occur in the main veins of the calf and above the knee (iliac veins, popliteal veins, and femoral veins); thrombosis of the deep venous system, compared to thrombosis of the superficial vessels, is more clinically relevant because it can represent a source of distant embolism. The incidence of pulmonary embolism (PE) determined by DVT of the upper limbs is about 5%–10% of the cases. Moreover, the increasing use of intravenous catheters is associated with an increased risk of DVT of the upper limbs. The sites of thrombosis most frequently causing embolism are the subclavian and the brachiocephalic veins.

Less frequently, distant embolism may arise from venous vessels of the periprostatic plexus, the ovaric veins, and the periuterine veins.

Once the thrombus is formed, it can have one of the following outcomes:

- *Propagation*: the thrombus grows in dimension with occlusion of the vessel's lumen.
- *Embolization*: it occurs when a thrombus breaks free from the vascular wall and becomes mobile, reaching a distant localization.
- *Dissolution*: fibrinolytic mechanisms break up the thrombus and blood flow is restored to the vessel.
- *Organization and recanalization*: ingrowth of smooth muscle cells, fibroblasts, and endothelium into the fibrin-rich thrombus: the thrombus is incorporated in the vessel wall with restored blood flow.

Chronic thrombosis is characterized by a reduction of the caliber of the vessel lumen; in most reiterated cases, the affected vessel can evolve in a fibrotic cordon. The formation of surrounding collateral circles represents a secondary effect of the thrombosis, and its presence can be a sign of chronic or subacute vessel occlusion. Over time, the thrombus changes its constitution with "organization" of its structure, which can lead to restoration of blood flow. At the end of the organization process, the residual thrombus is circumferentially displaced along the vessel's walls.

CT accuracy in the differentiation between acute and chronic thrombosis is still unknown; unenhanced scans can help in the identification of an acute thrombosis, showing hyperdense clots inside the vessel lumen. Chronic thrombi can show inner calcification and they can be associated with recanalization; the affected vessels are typically small and narrowed, with multiple collateral circles.

20.5.8 May–Thurner Syndrome

May–Thurner syndrome is a rare condition that is caused by the compression of the left common iliac veins by the right common iliac artery, with obstruction to the venous outflow tract of the left lower extremity. Its clinical manifestations are discomfort, swelling, or DVT in the iliofemoral vein. Compared to the right common iliac vein, the left common iliac vein takes a more transverse course, crossing posteriorly the right common iliac artery, which may compress it against the lumbar spine. When suspected, CT venography can confirm the diagnosis, showing the venous compression [11].

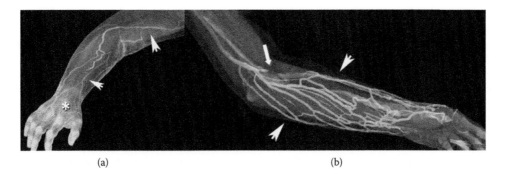

(a)   (b)

FIGURE 20.15
CT venography of the upper extremity showing the superficial veins of the forearm (a) showing the path of the cephalic vein from the radial side of the dorsal venous network (asterisk) and ascending in front of the elbow in the groove between the brachioradialis and the biceps brachii (small arrows). In subpart (b), direct CT venography of the upper extremity showing a dilatated tortuous superficial system of the forearm (radial side, small arrows) as a consequence of venous obstruction in the elbow (big arrow).

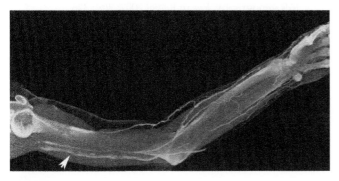

FIGURE 20.16
A 28-year-old patient with compression of the left anonymous vein and deep venous thrombosis of the homolateral basilic vein.

20.5.9 CT Venography of the Upper Limbs

CT venography continues to evolve as a state-of-the-art imaging modality in the diagnosis of upper extremity DVT [12]. Upper extremity DVT (Figure 20.15) is a rare thrombotic disorder (1%–4% of all DVT) that, in most of the cases, is caused by acquired or congenital conditions associated with hypercoagulability (as discussed for DVT of the lower limbs). Less frequently, DVT of the upper limbs may be secondary to pathological conditions, which determine a compression or obstruction of the venous blood flow in the deep veins of the arm (Figure 20.16); this compression may be caused by neoplastic diseases (SVC syndrome) or anatomical variants (thoracic outlet syndrome; Paget–von Schrötter disease).

The SVC syndrome is usually caused by a compression or obstruction of the SVC determined by different kinds of neoplasms localized in the superior mediastinum (right upper lobe tumors, thymoma, lymphoma, and/or mediastinal lymphadenopathy). This syndrome may cause venous distention in the neck and in the upper chest and limbs. The blood stasis in the deep veins of the arms may lead to DVT.

20.5.10 Paget–von Schrötter Disease

This condition (also known as "effort thrombosis of upper extremity"), relatively rare, is characterized by DVT of the axillary or subclavian vein. It usually presents in young and otherwise healthy patients, more often in males than females. It has been reported to occur after vigorous or repetitive activity, though it can also occur spontaneously or as consequence of thoracic outlet syndrome. CT venography can show a venous compression by the first rib or a cervical rib, a hypertrophic anterior scalene muscle or a hypertrophic subclavius muscle [13].

Symptoms may include sudden onset of pain, warmth, redness, blueness, and swelling in the arm. DVT related to Paget–von Schrötter disease can rarely cause PE.

References

1. Mavili E, Ozturk M, Akcali Y, Donmez H, Yikilmaz A, Tokmak TT, Ozcan N. Direct CT venography for evaluation of the lower extremity venous anomalies of Klippel-Trenaunay Syndrome. *Am J Roentgenol* 2009; 192(6): W311–316.
2. Oda S, Utsunomiya D, Awai K, Takaoka H, Nakaura T, Katahira K, Morishita S, Namimoto T, Yamashita Y. Indirect computed tomography venography with a low-tube-voltage technique: Reduction in the radiation and contrast material dose—A prospective randomized study. *J Comput Assist Tomogr* 2011; 35(5): 631–636.
3. Escott EJ, Branstetter BF. It's not a cervical lymph node, it's a vein: CT and MR imaging findings in the veins of the head and neck. *Radiographics* 2006; 26(5): 1501–1515.
4. Burney K, Young H, Barnard SA, McCoubrie P, Darby M. CT appearances of congential and acquired abnormalities of the superior vena cava. *Clin Radiol* 2007; 62(9): 837–842.

5. Demondion X, Herbinet P, Van Sint Jan S, Boutry N, Chantelot C, Cotten A. Imaging assessment of thoracic outlet syndrome. *Radiographics* 2006; 26(6): 1735–1750. Review.
6. Malaki M, Willis AP, Jones RG. Congenital anomalies of the inferior vena cava. *Clin Radiol.* 2012; 67(2): 165–171.
7. Kim KW, Cho JY, Kim SH, Yoon JH, Kim DS, Chung JW, Park JH. Diagnostic value of computed tomographic findings of nutcracker syndrome: Correlation with renal venography and renocaval pressure gradients. *Eur J Radiol* 2011; 80(3): 648–654.
8. Rossi S, Ghittoni G, Ravetta V, Torello Viera F, Rosa L, Serassi M, Scabini M, Vercelli A, Tinelli C, Dal Bello B et al. Contrast-enhanced ultrasonography and spiral computed tomography in the detection and characterization of portal vein thrombosis complicating hepatocellular carcinoma. *Eur Radiol* 2008; 18(8): 1749–1756.
9. Lee W, Chung JW, Yin YH, Jae HJ, Kim SJ, Ha J, Park JH. Three-dimensional CT venography of varicose veins of the lower extremity: Image quality and comparison with doppler sonography. *Am J Roentgenol* 2008; 191(4): 1186–1191.
10. Ho VB, van Geertruyden PH, Yucel EK, Rybicki FJ, Baum RA, Desjardins B, Flamm SD, Foley WD, Jaff MR, Koss SA et al. ACR Appropriateness Criteria(®) on suspected lower extremity deep vein thrombosis. *J Am Coll Radiol* 2011; 8(6): 383–387.
11. Jeon UB, Chung JW, Jae HJ, Kim HC, Kim SJ, Ha J, Park JH. May-Thurner syndrome complicated by acute iliofemoral vein thrombosis: Helical CT venography for evaluation of long-term stent patency and changes in the iliac vein. *AJR Am J Roentgenol* 2010; 195(3): 751–757.
12. Sabharwal R, Boshell D, Vladica P. Multidetector spiral CT venography in the diagnosis of upper extremity deep venous thrombosis. *Australas Radiol* 2007; 51 Suppl: B253–B256.
13. Pedrosa I, Aschkenasi C, Hamdan A, Rofsky NM. Effort-induced thrombosis: Diagnosis with three-dimensional MR venography. *Emerg Radiol* 2002; 9(6): 326.

Section IV

Thorax and Mediastinum

21

Infective Pathology of the Lung

Jeffrey P. Kanne

CONTENTS

21.1 Introduction

Lower respiratory tract infections are a major cause of morbidity and mortality worldwide and have a significant economic impact on societies. In the United States, community-acquired pneumonia (CAP) has an estimated $16 billion worth of adverse economic impact annually [1].

Pneumonia is the eighth leading cause of death in the United States and is the number one cause of infection-related mortality [2]. Precise numbers are difficult to determine because of great variations in population makeup, inconsistencies in confirming the diagnosis of pneumonia, and lack of a central data repository as pneumonia is not a reportable disease in the United States [3]. Nevertheless, in the geriatric population, pneumonia accounts for approximately half of all infection-related deaths. The reported incidence across multiple studies ranges from 2.6 to 16.8 cases per 1000 adults annually [4] and is greater in women, the elderly, and members of lower socioeconomic groups [5–8]. Mortality rates range from 0.1% for patients not requiring hospitalization [9] to 40% for patients requiring hospital care [5,10,11]. Healthcare-acquired pneumonia (HCAP) affects 0.5%–1.0% of patients [12], but is more common following surgery [13] and in patients requiring mechanical ventilation [14]. HCAP has the highest mortality rate of any nosocomial infection [15], increases length of stay, and negatively impacts healthcare cost containment measures.

Imaging plays a central role in the diagnosis of pulmonary infection as well as in identifying complications or underlying causes. Chest radiography remains the primary examination for establishing the diagnosis of pneumonia and for assessing the response to treatment. Computed tomography (CT) of the chest is generally reserved for evaluating patients with suspected complications of infection or for detecting the structural causes of recurrent infection, such as obstructing neoplasm, or a congenital malformation, such as a bronchopulmonary sequestration [16–19]. Occasionally, CT can help narrow the differential diagnosis of the causative agent, although few CT features distinguish among bacterial pneumonias. CT may also be used in evaluating immunocompromised patients with normal or near-normal radiographs in whom the index of suspicion for pneumonia is high.

Pulmonary infections are traditionally categorized by type of causative organism as this guides appropriate treatment. However, imaging performs poorly in predicting even the broad category of infective agents. Pulmonary infections are sometimes classified by their respective radiology patterns, but this, too, suffers from lack of specificity and the frequent coexistence of several patterns in the same patient. Currently, a clinical classification system based on the source of infection and underlying host factors is preferred [7,20,21].

Modern CT scanners can perform rapid volumetric helical acquisitions during a single breath-hold. Although most routine thoracic CT scans are reconstructed with a 5 mm slice thickness, a dataset of thin section (1.0–1.5 mm) images using a high spatial frequency kernel can be reconstructed from the same dataset while employing low radiation dose technique, obviating the need for separate "step-and-shoot" high-resolution imaging through the chest. A kilovoltage peak (kVp) of 120 kV with a tube output of 40–80 mAs is sufficient to image the chest in most adults. Lower kVp may be preferable in children and small adults, and higher kVp may be required in severely obese patients. Newer CT scanner models provide added radiation dose reduction options using a variety of tube current modulation strategies and iterative reconstruction techniques.

Prone and expiratory images are not necessary in the vast majority of patients. Coronal and sagittal reformations can be useful in select cases and can be generated "on-the-fly" in many picture archiving and communication systems (PACS).

In the vast majority of cases, intravenous contrast administration is not necessary to evaluate patients with suspected pulmonary infection. Contrast administration may be useful in patients with extensive lung consolidation, helping distinguish intensely and uniformly enhancing atelectatic lung from heterogeneous areas of consolidation due to pneumonia or obstruction. Furthermore, unenhancing a consolidated lung may reflect areas of pulmonary necrosis or abscess formation.

21.2 Imaging Techniques

Chest radiography should be the first imaging test performed in patients suspected of having pneumonia and is usually sufficient for establishing or excluding a diagnosis of pneumonia. However, false-positive interpretations may occur in the setting of chronic obstructive lung disease, atelectasis, or congestive heart failure [22–24]. The extent of infection (e.g., number of lobes involved) and the presence of associated pleural disease portend more severe infection and increase the likelihood that critical care unit admission may be required [25].

CT scanning is more sensitive and specific than radiography for detecting and characterizing pulmonary infections. However, like radiography, CT is limited in its ability to predict the causative organism, although some findings of CT may favor a limited number of possible causative organisms.

21.3 Patterns of Lower Respiratory Tract Infection

21.3.1 Tracheobronchitis

Acute tracheobronchitis occurs primarily in children and manifests most notably as croup related to parainfluenza virus infection. Adult infections are uncommon and are usually associated with an underlying immune deficiency [26]. In this population, fungi, particularly belonging to *Aspergillus* species, may be involved. CT findings are not well described, but include diffuse tracheal wall thickening and edema of the adjacent mediastinal fat [27].

Causes of chronic tracheobronchitis include *Mycobacterium tuberculosis* [28,29] and *Klebsiella rhinoscleromatis* [30–32], the latter being the cause of rhinoscleroma. Rhinoscleroma is a relapsing and remitting chronic granulomatous infection of the respiratory tract that, if untreated, can progress from disease limited to the nasal mucosa to involvement of the tracheobronchial tree. It is endemic in tropical and subtropical areas, particularly Eastern and Central Europe, Africa, India, Indonesia, and Central and South America [33]. Granulomatous inflammation, similar to that encountered with *M. tuberculosis*, can lead to scarring and airway wall thickening. The CT findings correspond to the histopathologic findings, and include smooth or nodular diffuse tracheobronchial wall thickening, focal stricture, and diffuse luminal stenosis [34–36].

21.3.2 Lobar Pneumonia

Lobar (air space) pneumonia begins in the subpleural region of the lung periphery, and infection spreads to the adjacent alveoli through the pores of Kohn, resulting in confluent consolidation. It is characterized by rapid tissue edema and little cellular response. Infection spreads from one acinus to the next via direct flow of edema fluid laden with organisms, confined only by pleural boundaries, and eventually the host immune response [37]. Total lobar consolidation is uncommon because most patients present earlier in the course of disease with signs and symptoms of pneumonia and are started on therapy. Consolidation may be confined to one lobe, but other lobes too can be affected. Direct spread to adjacent lobes can occur through incomplete pulmonary fissures (Figure 21.1). Because airway involvement is usually limited, lobar volume is typically preserved, and air bronchograms are usually

present [38]. Ground-glass opacity may be located adjacent to the consolidated lung, reflecting incomplete acinar filling [39].

Streptococcus pneumonia is the most common cause of lobar pneumonia. Other common bacterial causes of lobar pneumonia include *Klebsiella pneumonia*, *Haemophilus influenzae*, and occasionally, *M. tuberculosis*. *Legionella pneumophila* can cause a lobar pattern of pneumonia early in the course of infection, but there is often a rapid spread of infection to other lobes.

21.3.3 Bronchopneumonia

Bronchopneumonia is characterized by multifocal inflammatory exudates centered on the affected airways with involvement of adjacent pulmonary lobules and acini. In contrast to lobar pneumonia, fluid production with bronchopneumonia is low and the cellular (neutrophilic) response is robust, resulting in a patchy distribution of infection. Associated volume loss may be present, and the affected airways may contain inflammatory secretions and debris, which can spread through the airways to other sites in the lungs. Progressive infection can lead to a confluence of the affected areas, often accompanied by hemorrhage and necrosis.

The most common causes of bronchopneumonia include *Staphylococcus aureus*, *H. influenzae*, and fungi. Aspiration can also result in a bronchopneumonia pattern and favors the posterior and basal portions of the lungs.

The primary CT finding of bronchopneumonia is peribronchial lung consolidation (Figure 21.2). Ground-glass opacity may be located adjacent to consolidation.

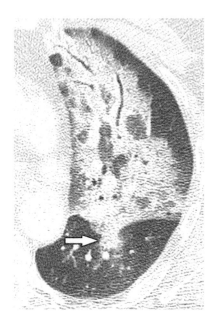

FIGURE 21.1
Male patient with *Streptococcus pneumonia* infection. HRCT image shows a lobar pattern of pneumonia characterized by extensive consolidation and ground-glass opacity in the left upper lobe. The pneumonic process has spread into the superior segment of the left lower lobe (arrow) through an incomplete major fissure.

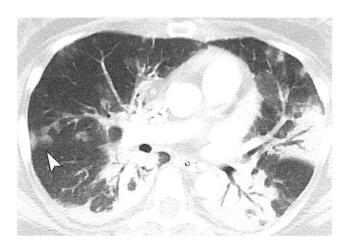

FIGURE 21.2
45-year-old woman with H1N1 influenza pneumonia. HRCT shows a bronchopneumonia pattern of infection characterized by multifocal peribronchial consolidation with air bronchograms. A few nodular foci of ground-glass opacity (arrowhead) are present.

Additionally, centrilobular or acinar nodules may be present around the areas of consolidation. Volume loss is characterized by hypoinflation of the infected lobe(s), retraction of the fissures, and crowding of the bronchovascular structures [40].

21.3.4 Round Pneumonia

Round pneumonia describes early pulmonary infection presenting as a spherical nodular or mass-like area of lung consolidation. Air bronchograms are sometimes present, and infection can evolve into a lobar pattern. Round pneumonia occurs most commonly in children and is usually caused by *S. pneumoniae* [41,42]. Q fever and endemic fungal pneumonia (Figure 21.3) should be considered when round pneumonia develops in an adult [43].

21.3.5 Interstitial Pneumonia

Interstitial pneumonia most commonly results from viral infection (Figure 21.4), *Mycoplasma pneumoniae*, and *Pneumocystis jiroveci*. Histopathologically, infection may be a smoldering lymphocyte-predominant process affecting the alveolar septa or a rapidly progressive process characterized by diffuse alveolar damage. *M. pneumoniae* and viruses typically cause bronchiolitis and bronchitis, as well. The interstitial pattern on chest

radiography comprises peribronchial thickening and reticulonodular opacities. On CT, ground-glass opacity, centrilobular nodules, tree-in-bud opacities, and septal thickening may be present.

21.3.6 Acute Infectious Bronchiolitis

Acute infectious bronchiolitis occurs most commonly in children. The most common infectious agents are respiratory tract viruses, particularly respiratory syncytial virus, adenovirus, influenza virus, parainfluenza virus, and human metapneumovirus. *M. pneumoniae*, *Chlamydia pneumoniae*, and fungi can also cause acute infectious bronchiolitis.

Bronchiolar wall inflammation and the accumulation of mucus and a neutrophil-predominant inflammatory exudate in the airway lumen characterize infectious bronchiolitis. Bronchiolar epithelial necrosis can develop in severe cases.

The clinical presentation of acute infectious bronchiolitis is typically more severe in children. Young children commonly develop acute onset dyspnea, tachypnea, and fever several days after an upper respiratory tract infection. Wheezing is frequently present on chest auscultation. Adults usually have milder signs and symptoms because of the relatively larger cross-sectional areas of the small airways, presumably accounting for a smaller contribution of small airways to overall pulmonary resistance. Severe or fatal disease in adults is uncommon.

Acute infectious bronchiolitis is characterized on CT by the presence of centrilobular nodules

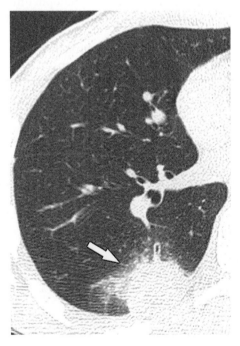

FIGURE 21.3
24-year-old man with North American blastomycosis. HRCT image shows a rounded, mass-like focus of consolidation with peripheral ground-glass opacity (arrow) in the right lower lobe.

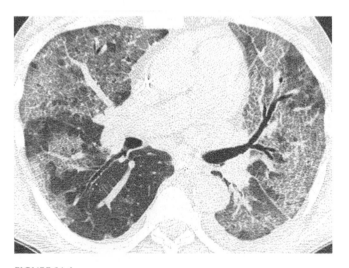

FIGURE 21.4
55-year-old woman with H1N1 influenza pneumonia. HRCT image demonstrates an "interstitial" pneumonia pattern characterized by extensive ground-glass opacity with superimposed septal thickening ("crazy-paving") and small pleural effusions.

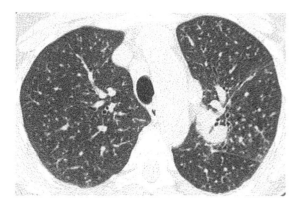

FIGURE 21.5
54-year-old woman with viral bronchiolitis. HRCT image shows scattered, well-defined centrilobular nodules.

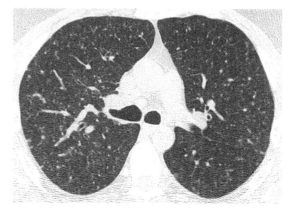

FIGURE 21.6
36-year-old male renal transplant recipient with disseminated histoplasmosis. HRCT image shows numerous tiny (1 mm–3 mm) lung nodules in a random distribution.

(Figure 21.5) and tree-in-bud opacities, either in one or both lungs. The extent is typically patchy, and when bilateral, disease is usually asymmetric. The centrilobular nodules and tree-in-bud opacities correspond to the bronchiolar inflammation and intraluminal exudates and mucus, respectively. Infection can progress to bronchopneumonia, characterized by the development of larger (5–10 mm) acinar nodules and patchy areas of lung consolidation or ground-glass opacity.

21.3.7 Miliary Pattern

A miliary pattern consists of innumerable tiny (1–3 mm) nodules distributed randomly throughout the lungs. Hematogenous dissemination of *M. tuberculosis* is the most common infectious cause of miliary nodules. Less commonly, some viruses, such as the varicella-zoster virus, and endemic fungal infections, such as histoplasmosis (Figure 21.6), North American blastomycosis, and coccidioidomycosis can cause a miliary pattern of disease. The disseminated infections usually occur in immunosuppressed patients with impaired cell-mediated immunity.

21.3.8 Septic Pulmonary Emboli and Septic Pulmonary Infarcts

Septic pulmonary emboli are microabscesses that develop following embolization of microorganisms or infected thrombus into the lung periphery. *S. aureus* is the most common cause of septic pulmonary emboli. Common sources of septic emboli include infected indwelling venous catheters, implanted cardiac pacers and defibrillators, and other infected prosthesis. Bacterial endocarditis from intravenous drug use can

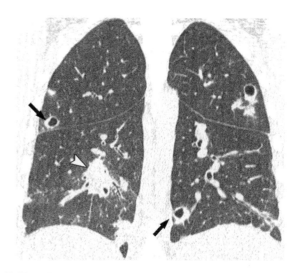

FIGURE 21.7
22-year-old woman with septic emboli from intravenous drug abuse. Coronal reformatted HRCT image demonstrates multiple peripheral and basal predominant nodules of varying size, some of which are cavitary (arrows). A large focus of peribronchial consolidation (arrowhead) is in the right lower lobe.

also result in septic pulmonary emboli. The occlusion of small arterioles by infected emboli can result in septic infarcts.

CT findings of septic pulmonary emboli are fairly characteristic and include multiple nodules of varying sizes, typically 1–3 cm in diameter, located in a predominantly peripheral and basal distribution (Figure 21.7). Approximately 50% of these nodules will cavitate. Septic infarcts are indistinguishable from bland infarcts and consist of subpleural wedge-shaped foci of consolidation, frequently containing central ground-glass opacity, absent air bronchograms, and occasionally, frank necrosis.

21.4 Specific Infections

21.4.1 Mycobacteria Tuberculosis

Pulmonary tuberculosis (TB) continues to be a significant cause of morbidity and mortality worldwide [44]. Southeast Asia and sub-Saharan Africa account for the majority of cases. Cell-mediated immune deficiency, particularly HIV infection, is a significant risk factor for developing active pulmonary TB. In endemic areas, reinfection may account for 50% of cases [45].

The imaging findings of TB traditionally have been categorized into two distinct patterns—acute tuberculosis and reactivation or post-primary tuberculosis. However, host immune factors better predict the radiographic findings of pulmonary TB [46].

CT findings of pulmonary TB include tree-in-bud opacities (Figures 21.8 and 21.9), lung consolidation, septal thickening, bronchial wall thickening, and bronchial distortion (Figures 21.10 and 21.11) [47]. Centrilobular nodules and tree-in-bud opacities reflect inflammation and necrosis in the distal small airways. A large volume of these small airway opacities indicates the endobronchial spread of *M. tuberculosis* [47]. In the majority of patients with reactivation or reinfection, CT accurately distinguished scars from previous infection from centrilobular nodules and tree-in-bud opacities related to active disease [47]. Other studies have shown that the presence of centrilobular nodules and tree-in-bud opacities are present only in patients with active TB [48,49].

Cavitation, traditionally associated with reactivated infection, can occur in both primary infection and reinfection (Figure 21.12) [50]. Cavities tend to have thick walls, but thin-walled cavities may also be seen. Cavitary disease is associated with an increased load of *M. tuberculosis*, worse treatment outcome, increased risk of drug resistance, and increased risk of spread of infection to other individuals.

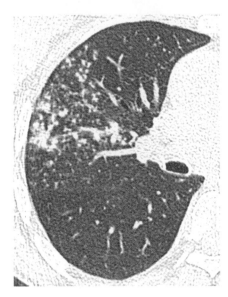

FIGURE 21.9
59-year-old woman with active tuberculosis. HRCT image shows extensive tree-in-bud opacities in the right upper lobe, coalescing laterally.

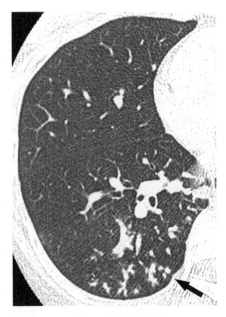

FIGURE 21.8
26-year-old woman with active tuberculosis. HRCT image shows clusters tree-in-bud opacities (arrow) in the right lower lobe.

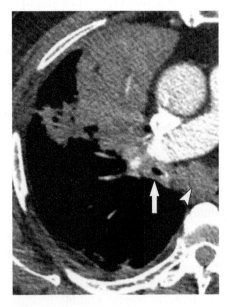

FIGURE 21.10
80-year-old man with active tuberculosis. Contrast-enhanced CT image shows circumferential thickening of the bronchus intermedius (arrow) and right lung consolidation. Subcarinal lymphadenopathy (arrowhead) is present.

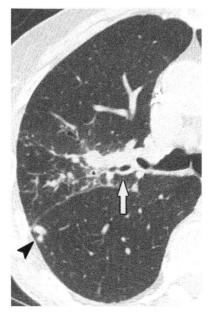

FIGURE 21.11
79-year-old man with active tuberculosis. HRCT image shows bronchial wall thickening and narrowing (arrow) with peripheral nodules (arrowhead).

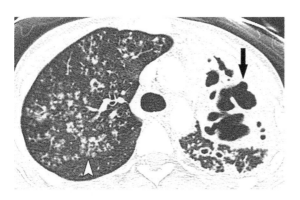

FIGURE 21.12
18-year-old woman with active tuberculosis. HRCT image demonstrates a large, complex left upper lobe cavity (arrow). Bronchial dilation and wall thickening are in the superior segment of the left lower lobe, and numerous tree-in-bud opacities (arrowhead) are present, consistent with spread of infection throughout the airways.

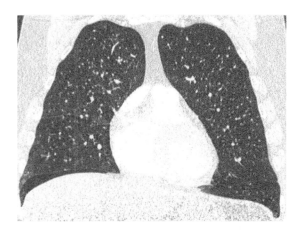

FIGURE 21.13
57-year-old man with miliary tuberculosis. Coronal reformatted HRCT image shows innumerable tiny nodules distributed throughout the lungs.

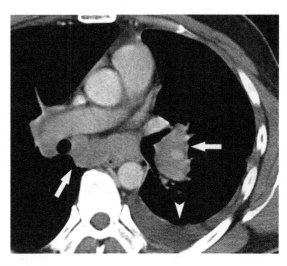

FIGURE 21.14
38-year-old man with active tuberculosis. Contrast-enhanced CT image demonstrates mediastinal and hilar lymphadenopathy (arrows) and a small pleural effusion (arrowhead).

A miliary pattern of lung nodules is seen with hematogenous dissemination of TB and usually occurs in immune suppressed patients [51]. These nodules range from 1 to 3 mm and are randomly distributed throughout the lungs (Figure 21.13). Septal lines may accompany the miliary nodules [47].

Lung consolidation is typically homogeneous with no zonal predominance [52], but can also be mass-like or linear [52,53]. In some patients with reactivation or reinfection, a dominant nodule or mass measuring 5–40 mm develops, usually in the upper lobes. These tuberculomas consist of central caseous necrosis and peripheral histiocytes and giant cells with varying degrees of collagen. Tuberculomas may be multiple in 20% of patients. Satellite nodules of up to 5 mm in diameter are usually apparent on CT [54,55].

Hilar and mediastinal lymph node enlargement is present in up to one-third of patients with active tuberculosis (Figure 21.14) [47,56,57]. On contrast-enhanced CT, infected lymph nodes may show central low attenuation with peripheral enhancement (Figure 21.15), the former reflecting caseous necrosis and the latter inflammation [58].

TB can cause both acute and chronic inflammation in the central airways. Typically, both the trachea and the proximal main bronchi are involved as isolated tracheal disease is rare [28,29]. The exact mechanism of development of tuberculous tracheobronchitis is unknown, but it may result from direct inoculation of the mucosa, direct extension from adjacent infected lymph nodes, or lymphatic or hematogenous dissemination from other

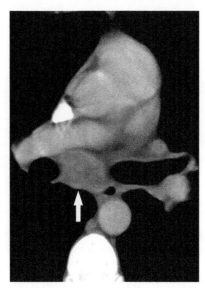

FIGURE 21.15
Male patient with tuberculous lymphadenitis. Contrast-enhanced CT image shows an enlarged, peripherally enhancing subcarinal lymph node with central low attenuation, the latter finding suggesting caseous necrosis.

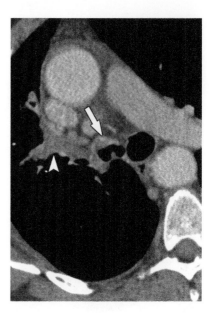

FIGURE 21.16
52-year-old man with tuberculous bronchitis. Contrast-enhanced CT image demonstrates thickening and enhancement of the right main bronchus (arrow) with luminal narrowing and irregularity. The right upper lobe segmental bronchi are distended with mucinous secretions (arrowhead) secondary to obstruction.

sites of disease [59]. In the acute phase, lymphocytes infiltrate the mucosa and lead to caseous necrosis and ulceration. With chronic infection, fibrosis can develop in the lamina propria and at sites of healing mucosal ulcers.

The CT findings of tuberculous tracheobronchitis reflect the histologic findings. Initially, the affected airway walls, usually the distal trachea and the proximal main bronchi, become thickened, sometimes nodular, and the definition of the wall diminishes as the result of confluence with adjacent inflammatory lymphadenopathy. Luminal narrowing is variable and may result in downstream obstruction when extensive (Figure 21.16). Enhancement of the tracheobronchial wall and the periphery of affected lymph nodes may be evident following the administration of intravenous contrast material [29,60]. Rare complications of acute tuberculous tracheobronchitis include erosion of an adjacent infected lymph node in the airway with subsequent cavitation [59] and tracheobronchial cartilage fragment expectoration [61]. With ongoing inflammation, long segment (>3 cm) strictures can form as a consequence of mural fibrosis. The left main bronchus is the most commonly affected. The bronchial wall is concentrically narrowed and can be smooth or nodular [28,29]. Bronchogenic carcinoma and other causes of tracheobronchitis can mimic tracheobronchial tuberculosis. Organisms may not be recovered on sputum sampling, and tissue sampling may be required to confirm the diagnosis. With appropriate therapy, infection usually clears with varying degrees of residual inflammation and fibrosis.

21.4.2 Nontuberculous Mycobacteria

The incidence of infection attributed to nontuberculous mycobacteria (NTM) has been increasing worldwide [62]. NTM are ubiquitous throughout the environment, and human infection is common. However, disease is quite rare, given the widespread extent of NTM in the environment. It is believed that most humans are infected through soil and water [63]. The *M. avium* complex (MAC) comprises *M. avium* and *M. intracellulare* and accounts for the vast majority of cases of NTM pulmonary disease [62]. Infection incidence by other species of NTM varies, depending on the patient population [64–66].

Three patterns of lung disease have been described with MAC in immunocompetent hosts. However, the "classic" and "non-classic" patterns may represent a spectrum of the same process, with the former representing a more advanced form of the disease. The term "classic" alludes to the similar appearance to TB.

Fibrocavitary or "classic" disease most commonly occurs in middle-aged and older men with underlying structural lung disease, such as emphysema, bronchiectasis, and sarcoidosis (Figure 21.17) [67,68]. The apical and posterior segments of the upper lobes are typically involved, but any segment can be affected. Cavities tend to have thick walls and are associated with pleural thickening [69].

The most common pattern of NTM pulmonary infection is nodular bronchiectasis or "non-classical" pattern. This pattern most commonly occurs in older female nonsmokers [62]. The most common CT finding in early

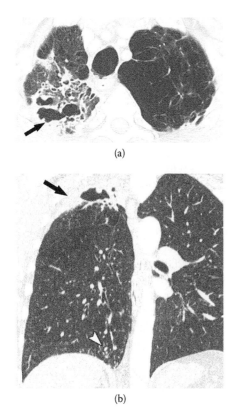

(a)

(b)

FIGURE 21.17
48-year-old man with fibrocavitary *Mycobacterium avium* complex infection. (a) Transverse HRCT image shows an irregular right upper lobe cavity (arrow) with adjacent ectatic and thickened bronchi. (b) Coronal reformatted HRCT image shows thickening of the pleural and extrapleural tissues (arrow) adjacent to the cavity.

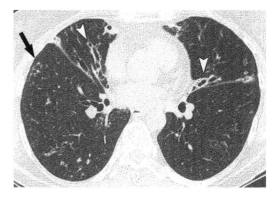

FIGURE 21.18
60-year-old woman with *Mycobacterium avium* complex infection. HRCT image shows right middle lobe and lingular bronchiectasis (arrowheads). Scattered tree-in-bud opacities (arrow) are present.

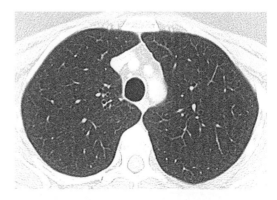

FIGURE 21.19
56-year-old woman with hypersensitivity pneumonitis from an indoor lap pool contaminated with *Mycobacterium avium* complex. HRCT image shows diffuse tiny, poorly defined centrilobular nodules.

disease is tree-in-bud opacities, reflecting bronchiolitis. Bronchiectasis is often present and has a predilection for the right middle lobe, lingula, and anterior segments of the upper lobes; however, any segment can be involved (Figure 21.19) [70]. Randomly scattered nodules measuring up to 2 cm, with or without cavitation, and scattered foci of consolidation may also be present. This constellation of findings (Figure 21.18) is highly suggestive of MAC infection in elderly women and should prompt further investigation [71–73]. In some patients, a mosaic pattern of attenuation may be present, reflecting small airways obstruction [74]. It remains unclear as to whether this is a direct result of MAC infection or a result of bronchiectasis. In contrast to TB, empyema and significant lymphadenopathy are uncommon with NTM infection [68,75,76].

NTM colonizing hot tubs and other water sources can be aerosolized and inhaled, resulting in a form of hypersensitivity pneumonitis termed "hot tub lung" [77,78]. Whether the ensuing host response is a hypersensitivity reaction, granulomatous reaction, or a combination of the two remains to be resolved. The usual HRCT findings are indistinguishable from other causes of hypersensitivity pneumonitis and include poorly defined centrilobular nodules (Figure 21.19), patchy ground-glass opacity, and air trapping on expiratory CT [79,80]. Peripheral tree-in-bud opacities may also be present, a finding not typically associated with other causes of hypersensitivity pneumonitis [80].

21.4.3 Aspergillosis

The spectrum of pulmonary aspergillosis ranges from the hyperimmune allergic bronchopulmonary aspergillosis (ABPA) to angioinvasive infection in immunocompromised patients. Furthermore, several manifestations of the disease can coexist in the same patient, such as aspergilloma in a patient with ABPA.

ABPA is a hyperimmune response to *Aspergillus* and is both IgE (type-I) and immune complex (type-III) mediated. A cell-mediated (type-IV) response may develop in some patients in the form of bronchocentric granulomatosis. Most patients with ABPA have asthma [81,82], and a smaller percentage of patients have cystic fibrosis [83,84].

Early in the disease course, patients may have patchy, fleeting or migratory areas of lung consolidation or ground-glass opacity, presumably foci of eosinophilic pneumonia [85]. Later in the course of the disease, central bronchiectasis with normal distal airways and fibrosis develop with upper lobe predominance [86–88]. Peripheral bronchiectasis may also be present, and a small minority of patients may have cylindrical bronchiectasis in the lower lobes, similar to that encountered in idiopathic bronchiectasis [89]. Varying degrees of mucoid impaction may be present; high attenuation mucoid impaction, believed to reflect calcium and metal ions in the mucus, occurs in up to 30% of patients and is highly suggestive of ABPA (Figure 21.20) [90,91]. Other CT findings include centrilobular nodules and

tree-in-bud opacities, lung consolidation, scar, and small pleural effusions or mild pleural thickening [87,88,92].

Aspergilloma is a saprophytic infection caused by *Aspergillus* and consists of a mobile fungus ball located in a pre-existing cavity. Any cystic space in the lung is a potential site for aspergilloma formation, but cavities from tuberculosis are the common predisposing factor worldwide [93]. Sarcoidosis is another common cause, particularly in North America, with approximately half of patients with advanced fibrosis from sarcoidosis developing aspergilloma [94]. Aspergilloma can also develop in a bronchiectatic airway [95]. Bronchial blood supply to the cavity wall is extensive with friable vessels, resulting in a propensity to bleed, with subsequent hemoptysis, which can be life threatening [96].

The typical CT appearance of aspergilloma is an intracavitary mass, often containing pockets of gas, surrounded by air (air crescent sign) (Figure 21.21). The aspergilloma usually layers dependently and can change position concomitantly with changes in patient position. Foci of high attenuation resulting from calcification may be evident within the intracavitary mass [97]. The cavity wall is usually thick because of chronic inflammation and fibrosis. The adjacent pleura is usually thickened, and this finding may precede the appearance

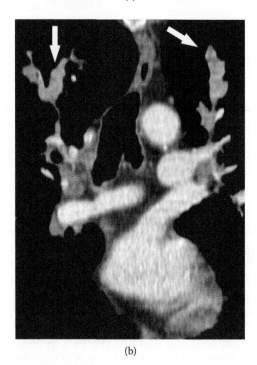

(a)

(b)

FIGURE 21.20
49-year-old man with asthma and allergic bronchopulmonary aspergillosis. (a) HRCT image shows central varicose bronchiectasis (arrows) with bronchial wall thickening. (b) Coronal-reformatted contrast-enhanced CT image demonstrates high attenuation mucoid impaction (arrows), a finding highly suggestive of ABPA.

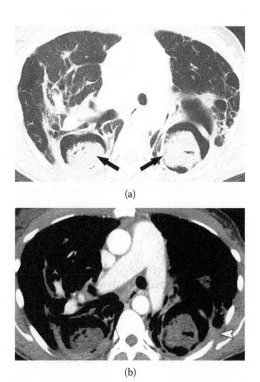

(a)

(b)

FIGURE 21.21
48-year-old woman with advanced pulmonary sarcoidosis and bilateral aspergillomas. (a-b) Contrast-enhanced CT images show bilateral upper lobe cavities with intracavitary masses (arrows) containing pockets of gas. The adjacent pleural and extrapleural tissues are thickened (arrowhead), reflecting the chronic inflammatory process.

of the aspergilloma [98]. Fungal fronds arising from the cavitary wall may be apparent [97].

Invasive aspergillosis can be classified as angioinvasive or airways invasive, although both patterns frequently coexist because of the close proximity of the small airways and small pulmonary arteries [96]. Usually, invasive aspergillosis occurs in heavily immune compromised patients, particularly those who are neutropenic, such as transplant recipients, patients with leukemia, and patients on chemotherapy [96,97,99]. Angioinvasive aspergillosis manifests as a hemorrhagic bronchopneumonia, and up to 25% of patients will have findings of disseminated disease at autopsy [96]. HRCT findings of angioinvasive aspergillosis include nodules, sometimes surrounded by ground-glass opacity (CT halo sign), the latter reflecting the surrounding hemorrhage and infarction (Figure 21.22) [100–102]. Multiple foci of consolidation with or without the surrounding ground-glass opacity are also observed. In the correct clinical setting, the CT halo sign is highly suggestive of angioinvasive aspergillosis, but it can also occur in other infections, such as invasive candidiasis, cytomegalovirus and herpes virus infection, and mucormycosis. Noninfectious causes include hemorrhagic metastases, Kaposi sarcoma, organizing pneumonia, and granulomatosis with polyangiitis (Wegener granulomatosis) [99].

Airways-invasive aspergillosis accounts for less than one-third of invasive *Aspergillus* infections and includes bronchiolitis and bronchopneumonia [103]. In addition to invading beyond the basement membrane of the affected airways, *Aspergillus* organisms are typically present in the airway lumen, resulting in a high diagnostic yield on bronchoalveolar lavage [104]. HRCT findings include peribronchial consolidation and ground-glass opacity, centrilobular nodules, and tree-in-bud opacities (Figure 21.23) [99,105].

Aspergillus accounts for the majority of cases of fungal tracheobronchitis and occurs primarily in severely immunosuppressed patients, particularly patients with AIDS, solid organ and hematopoietic stem cell transplant recipients, and patients with hematologic malignancies [106,107]. CT findings are similar to other causes of tracheobronchitis and include smooth or nodular wall thickening with varying degrees of luminal stenosis (Figure 21.24). Infiltration of the paratracheal fat and pneumomediastinum may develop. Prognosis is poor [96,107].

Chronic airway-invasive aspergillosis (formerly chronic necrotizing or semi-invasive aspergillosis) is a chronic form of airways-invasive aspergillosis and occurs in older men with chronic obstructive lung disease. Other structural lung disease, such as fibrosis and previous resection, in addition to immune suppressing conditions such as alcoholism, diabetes, and chronic corticosteroid therapy, predispose patients to chronic airway-invasive aspergillosis [99]. The initial CT finding is consolidation (typically upper lobe) that slowly becomes cavitary, similar to reactivation or reinfection tuberculosis. Intracavitary aspergilloma formation ensues with associated pleural thickening (Figure 21.25) [108]. Mortality rates of up to 34% are reported; however, underlying pulmonary or systemic disease is likely to be the major contributing factor in a majority of these patients [109]. Coexistent NTM infection may occur in some patients with chronic airways-invasive aspergillosis, presumably given the similarity in underlying risk factors in these patients [110].

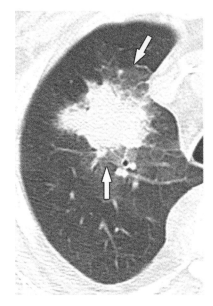

FIGURE 21.22
63-year-old man with acute myelogenous leukemia and angioinvasive aspergillosis. HRCT image demonstrates mass-like consolidation in the right upper lobe surrounded by a halo of ground-glass opacity (arrows).

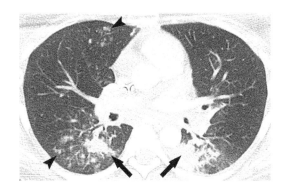

FIGURE 21.23
36-year-old immunocompromised woman with airways invasive aspergillosis. HRCT image shows bilateral peribronchial consolidation (arrows) and tree-in-bud opacities (arrowheads). (Courtesy of Sudhakar Pipavath, M.D. [Seattle, WA].)

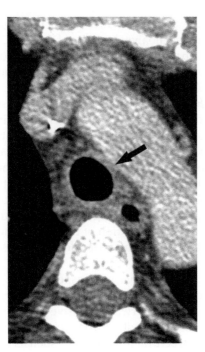

FIGURE 21.24
36-year-old immunocompromised woman with tracheal aspergillosis. Contrast-enhanced CT image shows tracheal wall thickening and enhancement (arrow). The adjacent mediastinal fat is somewhat hazy. Courtesy of Sudhakar Pipavath, M.D. (Seattle, WA).

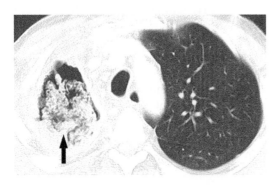

FIGURE 21.25
58-year-old man with chronic airways invasive (chronic necrotizing) aspergillosis. HRCT image shows a large, thick-walled cavity in the right upper lobe containing a large aspergilloma (arrow).

21.4.4 Pneumocystis Jiroveci

Pneumocystis jiroveci pneumonia (PJP) occurs almost exclusively in immunocompromised patients. PJP remains the most common opportunistic infection in patients with AIDS in developed nations despite widespread use of highly active antiretroviral therapy (HAART) and chemoprophylaxis. However, non-HIV-infected immunosuppressed patients now account for the majority of cases of PJP because of increases in solid organ and blood stem cell transplantation and the increased use of immunosuppressive therapy for systemic diseases [78,111].

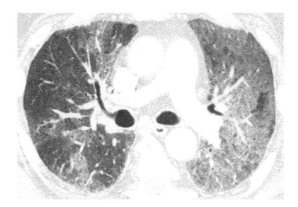

FIGURE 21.26
68-year-old man with HIV infection and *Pneumocystis jiroveci* pneumonia. HRCT image demonstrates extensive ground-class opacity in both lungs.

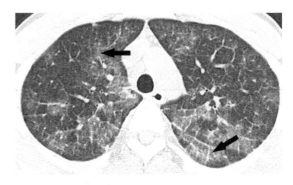

FIGURE 21.27
29-year-old man with HIV infection and *Pneumocystis jiroveci* pneumonia. HRCT image shows patchy ground-glass opacity and interlobular septal thickening (arrows).

Approximately one-third of patients with PJP have a normal chest radiograph. The principal finding of PJP on HRCT is extensive ground-glass opacity resulting from organisms, fibrin, and inflammatory debris accumulating in the alveoli (Figure 21.26). Ground-glass opacity may be diffuse, have relative peripheral sparing, or be heterogeneous with a mosaic pattern of attenuation [112]. The upper lobes are more often involved [113,114]. The extent of ground-glass opacity is often wider in patients without HIV infection [115]. Septal lines, crazy-paving [112], and lung consolidation can develop with more advanced disease (Figure 21.27) [113,116]. Lung consolidation is a manifestation of tissue damage from the host immune response and is more common and develops more rapidly in non-HIV-infected patients [117].

Cysts develop in up to one-third of patients with PJP and have a higher incidence in patients with HIV infection (Figure 21.28). Cysts vary in size and morphology and are associated with a higher incidence of spontaneous pneumothorax. Cysts may or may not resolve with treatment and clearing of infection [112–114].

Lung nodules are uncommon in PJP and tend to occur in HIV-infected patients with only slightly impaired

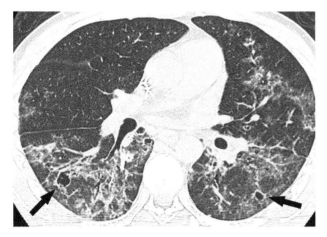

FIGURE 21.28
41-year-old man with HIV infection and *Pneumocystis jiroveci* pneumonia. HRCT image shows patchy ground-glass opacity, minimal consolidation, and small cysts (arrows).

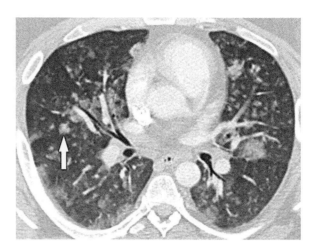

FIGURE 21.29
Patient with *Mycoplasma* pneumonia. Contrast-enhanced CT image shows lobular foci of consolidation (arrow) and patchy ground-glass opacity. Courtesy of Loren Ketai, M.D. (Albuquerque, NM).

cell-mediated immunity when a granulomatous response is still possible [116]. The presence of centrilobular nodules with or without tree-in-bud opacities favors infectious bronchiolitis from other organisms [118].

21.4.5 Mycoplasma Pneumoniae

Mycoplasma pneumoniae is a small bacterium that is a common cause of CAP, particularly in young adults, accounting for up to one-third of infections. Patients with *Mycoplasma* pneumonia present similarly to patients with other causes of CAP, although the clinical manifestations are often milder. The mortality rate is quite low [4,119]. Typical CT findings of *Mycoplasma* pneumonia include patchy lobar or lobular consolidation and ground-glass opacity, centrilobular nodules, tree-in-bud opacities, and bronchial wall thickening (Figure 21.29) [40,120].

21.4.6 Nocardia

Nocardia is a filamentous gram positive, weakly acid fast aerobic genus of bacteria that resides in soil throughout the world [121]. Most human nocardial infections are related to *Nocardia asteroids* complex, occurring primarily in immunocompromised patients, particularly in the settings of AIDS and transplants [121,122].

The CT findings of nocardiosis are similar to many other infections and include lung consolidation, nodules and masses (Figure 21.30), and pleural effusion or empyema [123–125]. Multifocal lung consolidation is reported to be the most common findings in a small series of patients [124]. Areas of low attenuation within consolidation suggest abscess formation. Cavitation may develop in one-third of patients (Figure 21.31). Multiple nodules,

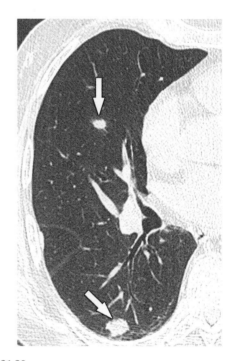

FIGURE 21.30
73-year-old male renal transplant recipient with nocardiosis. HRCT image shows two large nodules (arrows) in the right lung.

masses, or both may also be apparent with or without central low attenuation or cavitation. Endobronchial spread of infection results in small centrilobular nodules and tree-in-bud opacities. Hematogenous dissemination can cause a miliary pattern of disease [125]. In contrast to other infections, lymphadenopathy is uncommon. Direct pleural and chest wall extension [124] as well as spread to extrathoracic sites, such as the central nervous system and skin, can occur [126].

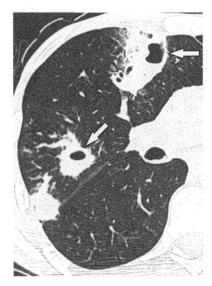

FIGURE 21.31
42-year-old man with HIV infection and nocardiosis. HRCT image demonstrates large nodular and mass like foci of consolidation, some of which have central cavitation (arrows) and fluid levels.

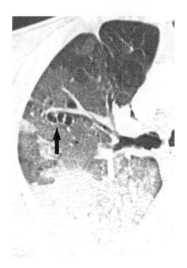

FIGURE 21.32
Patient with methicillin-resistant *Staphylococcal pneumoniae* pneumonia and pneumatoceles. Unenhanced CT image shows dense consolidation and extensive ground-glass opacity. Several pneumatoceles (arrow) have formed in the right upper lobe.

21.5 Complications of Pulmonary Infection

A variety of thoracic complications can develop as a direct result of lower respiratory tract infections, ranging from abscess formation to empyema. CT is frequently used to identify suspected complications, particularly in patients who do not respond to therapy.

21.5.1 Pneumatoceles

Pneumatoceles are thin-walled gas-filled spaces occurring in areas of ground-glass opacity or lung consolidation [127]. Drainage of a focal area of necrotic lung and the subsequent check-valve obstruction of the associate airway are thought to lead to pneumatocele formation [128]. Pneumatoceles are most commonly associated with *S. aureus* in children and PJP in immunocompromised adults [113], but can occur with many other infections.

Pneumatoceles manifest on CT in patients with pneumonia as thin-walled, rounded gas-filled foci surrounded by consolidation or ground-glass opacity (Figure 21.32). Emphysematous bullae within an area of pneumonia can mimic pneumatoceles. However, while emphysematous bullae expand slowly over time and are permanent, pneumatoceles can enlarge over days to weeks and generally resolve slowly as pneumonia clears. Pneumatocele rupture can lead to pneumothorax, particularly in PJP.

21.5.2 Lung Abscess

An inflammatory pulmonary mass containing central liquefaction necrosis defines a lung abscess [127].

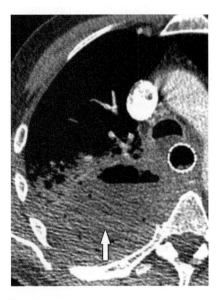

FIGURE 21.33
62-year-old man with esophageal carcinoma and a polymicrobial lung abscess. Contrast-enhanced CT image shows a large low attenuation collection (arrow) in the right lung with a fluid level and surrounding consolidation.

Anaerobic bacteria (Figure 21.33), particularly *Fusobacterium nucleatum* and *Bacteroides* species, are responsible for the majority of lung abscesses, but *S. aureus*, *Pseudomonas aeruginosa* (Figure 21.34), and *K. pneumoniae* are also associated with abscess formation [129]. On CT, lung abscesses may be single or multiple spherical masses with central low attenuation. Cavitation occurs when abscesses erode into an adjacent airway. Cavity walls tend to be irregular and thick, but smooth, and usually enhance following intravenous contrast material administration. The posterior

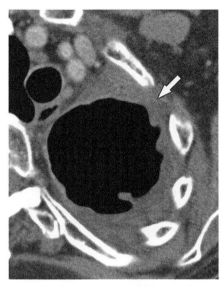

FIGURE 21.34
62-year-old woman with a chronic lung abscess from *Pseudomonas aeruginosa*. Contrast-enhanced CT image shows a thick walled cavity (arrow) in the left upper lobe.

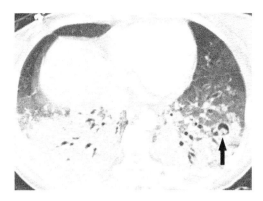

FIGURE 21.35
23-year-old woman with methicillin-resistant *Staphylococcal pneumoniae* pneumonia and pulmonary gangrene. Unenhanced CT image shows a small cavity in the left lower lobe containing a pulmonary sequestrum (arrow). The patient died from severe necrotizing pneumonia.

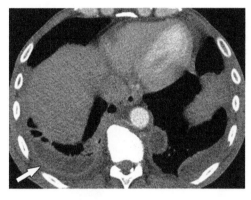

FIGURE 21.36
59-year-old man with bilateral empyema. Contrast-enhanced CT shows bilateral complex pleural fluid collections. Note enhancement of the parietal pleura (arrow) on the right.

segments of the upper lobes and the superior segments of the lower lobes are most commonly involved [130].

21.5.3 Necrotizing Pneumonia and Pulmonary Gangrene

Necrotizing pneumonia is usually the sequela of severe bacterial pneumonia or tuberculosis [131,132]. *S. aureus*, *K. pneumoniae*, and *P. aeruginosa* are most commonly implicated and are associated with higher mortality rates [133]. In particular, Panton-Valentine leukocidin (PVL) positive community-acquired methicillin-resistant *S. aureus* (MRSA) is associated with a rapidly progressive necrotizing pneumonia in otherwise healthy individuals [134].

Necrotizing pneumonia is characterized on CT by the development of cavitation within areas of lung consolidation. On contrast-enhanced CT, consolidation is often heterogeneous with areas of decreased attenuation and attenuated vessels, reflecting decreased perfusion [131].

Direct cytotoxic effects of bacterial toxins, thrombosis of vessels in an area of necrotizing pneumonia, or both can lead to pulmonary gangrene, a rare and potentially life-threatening complication of pneumonia [135]. CT shows sloughed lung within a cavity, sometimes with an air-crescent sign (Figure 21.35) [135,136].

21.5.4 Pleural Effusion and Empyema

Parapneumonic effusion develops in 20%–60% of patients with bacterial pneumonia and is less common with fungal and viral infections [137,138]. Most effusions resolve as the adjacent pneumonia clears with treatment. However, some patients develop empyema, a frank infection of the pleural space. Distinguishing loculated pleural fluid from consolidated lung or lung abscess on chest radiography can be difficult or impossible in some cases. Thus, CT can be valuable in further evaluation [130].

Features of empyema on CT include a round or lenticular-shaped pleural collection forming an obtuse angle with the chest wall. A uniformly enhancing wall and separation of the pleural layers ("split pleura sign") are often visible. Compressive atelectasis of the adjacent lung may be present [139,140]. Haziness or edema of the adjacent extrapleural fat is also highly suggestive of exudative pleural effusion or empyema [141]. Hypertrophy of the adjacent pleural fat usually suggests a more long-standing inflammatory process in the pleura and is most often associated with tuberculous empyema [142]. Finally, the presence of pleural gas in the absence of pleural instrumentation is highly suggestive of empyema (Figures 21.36 through 21.38).

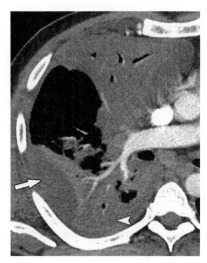

FIGURE 21.37
45-year-old man with pneumococcal pneumonia and empyema. Contrast-enhanced CT image demonstrates dense consolidation in the right lung. A small area of subtle decreased attenuation (arrowhead) is present, suggesting developing necrosis. A small biconvex pleural collection (arrow) displacing lung is present and proved to be an empyema.

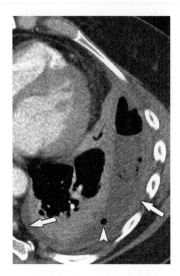

FIGURE 21.38
55-year-old woman with empyema. Contrast-enhanced CT image shows a complex left pleural collection containing small pockets of gas (arrowhead) and with mild parietal pleural enhancement (arrows).

21.5.5 Bronchopleural Fistula

Bronchopleural fistula occurs when the inflamed or necrotic lung or airway ruptures into the pleural space. Inflammatory exudates and organisms can spill into the pleural space and lead to empyema formation. The characteristic finding of a bronchopleural fistula on CT is the presence of a visible direct communication between an airway or lung parenchyma and the adjacent pleural space (Figure 21.39). The development of gas in the pleural space, particularly adjacent to an area of pneumonia, in the absence of instrumentation, should also raise the specter

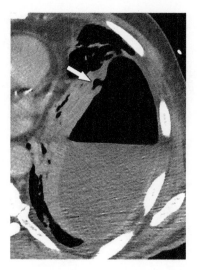

FIGURE 21.39
57-year-old man with polymicrobial empyema resulting from aspiration pneumonia and subsequent bronchopleural fistula. Contrast-enhanced CT image shows a biconvex complex left pleural collection. A small communication (arrow) exists between the pleural cavity and the adjacent lung, indicative of a bronchopleural fistula.

of bronchopleural fistula [143,144]. Multiplanar reformations may help in identifying bronchopleural fistulas.

21.6 Nonresolving Pneumonia

Nonresolving pneumonia defines the clinical scenario in which a patient with pneumonia does not achieve adequate therapeutic response despite appropriate antibiotic administration [17]. Failure of radiographic abnormalities to decrease by at least 50% at two weeks or to resolve by four weeks has been suggested to indicate nonresolving or slowly resolving pneumonia [145].

Causes of nonresolving pneumonia include antibiotic resistance or incorrect coverage (e.g., treating endemic fungal pneumonia [Figure 21.40] with antibacterial agents), empyema, and underlying obstructing lesions, such as bronchial neoplasm. However, the most common reason that patients undergo workup for nonresolving pneumonia is the failure to understand the normal time course of resolution of abnormalities on imaging [146]. Older patients and patients with more extensive infections may require months for radiographic abnormalities to clear. Furthermore, pulmonary infection may result in scar, bronchiectasis, and pleural thickening that remain on follow-up imaging. For example, patients with pneumococcal pneumonia and bacteremia may require three to five months for radiographic clearing, and patients with *Legionella* may require up to six months for radiographic clearing. Signs and symptoms may resolve slowly as well, but radiographic clearance

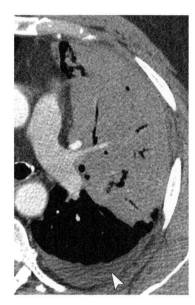

FIGURE 21.40
53-year-old man with nonresolving lobar pneumonia subsequently determined to represent North American blastomycosis. Contrast-enhanced CT image shows dense left upper lobe consolidation and a small pleural effusion (arrowhead).

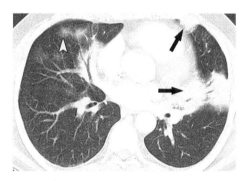

FIGURE 21.41
54-year-old man with nonresolving bronchopneumonia subsequently shown to be primary pulmonary lymphoma. Contrast-enhanced CT image shows multiple foci of peribronchial consolidation (arrows) and ground-glass opacity (arrowhead).

tends to lag behind. In one study of 2287 patients with pneumonia, 76% of outpatients had persistent symptoms after 30 days and 86.1% of hospitalized patients had persistent symptoms after 30 days [147].

Noninfectious causes of a febrile lower respiratory tract illness can mimic pneumonia and include granulomatosis with polyangiitis, eosinophilic pneumonia, organizing pneumonia, and other tissue reactions [148]. Neoplasm, in particular, should be suspected when findings of obstruction such as lobar atelectasis or bronchial occlusion are evident. Pulmonary lymphoma (Figure 21.41) and invasive mucinous adenocarcinoma (formerly classified as a subtype of bronchioloalveolar carcinoma) (Figure 21.42) can also result in chronic and progressive lung consolidation.

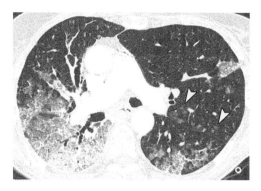

FIGURE 21.42
74-year-old man with nonresolving pneumonia shown to represent invasive mucinous adenocarcinoma of the lung. HRCT image shows patchy ground-glass opacity with some foci of septal thickening and consolidation. Small ground-glass attenuation nodules (arrowheads) are scattered throughout.

21.7 Conclusion

While chest radiography usually suffices for establishing the diagnosis of pneumonia and monitoring response to therapy, chest CT is a useful adjunct test in patients with atypical presentations, immune compromise, and suspected complications of pulmonary infection. Although the radiographic and CT patterns of infection, in conjunction with the clinical presentation of the patient, may narrow the potential list of causative organisms, in reality, imaging continues to perform poorly in precisely determining the etiology of pneumonia. Failure to recognize these limitations may result in an inaccurate diagnosis and inappropriate failure to further evaluate a patient with suspected pneumonia.

References

1. File TM, Jr., Marrie TJ. Burden of community-acquired pneumonia in North American adults. *Postgraduate Medicine*. 2010;122(2):130–41.
2. Centers for Disease Control and Prevention. Fast Stas. Deaths and mortality. 2010 [updated 10/27/2010; cited 2012 1/16/2012]; Available from: http://www.cdc.gov /nchs/fastats/pneumonia.htm.
3. Attridge RT, Frei CR. Health care-associated pneumonia: an evidence-based review. *The American Journal of Medicine*. 2011;124(8):689–97.
4. Bochud PY, Moser F, Erard P, Verdon F, Studer JP, Villard G et al. Community-acquired pneumonia. A prospective outpatient study. *Medicine*. 2001;80(2):75–87.
5. Kaplan V, Angus DC, Griffin MF, Clermont G, Scott Watson R, Linde-Zwirble WT. Hospitalized community-acquired pneumonia in the elderly: age- and sex-related

patterns of care and outcome in the United States. *American Journal of Respiratory and Critical Care Medicine.* 2002;165(6):766–72.

6. Macfarlane J. An overview of community acquired pneumonia with lessons learned from the British Thoracic Society study. *Seminars in Respiratory Infections.* 1994;9(3):153–65.

7. Mandell LA. Community-acquired pneumonia. Etiology, epidemiology, and treatment. *Chest.* 1995;108(2 Suppl): 35S–42S.

8. Marston BJ, Plouffe JF, File TM, Jr., Hackman BA, Salstrom SJ, Lipman HB et al. Incidence of community-acquired pneumonia requiring hospitalization. Results of a population-based active surveillance study in Ohio. The community-based pneumonia incidence study group. *Archives of Internal Medicine.* 1997;157(15):1709–18.

9. Fine MJ, Auble TE, Yealy DM, Hanusa BH, Weissfeld LA, Singer DE et al. A prediction rule to identify low-risk patients with community-acquired pneumonia. *The New England Journal of Medicine.* 1997;336(4):243–50.

10. Fine MJ, Smith MA, Carson CA, Mutha SS, Sankey SS, Weissfeld LA et al. Prognosis and outcomes of patients with community-acquired pneumonia. A meta-analysis. *JAMA: The Journal of the American Medical Association.* 1996;275(2):134–41.

11. Leeper KV, Jr. Severe community-acquired pneumonia. *Seminars in Respiratory Infections.* 1996;11(2):96–108.

12. Craven DE, Steger KA. Nosocomial pneumonia in mechanically ventilated adult patients: epidemiology and prevention in 1996. *Seminars in Respiratory Infections.* 1996;11(1):32–53.

13. Baker AM, Meredith JW, Haponik EF. Pneumonia in intubated trauma patients. Microbiology and outcomes. *American Journal of Respiratory and Critical Care Medicine.* 1996;153(1):343–9.

14. Craven DE. Epidemiology of ventilator-associated pneumonia. *Chest.* 2000;117(4 Suppl 2):186S–7S.

15. Craven DE, De Rosa FG, Thornton D. Nosocomial pneumonia: emerging concepts in diagnosis, management, and prophylaxis. *Current Opinion in Critical Care.* 2002;8(5):421–9.

16. Primack SL, Muller NL. High-resolution computed tomography in acute diffuse lung disease in the immunocompromised patient. *Radiologic Clinics of North America.* 1994;32(4):731–44.

17. Kuru T, Lynch JP, 3rd. Nonresolving or slowly resolving pneumonia. *Clinics in Chest Medicine.* 1999;20(3):623–51.

18. Brown MJ, Miller RR, Muller NL. Acute lung disease in the immunocompromised host: CT and pathologic examination findings. *Radiology.* 1994;190(1):247–54.

19. Tomiyama N, Muller NL, Johkoh T, Honda O, Mihara N, Kozuka T et al. Acute parenchymal lung disease in immunocompetent patients: diagnostic accuracy of high-resolution CT. *AJR American Journal of Roentgenology.* 2000;174(6):1745–50.

20. Hospital-acquired pneumonia in adults: diagnosis, assessment of severity, initial antimicrobial therapy, and preventive strategies. A consensus statement, American Thoracic Society, November 1995. *American Journal of Respiratory and Critical Care Medicine.* 1996;153(5):1711–25.

21. Torres A. The new American Thoracic Society/Infectious Disease Society of North America guidelines for the management of hospital-acquired, ventilator-associated and healthcare-associated pneumonia: a current view and new complementary information. *Current Opinion in Critical Care.* 2006;12(5):444–5.

22. Boersma WG, Daniels JM, Lowenberg A, Boeve WJ, van de Jagt EJ. Reliability of radiographic findings and the relation to etiologic agents in community-acquired pneumonia. *Respiratory Medicine.* 2006;100(5):926–32.

23. Basi SK, Marrie TJ, Huang JQ, Majumdar SR. Patients admitted to hospital with suspected pneumonia and normal chest radiographs: epidemiology, microbiology, and outcomes. *The American Journal of Medicine.* 2004;117(5):305–11.

24. Hopstaken RM, Witbraad T, van Engelshoven JM, Dinant GJ. Inter-observer variation in the interpretation of chest radiographs for pneumonia in community-acquired lower respiratory tract infections. *Clinical Radiology.* 2004;59(8):743–52.

25. Woodhead M, Blasi F, Ewig S, Huchon G, Ieven M, Ortqvist A et al. Guidelines for the management of adult lower respiratory tract infections. *The European Respiratory Journal: Official Journal of the European Society for Clinical Respiratory Physiology.* 2005;26(6):1138–80.

26. Valor RR, Polnitsky CA, Tanis DJ, Sherter CB. Bacterial tracheitis with upper airway obstruction in a patient with the acquired immunodeficiency syndrome. *The American Review of Respiratory Disease.* 1992;146(6):1598–9.

27. Naidich DP, Webb WR, Grenier PA, Harkin TJ, Gefter WB. *Imaging of the Airways.* Philadelphia: Lippincott Williams & Wilkins; 2005.

28. Kim Y, Lee KS, Yoon JH, Chung MP, Kim H, Kwon OJ et al. Tuberculosis of the trachea and main bronchi: CT findings in 17 patients. *AJR American Journal of Roentgenology.* 1997;168(4):1051–6.

29. Moon WK, Im JG, Yeon KM, Han MC. Tuberculosis of the central airways: CT findings of active and fibrotic disease. *AJR American Journal of Roentgenology.* 1997;169(3):649–53.

30. Yigla M, Ben-Izhak O, Oren I, Hashman N, Lejbkowicz F. Laryngotracheobronchial involvement in a patient with nonendemic rhinoscleroma. *Chest.* 2000;117(6):1795–8.

31. Sedano HO, Carlos R, Koutlas IG. Respiratory scleroma: a clinicopathologic and ultrastructural study. *Oral Surgery, Oral Medicine, Oral Pathology, Oral Radiology, and Endodontics.* 1996;81(6):665–71.

32. Amoils CP, Shindo ML. Laryngotracheal manifestations of rhinoscleroma. *The Annals of Otology, Rhinology, and Laryngology.* 1996;105(5):336–40.

33. Hart CA, Rao SK. Rhinoscleroma. *Journal of Medical Microbiology.* 2000;49(5):395–6.

34. Abou-Seif SG, Baky FA, el-Ebrashy F, Gaafar HA. Scleroma of the upper respiratory passages: A CT study. *The Journal of Laryngology and Otology.* 1991;105(3):198–202.

35. Prince JS, Duhamel DR, Levin DL, Harrell JH, Friedman PJ. Nonneoplastic lesions of the tracheobronchial wall: radiologic findings with bronchoscopic correlation. *Radiographics: A Review Publication of the Radiological Society of North America, Inc.* 2002;22 Spec No:S215–30.

36. Fawaz S, Tiba M, Salman M, Othman H. Clinical, radiological and pathological study of 88 cases of typical and complicated scleroma. *The Clinical Respiratory Journal.* 2011;5(2):112–21.

37. Loosli CG. Pathogenesis and pathology of lobar pneumonia. *Lancet.* 1940;60:49–54.

38. Katz DS, Leung AN. Radiology of pneumonia. *Clinics in Chest Medicine.* 1999;20(3):549–62.

39. Reittner P, Ward S, Heyneman L, Johkoh T, Muller NL. Pneumonia: high-resolution CT findings in 114 patients. *European Radiology.* 2003;13(3):515–21.

40. Tanaka N, Matsumoto T, Kuramitsu T, Nakaki H, Ito K, Uchisako H et al. High resolution CT findings in community-acquired pneumonia. *Journal of Computer Assisted Tomography.* 1996;20(4):600–8.

41. Eggli KD, Newman B. Nodules, masses, and pseudomasses in the pediatric lung. *Radiologic Clinics of North America.* 1993;31(3):651–66.

42. Hershey CO, Panaro V. Round pneumonia in adults. *Archives of Internal Medicine.* 1988;148(5):1155–7.

43. Anton E. A frequent error in etiology of round pneumonia. *Chest.* 2004;125(4):1592–3.

44. Dye C, Scheele S, Dolin P, Pathania V, Raviglione MC. Consensus statement. Global burden of tuberculosis: estimated incidence, prevalence, and mortality by country. WHO Global Surveillance and Monitoring Project. *JAMA: The Journal of the American Medical Association.* 1999;282(7):677–86.

45. Verver S, Warren RM, Beyers N, Richardson M, van der Spuy GD, Borgdorff MW et al. Rate of reinfection tuberculosis after successful treatment is higher than rate of new tuberculosis. *American Journal of Respiratory and Critical Care Medicine.* 2005;171(12):1430–5.

46. Pastores SM, Naidich DP, Aranda CP, McGuinnes G, Rom WN. Intrathoracic adenopathy associated with pulmonary tuberculosis in patients with human immunodeficiency virus infection. *Chest.* 1993;103(5):1433–7.

47. Im JG, Itoh H, Shim YS, Lee JH, Ahn J, Han MC et al. Pulmonary tuberculosis: CT findings—early active disease and sequential change with antituberculous therapy. *Radiology.* 1993;186(3):653–60.

48. Hatipoglu ON, Osma E, Manisali M, Ucan ES, Balci P, Akkoclu A et al. High resolution computed tomographic findings in pulmonary tuberculosis. *Thorax.* 1996;51(4):397–402.

49. Poey C, Verhaegen F, Giron J, Lavayssiere J, Fajadet P, Duparc B. High resolution chest CT in tuberculosis: evolutive patterns and signs of activity. *Journal of Computer Assisted Tomography.* 1997;21(4):601–7.

50. Marais BJ, Gie RP, Schaaf HS, Hesseling AC, Obihara CC, Starke JJ et al. The natural history of childhood intra-thoracic tuberculosis: a critical review of literature from the pre-chemotherapy era. *The International Journal of Tuberculosis and Lung Disease: The Official Journal of the International Union against Tuberculosis and Lung Disease.* 2004;8(4):392–402.

51. Kwong JS, Carignan S, Kang EY, Muller NL, FitzGerald JM. Miliary tuberculosis. Diagnostic accuracy of chest radiography. *Chest.* 1996;110(2):339–42.

52. Leung AN. Pulmonary tuberculosis: The essentials. *Radiology.* 1999;210(2):307–22.

53. Lee KS, Song KS, Lim TH, Kim PN, Kim IY, Lee BH. Adult-onset pulmonary tuberculosis: findings on chest radiographs and CT scans. *AJR American Journal of Roentgenology.* 1993;160(4):753–8.

54. Woodring JH, Vandiviere HM, Fried AM, Dillon ML, Williams TD, Melvin IG. Update: the radiographic features of pulmonary tuberculosis. *AJR American Journal of Roentgenology.* 1986;146(3):497–506.

55. Krysl J, Korzeniewska-Kosela M, Muller NL, FitzGerald JM. Radiologic features of pulmonary tuberculosis: an assessment of 188 cases. *Canadian Association of Radiologists Journal = Journal l'Association Canadienne Des Radiologistes.* 1994;45(2):101–7.

56. Codecasa LR, Besozzi G, De Cristofaro L, Miradoli A, Sabolla L, Tagliaferri B. Epidemiological and clinical patterns of intrathoracic lymph node tuberculosis in 60 human immunodeficiency virus-negative adult patients. *Monaldi archives for chest disease = Archivio Monaldi per le malattie del torace.* 1998;53(3):277–80.

57. Lee KS, Im JG. CT in adults with tuberculosis of the chest: characteristic findings and role in management. *AJR American Journal of Roentgenology.* 1995;164(6):1361–7.

58. Im JG, Song KS, Kang HS, Park JH, Yeon KM, Han MC et al. Mediastinal tuberculous lymphadenitis: CT manifestations. *Radiology.* 1987;164(1):115–9.

59. Lee JH, Park SS, Lee DH, Shin DH, Yang SC, Yoo BM. Endobronchial tuberculosis. Clinical and bronchoscopic features in 121 cases. *Chest.* 1992;102(4):990–4.

60. Choe KO, Jeong HJ, Sohn HY. Tuberculous bronchial stenosis: CT findings in 28 cases. *AJR American Journal of Roentgenology.* 1990;155(5):971–6.

61. Park MJ, Woo IS, Son JW, Lee SJ, Kim DG, Mo EK et al. Endobronchial tuberculosis with expectoration of tracheal cartilages. *The European Respiratory Journal: Official Journal of the European Society for Clinical Respiratory Physiology.* 2000;15(4):800–2.

62. Taiwo B, Glassroth J. Nontuberculous mycobacterial lung diseases. *Infectious Disease Clinics of North America.* 2010;24(3):769–89.

63. Falkinham JO, 3rd. Nontuberculous mycobacteria in the environment. *Clinics in Chest Medicine.* 2002;23(3):529–51.

64. Bodle EE, Cunningham JA, Della-Latta P, Schluger NW, Saiman L. Epidemiology of nontuberculous mycobacteria in patients without HIV infection, New York City. *Emerging Infectious Diseases.* 2008;14(3):390–6.

65. Koh WJ, Kwon OJ, Jeon K, Kim TS, Lee KS, Park YK et al. Clinical significance of nontuberculous mycobacteria isolated from respiratory specimens in Korea. *Chest.* 2006;129(2):341–8.

66. Corbett EL, Hay M, Churchyard GJ, Herselman P, Clayton T, Williams BG et al. Mycobacterium kansasii and M. scrofulaceum isolates from HIV-negative South African gold miners: incidence, clinical significance and radiology. *The International Journal of Tuberculosis and Lung Disease: The Official Journal of the International Union against Tuberculosis and Lung Disease.* 1999;3(6):501–7.

67. Christensen EE, Dietz GW, Ahn CH, Chapman JS, Murry RC, Anderson J et al. Pulmonary manifestations of Mycobacterium intracellularis. *AJR American Journal of Roentgenology*. 1979;133(1):59–66.

68. Woodring JH, Vandiviere HM, Melvin IG, Dillon ML. Roentgenographic features of pulmonary disease caused by atypical mycobacteria. *Southern Medical Journal*. 1987;80(12):1488–97.

69. Tanaka D, Niwatsukino H, Oyama T, Nakajo M. Progressing features of atypical mycobacterial infection in the lung on conventional and high resolution CT (HRCT) images. *Radiation Medicine*. 2001;19(5):237–45.

70. Huang JH, Kao PN, Adi V, Ruoss SJ. Mycobacterium avium-intracellulare pulmonary infection in HIV-negative patients without preexisting lung disease: diagnostic and management limitations. *Chest*. 1999;115(4):1033–40.

71. Tanaka E, Amitani R, Niimi A, Suzuki K, Murayama T, Kuze F. Yield of computed tomography and bronchoscopy for the diagnosis of Mycobacterium avium complex pulmonary disease. *American Journal of Respiratory and Critical Care Medicine*. 1997;155(6):2041–6.

72. Hartman TE, Swensen SJ, Williams DE. Mycobacterium avium-intracellulare complex: evaluation with CT. *Radiology*. 1993;187(1):23–6.

73. Swensen SJ, Hartman TE, Williams DE. Computed tomographic diagnosis of Mycobacterium avium-intracellulare complex in patients with bronchiectasis. *Chest*. 1994;105(1):49–52.

74. Kubo K, Yamazaki Y, Masubuchi T, Takamizawa A, Yamamoto H, Koizumi T et al. Pulmonary infection with Mycobacterium avium-intracellulare leads to air trapping distal to the small airways. *American Journal of Respiratory and Critical Care Medicine*. 1998;158(3):979–84.

75. Reich JM, Johnson RE. Mycobacterium avium complex pulmonary disease. Incidence, presentation, and response to therapy in a community setting. *The American Review of Respiratory Disease*. 1991;143(6):1381–5.

76. Albelda SM, Kern JA, Marinelli DL, Miller WT. Expanding spectrum of pulmonary disease caused by nontuberculous mycobacteria. *Radiology*. 1985;157(2):289–96.

77. Khoor A, Leslie KO, Tazelaar HD, Helmers RA, Colby TV. Diffuse pulmonary disease caused by nontuberculous mycobacteria in immunocompetent people (hot tub lung). *American Journal of Clinical Pathology*. 2001;115(5):755–62.

78. Respiratory illness in workers exposed to metalworking fluid contaminated with nontuberculous mycobacteria— Ohio, 2001. *MMWR Morbidity and Mortality Weekly Report*. 2002;51(16):349–52.

79. Pham RV, Vydareny KH, Gal AA. High-resolution computed tomography appearance of pulmonary Mycobacterium avium complex infection after exposure to hot tub: case of hot-tub lung. *Journal of Thoracic Imaging*. 2003;18(1):48–52.

80. Chalermskulrat W, Gilbey JG, Donohue JF. Nontuberculous mycobacteria in women, young and old. *Clinics in Chest Medicine*. 2002;23(3):675–86.

81. Grammer LC, Greenberger PA, Patterson R. Allergic bronchopulmonary aspergillosis in asthmatic patients presenting with allergic rhinitis. *International Archives of Allergy and Applied Immunology*. 1986;79(3):246–8.

82. Basich JE, Graves TS, Baz MN, Scanlon G, Hoffmann RG, Patterson R et al. Allergic bronchopulmonary aspergillosis in corticosteroid-dependent asthmatics. *The Journal of Allergy and Clinical Immunology*. 1981;68(2):98–102.

83. Laufer P, Fink JN, Bruns WT, Unger GF, Kalbfleisch JH, Greenberger PA et al. Allergic bronchopulmonary aspergillosis in cystic fibrosis. *The Journal of Allergy and Clinical Immunology*. 1984;73(1 Pt 1):44–8.

84. Skov M, Koch C, Reimert CM, Poulsen LK. Diagnosis of allergic bronchopulmonary aspergillosis (ABPA) in cystic fibrosis. *Allergy*. 2000;55(1):50–8.

85. Bosken CH, Myers JL, Greenberger PA, Katzenstein AL. Pathologic features of allergic bronchopulmonary aspergillosis. *The American Journal of Surgical Pathology*. 1988;12(3):216–22.

86. Panchal N, Pant C, Bhagat R, Shah A. Central bronchiectasis in allergic bronchopulmonary aspergillosis: comparative evaluation of computed tomography of the thorax with bronchography. *The European Respiratory Journal: Official Journal of the European Society for Clinical Respiratory Physiology*. 1994;7(7):1290–3.

87. Panchal N, Bhagat R, Pant C, Shah A. Allergic bronchopulmonary aspergillosis: the spectrum of computed tomography appearances. *Respiratory Medicine*. 1997;91(4):213–9.

88. Ward S, Heyneman L, Lee MJ, Leung AN, Hansell DM, Muller NL. Accuracy of CT in the diagnosis of allergic bronchopulmonary aspergillosis in asthmatic patients. *AJR American Journal of Roentgenology*. 1999;173(4):937–42.

89. Reiff DB, Wells AU, Carr DH, Cole PJ, Hansell DM. CT findings in bronchiectasis: limited value in distinguishing between idiopathic and specific types. *AJR American Journal of Roentgenology*. 1995;165(2):261–7.

90. Goyal R, White CS, Templeton PA, Britt EJ, Rubin LJ. High attenuation mucous plugs in allergic bronchopulmonary aspergillosis: CT appearance. *Journal of Computer Assisted Tomography*. 1992;16(4):649–50.

91. Logan PM, Muller NL. High-attenuation mucous plugging in allergic bronchopulmonary aspergillosis. *Canadian Association of Radiologists journal = Journal l'Association Canadienne Des Radiologistes*. 1996;47(5):374–7.

92. Neeld DA, Goodman LR, Gurney JW, Greenberger PA, Fink JN. Computerized tomography in the evaluation of allergic bronchopulmonary aspergillosis. *The American Review of Respiratory Disease*. 1990;142(5):1200–5.

93. Aspergilloma and residual tuberculous cavities—the results of a resurvey. *Tubercle*. 1970;51(3):227–45.

94. Wollschlager C, Khan F. Aspergillomas complicating sarcoidosis. A prospective study in 100 patients. *Chest*. 1984;86(4):585–8.

95. Jewkes J, Kay PH, Paneth M, Citron KM. Pulmonary aspergilloma: analysis of prognosis in relation to haemoptysis and survey of treatment. *Thorax*. 1983;38(8):572–8.

96. Buckingham SJ, Hansell DM. Aspergillus in the lung: diverse and coincident forms. *European Radiology*. 2003;13(8):1786–800.

97. Roberts CM, Citron KM, Strickland B. Intrathoracic aspergilloma: role of CT in diagnosis and treatment. *Radiology*. 1987;165(1):123–8.

98. Libshitz HI, Atkinson GW, Israel HL. Pleural thickening as a manifestation of aspergillus superinfection. *The American Journal of Roentgenology, Radium Therapy, and Nuclear Medicine.* 1974;120(4):883–6.

99. Franquet T, Muller NL, Gimenez A, Guembe P, de La Torre J, Bague S. Spectrum of pulmonary aspergillosis: histologic, clinical, and radiologic findings. *Radiographics: A Review Publication of the Radiological Society of North America, Inc.* 2001;21(4):825–37.

100. Hruban RH, Meziane MA, Zerhouni EA, Wheeler PS, Dumler JS, Hutchins GM. Radiologic-pathologic correlation of the CT halo sign in invasive pulmonary aspergillosis. *Journal of Computer Assisted Tomography.* 1987;11(3):534–6.

101. Kuhlman JE, Fishman EK, Siegelman SS. Invasive pulmonary aspergillosis in acute leukemia: characteristic findings on CT, the CT halo sign, and the role of CT in early diagnosis. *Radiology.* 1985;157(3):611–4.

102. Kuhlman JE, Fishman EK, Burch PA, Karp JE, Zerhouni EA, Siegelman SS. Invasive pulmonary aspergillosis in acute leukemia. The contribution of CT to early diagnosis and aggressive management. *Chest.* 1987;92(1):95–9.

103. Orr DP, Myerowitz RL, Dubois PJ. Patho-radiologic correlation of invasive pulmonary aspergillosis in the compromised host. *Cancer.* 1978;41(5):2028–39.

104. Brown MJ, Worthy SA, Flint JD, Muller NL. Invasive aspergillosis in the immunocompromised host: utility of computed tomography and bronchoalveolar lavage. *Clinical Radiology.* 1998;53(4):255–7.

105. Logan PM, Primack SL, Miller RR, Muller NL. Invasive aspergillosis of the airways: radiographic, CT, and pathologic findings. *Radiology.* 1994;193(2):383–8.

106. Franquet T, Serrano F, Gimenez A, Rodriguez-Arias JM, Puzo C. Necrotizing Aspergillosis of large airways: CT findings in eight patients. *Journal of Computer Assisted Tomography.* 2002;26(3):342–5.

107. Franquet T, Muller NL, Oikonomou A, Flint JD. Aspergillus infection of the airways: computed tomography and pathologic findings. *Journal of Computer Assisted Tomography.* 2004;28(1):10–6.

108. Franquet T, Muller NL, Gimenez A, Domingo P, Plaza V, Bordes R. Semiinvasive pulmonary aspergillosis in chronic obstructive pulmonary disease: radiologic and pathologic findings in nine patients. *AJR American Journal of Roentgenology.* 2000;174(1):51–6.

109. Saraceno JL, Phelps DT, Ferro TJ, Futerfas R, Schwartz DB. Chronic necrotizing pulmonary aspergillosis: approach to management. *Chest.* 1997;112(2):541–8.

110. Hafeez I, Muers MF, Murphy SA, Evans EG, Barton RC, McWhinney P. Non-tuberculous mycobacterial lung infection complicated by chronic necrotising pulmonary aspergillosis. *Thorax.* 2000;55(8):717–9.

111. Catherinot E, Lanternier F, Bougnoux ME, Lecuit M, Couderc LJ, Lortholary O. Pneumocystis jirovecii Pneumonia. *Infectious Disease Clinics of North America.* 2010;24(1):107–38.

112. Fujii T, Nakamura T, Iwamoto A. Pneumocystis pneumonia in patients with HIV infection: clinical manifestations, laboratory findings, and radiological features. *Journal of Infection and Chemotherapy.* 2007;13(1):1–7.

113. Boiselle PM, Crans CA, Jr., Kaplan MA. The changing face of Pneumocystis carinii pneumonia in AIDS patients. *AJR American Journal of Roentgenology.* 1999;172(5):1301–9.

114. Kuhlman JE, Kavuru M, Fishman EK, Siegelman SS. Pneumocystis carinii pneumonia: spectrum of parenchymal CT findings. *Radiology.* 1990;175(3):711–4.

115. Hardak E, Brook O, Yigla M. Radiological features of Pneumocystis jirovecii Pneumonia in immunocompromised patients with and without AIDS. *Lung.* 2010;188(2):159–63.

116. Marchiori E, Muller NL, Soares Souza A, Jr., Escuissato DL, Gasparetto EL, Franquet T. Pulmonary disease in patients with AIDS: high-resolution CT and pathologic findings. *AJR American Journal of Roentgenology.* 2005;184(3):757–64.

117. Tasaka S, Tokuda H, Sakai F, Fujii T, Tateda K, Johkoh T et al. Comparison of clinical and radiological features of pneumocystis pneumonia between malignancy cases and acquired immunodeficiency syndrome cases: a multicenter study. *Internal Medicine.* 2010;49(4):273–81.

118. Mayaud C, Parrot A, Cadranel J. Pyogenic bacterial lower respiratory tract infection in human immunodeficiency virus-infected patients. *The European Respiratory Journal. Supplement.* 2002;36:28s–39s.

119. Marrie TJ. Mycoplasma pneumoniae pneumonia requiring hospitalization, with emphasis on infection in the elderly. *Archives of Internal Medicine.* 1993;153(4):488–94.

120. John SD, Ramanathan J, Swischuk LE. Spectrum of clinical and radiographic findings in pediatric mycoplasma pneumonia. *Radiographics: A Review Publication of the Radiological Society of North America, Inc.* 2001;21(1):121–31.

121. McNeil MM, Brown JM. The medically important aerobic actinomycetes: epidemiology and microbiology. *Clinical Microbiology Reviews.* 1994;7(3):357–417.

122. Brown-Elliott BA, Brown JM, Conville PS, Wallace RJ, Jr. Clinical and laboratory features of the Nocardia spp. based on current molecular taxonomy. *Clinical Microbiology Reviews.* 2006;19(2):259–82.

123. Buckley JA, Padhani AR, Kuhlman JE. CT features of pulmonary nocardiosis. *Journal of Computer Assisted Tomography.* 1995;19(5):726–32.

124. Yoon HK, Im JG, Ahn JM, Han MC. Pulmonary nocardiosis: CT findings. *Journal of Computer Assisted Tomography.* 1995;19(1):52–5.

125. Kanne JP, Yandow DR, Mohammed TL, Meyer CA. CT findings of pulmonary nocardiosis. *AJR American Journal of Roentgenology.* 2011;197(2):W266–72.

126. Ambrosioni J, Lew D, Garbino J. Nocardiosis: updated clinical review and experience at a tertiary center. *Infection.* 2010;38(2):89–97.

127. Hansell DM, Bankier AA, MacMahon H, McLoud TC, Muller NL, Remy J. Fleischner Society: glossary of terms for thoracic imaging. *Radiology.* 2008;246(3):697–722.

128. Quigley MJ, Fraser RS. Pulmonary pneumatocele: pathology and pathogenesis. *AJR American Journal of Roentgenology.* 1988;150(6):1275–7.

129. Mori T, Ebe T, Takahashi M, Isonuma H, Ikemoto H, Oguri T. Lung abscess: analysis of 66 cases from 1979 to 1991. *Internal Medicine.* 1993;32(4):278–84.

130. Stark DD, Federle MP, Goodman PC, Podrasky AE, Webb WR. Differentiating lung abscess and empyema: radiography and computed tomography. *AJR American Journal of Roentgenology*. 1983;141(1):163–7.
131. Moon WK, Im JG, Yeon KM, Han MC. Complications of Klebsiella pneumonia: CT evaluation. *Journal of Computer Assisted Tomography*. 1995;19(2):176–81.
132. Khan FA, Rehman M, Marcus P, Azueta V. Pulmonary gangrene occurring as a complication of pulmonary tuberculosis. *Chest*. 1980;77(1):76–80.
133. Hirshberg B, Sklair-Levi M, Nir-Paz R, Ben-Sira L, Krivoruk V, Kramer MR. Factors predicting mortality of patients with lung abscess. *Chest*. 1999;115(3):746–50.
134. Nguyen ET, Kanne JP, Hoang LM, Reynolds S, Dhingra V, Bryce E et al. Community-acquired methicillin-resistant Staphylococcus aureus pneumonia: radiographic and computed tomography findings. *Journal of Thoracic Imaging*. 2008;23(1):13–9.
135. Reich JM. Pulmonary gangrene and the air crescent sign. *Thorax*. 1993;48(1):70–4.
136. Curry CA, Fishman EK, Buckley JA. Pulmonary gangrene: radiological and pathologic correlation. *Southern Medical Journal*. 1998;91(10):957–60.
137. Taryle DA, Potts DE, Sahn SA. The incidence and clinical correlates of parapneumonic effusions in pneumococcal pneumonia. *Chest*. 1978;74(2):170–3.
138. Light RW, Girard WM, Jenkinson SG, George RB. Parapneumonic effusions. *The American Journal of Medicine*. 1980;69(4):507–12.
139. Waite RJ, Carbonneau RJ, Balikian JP, Umali CB, Pezzella AT, Nash G. Parietal pleural changes in empyema: appearances at CT. *Radiology*. 1990;175(1):145–50.
140. Aquino SL, Webb WR, Gushiken BJ. Pleural exudates and transudates: diagnosis with contrast-enhanced CT. *Radiology*. 1994;192(3):803–8.
141. Takasugi JE, Godwin JD, Teefey SA. The extrapleural fat in empyema: CT appearance. *The British Journal of Radiology*. 1991;64(763):580–3.
142. Im JG, Webb WR, Han MC, Park JH. Apical opacity associated with pulmonary tuberculosis: high-resolution CT findings. *Radiology*. 1991;178(3):727–31.
143. Ricci ZJ, Haramati LB, Rosenbaum AT, Liebling MS. Role of computed tomography in guiding the management of peripheral bronchopleural fistula. *Journal of Thoracic Imaging*. 2002;17(3):214–8.
144. Westcott JL, Volpe JP. Peripheral bronchopleural fistula: CT evaluation in 20 patients with pneumonia, empyema, or postoperative air leak. *Radiology*. 1995;196(1):175–81.
145. Rome L, Murali G, Lippmann M. Nonresolving pneumonia and mimics of pneumonia. *The Medical Clinics of North America*. 2001;85(6):1511–30, xi.
146. Kyprianou A, Hall CS, Shah R, Fein AM. The challenge of nonresolving pneumonia. Knowing the norms of radiographic resolution is key. *Postgraduate Medicine*. 2003;113(1):79–82, 5–8, 91–2.
147. Fine MJ, Stone RA, Singer DE, Coley CM, Marrie TJ, Lave JR et al. Processes and outcomes of care for patients with community-acquired pneumonia: results from the Pneumonia Patient Outcomes Research Team (PORT) cohort study. *Archives of Internal Medicine*. 1999;159(9):970–80.
148. Boiselle PM, Tocino I, Hooley RJ, Pumerantz AS, Selwyn PA, Neklesa VP et al. Chest radiograph interpretation of Pneumocystis carinii pneumonia, bacterial pneumonia, and pulmonary tuberculosis in HIV-positive patients: accuracy, distinguishing features, and mimics. *Journal of Thoracic Imaging*. 1997;12(1):47–53.

22

Interstitial Lung Disease

Irene Ariozzi, Carmelinda Manna, Eleonora Zambrini, Antonio Pavarani, and Nicola Sverzellati

CONTENTS

22.1 Technical Features

Thin collimation and high spatial frequency reconstruction algorithm are the two most important factors that affect the spatial resolution and the quality of high-resolution computed tomography (HRCT) images.

Spatial resolution is usually optimized by using 1-mm-thick section images. Thinner sections (<0.5 mm) do not improve spatial resolution and reduce the signal-to-noise ratio, whereas thicker images (>1.5 mm) may reduce the detection power of subtle density differences in lung parenchyma and also compromise the correct evaluation of small abnormalities such as lung nodules, bronchiectasis, cyst walls, and interlobular septa [1].

The use of high spatial frequency reconstruction algorithm (sharp or ultra sharp) is needed to optimize anatomic details as it makes both structure margins and tissue interfaces sharper The smallest possible field of view that encompasses both lungs and the largest available matrix in the reconstruction of scan data (usually 512 × 512) should be used to decrease the pixel size.

Standard HRCT is a sampling technique, with interspacing between each section of the order of 10 mm; each image being obtained independently during breath-hold at end inspiration. Owing to the diffuse nature of interstitial lung disease (ILD), this discontinuous sample provided a reasonably accurate diagnosis of diffuse lung diseases without exposing patients to high levels of radiation dose. However, the discontinuous sampling does not allow a full assessment of focal lung abnormalities such as bronchiectasis, air trapping, mucous plugging, nodules, and abnormal vascular structures. In addition, it is difficult to compare repeated HRCT images if the patients perform different levels of inspiration. The use of a thin-section volumetric protocol allows a perfect matching of baseline and follow-up computed tomography (CT) images to monitor the evolution of ILD. The development of multi-detector CT (MDCT) scanners allowed the entire chest to be scanned using thin-section collimation in a single breath-hold with spiral technique (volumetric HRCT). In repeated measures experimental design comparing gapped high-resolution single section CT images with MDCT high-resolution images, MDCT showed improved accuracy for vessels, bronchiectasis, air trapping, and lung nodules [2].

MDCT protocols continue to be developed and refined, and currently, particular attention is being directed at dose-reducing strategies. The easiest way to reduce the dose in spiral CT of the lung is to reduce tube current and take advantage of dose modulation systems available on new MDCT scanners. Different studies show no significant difference in the detection of lung parenchyma structures between low-dose image (i.e., 40 mAs) and high-dose image (i.e., 400 mAs) [3,4]. However, although the observed differences were not significant, mild ground-glass opacity (GGO) was difficult to be assessed at low-dose CT because of the increased image noise. Therefore, the investigators recommended that 200 mAs should be used for initial thin-section CT and lower doses (i.e., 40 to 100 mAs) for follow-up examinations [5].

For younger patients being investigated for suspected ILD, noncontiguous standard HRCT should be used for reducing the radiation exposure.

Although there is not a single ideal window setting for the evaluation of lung parenchyma, a window level of −500 to −600 Hounsfield units (HU) and a width of between 1500 and 1600 HU is generally satisfactory. However, different window settings may be applied for enhancing the visualization of specific abnormalities such as bronchial wall thickening or the mosaic attenuation pattern. Further technical details are summarized in Table 22.1.

HRCT is obtained at full inspiration, with the patient in the supine position. However, when early

TABLE 22.1

Suggest Tecnique for Volumetric High-Resolution Computed Tomography in Intestitial Lung Disease

Acquisition Parameters	
Obtain scan at maximal inspiration, without respiratory motion	
kVp	80–120 kVp depending on patient size
mA	Less than 250 mA, using three-dimensional tube current modulation
Rotation time	0.5–1 s or less gantry revolution time
Beam pitch	1.0–1.5
Reconstruction Parameters	
Lung reconstruction	High spatial frequency kernel (e.g., GE Bone, Philips D. Siemens B45 OR 60, Toshiba FC51)
Mediastinum, soft tissue	Intermediate spatial frequency kernel (e.g., GE Soft Tissue, Philips B, Siemens B31 or 35, Toshiba FC18)
Reformatting Parameters	
Field of view no larger than the lung	
Transaxial reconstruction slice thickness	≤2 mm
Coronal reconstruction slice thickness	3–5 mm thickness
Sagittal reconstruction slice thickness	3–5 mm thickness
Axial MIP thickness	5–8 mm thickness (for nodule detection)
Viewing Parameters	
Lung window	Width 1200–1500 HU, level −600 to 750 HU
Mediastinal window	Width 350–500 HU, level 35.50 HU
Additional Scan Indications	
All additional scans should be obtained using low dose, <60 mA	
Prone	To redistribute dependent atelectasis
End-expiratory	To assess for regional air trapping
Dynamic expiratory	To assess for dynamic narrowing of airways

Source: Adapted from CT Evaluation of Diffuse Infiltrative Lung Disease Dose Considerations and Optimal Technique, John R. Mayo, MD (*J Thorac Imaging* 2009; 24: 252–259).

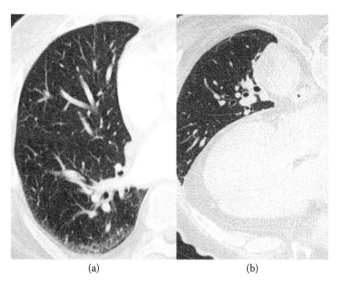

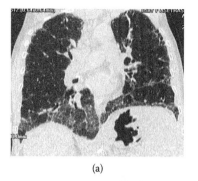

(a)

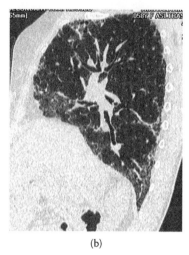

(b)

(a)　　　　　　　　(b)

FIGURE 22.1

(a) Supine computed tomography (CT) image shows ground-glass opacity limited to subleural regions of the lower right lobe. (b) Prone high-resolution computed tomography (HRCT) scanning revealed that such abnormality represented dependent atelectasis, namely no significant interstitial lung disease (ILD).

interstitial fibrosis is suspected, HRCT is often performed in the prone position to avoid the misinterpretation of mild GGO in the dependent posterobasal segments, which may mimic true ILD (Figure 22.1). Additional expiratory HRCT scanning may be helpful in establishing the nature of a mosaic pattern (small airway disease vs. occlusive vascular disease vs. ILD).

FIGURE 22.2

Usual interstitial pneumonia. (a) Coronal HRCT image shows abnormalities predominating in the posterior, subpleural regions of the lower lobes. (b) Sagittal reformation shows the abnormalities creeping up the periphery into the anterior zones of the upper lobes.

22.2 Postprocessing

Thin-section volumetric HRCT allows a retrospective reconstruction of the images in any desired plane.

Coronal and sagittal reconstructions produced from "isotropic" data can be of high quality. Such reconstructions may improve the interpretation of the abnormalities distribution and extent of ILD (Figure 22.2a and b). The use of minimum-intensity projections (MinIP) can improve the detection of regional density differences and may help identify airway involvement and concomitant mild emphysema in some ILDs (Figure 22.3). In contrast, maximum-intensity projection (MIP) is generally less used than the MinIP technique in the context of ILD, but MIP images may allow a better distinction between micronodules and vessels and between perilymphatic and centrilobular distribution of the nodules (Figure 22.4a and b).

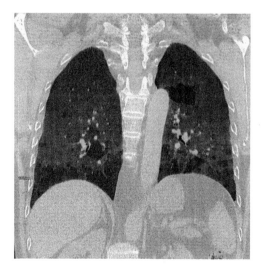

FIGURE 22.3

Expiratory coronal HRCT image reformatted by the minimum-intensity projection MinIP algorithm. Such algorithm enhances the density differences in the lungs, revealing some patchy decreased attenuation areas (in the basal regions as well as in the upper left lobe) because of air trapping.

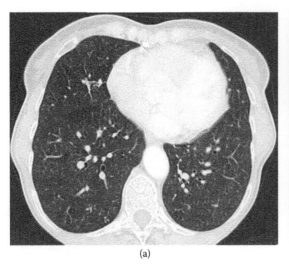 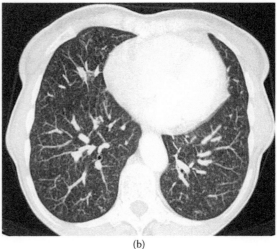

(a)   (b)

FIGURE 22.4
Tubercolosis. (a) This HRCT image shows random nodules in a patient with miliary tuberculosis. (b) Maximum-intensity projection (MIP) reformation clearly improves the visualization of the nodules profusion.

22.3 Basic Patterns in Interstitial Lung Disease

22.3.1 Nodular Pattern

According to the Fleishner Glossary, the nodular pattern is characterized on HRCT by the presence in the lungs of several small rounded opacities (nodules), from 2 mm to 10 mm of diameter [6]. By assessing both anatomic distribution and morphology of the nodules, it is possible to suggest a final diagnosis or, at least, substantially narrow the differential diagnosis.

First, lung nodules need to be characterized by their relation to secondary lobular anatomy, allowing a distinction between centrilobular nodules and those that predominantly involve the lobular periphery, including the interlobular septa and the fissural surfaces. Accordingly, the nodular pattern can be classified into centrilobular, random, or perilymphatic [6–8]. Indeed, radiologists have to establish the presence or the absence of any pleural or perifissural involvment. Once nodules are characterized as being primarily centrilobular, that is, there is no pleural or perifissural involvement, a differential diagnosis among different small airway diseases should be performed. If the nodules have a tree-in-bud configuration, an infectious bronchiolitis should be first suspected. Hazy centrilobular nodules are keeping in with subacute hypersitivity pneumonitis or smoking-related respiratory bronchiolitis (RB) (Figure 22.5).

If nodules are clustered along the interlobular septa, pleural, or perifissural surfaces, their distribution can be categorized as perilymphatic. This distribution is seen most frequently in sarcoidosis (Figure 22.6). The most

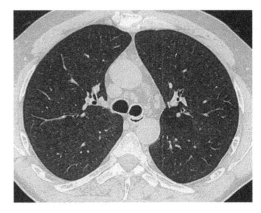

FIGURE 22.5
Centrilobular nodules. HRCT shows numerous poorly defined, relatively low attenuation nodules and ground glass opacification in the upper lobes.

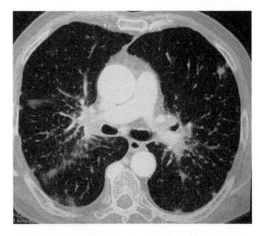

FIGURE 22.6
Perilymphatic nodules. Typical features are nodular opacities mainly distributed along the vessels and the interlobar fissures.

important differential diagnoses for this pattern of disease are silicosis and coal worker pneumoconiosis and more rarely lymphangitis carcinomatosa.

If nodules prove to be diffusing instead of clustered, they are properly considered to be random in distribution. A random distribution of very small well-defined nodules is seen in patients with hematogenous spread of tuberculosis and pulmonary metastases (Figure 22.7) (Table 22.2).

22.3.2 Cystic Pattern

On CT scans, a cyst appears as a round parenchymal lucency (or low-attenuating area) with a well-defined interface with normal lung (Figure 22.8) [9]. Both the

presence of a definable wall and the absence of residual centrilobular artery differentiate cysts from centrilobular emphysema. The most important cystic lung diseases are as follows: lymphangioleiomyomatosis (LAM), Langherans's cell hisyiocytosis, and lymphoid interstitial pneumonia (LIP) [10] (Table 22.2).

22.3.3 Reticular Pattern

At HRCT, a reticular pattern may be caused by thickened interlobular or intralobular septa or honeycomb destruction. The identification of the predominance of one of those types of abnormalities allows separating different groups of ILD [6,11].

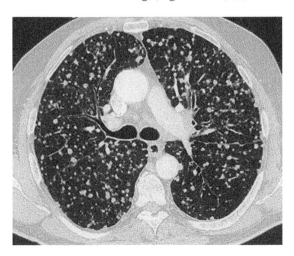

FIGURE 22.7
Random nodules. HRCT image shows variable size nodules distributed randomly through both lungs.

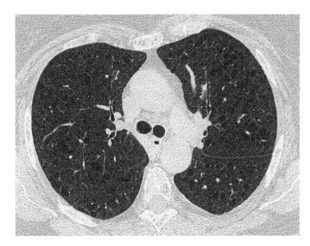

FIGURE 22.8
Lung cysts. There is a profusion of thin-walled cystic airspaces scattered evenly throughout the lungs.

TABLE 22.2

Basic Patterns in Interstitial Lung Disease

HRCT Pattern	Associated Diseases
Nodular	
Perilymphatic	Sarcoidosis, silicosis, pneumoconiosis
Random	Metastasis, miliary infections
Centrilobular	Infectious bronchiolitis, RB, subacute HP, LIP
Reticular	
Interlobular septal thickening	
Smooth	Dominant: pulmonary edema, lymphangitis carcinomatosis, PAP, amyloidosis, leukemia, rare diffuse lung diseases (e.g., Erdhem Chester disease)
	Not dominant: sarcoidosis, pneumoconiosis, acute lung injury, Churg–Strauss, LIP, Sjogren syndrome, chronic HP
Nodular	Sarcoidosis, lymphangitis carcinomatosis
Irregular	Lung fibrosis
Intralobular thickening	Lung fibrosis (UIP, NSIP)
Parenchymal band	Asbestosis, OP, scar from pleura disease
Cystic	PLCH, LAM, LIP, Birt–Hoog Dubè syndrome
Ground glass	DIP, HP, PAP, diffuse alveolar damage, NSIP, drug toxicity
Consolidation	OP, chronic eosinophilic pneumonia, sarcoidosis

Interlobular septa thickened by cells, fluid infiltration, or fibrosis appear as lines outlining partially or completely the secondary lobule, those resembling polygonal arcades with a polygonal shape or perpendicular to the pleura (Figure 22.9).

Interlobular septa thickening may be smooth, nodular, or irregular. Smooth septal thickening is seen most commonly in patients with pulmonary edema or lymphangitic carcinomatosis. Nodular septal thickening occurs most commonly in patients with lymphangitic carcinomatosis [12]. Irregular interlobular thickening is generally seen in different types of lung fibrosis, though this never constitutes the dominant pattern.

Thus, lung fibrosis, particularly usual interstitial pneumonia (UIP), is characterized by fine thickened intralobular septa in association with other signs of architectural distortion such as traction bronchiectasis and honeycombing. The identification of honeycombing is of particular relevance as it may directly impact patient care [6]. Honeycombing consists of clustered cystic airspaces surrounded by irregular walls and should be differentiated from emphysema (Figure 22.10) (Table 22.2).

22.3.4 Ground-Glass Pattern

The term GGO is a common and nonspecific finding on HRCT, characterized by areas of increased hazy attenuation of the lung of variable intensity, with preserved visibility of the surrounding bronchial walls and vascular structures [6] (Figure 22.11).

This lesion is due to a partial filling of airspaces or considerable thickening of interstitium or a combination of the two [13]. GGO may represent either a dominant pattern or an ancillary finding frequently associated with other diffuse abnormalities. Indeed, a correct assessment of ground-glass pattern should be corroborated by the evaluation of the associated findings and, when possible, by clinical clues (acute vs. subacute/chronic) to narrow the differential diagnosis as much as possible. It is also important to identify any bronchial dilatation or distortion within ground-glass, which may represent subtle interstitial lung fibrosis [7–10] (Table 22.2).

22.3.5 Consolidation

It is an abnormal opacification of the lung parenchyma in which vessels are obscured by consolidated (white) lung, and an air bronchogram may, or may not, be present [6,11] (Figure 22.12). The approach to diagnosis is

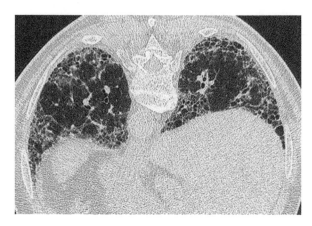

FIGURE 22.10
Honeycombing. HRCT image shows subpleural basal clustered cysts in a patient with usual interstitial pneumonia.

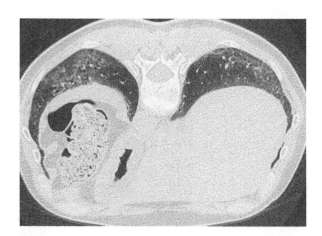

FIGURE 22.11
Ground-glass opacification in a patient with nonspecific interstitial pneumonia.

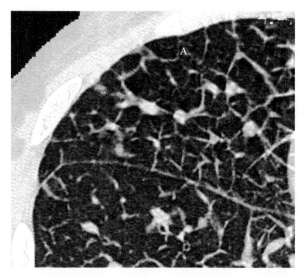

FIGURE 22.9
Interlobular septal thickening. In the magnified HRCT view of the right lung, thickened interlobular septa appear as lines outlining partially or completely the secondary lobules.

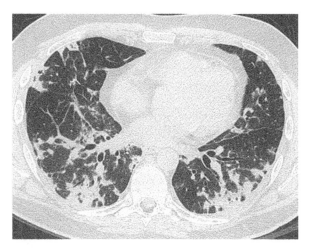

FIGURE 22.12
Consolidation. Patchy multifocal consolidation and ground-glass opacity in the lower zones of the lung of a patient with organizing pneumonia.

potentially daunting since consolidation is a nonspecific radiological pattern, being present in other common conditions such as infections and neoplasms. An appreciation of the clinical features, the distribution of the abnormalities, and the changes on serial examination are often invaluable. A review of the radiology together with the clinical features may also be diagnostic in some instances. Predominant consolidation is more commonly seen in the following diffuse lung diseases: organizing pneumonia, chronic eosinophilic pneumonia, and Wegener's granulomatosis. [6–10] (Table 22.2).

22.4 Interstitial Lung Diseases: Unknown Etiology

22.4.1 Idiopathic Pulmonary Fibrosis

Idiopathic pulmonary fibrosis is associated with the histopathological finding of UIP, a chronic fibrosing lung disease characterized by a heterogeneous picture of fibrosis, inflammatory infiltrate, and honeycombing [14]. IPF is the most common ILD and is associated with a fatal prognosis. Familiarity with the typical appearances of IPF on HRCT is important, as in the appropriate clinical setting, it is often sufficient for establishing a confident diagnosis of IPF without the need for surgical biopsy [15–17].

The characteristic HRCT features of UIP are a reticular pattern with honeycombing, often associated with traction bronchiectasis; ground glass may be present, but is less extensive than reticular abnormality

(Figures 22.1 and 22.10). Such abnormalities are characteristically basal and peripheral, though often patchy. Less frequently, an HRCT UIP pattern may be also seen in other conditions associated with known etiology such as chronic hypersensitivity pneumonitis (HP) and connective tissue diseases, thus making the differential diagnosis more difficult by the sole evaluation of the HRCT findings [18].

Furthermore, up to 50% of patients with UIP do not show any typical HRCT pattern owing to either the absence of typical findings of UIP (e.g., evident honeycombing) or the presence of findings suggestive of other diagnoses such as predominant GGO. Generally, such UIP cases associated with an atypical HRCT pattern are very similar or identical to the nonspecific interstitial pneumonia (NSIP) pattern [19].

Important complications of IPF include infection, lung cancer, and accelerated deterioration [20].

An acute clinical deterioration may represent the so-called acute exacerbation because of superimposed diffuse alveolar damage and/or organizing pneumonia. The HRCT signs of acute exacerbations consist of newly developed GGO and/or consolidation. Such abnormalities are virtually identical to those of other causes of acute clinical worsening such as opportunistic superinfections and heart failure [21].

22.4.2 Nonspecific Interstitial Pneumonia

NSIP was initially proposed to identify a group of patients with interstitial pneumonia that had a more favorable prognosis than IPF and that also differ from the other major idiopathic interstitial pneumonias including desquamative interstitial pneumonitis (DIP), acute interstitial pneumonia, and cryptogenic organizing pneumonia (COP). As such, it was originally a diagnosis of exclusion. However, now it is accepted that NSIP is a distinct form of IIP. However, it occurs not only as an idiopathic condition, but also in a variety of settings including collagen vascular disease [22,23], HP [24], and drug toxicity [15]. It also has been reported in patients with familial pulmonary fibrosis [25]. The HRCT features of NSIP consist mainly of GGO [26–28] and reticular abnormalities involving the lower zones with a peripheral and/ or a peribronchovascular distribution (Figure 22.13). Sometimes NSIP may spare the subpleural lung [29,30]. In most cases, traction bronchiectasis is present in areas of ground glass attenuation or reticular abnormality. Honeycombing is not usually observed in NSIP and, when present, is usually of limited extension [18].

NSIP may be classified on the basis of the relative amounts of lung fibrosis and inflammation. Patients with predominant fibrosis (fibrotic NSIP) have a poorer prognosis than do those with inflammatory histological findings (cellular NSIP) [31,32].

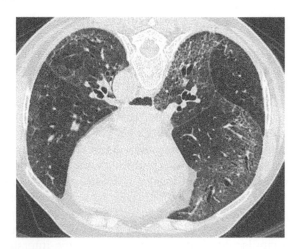

FIGURE 22.13
Nonspecific interstitial pneumonia pattern. In this case, ground-glass opacification admixed with fine reticular opacities are associated with mild traction bronchiectasis.

Differentiation between UIP and fibrotic NSIP is sometimes quite difficult, especially in cigarette smokers with emphysema [32]. It is important to realize that an HRCT pattern consistent with NSIP does not necessarily match the histological findings, which may reveal UIP or additional abnormalities suggesting a more specific diagnosis such as HP [29].

22.4.3 Lymphoid Interstitial Pneumonia

LIP is a rare disease characterized by a diffuse pulmonary lymphoid proliferation with predominant interstitial involvement [6]. It occurs commonly in middle-aged women, rare as idiopathic, more frequently secondary to Sjogren syndrome, dysproteinemia, HIV, bone marrow transplantation, and intrathoracic Castlemans' disease. Hystologically, it is characterized by an expansion of the lung interstitium because of a diffuse infiltration of lymphocites, plasma cell, and hystiocites [33,34].

HRCT shows areas of GGO, ill-defined nodules of varying sizes, interlobular septal thickening, and cysts. The cysts, when present, are usually characteristic. They are thin-walled, usually of 1–30 mm, and randomly distributed within the lung parenchyma in the mid-lung zone [35,36].

22.4.4 Cryptogenic Organizing Pneumonia

Organizing pneumonia (OP) is a nonspecific form of reparative reaction of the lung to an acute injury, in which there is an incomplete resolution of inflammation within the alveoli and the distal bronchioles. OP is associated with many conditions: infections, drugs, connective tissue disorders, hypersensitivity pneumonia, immunological disorders, and so on. However, OP may be idiopathic and indeed termed as COP [37,38].

COP is a subacute disease, with equal sex distribution on VI decade. The onset is of a flu-like illness with fever, malaise, cough, and mild dyspnea.

The histopathology of organizing pneumonia is characterized by the presence of plugs of organized granulation tissue within the alveoli and the distal bronchioles, consisting in fibroblast, myofibroblast, and inflammatory cells in a connective matrix (Masson bodies) 1; these buds may extend to adjacent alveoli through Kohn pores.

The classic HRCT findings consist of patchy areas of consolidation, usually bilateral, peripheral, and migrating. A predilection for subpleural regions of the lower zones has been reported (Figure 22.12). Other findings include GGO, small centrilobular nodules, perilobular densities (arcade-like opacities near to the pleura surface surrounded by normal lung parenchyma), and band-like opacities.

Unusual patterns include crazy paving, bronchocentric pattern, solitary focal mass (usually in the upper lobes), and the "atollo sign" (or reversed halo sign) constituted by peripheral consolidation with inner GGO [38,10].

COP has usually a complete response to high dose of corticosteroids; however, recurrence is not infrequent and in a minority of cases may be a progression to fibrosis, probably representing an overlap between OP and NSIP [39,40].

22.4.5 Sarcoidosis

Sarcoidosis is a multisystem disorder of unknown cause characterized by noncaseous epithelioid cell granulomas. Thoracic manifestations occur in 90% of the patients, and the classic presentation consists of enlarged hilar and mediastinal lymph nodes, with or without parenchymal involvement [41].

Granulomas in the lung have a characteristic distribution along the lymphatics in the bronchovasculars health and, to a lesser extent, in the interlobular septa and subpleural lung regions [42].

Frequently, the diagnosis is first brought to attention by chest radiography, and thus the staging of the disease is traditionally based on chest x-ray findings (Siltzbach staging Table 22.3) [43]. This classification scheme has substantial prognostic significance.

Intrathoracic lymphadenopathy occurs in 75%–85% of patients with sarcoidosis at sometime during the course of the disease. The most common pattern is well-defined, bilateral, symmetric hilar, and right paratracheal lymph node enlargement. Differential diagnosis of bilateral hilar lymph node enlargement are infection (fungal or mycobacterial) or malignancy (lymphoma).

The enlarged nodes eventually may become calcified with different pattern. Usually, calcified lymph nodes

TABLE 22.3

Siltzbach Staging

Stage 0	No demonstrable abnormality
Stage I	Hilar and mediastinal lymph node enlargement unassociated with pulmonary abnormality
Stage II	Hilar and mediastinal lymph node enlargement associated with pulmonary abnormality
Stage III	Diffuse pulmonary disease unassociated with node enlargement
Stage IV	Significant lung fibrosis with architectural distortion or bulla

are evenly distributed throughout the mediastinum and hila, but sometimes that may be indistinguishable from other disease (silicosis or pulmonary tuberculosis) (Figure 22.14).

Parenchymal abnormalities are seen on chest radiograph at presentation in approximately 40% of patients with sarcoidosis [44]. Nodular or reticulonodular opacities are the most frequent pulmonary pattern. At HRCT, the nodules are clustered along the bronchovascular bundles, interlobular septa, interlobar fissures, adjacent to the costal pleura (often mimicking small pleural plaques) [45], and also in the centrilobular regions (Figure 22.6) [46]. Nodules usually tend to predominate in perihilar with relative sparing of the lung periphery and may be grouped in small areas. Nodules typically measure 1–5 mm, but larger parenchymal nodules (>1 cm in diameter) may also be seen in sarcoidosis. On HRCT, innumerable small satellite nodules may be adjacent to the larger nodules, a finding termed "the CT galaxy sign" [47].

In approximately 10% of patients with sarcoidosis, a confluence of granulomas may cause compression of the alveoli and result in poorly defined bilateral parenchymal consolidations containing an air bronchogram, which may mimic tuberculosis, pneumonia, or bronchiolitis obliterans organizing pneumonia. Innumerable small interstitial granulomas (beyond the resolution of CT) may cause patchy GGOs on HRCT [48].

All these aforementioned parenchymal abnormalities may be reversible and, sometimes, may resolve spontaneously. However, they might evolve into pulmonary fibrosis in 20–25% of cases. The classic irreversible changes seen in fibrotic sarcoidosis generally consist of reticular opacities and traction bronchiectasis, radiating from the hilum to the dorsal regions of the upper lobes (Figure 22.15). Honeycombing, when present, may be constituted by large cysts in which fungal infection may get superimposed in more advanced disease.

High-resolution CT may be particularly helpful for distinguishing active inflammation from irreversible fibrosis in selected patients with Stage 2 or 3 sarcoidosis. It can also help to show specific complications

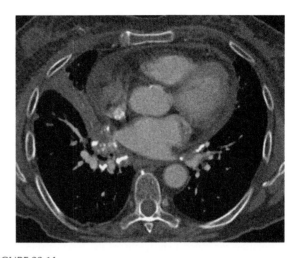

FIGURE 22.14
Egg-shell lymph nodes calcification of lymph nodes in a patient with sarcoidosis.

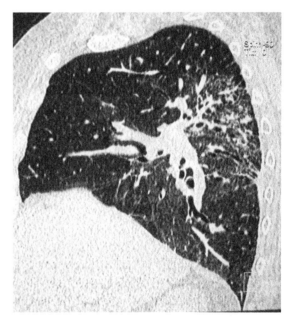

FIGURE 22.15
Fibrotic sarcoidosis. The sagittal HRCT image shows areas of conglomerate fibrosis in a perihilar distribution with associated bronchial distortion and volume loss.

(pulmonary hypertension, bronchial stenosis, etc.) and comorbidities (e.g., aspergilloma colonization of the cavities).

Besides the typical manifestation of pulmonary sarcoidosis, there may be several less common abnormalities: it is not by chance that the literature often describes sarcoidosis "the great mimic."

22.4.6 Pulmonary Alveolar Proteinosis

The idiopathic primary form of pulmonary alveolar proteinosis (PAP) is a chronic disease, probably

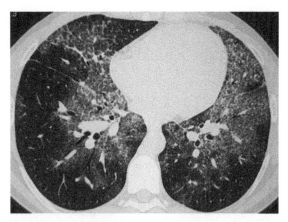

FIGURE 22.16
High-resolution computed tomography of the "crazy paving" pattern in alveolar proteinosis. Patchy ground-glass opacification is seen, and there are numerous thickened interlobular septa in areas of ground-glass opacification.

substained by an autoimmune disorder that causes dysfunction of alveolar macrophages and lower surfactant clearance in adults. The more common secondary form is caused by inhalation syndromes (smoke and dusts), immunodeficiency syndromes, and hematolymphoid neoplasms.

PAP is histopathologically characterized by areas of pulmonary alveoli filled with granular, eosinophilic, proteinaceous material that is rich in lipid and positive for periodic acid-Shiff stain. The interlobular and intralobular intestitium adjacent to the pathological alveoli often show an edematous inflammatory reaction [49,50].

The HRCT findings well correlate with the histopathologic findings. There is a variable combination of GGO intermingled with interlobular septal thickening, thus constituting the so-called crazy-paving pattern [51,52] (Figure 22.16). Usually the abnormalities are patchy, sometimes predominantly distributed in the perihilar regions. The final diagnosis is established by bronchoalveolar lavage [53].

22.4.7 Chronic Eosinophilic Pneumonia

Chronic eosinophilic pneumonia is an idiophatic pulmonary disease characterized by eosinophilic infiltrates in lung parenchyma and peripheral blood eosinophilia.

HRCT findings show characteristic patchy and peripheral consolidations, which may relatively spare the subpleural regions ("photographic negative" of pulmonary edema on chest radiograph) [49,54].

Consolidation may predominate in the middle zones and are frequently bilateral. The major differential diagnosis is with organizing pneumonia [53,54]. However, sarcoidosis with uncommon pattern, chronic infections (tubercolosis and fungal), lymphoma, avanced bronchioloalveolar carcinoma, multiple and extensive pulmonary

infarcts may also resemble the HRCT appearance of chronic eosinophilic pneumonia.

22.4.8 Lymphangioleiomyomatosis

Lymphangioleiomyomatosis is a rare multisystem disease that occurs almost exclusively in women of childbearing age, characterized by a cystic degeneration of the lungs, renal angiomyolipomas, and lymphatic spread [55].

LAM could be sporadic or associated with tuberous sclerosis complex (TSC), namely an autosomal dominant disorder. Patients with TSC develop pulmonary LAM in about 25%–35% of cases [56,57].

HRCT findings are typical and reflect the histological lesions: there are numerous thin-wall, round cysts, ranging in diameter from 2 mm to 50 mm, randomly distributed with intervening normal lung tissue, and with no lung zone preference. Usually there is no sparing of costophrenic recesses and such a finding should be identified to differentiate LAM from Langerhans cells' hystiocytosis [58,50] (Figure 22.8).

Less commonly, it could be seen as thickening of interlobular septa because of pulmonary lymphatics obstruction or patchy areas of GGO that result from pulmonary hemorrhage or hemosiderosis.

Additional findings are chylous pleural effusion, mediastinal lymphonodes enlargement, or pneumothorax; abdominal manifestations are renal angiomyolipomas (50% of patients TSC: 67% sLAM: 60% chylous ascites and lymphangioma).

22.5 Interstitial Lung Diseases: Known Causes and Associations

22.5.1 Hypersensitivity Pneumonitis

HP is an immunologically induced inflammatory disease of the lung parenchyma and terminal airways caused by inhalation of various antigenic organic particles or other agent in a sensitized host [59].

The cell-mediated response results in a delayed hypersensitivity with granulomatous inflammation within the pulmonary interstitium with a classic histopathology feature of cellular bronchiolitis, bronchiolocentric interstitial pneumonitis with a predominance of lymphocytes, and poorly formed non-necrotizing granulomas. However, pathologic features may vary with disease stage.

Traditionally, HP has been classified as manifesting in three phases, acute, subacute, and chronic, on the strength of duration of patient's symptoms and antigen's exposure.

Significant clinical and radiological overlap can often occur between these nominal phases.

The most typical HRCT finding in patients with acute/subacute HP are the presence of nodules, GGO, and areas of decreased attenuation, which turn to be air-trapping areas at expiratory CT scanning (Figure 22.5). The nodules are the most distinctive HRCT feature: they are centrilobular and poorly defined and of ground-glass (GG) attenuation [60,61].

Pulmonary cysts were reported in 13% of patients with subacute HP.

Chronic HP is characterized by the presence of reticulation and traction bronchiectasis because of fibrosis. Reticulation are usually patchy or peribronchovascular and tends more frequently to spare the lung bases [62]. At this stage, the predominant midlung distribution of the abnormalities, the presence of centrilobular nodules, and lobular areas of air trapping help to differentiate chronic HP from other fibrotic lung diseases such as idiopathic NSIP and UIP.

22.5.2 Smoking-Related Interstitial Lung Disease

Cigarette smoking is related to the development of RB associated with ILD (RB-ILD), DIP, and pulmonary Langerhans cell histiocytosis (PLCH), which form a spectrum of interstitial patterns in response to smoking-related lung injury. These clinicopathologic entities may coexist in the same patient with an overlap of radiologic pattern [63].

RB is a histopathologic finding frequently observed in asymptomatic smokers. It is characterized by the presence of pigmented intraluminal macrophages within RB and mild interstitial inflammatory changes on neighboring alveoli. The symptomatic form of RB is termed as RB-ILD, which is also characterized by abnormal pulmonary function test results [64].

HRCT findings of RB-ILD consist of hazy centrilobular nodules and small patches of GG attenuation predominating in the upper lobes (Figure 22.17). Either bronchial wall thickening or mild emphysema is commonly seen in RB-ILD. Mild interlobular septal thickening may be observed, but is exceptionally a dominate feature. Knowledge of a smoking history is clearly important and may help to distinguish RB/RB-ILD from HP, which is usually not associated with this habit [65].

In DIP, there is an intra-alveolar accumulation of pigmented macrophages. Thereby, the predominant HRCT feature is GGO, which is generally more extensive than in RB-ILD. In DIP, GGO may be peripheral or diffuse, and a basal distribution predominance has been reported.

Chest radiography in Langerhans cell histiocytosis shows nodular, cystic, reticular, or reticulonodular lesions, predominantly in the upper lung. Pneumothorax

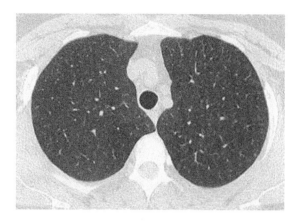

FIGURE 22.17
Respiratory bronchiolitis–interstitial lung disease. High-resolution computed tomography shows hazy centrilobular nodules.

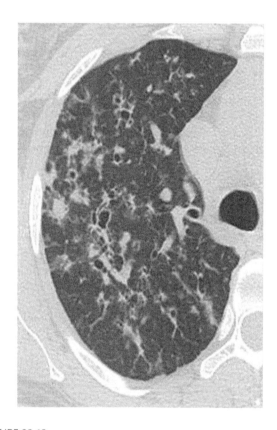

FIGURE 22.18
Langerhans cell histiocytosis. Magnified high-resolution computed tomography image shows the characteristic combination of thin-walled cysts and irregular nodules.

is a recognized feature of Langerhans cell histiocytosis. HRCT typically shows a variable combination of nodules and cysts, mainly involving the upper lobes with spare of the costophrenic angles. Nodules are usually <5 mm in diameter, have a peribronchiolar and centrilobular distribution, and may cavitate (Figure 22.18). Cysts are usually <10 mm in diameter but may coalesce becoming >20 mm and leading to bizarre-shaped spaces [66]. Occasionally, patchy or diffuse GGOs may be seen, probably related to areas of RB and DIP.

22.5.3 Vasculitis

22.5.3.1 Wegener Granulomatosis

Wegener granulomatosis (WG) is an idiopathic multisystem disorder characterized by necrotizing extravascular granulomas and granulomatous necrotizing vasculitis involving small arteries and veins of the upper and lower respiratory tract and glomerulonephritis.

The most common HRCT pattern in WG is that of multiple, bilateral, peribronchovascular nodules, or masses, typically ill-defined or surrounded by a zone of GG attenuation ("halo-sign") and often cavitary [67,51] (Figure 22.19). Other relatively common manifestations are tracheal narrowing and bronchial abnormalities, including bronchiectasis and bronchial wall thickening. Bilateral air-space consolidation owing to pulmonary hemorrhage is an infrequent but serious complication [68].

The differential diagnosis usually includes sarcoidosis, infectious granulomatous disease (tubercolosis, fungal), early stage of PLCH, and lung metastases.

22.5.3.2 Churg–Strauss Syndrome

Churg–Strauss syndrome is a chronic, idiophathic disease characterized by eosinophil-rich granulomas and infiltrates involving the respiratory tract, necrotizing vasculitis affecting small and medium vessels, and associated with asthma and eosinophilia.

The most common HRCT features of Churg–Strauss syndrome consist of GGO, air-space consolidation,

and nodules with a patchy or predominatly periphreal distribution and interlobular septal thickening with or without pleural effusions: these findings reflect the presence in the pulmonary parenchyma of eosinophilic infiltrates as well as foci of organizing pneumonia and interstitial edema, which may be secondary to cardiac dysfunction. Less common findings are pericardial effusion and enlarged mediastinal lymph nodes. Airway changes, in particular bronchial wall thickening, may be ascribed to the underlying asthma [68,69].

References

1. Mayo JR. Evaluation of diffuse infiltrative lung disease dose considerations and optimal technique. *J Thorac Imaging* 2009; 24: 252–259.
2. Dodd JD, de Jong PA, Levy RD et al. Conventional high resolution CT versus contiguous multidetector CT in the detection of bronchiolitis obliterans syndrome in lung transplant recipients. *J Thorac Imaging* 2008; 23:235–243.
3. Lee KS, Primack SL, Staples CA et al. Chronic infiltrative lung disease: Comparison of diagnostic accuracies of radiography and low- and conventional-dose thin-section CT. *Radiology* 1994; 191: 669–673.
4. Zwirewich CV, Mayo JR, Muller NL. Low-dose high-resolution CT of lung parenchyma. *Radiology* 1991; 180:413–417.
5. Bankier AA, Tack D. Reduction strategies for thoracic multidetector computed tomography background, current issues, and recommendations. *J Thorac Imaging* 2010; 25: 278–288.
6. Hansell DM, Bankier AA, MacMahon H et al. Fleishner society: Glossary of terms for thoracic imaging. *Radiology* 2008; 246: 697–724.
7. Gotway MB, Reddy GP, Webb WR et al. High-resolution ct of the lung: patterns of disesase and differential diagnoses. *Radiol Clin N Am* 2005; 43: 513–542.
8. Raoof S, Amchentsev A, Vlahos I et al. Pictorial essay: Multinodular disease: a high-resolution CT scan diagniostic algorithm. *Chest* 2006; 129: 805–815.
9. Collins J. CT signs and patterns of lung disease. *Radiol Clin North Am* 2001; 39: 1115–1135.
10. Zompatori M, Sverzellati N, Poletti V et al. High-resolution CT in diagnosis of diffuse infintrative lung disease. *Semin Ultrasound CT MR* 2005; 26: 332–347.
11. Hansell DM, Armstrong P, Lynch DA et al. *Basic HRCT Patterns of Lung Disease. Imaging of Diseases of the Chest.* Amsterdam, Elsevier, 2005, pp 143–181.
12. Kang EY, Grenier P, Laurent F et al. Interlobular septal thickening: patterns at high-resolution computed tomography. *J Thorac Imaging* 1996; 11: 260–264.
13. Battista G, Sassi C, Zompatori M et al. Ground-glass opacity: Interpretation of high resolution CT findings. *Radiol Med* 2003; 106: 425–442.

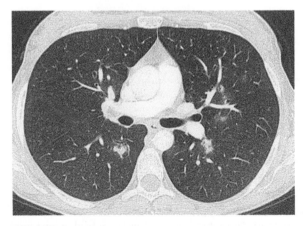

FIGURE 22.19
Wegener's granulomatosis. HRCT through the middle zones also shows multiple irregular nodules.

14. Sverzellati N, De Filippo M, Bartalena T et al. High-resolution computed tomography in the diagnosis and follow-up of idiopathic pulmonary fibrosis. *Radiol Med* 2010; 115: 526–538.

15. Raghu G, Collard HR, Egan JJ et al. An official ATS/ERS/JRS/ALAT statement: Idiopathic pulmonary fibrosis: Evidence-based guidelines for diagnosis and management. *Am J Respir Crit Care Med* 2011; 183: 788–824.

16. Hunninghake GW, Zimmerman MB, Schwartz DA et al. Utility of a lung biopsy for the diagnosis of idiopathic pulmonary fibrosis. *Am J Respirat Crit Care Med* 2001; 164: 193–196.

17. American Thoracic Society. Idiopathic pulmonary fibrosis: Diagnosis and treatment international consensus statement: American Thoracic Society (ATS) and the European Respiratory Society (ERS). *Am J Respir Crit Care Med* 2000; 161: 646–664.

18. Lynch DA, Travis WD, Muller NL et al. Idiopathic interstitial pneumonias: CT features. *Radiology* 2005; 236: 10–21.

19. Flaherty KR, Thwaite EL, Kazerooni EA et al. Radiological versus histological diagnosis in UIP and NSIP: Survival implications. *Thorax* 2003; 58: 143–148.

20. Panos RJ, Mortenson RL, Niccoli SA et al. Clinical deterioration in patients with idiopathic pulmonary fibrosis: Causes and assessment. *Am J Med* 1990; 88: 396–404.

21. Collard HR, Moore BB, Flaherty KR et al. Acute exacerbations of idiopathic pulmonary fibrosis. *Am J Respir Crit Care Med* 2007; 176: 636–643.

22. Park JH, Kim DS, Park IN et al. Prognosis of fibrotic interstitial pneumonia: Idiopathic versus collagen vascular disease-related subtypes. *Am J Respir Crit Care Med* 2007; 175: 705–711.

23. Sato T, Fujita J, Yamadori I et al. Non-specific interstitial pneumonia; as the first clinical presentation of various collagen vascular disorders. *Rheumatol Int* 2006; 26: 551–555.

24. Trahan S, Hanak V, Ryu JH et al. Role of surgical lung biopsy in separating chronic hypersensitivity pneumonia from usual interstitial pneumonia/idiopathic pulmonary fibrosis: Analysis of 31 biopsies from 15 patients. *Chest* 2008; 134: 126–132.

25. Yang IV, Burch LH, Steele MP et al. Gene expression profiling of familial and sporadic interstitial pneumonia. *Am J Respir Crit Care Med* 2007; 175: 45–54.

26. Kim T, Lee K, Chung M et al. Nonspecific interstitial pneumonia with fibrosis: High resolution CT and pathologic findings. *AJR Am J Roentgenol* 1998; 171: 1645–1650.

27. Nagai S, Kitaichi M, Itoh H et al. Idiopathic nonspecific interstitial pneumonia/fibrosis: Comparison with idiopathic pulmonary fibrosis and BOOP. *Eur Respir J* 1998; 12: 1010–1019.

28. Hartman TE, Swensen SJ, Hansell DM et al. Nonspecific interstitial pneumonia: Variable appearance at high-resolution chest CT. *Radiology* 2000; 217: 701–705.

29. Travis WD, Hunninghake G, King TE, Jr. et al. Idiopathic nonspecific interstitial pneumonia: Report of an American Thoracic Society project. *Am J Respir Crit Care Med* 2008; 177: 1338–1347.

30. Silva CI, Muller NL, Hansell DM et al. Nonspecific interstitial pneumonia and idiopathic pulmonary fibrosis: Change in pattern and distribution of disease over time. *Radiology* 2008; 247: 251–259.

31. Johkoh T, Muller NL, Colby TV et al. Nonspecific interstitial pneumonia: Correlation between thin-section CT findings and pathologic subgroups in 55 patients. *Radiology* 2002; 225: 199–204.

32. Akira M, Inoue Y, Kitaichi M et al. Usual interstitial pneumonia and nonspecific interstitial pneumonia with and without concurrent emphysema: Thin-section CT findings. *Radiology* 2009; 251: 271–279.

33. Gal AA, Staton GW, Jr. Current concepts in the classification of interstitial lung disease. *Am J Clin Pathol* 2005; 123(Suppl 1): S67–S81.

34. Mueller-Mang C, Grosse C, Schmid K et al. What every radiologist should know about idiopathic interstitial pneumonias. *Radiographics* 2007; 27: 595–615.

35. Swigris JJ, Berry GJ, Raffin TA et al. Lymphoid interstitial pneumonia: A narrative review. *Chest* 2002; 122: 2150–2164.

36. Johkoh T, Müller NL, Pickford HA et al. Lymphocytic interstitial pneumonia: Thin-section CT findings in 22 patients. *Radiology* 1999; 212: 567–572.

37. American Thoracic Society, European Respiratory Society. American Thoracic Society/European Respiratory Society International Multidisciplinary Consensus Classification of the Idiopathic Interstitial Pneumonias. This joint statement of the American Thoracic Society (ATS), and the European Respiratory Society (ERS) was adopted by the ATS board of directors, June 2001 and by the ERS Executive Committee, June 2001. *Am J Respir Crit Care Med* 2002; 165: 277–304.

38. Roberton BJ, Hansell DM. Organizing pneumonia: A kaleidoscope of concepts and morphologies. *Eur Radiol* 2011; 21: 2244–2254.

39. Wells AU, Hirani N. Interstitial lung disease guideline: The British Thoracic Society in collaboration with the Thoracic Society of Australia and New Zealand and the Irish Thoracic Society. *Thorax* 2008; 63: 1–58.

40. Drakopanagiotakis F, Palaschalaki K, Abu-Hijlei M et al. Cryptogenic and secondary organizing pneumonia: Clinical presentation, radiographics findings, treatment response, and prognosis. *Chest* 2011; 139: 839–900.

41. Statement on sarcoidosis. Joint Statement of the American Thoracic Society (ATS), the European Respiratory Society (ERS) and the World Association of Sarcoidosis and Other Granulomatous Disorders (WASOG) adopted by the ATS Board of Directors and by the ERS Executive Committee, February 1999. *Am J Respir Crit Care Med* 1999; 160: 736–755.

42. Nishimura K, Itoh H, Kitaichi M et al. Pulmonary sarcoidosis: Correlation of CT and histopathologic findings. *Radiology* 1993; 189: 105–109.

43. Siltzbach LE. Sarcoidosis: Clinical features and management. *Med Clin North Am* 1967; 51: 483–502.

44. McLoud TC, Epler GR, Gaensler EA et al. A radiographic classification for sarcoidosis: Physiologic correlation. *Invest Radiol* 1982; 17: 129–138.

45. Nishimura K, Itoh H, Kitaichi M et al. Pulmonary sarcoidosis: correlation of CT and histopathologic findings. *Radiology* 1993; 189: 105–109.

46. Gruden JF, Webb WR, Warnock M. Centrilobular opacities in the lung on high-resolution CT: Diagnostic considerations and pathologic correlation. *AJR Am J Roentgenol* 1994; 162: 569–574.

47. Nakatsu M, Hatabu H, Morikawa K et al. Large coalescent parenchymal nodules in pulmonary sarcoidosis: "Sarcoid galaxy" sign. *AJR Am J Roentgenol* 2002; 178: 1389–1393.

48. Muller NL, Miller RR. Ground-glass attenuation, nodules, alveolitis, and sarcoid granulomas. *Radiology* 1993; 189: 31–32.

49. Leslie KO, Gruden JF, Parish JM et al. Transbronchial biopsy interpretation in the patient with diffuse parenchymal lung disease. *Arch Pathol Lab Med* 2007; 131: 407–423.

50. Pipavath S. Imaging of interstitial lung disease. *Radiol Clin N Am* 2005; 43: 589–599.

51. Marshall GB, Farnquist BA, MacGregor JH et al. Signs in thoracic imaging. *J Thorac Imaging* 2006; 21: 76–90.

52. Hansell DM. High-resolution CT of diffuse lung disease: Value and limitations. *Radiol Clin North Am* 2001; 39: 1091–1113.

53. Rossi SE, Erasmus JJ, Volpacchio M et al. "Crazy-paving" pattern at thin-section ct of the lungs: Radiologic-pathologic overview. *Radiographics* 2003; 23: 1509–1519.

54. Gotway MB, Reddy GP, Webb WR et al. High-resolution CT of the lung: Patterns of disease and differential diagnoses. *Radiol Clin N Am* 2005; 43: 513–542.

55. Talmadge E. King Clinical Advances in the diagnosis and therapy of interstitial lung disease. *Am J Respir Crit Care Med* 2005; 172: 268–279.

56. Cormack FX. Lymphangioleiomyomatosis: a clinical update. *Chest* 2008; 133: 507–516.

57. Bissler JJ, Kingswood JC. Renal angiomyolipomata. *Kidney Int* 2004; 66: 924–934.

58. Seaman DM, Meyer CA, Gilman MD et al. Diffuse cystic lung disease at high-resolution CT. *AJR Am J Roentgenol* 2011; 196: 1305–1311.

59. Mohr LC. Hypersensitivity pneumonitis. *Curr Opin Pulm Med* 2004; 10: 401–411.

60. Silver SF, Müller NL, Miller RR et al. Hypersensitivity pneumonitis: Evaluation with CT. *Radiology* 1989; 173: 441–445.

61. Hansell DM, Wells AU, Padley SP et al. Hypersensitivity pneumonitis: Correlation of individual CT patterns with functional abnormalities. *Radiology* 1996; 199: 123–128.

62. Patel RA, Sellami D, Gotway MB et al. Hypersensitivity pneumonitis: patterns on high-resolution CT. *J Comput Assist Tomogr* 2000; 24: 965–970.

63. Vassallo R, Jensen EA, Colby TV et al. The overlap between respiratory bronchiolitis and desquamative interstitial pneumonia in pulmonary Langerhans cell histiocytosis: High-resolution CT, histologic, and functional correlations. *Chest* 2003; 124: 1199–1205.

64. Hansell DM, Nicholson AG. Smoking-related diffuse parenchymal lung disease: HRCT-pathologic correlation. *Semin Respir Crit Care Med* 2003; 24: 377–392.

65. Attili AK, Kazerooni EA, Gross BH et al. Smoking-related interstitial lung disease: Radiologic-clinical-pathologic correlation. *Radiographics* 2008; 28: 1383–1396.

66. Brauner MW, Grenier P, Tijani K et al. Pulmonary Langerhans cell histiocytosis: Evolution of lesions on CT scans. *Radiology* 1997; 204: 497–502.

67. Pinto PS. The CT Halo Sign. *Radiology* 2004; 230: 109–110.

68. Castañer E, Alguersuari A, Gallardo X et al. When to suspect pulmonary vasculitis: Radiologic and clinical clues. *Radiographics* 2010; 30: 33–53.

69. Silva CI, Muller NL, Fujimoto K et al. Churg-Strauss syndrome: High resolution CT and pathologic findings. *J Thorac Imaging* 2005; 20: 74–80.

23

Pulmonary Neoplasms of the Lung

Jin Mo Goo

CONTENTS

23.1 Introduction

Among various pulmonary neoplasms, identification of lung cancer is important because lung cancer is the leading cause of cancer-related mortality in many countries. In the detection, characterization, staging, and monitoring of treatment response of lung neoplasms, imaging plays an essential role. However, the radiological evaluation of pulmonary neoplasms is complex.

Management decisions are based on clinical history, radiological findings of the lesion, and feasibility of obtaining a tissue diagnosis.

23.2 Radiological Manifestations

23.2.1 Masses and Nodules

A nodule is a rounded opacity, well or poorly defined, measuring up to 3 cm in diameter, whereas a mass is an opacity greater than 3 cm in diameter [1]. With the increased detection of solitary pulmonary nodules (SPNs), their characterization is a major concern because malignant lesions account for only 60%–80% of resected pulmonary nodules [2,3]. Several morphologic features are often diagnostically helpful although they may not be specific for lung cancer.

23.2.1.1 Characterization

23.2.1.1.1 Size and Shape

Lung cancer can manifest as a solitary nodule of any size; however, cancer probability has been shown to be closely related to size. Generally, a nodule smaller than 5 mm in diameter has a very low probability of cancer [4]. In the cases of masses of 30 mm or larger, cancer probability is considerably high. Masses that are not primary or metastatic cancers prove to be lung abscess, Wegener's granulomatosis, lymphoma, round pneumonia, and round atelectasis (Figure 23.1).

Certain shapes have been shown to provide important diagnostic information. Irregular edges are known to be highly probable in lung cancer, and a spiculated border in which numerous strands radiate into the surrounding lung is almost specific of lung cancer (Figure 23.2). Furthermore, it has been shown that the more pronounced the lobulation or notching, the greater the likelihood that the lesion is lung cancer (Figure 23.3). In contrast, a well-defined, smooth border has been shown to be most compatible with a benign lesion, such as hamartoma or granuloma, and has been rarely seen in lung cancer (Figure 23.4). However, this shape is also frequently seen in pulmonary metastasis (Figure 23.5).

23.2.1.1.2 Cavitation

A cavity is defined as "gas-filled space within pulmonary consolidation, nodule, or mass" [1] and is usually produced by expulsion of necrotic part of the lesion via the bronchial tree. As many pathological processes appearing as SPNs can show cavitation, the presence of cavitation does not indicate any specific disease. However, the morphology of a cavity may yet be helpful. Benign lesions including lung abscess generally show a thinner, smoother wall, whereas cavitary lung cancer usually shows a thick wall with uneven thickness (Figure 23.6). Woodring and Fried [5] reported that among 32 cases with a maximum wall thickness

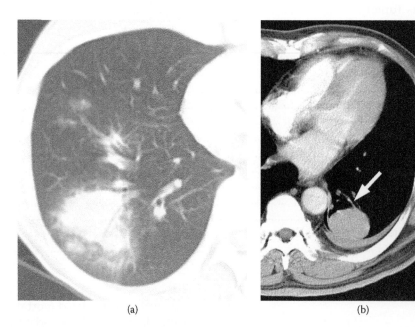

(a)   (b)

FIGURE 23.1

(a) Wegener's granulomatosis. Contrast-enhanced computed tomography (CT) showing a 4.4 cm large lobulating mass with an air bronchogram and peripheral halo in the right lower lobe. Biopsy revealed Wegener's granulomatosis. (b) Round atelectasis. Contrast-enhanced computed tomography showing a 4 cm well-enhancing mass in the left lower lobe. Note the curvilinear configuration of the vessels around the mass (arrow) and pleural thickening adjacent to the mass.

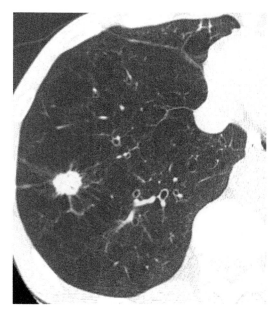

FIGURE 23.2
Squamous cell carcinoma showing a spiculated border. Note emphysema in the lung.

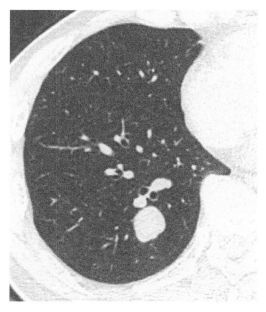

FIGURE 23.4
Hamartoma with a well-defined border. Because of the slow growth of the nodule over 7 years, surgical resection of the nodules was performed and pathology revealed hamartoma.

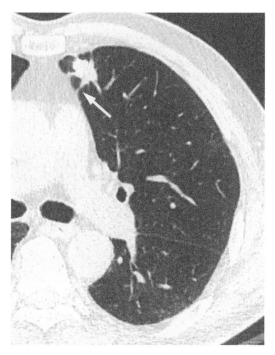

FIGURE 23.3
Adenocarcinoma with a lobulated border and pleural tails (arrow).

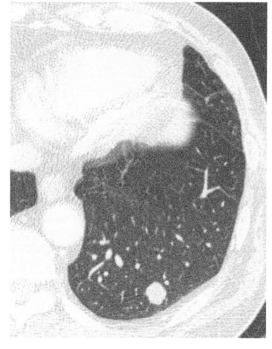

FIGURE 23.5
Metastatic nodule from colon cancer showing a well-defined border.

of 4 mm or less, only 2 were malignant neoplasms and 30 were benign. In practice, the diagnosis of acute lung abscess can usually be made with the clinical features along with morphologic features such as a cavitary lesion occurring in an area of undoubted pneumonia. The more difficult problem is to distinguish a cavitary neoplasm from chronic inflammatory processes. Tuberculosis, fungal pneumonia such as cryptococcosis, Wegener's granulomatosis, and rheumatoid arthritis are several conditions in which cavitary lesions may mimic cavitary lung cancer, and may sometimes be clinically indistinguishable.

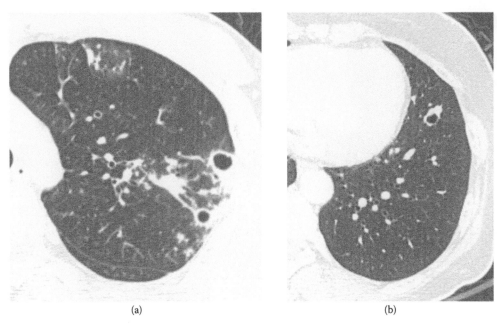

(a)   (b)

FIGURE 23.6
(a) Cavitary nodules. Active pulmonary tuberculosis showing multiple thin-walled cavities, nodule, and tree-in-bud lesions. (b) Cavitary adenocarcinoma. Although the nodule size is small, the nodule has a lobulated border and the cavity wall has uneven thickness.

23.2.1.1.3 Calcification

SPNs may present with various kinds of calcifications, which can aid in deducing a more specific diagnosis: concentric (laminated), popcorn, uniform homogeneous, and punctate. Concentric (laminated) calcification suggests tuberculosis or fungal granulomas (Figure 23.7). Popcorn calcifications, seen as small randomly distributed ring- and arc-shaped calcifications, are specific to hamartoma and cartilage tumors (Figure 23.8). Uniform homogeneous calcification within an SPN is nearly diagnostic of calcified granuloma and excludes the diagnosis of lung cancer (Figure 23.9) [6]. Punctate calcification can occur in both benign and malignant lesions (Figure 23.10). Granulomas, hamartomas, and amyloid deposits may contain punctate calcifications, but malignancies such as carcinoids or metastases particularly osteosarcoma may also have punctate calcifications. It should be kept in mind that lung cancer can show calcification by engulfing preexisting calcified granulomas, producing mucin or forming dystrophic calcification in intratumoral necrosis. Osteosarcoma and chondrosarcoma are the best known malignant tumors that give rise to calcification or ossification by bone formation in tumor osteoid and ossification of tumor cartilage. Calcified pulmonary metastatic nodules may also arise in papillary carcinomas of the thyroid and the ovary or mucinous adenocarcinomas of the gastrointestinal (GI) tract and breast [7]. After chemotherapy or radiotherapy, dystrophic calcification may also develop within areas of necrosis, degeneration, or hemorrhage of tumors. If lesion is larger than 3 cm,

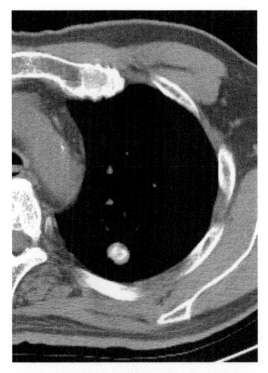

FIGURE 23.7
Concentric calcification within a nodule suggesting benign granuloma.

shows an irregular or spiculated border, or grows at a rate compatible with lung cancer, we should not assume nodules to be benign solely for the reason that they show calcification [6]. For the detection of calcification within a nodule, computed tomography (CT) has shown

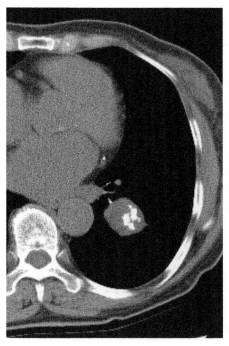

FIGURE 23.8
Popcorn calcification within a nodule that is consistent with chondroid hamartoma.

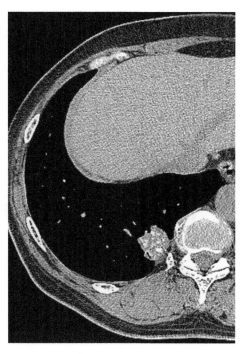

FIGURE 23.10
Metastatic rectal cancer showing punctate calcifications within the nodule.

23.2.1.1.4 Growth Rate

The volume doubling time of lung cancer (an increase in diameter of 26%) is 1–18 months with an average of 4.2–7.3 months, depending on cell type. Therefore, if the doubling time of a certain nodule is faster than 1 month or slower than 18 months, the diagnosis of lung cancer is usually unlikely. The absence of detectable growth over a 2-year period of observation is a reliable criterion for establishing that a nodule is benign [8] except for ground-glass nodules (GGNs).

Determining growth in small subcentimeter nodule is difficult. Recent studies revealed that computer-aided volumetry can provide more accurate and reproducible measurement of nodules than manual measurements [9]. By calculating doubling time using these tools, malignant nodules can be effectively differentiated from benign nodules [10], and the NELSON randomized lung cancer screening trial employed the volumetric nodule assessment in the nodule management protocol [11]. However, it is important to understand that there can be measurement variability in applying this technique. Several studies that used a same-day repeat CT protocol in patients with lung nodules revealed that the 95% confidence intervals for the difference in measured volumes can be up to 26% [9].

23.2.1.1.5 Dynamic Contrast Enhancement

Malignant nodules show a greater degree of contrast enhancement with iodinated contrast media than benign

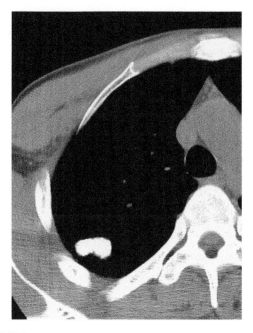

FIGURE 23.9
Uniform homogeneous calcification within the nodule that is consistent with calcified granuloma.

far better performance than chest radiograph. However, care should be taken so as not to misdiagnose artificial high attenuation at the small nodule's edge as calcification on high-frequency reconstruction algorithms (Figure 23.11).

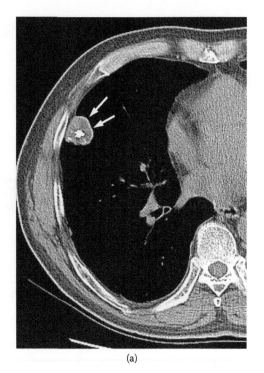
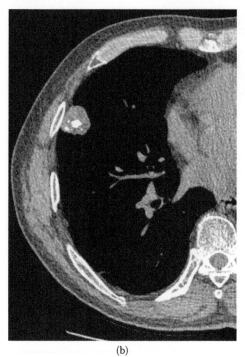

(a)   (b)

FIGURE 23.11
Thin high-attenuation rim (arrows) around a nodule is seen when CT scan is reconstructed with a high-frequency algorithm (a). When the CT scan is reconstructed with a standard algorithm, this high-attenuation rim disappears (b).

nodules. This enhancement is thought to be due to the phenomenon of angiogenesis. According to Swensen et al. [12], this enhancement of SPNs can be used as a very useful differentiation of lung cancer from a benign nodule. They reported that SPNs, which enhance less than 15 HU on each image obtained at 1, 2, 3, and 4 minutes, are indicative of a benign nodule. In studies using combined wash-in and washout characteristics on dynamic contrast-enhanced CT, when diagnostic criteria of a wash-in of ≥25 HU and a washout of 5–31 HU were applied for malignant nodules, sensitivity, specificity, and accuracy for malignancy were 81%–94%, 90%–93%, and 85%–92%, respectively [13,14].

23.2.1.1.6 Ground-Glass Nodules

A GGN is a focal hazy increased attenuation in the lung that does not obliterate the bronchial and vascular margins [1]. If a nodule has a combination of both ground-glass opacity (GGO) and solid components, it is called "part-solid" GGN. As a separate category from purely solid nodules, the term "subsolid" nodule can be used that includes both pure GGN and part-solid GGN (Figure 23.12).

A substantial proportion of GGNs has been reported to be transient [15]. Thus, when encountering a GGN on CT, it is necessary to rule out the possibility of transient lesion. Peripheral blood eosinophilia, ill-defined border, and newly occurring lesion on a follow-up scan

can be important features in suspecting transient lesion (Figure 23.13) [15].

Persistent GGNs on CT have shown a good correlation with lung adenocarcinoma, from atypical adenomatous hyperplasia (AAH) to invasive adenocarcinoma [16–18]. GGNs have higher malignant likelihood than solid nodules at screening CT [19], represent the lepidic component in adenocarcinoma on histology, and indicate a better prognosis in patients with lung adenocarcinoma [18]. In the Early Lung Cancer Action Project, Henschke et al. [19] reported that the malignancy rates of part-solid GGNs and pure GGNs were 64% and 18%, respectively, whereas the malignancy rate of solid nodule was 7%. GGNs, especially when ground-glass proportion is predominant, typically show a slow growth rate despite their high potential for malignancy. The relative proportion of ground glass is a good prognostic marker and also correlates well with recurrence, vascular invasion, nodal metastasis, and survival [18].

23.2.2 Atelectasis and Consolidation

Atelectasis is reduced inflation of the lung and is a frequent secondary sign of airway obstruction by lung malignancy. Obstructive atelectasis can result from the blockage of airway, by absorption of alveolar gas into circulating blood without replacement by inspired gas. Direct signs of atelectasis include increased

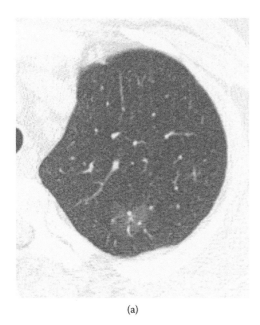

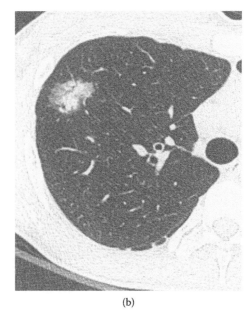

(a)	(b)

FIGURE 23.12
If there is no solid component within a ground-glass nodule, the nodule is called pure ground-glass nodule (a). If there is some solid component with a ground-glass nodule, it is called part-solid ground-glass nodule (b). They can be collectively called subsolid nodule.

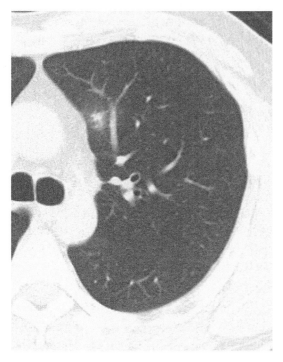

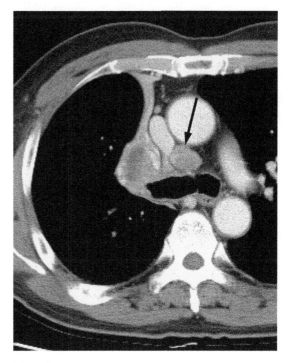

FIGURE 23.13
Transient ground-glass nodule. Part-solid ground glass nodule in the left upper lobe disappeared at 1-month follow-up CT scan. This patient had peripheral blood eosinophilia.

FIGURE 23.14
Atelectasis in the right upper lobe caused by squamous cell carcinoma obstructing lobar bronchus. Note the enlarged right paratracheal lymph node (arrow).

opacification of the airless lobe, displacement of the interlobar fissures, and crowding of bronchi and vessels with the area of atelectasis (Figure 23.14). Indirect signs are related to mechanisms that compensate for the reduction in intrapleural pressure—diaphragmatic elevation, mediastinal shift, approximation of ribs, and overinflation of the remainder of the lung.

Consolidation appears as an area of homogeneous increased attenuation that obscures the margins of vessels and airway walls [1]. In addition to

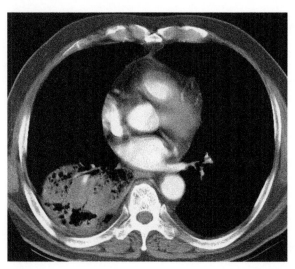

FIGURE 23.15
Consolidation in the right lower lobe due to adenocarcinoma. Airways are patent and the patient had no symptoms of pneumonia.

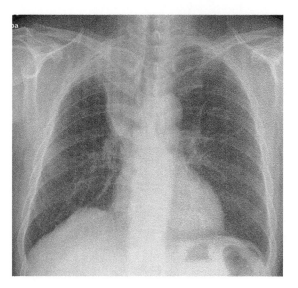

FIGURE 23.16
Inverted S-sign caused by atelectasis in the right upper lobe and a central bulging mass.

postobstructive consolidation due to malignancies, mucinous adenocarcinoma and lymphoma are malignant neoplasm that may present as chronic consolidations (Figure 23.15). Lymphangitic metastasis is a rare cause of the entity. Mucinous adenocarcinoma tumors grow along the alveolar wall without destroying the underlying architecture, so-called lepidic growth, combined with copious secretion of mucin, which results in consolidation. In the cases with areas of consolidation, lung cancer should be suspected if the clinical symptoms and signs of pneumonia are absent, and there is no radiological improvement despite appropriate antibiotic therapy over 2–4 weeks.

23.3 Lung Cancer

Lung cancer is the leading cause of cancer-related deaths worldwide, with a 5-year survival rate of only 15% [20]. The probability to develop lung cancer is strongly associated with certain risk factors and cigarette smoking is the most important one. Other risk factors include exposure to asbestos, radioactive radon, nickel, chromium, and arsenic.

23.3.1 Imaging Modalities

23.3.1.1 Chest Radiography

Despite the known diagnostic superiority and increasing availability of cross-sectional techniques, chest radiography is the mainstay of chest imaging. Chest radiographs still play an important role as a fast tool to detect and monitor various chest disease with low cost and low radiation exposure.

Lung cancers are often detected on a routine chest radiograph in a person without any symptoms. Lung cancer on chest radiography can be seen as nodules, masses, consolidation, or atelectasis (Figure 23.16). Other possible clues are enlarged lymph nodes and pleural effusion. However, chest radiography is an insensitive tool for detecting early and small lung cancers [21,22], and several randomized trials using chest radiographs failed to detect a significant reduction in lung cancer mortality [23–27].

In addition to the introduction of digital radiography and advanced techniques such as dual energy subtraction, digital tomosynthesis and computer-aided detection may play an increasing role in better detection and interpretation of chest radiographs [28].

23.3.1.2 Computed Tomography

CT provides the information regarding the location and features of the lesion and depicts associated findings to help document the extent of disease. Based on this information, appropriate surgical planning can be established. Important findings of tumors to note are whether tumor involves the major airways, fissures, chest wall, diaphragm, pericardium, and mediastinal structures.

In the evaluation of the chest wall and mediastinal invasion, the tumor extension into the tissues of the chest wall, rib destruction by the tumor (Figure 23.17), and encasement of the mediastinal structures by the tumor (Figure 23.18) are obvious sign for the

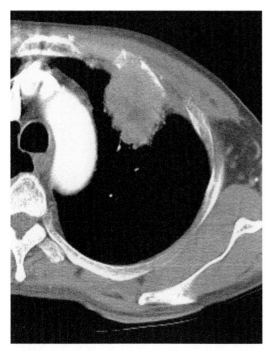

FIGURE 23.17
Contrast-enhanced CT scan showing a left upper lobe mass destructing the adjacent rib.

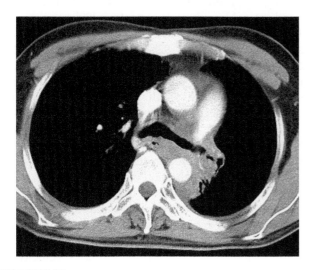

FIGURE 23.18
Descending aorta encased by the tumor, which is an obvious sign of mediastinal involvement.

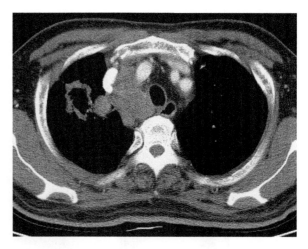

FIGURE 23.19
Cavitary lung cancer in the right upper lobe with extensive mediastinal lymph node enlargement.

chest wall or mediastinal invasion. In other cases, extent of tumors with chest wall or mediastinal structures can be considered for potential findings of invasion. In determining chest wall invasion, the sensitivity and specificity of CT are reported to range from 38% to 87% and 40% to 89%, respectively [29]. In identifying mediastinal invasion, the sensitivity, specificity, and accuracy of CT have been reported to vary from 40% to 84%, 57% to 94%, and 56% to 89%, respectively [30].

Nodal staging on CT requires identification of enlarged lymph nodes and assignment of these to particular stations. Lymph node size is the criterion most often used for distinguishing normal from abnormal nodes (Figure 23.19). A short-axis diameter of 10 mm is considered the upper limit of normal lymph node size [31]. Unfortunately, CT has a limited value in nodal staging, with reported sensitivities, specificities, and accuracies ranging between 46% and 87%, 69% and 89%, and 65% and 84%, respectively [29].

Among various sites of metastases from lung cancer, adrenal metastases can be easily identified on chest CT, with a reported detection rate as high as 20% at initial presentation [30]. CT is also an effective imaging modality that can exclude benign adrenal adenomas, which are a large proportion of cases of nodular adrenal enlargement. An adrenal mass is considered benign if it has an attenuation value of less than 10 HU on an unenhanced CT scan [32].

23.3.1.3 Magnetic Resonance

Despite advances in magnetic resonance (MR) techniques, the lung remains a challenge for MR. For lung cancer, evaluation of superior sulcus tumor and assessment of possible invasion of the spinal canal are established indications for chest MR. When the extent of tumor invasion is unclear by CT, MR can play an important role in defining degrees of invasion. Because MR is superior to CT in the visualization of cardiovascular structures, it can be used for assessing invasion of the major vessels and heart [33]. In addition to static MR images, tumor invasion to the mediastinum and chest wall can be assessed with cine MR images

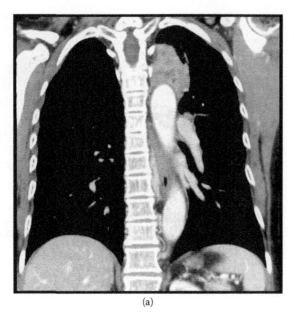
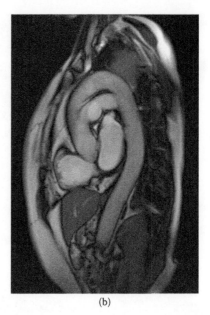

(a)   (b)

FIGURE 23.20
Because there is broad contact between the tumor and aortic arch on coronal reformatted CT, invasion of the aorta by the tumor is suspected (a). On oblique sagittal magnetic resonance, although there is broad contact between the tumor and aorta (b), sliding motion was preserved between two structures at cine MR. Surgical resection of the tumor was performed and there was no invasion of the aorta by the tumor.

(Figure 23.20) [34,35]. MR can distinguish the lung mass from the adjacent atelectasis or consolidation, and areas of changes after radiation therapy.

In assessment of mediastinal lymph node metastasis, MR with short tau inversion-recovery turbo spin-echo sequences showed better sensitivity and accuracy than positron emission tomography (PET)/CT [36]. In detection of brain metastasis, the sensitivity of MR (88%) is significantly higher than that of PET/CT (24%) [37].

23.3.1.4 Positron Emission Tomography

F-18 fluorodeoxyglucose (FDG) PET is effective for assessing the metabolic activity of primary tumor and may indicate tumor aggressiveness. Maximum standardized uptake value (SUV) has a prognostic value independent of clinical staging. Adenocarcinoma in situ (AIS), formerly bronchioloalveolar carcinoma (BAC), and carcinoid tumor may not be hypermetabolic on PET because of their low metabolic activity, and a false-negative rate of 40% has been reported in PET studies of patients with AIS (Figure 23.21) [38]. In addition, small lung cancers less than 1 cm in size do not show hot uptake on PET scan.

FDG-PET is an effective tool in identifying mediastinal lymph node metastasis, which is more accurate (reported accuracy, 81%–96%) than CT [30]. PET has a

high negative predictive value of 98.4% in the evaluation of mediastinal lymph node metastasis [39].

PET is effective for the identification of adrenal metastasis with greater than 92% accuracy (Figure 23.22). However, false-positive findings have been obtained with adenoma and pheochromocytoma, and false-negative results with small lesions, or lesions with hemorrhage or necrosis. In assessing brain metastasis, FDG-PET/CT has difficulty in differentiating FDG-avid focus from the normal hypermetabolic gray matter. PET imaging is more sensitive than traditional bone scintigraphy in the evaluation of bone metastasis, especially in cases of early marrow metastasis. PET/CT has limitation in the evaluation of liver and kidney metastases. Diagnostic accuracy of PET imaging for pleural metastasis is promising, with sensitivity of 92%–100%, negative predictive value of 100%, and specificity of 67%–71% [40]. Clinically unsuspected distant metastases have been found in up to 28% of patients who underwent PET studies [40].

23.3.2 Staging

Lung cancer stating is important for establishing effective treatment options and prognosis of lung cancer. Staging of lung cancer is based on the tumor, node, and metastasis (TNM) classification for describing the anatomical extent of disease. In 2009, the new TNM staging classification (7th edition) for lung cancer was

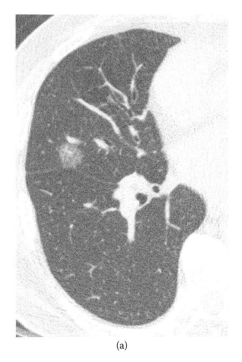
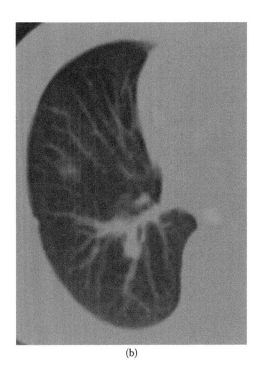

(a) (b)

FIGURE 23.21
(a) CT scan showing a pure ground-glass nodule in the right middle lobe that turned out to be adenocarcinoma. (b) FDG-PET/CT shows a mild FDG uptake (maximum SUV, 1.7) for this lesion.

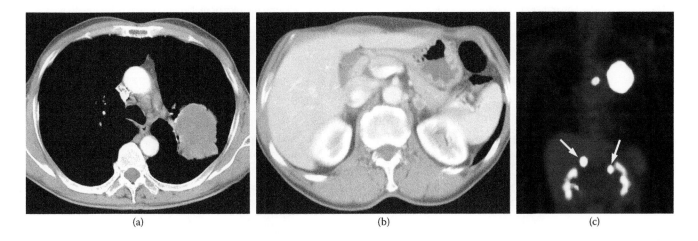

(a) (b) (c)

FIGURE 23.22
(a) Contrast-enhanced CT showing a mass in the left upper lobe with an enlarged left lower paratracheal lymph node. (b) CT scan of the upper abdomen showing bilateral adrenal nodular enlargement (only left adrenal gland is covered on this scan) with central area of low attenuation. (c) FDG-PET scan shows FDG uptake in the lung mass, mediastinal lymph node, and bilateral adrenal glands (arrows).

published by the Union Internationale Contre le Cancer and the American Joint Committee on Cancer [41] (Table 23.1). The new system is based on evidence obtained from large global database with extensive validation [42–44], and the major determinant chosen for development of subgroups of TNM descriptors as well as the stage grouping was the overall survival based on the best stage. In addition to non-small cell lung cancer

(NSCLC), this classification system will be used in staging both small cell lung cancer (SCLC) and bronchopulmonary carcinoid tumors.

The tumor (T) descriptor is determined by the size measured in the long-axis diameter, degree of locoregional invasion (Figure 23.23), endobronchial location (Figure 23.24), and the presence of separate tumor nodules (Figure 23.25). In cases with multiple tumors, if the

TABLE 23.1

Definitions for TNM Descriptors

Descriptors	Definitions
T	Primary tumor
T0	No primary tumor
T1	Tumor ≤3 cm, surrounded by lung or visceral pleura, not more proximal than the lobar bronchus
T1a	Tumor ≤2 cm
T1b	Tumor >2 cm but ≤3 cm
T2	Tumor >3 cm but ≤7 cm or tumor with any of the following: Invades visceral pleura, involves main bronchus ≥2 cm distal to the carina, atelectasis/obstructive pneumonia extending to hilum but not involving the entire lung
T2a	Tumor >3 cm but ≤5 cm
T2b	Tumor >5 cm but ≤7 cm
T3	Tumor >7 cm; or directly invading chest wall, diaphragm, phrenic nerve, mediastinal pleura, or parietal pericardium; or tumor in the main bronchus <2 cm distal to the carina; or atelectasis/obstructive pneumonitis of entire lung; or separate tumor nodules in the same lobe
T4	Tumor of any size with invasion of heart, great vessels, trachea, recurrent laryngeal nerve, esophagus, vertebral body, or carina; or separate tumor nodules in a different ipsilateral lobe
N	Regional lymph nodes
N0	No regional node metastasis
N1	Metastasis in ipsilateral peribronchial and/or perihilar lymph nodes and intrapulmonary nodes, including involvement by direct extension
N2	Metastasis in ipsilateral mediastinal and/or subcarinal lymph nodes
N3	Metastasis in contralateral mediastinal, contralateral hilar, ipsilateral, or contralateral scalene, or supraclavicular lymph nodes
M	Distant metastasis
M0	No distant metastasis
M1a	Separate tumor nodules in a contralateral lobe; or tumor with pleural nodules or malignant pleural dissemination
M1b	Distant metastasis

Source: Detterbeck FC, Boffa DJ, Tanoue LT, *Chest*, 2009, 136, 260–271.

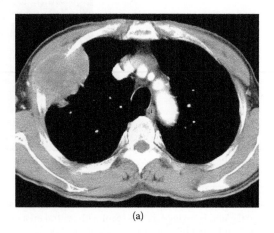 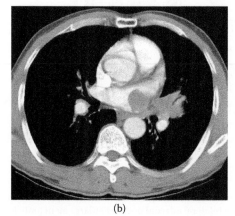

         (a)   (b)

FIGURE 23.23

CT evaluation of regional extent. Peripheral mass in the right upper lobe invading the chest wall with destruction of the adjacent rib indicate T3 lesion (a). Direct extension of the tumor into the left atrium through the left pulmonary vein indicates that this lesion is T4 (b).

tumors are of different histological cell types, they can be considered as synchronous primary lung cancers. If multiple tumors are of the same cell type, to make a diagnosis of synchronous primary lung cancers, histological subtypes should be different and there should be no evidence of mediastinal nodal metastases or nodal metastases within a common nodal drainage. Synchronous primary tumors are staged separately and the highest T category should be designated.

The nodal (N) descriptor refers to the involvement of the regional lymph nodes that extend from the supraclavicular region to the diaphragm. A nodal chart has been established to classify lymph nodes into seven specific zones: supraclavicular, upper, aortopulmonary, subcarinal,

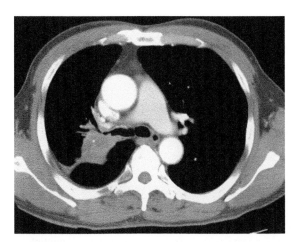

FIGURE 23.24
Contrast-enhanced computed tomography scan showing the extent of tumor involving the right main bronchus less than 2 cm distal to the carina (T3 lesion).

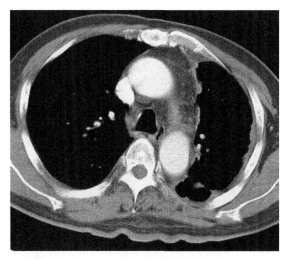

FIGURE 23.26
Multiple irregular nodular pleural thickening in the left hemithorax indicates M1a disease.

skeletal system are the most likely sites of metastatic disease in patients with lung cancer. Pleural metastasis and metastasis in the contralateral lung are also classified as M1a category (Figure 23.26).

23.3.3 Histological Subtypes

Lung cancer is classified as either NSCLC or SCLC. The prevalence of the various histological subtypes of NSCLC has changed in recent decades [47,48], and adenocarcinoma is the predominant type of lung cancer followed by squamous cell carcinoma.

23.3.3.1 Adenocarcinoma

Since Noguchi's classification [49], studies have been done on radiological-histological correlations of lung adenocarcinoma [16,17,50].

AAH is a preinvasive lesion for lung adenocarcinoma and appears as a well-defined, round or oval, pure GGN usually ≤5 mm in size (Figure 23.27) [51]. AIS, formerly BAC, is defined as a localized adenocarcinoma ≤3 cm that exhibits a lepidic pattern with neoplastic cells along the alveolar structures without stromal, vascular, or pleural invasion [52]. AIS presents typically as a pure GGN or a part-solid nodule (Figure 23.28) [18]. Recently, a new concept of minimally invasive adenocarcinoma (MIA) has been introduced, and patients with AIS or MIA subjected to complete resection may expect 100% or near 100% disease-specific survival [52]. MIA is defined as a solitary adenocarcinoma ≤3 cm, with a predominantly lepidic pattern and with an invasive component ≤5 mm in greatest dimension. CT features of pure GGN or part-solid nodules are suggestive of AIS, MIA, or lepidic predominant adenocarcinoma. Invasive adenocarcinoma is usually a solid nodule or mass with a variable

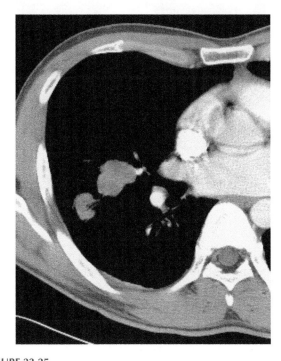

FIGURE 23.25
A separate nodule adjacent to the main tumor indicates that T stage for this tumor is T3.

lower, hilar-interlobar, and peripheral. More favorable outcome has been reported in patients with nodal skip metastases, particularly the presence of N2 disease in the absence of N1 disease, and upper-lobe tumors are thought to be most frequently associated with these [45].

The metastasis (M) descriptor is determined by the presence or absence of metastatic disease within or outside the thorax. Extrathoracic metastasis in NSCLC is common, occurring in 40% of patients, at the time of diagnosis [46]. The brain, liver, adrenal glands, and

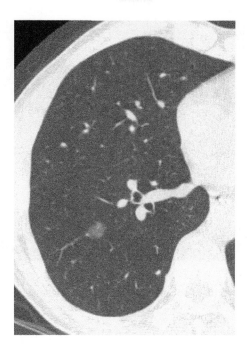

FIGURE 23.27
Atypical adenomatous hyperplasia shown as a well-defined pure ground-glass nodule.

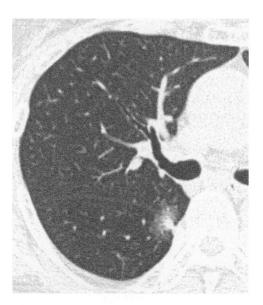

FIGURE 23.28
Adenocarcinoma in situ shown as a part-solid ground-glass nodule.

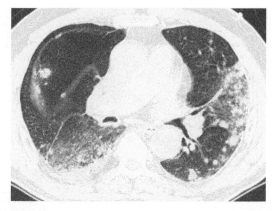

FIGURE 23.29
Adenocarcinoma with lepidic pattern shown as multiple poorly defined nodules and areas of ground-glass opacity in both lungs.

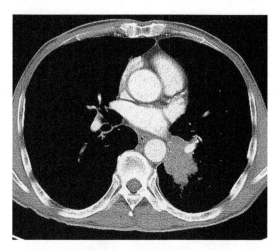

FIGURE 23.30
Squamous cell carcinoma obstructing the left lower lobar bronchus.

extent of GGO. The GGO component is correlated with a lepidic pattern and solid component with an invasive pattern. Therefore, the extent of GGO and favorable prognosis appear positively correlated and adenocarcinoma manifested as GGN usually shows a long doubling time [18]. A marginal characteristic of thick spiculation is associated with lymph node metastasis, vascular invasion, and subsequent decrease in survival [50]. Invasive mucinous adenocarcinoma can be seen as nodules to lobar consolidation with areas of low attenuation because of its mucoid component. CT angiogram sign, which is well visualization of pulmonary vessels in the areas of consolidation, has been described [53]. Adenocarcinoma sometimes spread through the airways and mimic pneumonia with patchy peribronchial or lobar consolidation (Figure 23.29).

23.3.3.2 Squamous Cell Carcinoma

Squamous cell lung cancer is found mainly among older males in close association with smoking [48,54]. Approximately, 60%–70% of squamous cell carcinomas originate from the central bronchi and are localized at the bronchial wall at the early stages, leading to difficulties in radiological detection [54,55]. As a result, malignant cells can be found in sputum cytology, even in cases where no definite mass is evident during radiological evaluation.

When squamous cell carcinoma involves the central bronchi, atelectasis is the most common secondary sign (Figure 23.30). The tumor itself or enlarged lymph nodes may appear on the chest radiography. Occasionally, the primary mass cannot be visualized since it is surrounded by the collapsed lung. The huge central tumor and atelectasis in the distal area are present as the typical Golden S sign (Figure 23.14). The Golden S sign is composed of the convex contour of the primary mass and concave contour of the elevated minor fissure.

The central tumor can expand toward the mediastinum, and can invade mediastinal and bony structures. Tumors invading the great vessels can induce superior vena cava (SVC) syndrome (Figure 23.31), and by invading the phrenic or recurrent laryngeal nerves, elevated diaphragm or hoarseness can occur.

Approximately 30%–40% of squamous cell carcinoma is located in the peripheral portion of the lung (Figure 23.2) [54]. The margin of this type of tumor is irregular or may show lobulating contours. Central necrosis is frequent and often extensive (Figure 23.32).

Drainage of necrotic material leads to cavitation in many cases. Cavitating cancer occurs more frequently in squamous cell carcinoma than other cell types. Most of the cavities have a relatively thick wall and sometimes show mass-like lesions protruding from the wall. This cavitating cancer can occur either in the central or peripheral area and varies in size from 1 to 10 cm in diameter with 0.5–3.0 cm thick walls. The inner surface is usually irregular as a result of variably sized nodules of neoplastic tissue projecting into the cavity and the patchy nature of necrosis. Cavitating cancer can be confused with lung abscess or occasionally with pulmonary tuberculosis. Occasionally, this cavitating cancer displays a very thin wall, simulating a bulla or bronchial cyst. Sometimes, free necrotic debris in the cavity can be separated from the cavity wall, simulating a fungus ball.

23.3.3.3 Large Cell Lung Cancer

Large cell carcinoma accounts for 10%–15% of lung cancers [56] and shows rapid growth with early metastasis. Large cell neuroendocrine carcinoma is a subtype of large cell carcinoma and is a high-grade, poorly differentiated neuroendocrine tumor. It usually presents as a large peripheral mass but may also be central tumors (Figure 23.33). Large cell neuroendocrine carcinoma usually appears as a well-defined, lobulated mass with necrosis [57].

23.3.3.4 Small Cell Lung Cancer

Small cell carcinoma is a neuroendocrine tumor and constitutes approximately 15% of all lung cancers [58]. Unlike NSCLC, SCLC is seen almost exclusively in

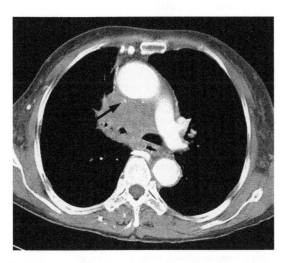

FIGURE 23.31
Squamous cell carcinoma encasing the right main bronchus extends into the mediastinum. The superior vena cava (arrow) is nearly obliterated by the mass.

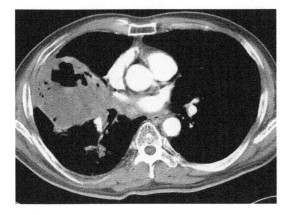

FIGURE 23.32
Large squamous cell carcinoma obstructing the right middle lobar bronchus shows extensive necrosis and cavitation.

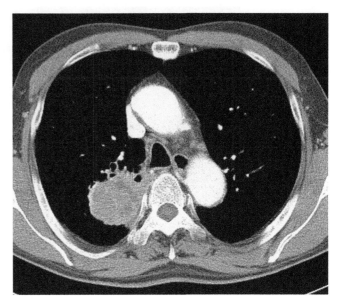

FIGURE 23.33
Large cell carcinoma shown as a heterogeneous mass.

smokers and is known for its rapid doubling time, early development of metastatic disease, and initial sensitivity to chemotherapy and radiation therapy [59]. Despite its initial response to treatment, the long-term survival of patients with SCLC is much worse than that of patients with NSCLC [59].

SCLC typically presents as a large central mass and bulky hilar and mediastinal lymphadenopathy (Figure 23.34) (90%–95%) while presentation as a

peripheral lung nodule is uncommon [60]. Along with compression of the central airways, SCLC can compress and invade mediastinal vascular structures causing SVC syndrome (Figure 23.35).

23.3.3.5 Carcinoid Tumors

Carcinoid tumors are malignant neuroendocrine tumors that are divided into typical and atypical subtypes based on pathological criteria. Carcinoid tumors are one of the neuroendocrine tumors of the lung that range from low-grade typical carcinoid tumors to intermediate-grade atypical carcinoid tumors and high-grade small cell carcinomas and large cell carcinomas.

Most carcinoid tumors arise centrally and appear as a round or ovoid hilar or perihilar soft tissue causing atelectasis or mucoid impaction. The endobronchial component may be relatively small compared to the bulk of the tumor resulting in so-called "iceberg" tumor (Figure 23.36). Most carcinoids are hypervascular and may demonstrate intense enhancement. Peripheral carcinoid tumors comprise 15%–40% of carcinoid tumors (Figure 23.37) [61]. Both the central and peripheral carcinoids show diffuse or punctuate calcifications in 30% of cases on CT [60,62]. Compared with typical carcinoid tumors, atypical carcinoids tend to be larger in diameter and show more frequent lymph node metastasis [60]. However, imaging features of typical and atypical carcinoids are hard to be separated. On FDG-PET, carcinoids usually have lower FDG uptake than usual malignant tumors.

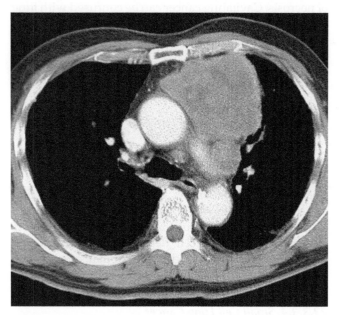

FIGURE 23.34
Small cell lung cancer shown as massive mediastinal lymphadenopathy.

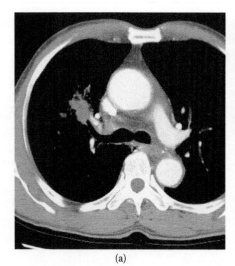

(a)

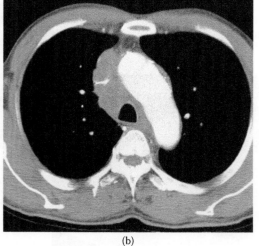

(b)

FIGURE 23.35
The anterior segmental bronchus of the right upper lobe obstructed by small cell lung cancer (a) and the superior vena cava compressed by extensive mediastinal lymph nodes (b).

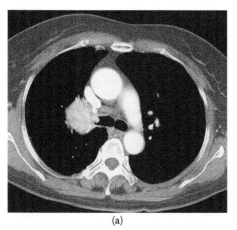
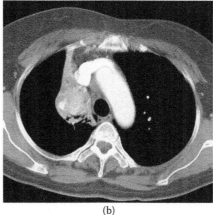
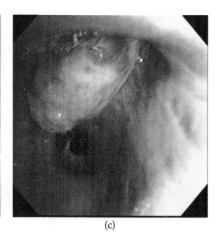

(a) (b) (c)

FIGURE 23.36
Carcinoid tumor shown as a well-enhanced mass with a small endobronchial component (a) and calcification (b). Bronchoscopy demonstrates an endobronchial tumor (c).

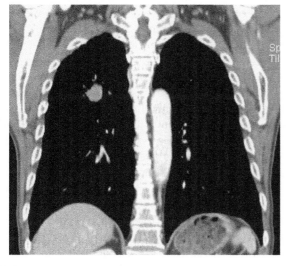

FIGURE 23.37
Atypical carcinoid tumor shown as a well-enhancing solitary pulmonary nodule.

23.3.3.6 Other Malignant Tumors

Adenosquamous cell carcinoma is usually peripherally located tumor and can show areas of necrosis, cavitation, and calcification [63,64]. Pleomorphic carcinoma usually manifests as a large peripheral mass with a central low-attenuation area and frequently invades the pleura and chest wall (Figure 23.38) [65].

23.3.4 Superior Sulcus Tumor

Lung cancer can invade the pleura and chest wall in the lung apical area, destroying the ribs and involving brachial plexus. Superior sulcus tumor (also known as Pancoast tumor) is characterized by pain, which may arise

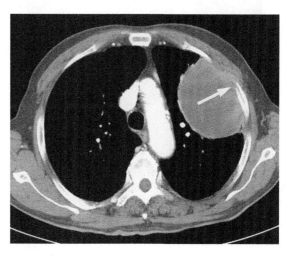

FIGURE 23.38
Pleomorphic carcinoma showing chest wall invasion and rib destruction (arrow).

in the shoulder or chest wall and can radiate to the neck. Characteristically, the pain radiates to the hand. Horner's syndrome, composed of ptosis, miosis, and anhidrosis, is from invasion of the paravertebral sympathetic chain. CT shows apical mass, bone abnormalities such as rib and vertebral bone destruction, and involvement of subclavian vessels (Figure 23.39). MR imaging is the optimal modality for evaluating the involvement of the chest wall, brachial plexus, subclavian vessels, and neural foramina [66]. Findings that prevent surgical resection of superior sulcus tumor include involvement of the brachial plexus and extension of the tumor into the spinal canal.

23.3.5 Superior Vena Cava Syndrome

Clinical manifestations of SVC syndrome include facial or neck swelling, arm swelling, cyanosis,

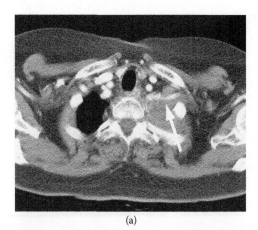

(a)

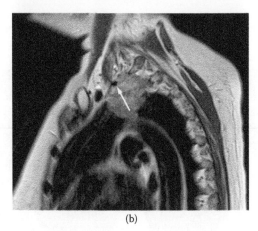

(b)

FIGURE 23.39
(a) Contrast-enhanced CT showing a left apical mass encasing the left subclavian artery (arrow). (b) T2-weighted coronal magnetic resonance shows a mass invading the chest wall and encasing the left subclavian artery (arrow).

plethora, and distension of subcutaneous vessels. Over 90% of SVC syndrome is caused by malignancies including lung cancer and lymphoma [67]. The presence of collateral vessels with compression of SVC on CT is a reliable indicator of the presence of SVC syndrome with good diagnostic performance (Figures 23.31 and 23.35).

23.3.6 Lung Cancer Screening

Early randomized controlled trials (RCTs) for lung cancer screening using chest radiography with or without sputum cytology were performed in the 1970s [23–27]. All trials disclosed increased incidence of earlier-stage lung cancers and improved 5-year survival rates in the screened groups, compared with the control groups (35% vs. 15%) [68]. However, no statistically significant decrease in lung cancer mortality was confirmed [68], which means ultimately equivalent number of patients in the two groups died of lung cancer.

From the late 1980s, low-dose CT has been reported as an effective tool for lung cancer screening because of its efficiency in detecting lung nodules despite low radiation dose compared to standard chest CT [69,70]. Several single-arm prevalence studies were performed and the fraction of participants with positive results from low-dose CT screening at base line ranged from 5.1% to 51.4%, and the rates of positive screening from low-dose CT at baseline were approximately three times higher than those for chest radiography [21,71–74]. According to the largest single-arm trial, International Early Lung Cancer Action Program, annual CT screening can be effectively used to detect curable lung cancer [75]. Among the 31,567 asymptomatic individuals at risk, lung cancer was detected in 484 participants. Of these participants, 412 (85%) were diagnosed with clinical stage I, with an estimated 10-year survival rate of 88%. These single-arm prevalence trials indicate the detection of more lung cancer cases, with more resectable cancers at CT screening.

The National Lung Screening Trial, a nationwide RCT involving more than 53,000 current and former heavy smokers aged 55–74, compared the effects of two screening procedures (low-dose CT and chest radiography) on lung cancer mortality and showed 20% fewer lung cancer-induced deaths among trial participants screened with low-dose CT [22]. Based on these results, low-dose CT screening of lung cancer can be recommended in older, heavy smokers.

Although CT is currently the best imaging modality for evaluating lung nodules in terms of spatial and contrast resolution, lung nodules on CT, especially those smaller than 5 mm, can be missed by readers. Many studies have revealed that radiologists' performance for detecting lung nodules can be improved by using a computer-aided diagnosis system [9].

23.3.7 Evaluation of Tumor Response to Treatment

Evaluation of tumor response to treatment is important to assess the efficacy of treatment and predict prognosis.

Application of PET after the initiation of chemotherapy or radiotherapy can facilitate assessment of the tumor via detection of a reduction in SUV of the primary tumor, which is a prognostic factor.

Recurrence after attempted curative treatment of lung cancer can be treated with repeat surgery, chemotherapy, or radiotherapy. Detection of recurrence with CT could be difficult after definitive treatment because of parenchymal scar, distortion of anatomy, and pleural thickening. In particular, radiotherapy can result in parenchymal distortion in the lung that may be nodular or mass-like and simulate recurrent tumor or infection.

23.4 Lymphoproliferative Disease

Most cases of pulmonary involvement by lymphoma are secondary in nature, and primary lymphomas in the lung are rare. Lung involvement of Hodgkin's lymphoma (HL) and non-Hodgkin's lymphoma (NHL) usually occurs in disseminated or recurrent lymphoma. The majority of the primary lymphomas in the lung are marginal zone lymphomas, also known as bronchus-associated lymphoid tissue (BALT) lymphoma.

At initial presentation, HL with lung involvement often occurs with enlarged mediastinal lymph nodes, whereas NHL can involve the lungs alone [76]. In comparison, recurrent HL and NHL can occur in the lung without enlarged mediastinal lymph nodes (Figure 23.40), and it may be difficult to differentiate other causes of consolidation such as infection, radiation pneumonitis, and drug-related pneumonitis. In BALT lymphoma, CT shows one or more nodules with or without air bronchograms (Figure 23.41), areas of consolidation or ground-glass attenuation, and bubble-like areas of hypoattenuation [77]. Mediastinal lymph node enlargement is seen in around 30% of cases. Prognosis of marginal zone lymphoma is excellent with a 5-year survival rate of almost 95% [78].

Lymphomatoid granulomatosis is an uncommon B-cell proliferative disease, which is associated with Epstein–Barr virus infection. In addition to the lung, it frequently involves the skin and central nervous system. Because it produces both pulmonary angiitis and granulomatosis, it can mimic Wegener's granulomatosis both clinically and radiologically. CT can show nodules or masses up to 10 cm in the peripheral lung, and bilateral involvement is frequent (Figure 23.42) [79].

Most common thoracic manifestation of extranodal lymphoma in AIDS-related lymphoma (ARL) and post-transplantation lymphoproliferative disorder are multiple, bilateral, circumscribed nodules or masses without cavitation [76]. In comparison to Kaposi's sarcoma, the pulmonary nodules in ARL tend to be more circumscribed and less likely to occur in a peribronchovascular distribution [80].

23.5 Benign Neoplasms

23.5.1 Hamartoma

Pulmonary hamartoma is the most common benign lung tumor accounting for 75% of all benign lung tumors and

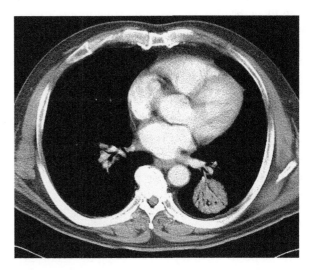

FIGURE 23.41
Bronchus-associated lymphoid tissue lymphoma shown as a well-defined mass with air bronchograms.

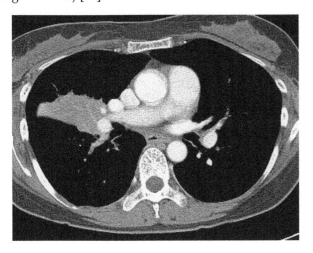

FIGURE 23.40
Recurrent Hodgkin's lymphoma shown as consolidation in the right middle lobe.

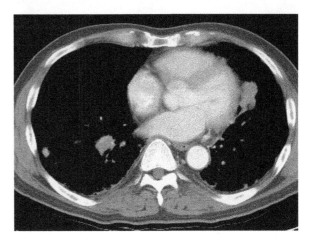

FIGURE 23.42
Lymphomatoid granulomatosis shown as multiple nodules in both lungs.

8% of all SPNs [81,82]. This tumor is composed of mesenchymal tissues that are normally present in the lung, including adipose, epithelial, fibrous, and cartilaginous tissues, and occasional bronchial glands. Hamartomas are most commonly diagnosed in patients between 30 and 60 years of age and 2–3 times more common in men than in women. They typically grow at a rate similar to normal tissue components.

Most hamartomas are shown as SPNs ranging from 1 to 3 cm in diameter, typically as smooth sharply outlined peripheral nodules, generally round to oval, often lobulated in appearances (Figure 23.4). Calcification is found in less than 10% with hamartomas less than 3 cm but is seen in 75% when larger than 5 cm [83]. When present, these calcifications are stippled, eccentric, conglomerate, or characteristically "popcorn" shape (Figure 23.8). Focal collection of fat can be seen within the tumor especially on thin-section CT. Findings of fat and calcification, at the same time in a nodule that appear only in 21% of cases, are specific for hamartomas (Figure 23.43), particularly when they are smaller than 2.5 cm [82]. On FDG-PET or PET/CT, most of hamartomas show FDG uptake less than mediastinum by visual assessment [82].

23.5.2 Inflammatory Myofibroblastic Tumor

Inflammatory myofibroblastic tumor of the lung, also known as inflammatory pseudotumor or plasma cell granuloma, is a rare disease entity, and 26% of patients are less than 18 years old [84]. Their clinical behavior may be unpredictable ranging from benign to locally invasive, to metastatic in spite of an apparently "benign" histology. The imaging features are nonspecific, but the diagnosis may be suggested in the presence of SPN or mass in children or young adults (Figure 23.44). Rarely, multiple masses occur, and calcification is unusual [85].

23.5.3 Sclerosing Hemangioma

Sclerosing hemangioma is a rare benign tumor of the lung and four or five times more frequently found in women than in men. The majority of lesions are discovered in patients between 30 and 50 years of age. Most cases are asymptomatic, but some patients present with hemoptysis, cough, and chest pain.

On CT, sclerosing hemangioma appears as a well-defined juxtapleural mass (Figure 23.45) [86,87]. Sclerosing hemangioma displays rapid and strong enhancement, and may contain calcifications. Because most sclerosing hemangiomas can show moderate to strong FDG uptake, this tumor can be falsely interpreted as malignancy on FDG-PET/CT [88].

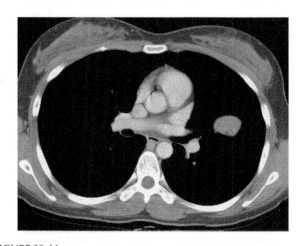

FIGURE 23.44
Inflammatory myofibroblastic tumor in a 22-year-old woman shown as a well-defined mass.

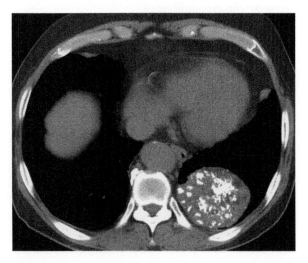

FIGURE 23.43
A large hamartoma in the left lower lobe showing both chondroid calcifications and small areas of fat.

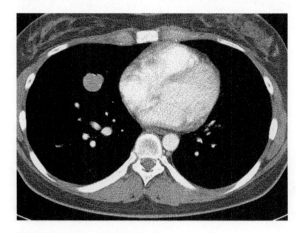

FIGURE 23.45
Sclerosing hemangioma shows as a well-defined juxtapleural mass with a strong enhancement.

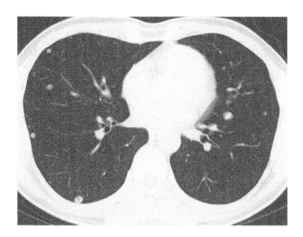

FIGURE 23.46
Epithelioid hemangioendothelioma shown as multiple well-defined nodules in both lungs that can mimic hematogenous metastasis.

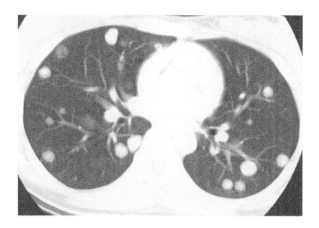

FIGURE 23.47
Hematogenous metastasis from salivary gland tumor showing multiple variable sized nodules in both lungs.

23.5.4 Epithelioid Hemangioendothelioma

Epithelioid hemangioendothelioma is a rare tumor of endothelial origin and four times more common in women than men. Although this tumor can occur at any age, 40% of patients are under 30 years of age [85]. Approximately 15%–20% of patients with pulmonary epithelioid hemangioendothelioma have hepatic involvement. The most common feature of this tumor on CT is multiple small discrete lung nodules with well-defined margins. This tumor can mimic hematogenous pulmonary metastases (Figure 23.46), but shows little or no growth [89].

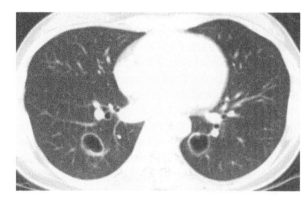

FIGURE 23.48
Metastasis from tongue cancer shown as multiple thin-walled cavitary nodules.

23.6 Metastatic Tumors

The lung is a common site of metastasis, and almost all cancer can metastasize to the lung. The incidence of pulmonary metastasis varies with the primary cancer and the stage of disease. In autopsy series, pulmonary metastases have been found in 20%–54% of patients dying of various malignancies [7,90,91].

Pulmonary metastasis can result from hematogenous spread, lymphatic spread, transbronchial spread, or direct extension.

23.6.1 Pathogenesis

The lung is an initial metastatic site for tumors of the head and neck, kidney, testis, choriocarcinoma, bone and soft tissue sarcoma, melanoma, thyroid, and adrenal glands because their venous drainage is primarily to the lung. The lung is the secondarily seeded after initial filtering of the liver for tumors of the GI tract (stomach,

pancreas, colon) and ovarian carcinomas. For carcinomas of the esophagus or rectum, either the lungs or the liver may be the first metastatic site [91].

23.6.2 Hematogenous Metastasis

Hematogenous pulmonary metastasis usually presents as multiple nodules or masses on chest radiography and CT scan. Nodules or masses are usually well-defined smooth margins. The size of metastatic lesions varies from a few millimeters to large masses. Multiple nodules are usually variable in size (Figure 23.47). Metastatic lesions are usually bilateral and more common in lower lung zones reflecting the effect of gravity on blood flow [7,90,91].

The possibility of cavitation in metastatic nodules varies with histology. Metastatic lesions showing cavitation suggest metastasis from tumors of the uterine cervix, colon, and head and neck and squamous cell carcinomas are the most common type of cavitating metastasis, comprising about 69% cases (Figure 23.48). Cavitation may also occur in metastatic adenocarcinoma, sarcoma, and transitional cell carcinoma, although this is relatively uncommon [7].

Metastasis from highly vascular primary tumors, such as choriocarcinoma, renal cell carcinoma, melanoma, and angiosarcoma, may have a surrounding halo of GGO due to hemorrhage into the adjacent parenchyma. Miliary metastasis is occasionally encountered and mostly from thyroid or renal carcinoma or melanoma (Figure 23.49) [7].

23.6.3 Lymphangitic Metastasis

Lymphangitic spread refers to tumor growth in the lymphatic system of the lungs. Although virtually any metastatic neoplasm can show lymphangitic spread, it occurs most commonly in patients with carcinoma of the lung, breast, stomach, colon, pancreas, prostate, cervix, or thyroid and metastatic adenocarcinoma of an unknown primary site [91].

Lymphangitic metastasis usually results from the hematogenous dissemination tumor microemboli and subsequent invasion of the vessel wall into the pulmonary interstitium, followed by spread through the lymphatic channels. Lymphangitic metastasis may uncommonly occur as a result of retrograde spread from tumor-laden hilar lymph nodes. The pathological findings of pulmonary lymphangitic metastasis are the presence of tumor thrombi in lymphatic vessels of bronchovascular bundles, interlobular septa, and pleura [92,93]. Neoplasms are often confined solely to the interstitium and lymphatic spaces but can spread outside these structures into the adjacent parenchyma, resulting in parenchymal nodules that alter the typical pattern.

The radiological findings of lymphangitic metastasis consist of fine reticulonodular opacities and/or coarsened bronchovascular markings, sometimes indistinct, simulating interstitial pulmonary edema. In addition, hilar and mediastinal lymphadenopathy and pleural effusion are observed. Septal lines (Kerley's B lines) are present in most cases. These findings are nonspecific, but the appearance of unilateral or asymmetric Kerley's B lines is particularly suggestive of lymphangitic metastasis.

Lymphangitic metastasis is characterized on CT by smooth or nodular thickening of the peribronchovascular interstitium in perihilar lung (peribronchial cuffing), interlobular septa, and subpleural interstitium, and thickening of the peribronchovascular axial interstitium in the centrilobular regions, with preservation of normal lung architecture at the lobular level (Figure 23.50). This pattern of distribution is termed "perilymphatic distribution." Pleural effusion and hilar or mediastinal lymph node enlargement is seen in about 40% of cases [94].

CT findings of typical lymphangitic metastasis are usually considered diagnostic in patients with known tumors and clinical symptoms, and lung biopsy is not performed in clinical practice. However, for patients without known tumors, CT can be helpful in indicating appropriate lung biopsy sites and identifying the appropriate procedure.

Differential diagnosis from pulmonary edema may be made on clinical grounds. Nodular septal thickening is not found in patients with pulmonary edema, fibrosis, and normal lungs, but is common in patients with sarcoidosis and coal worker's pneumoconiosis or silicosis. However, septal thickening is less extensive and distortion of lung architecture and pulmonary

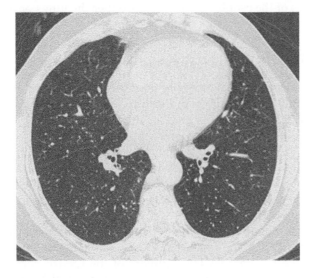

FIGURE 23.49
Metastasis from thyroid cancer shown as miliary nodules in both lungs.

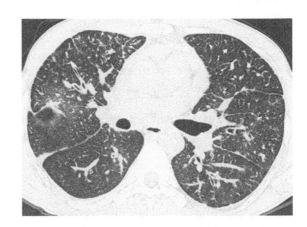

FIGURE 23.50
Lymphangitic metastasis showing interlobular septal thickening, peribronchial cuffing, and tiny nodules with perilymphatic distribution.

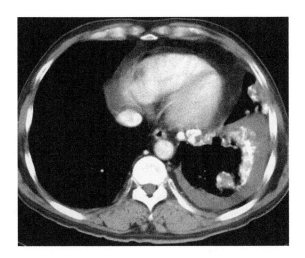

FIGURE 23.51
Osteosarcoma metastasis showing multiple calcified nodules in the lung and pleura with small left pleural effusion.

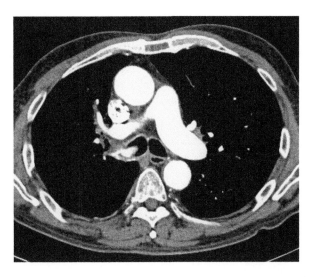

FIGURE 23.52
Metastasis from renal cell carcinoma showing a strongly enhancing endobronchial mass in the right main bronchus.

lobule is more evident in sarcoidosis and coal worker's pneumoconiosis.

23.6.4 Other Manifestations of Metastasis

Calcification in the pulmonary nodule is usually a reliable radiological finding of benign tumors, such as granulomas or hamartomas. However, metastatic malignant pulmonary nodules can also produce calcification by bone formation, dystrophic calcification, or mucoid calcification. Osteosarcoma and chondrosarcoma are the best known malignant tumors that give rise to calcification or ossification in metastatic pulmonary nodules (Figure 23.51). Other sarcomas such as giant cell tumor or synovial sarcoma can also produce calcification or ossification in metastatic pulmonary nodules. Calcified pulmonary metastatic nodules may also arise in papillary carcinomas or mucinous adenocarcinomas [7,95]. Calcification may also be present in successfully treated metastases.

Endobronchial metastasis is defined as bronchoscopically visible nonpulmonary metastatic tumors of the subsegmental or more proximal central bronchus [96]. The common sources of endobronchial metastases are kidney, breast, and colorectal cancers. Atelectasis is the most frequent radiological finding, and endobronchial lesion appears as diffuse concentric luminal narrowing, endobronchial mass (Figure 23.52), and diffuse bronchial wall thickening.

Pulmonary tumor embolism is rarely diagnosed before death. Primary malignancies frequently associated with pulmonary tumor emboli are hepatocellular carcinoma, breast and renal carcinoma, gastric and

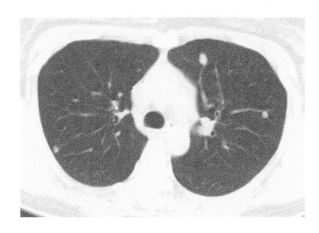

FIGURE 23.53
Benign metastasizing leiomyoma showing multiple nodules in both lungs. Patient had a history of hysterectomy 20 years ago and biopsy of lung nodule and pelvic mass revealed benign leiomyoma.

prostate cancer, and choriocarcinoma [97]. CT findings include peripheral wedge-shaped opacities, multifocal dilatation or beading of vessels, and enlarged central arteries [98].

Extrathoracic benign tumors rarely metastasize to the lung. Uterine leiomyoma has been reported to be the most frequent cause of benign metastasizing tumor to the lung, and other benign tumors such as a hydatidiform mole of the uterus, a giant cell tumor of the bone, a chondroblastoma, a pleormorphic adenoma of the salivary gland, or a meningioma can also metastasize to the lung [7]. CT findings of these benign metastasizing tumors are indistinguishable from those of hematogenous metastases from malignant tumors except for their slow growth (Figure 23.53).

Pneumothorax can occur in association with cavitary or cystic metastasis from sarcomas [7]. Osteosarcoma and angiosarcoma are the most common cause of pneumothorax due to metastasis. Necrosis of subpleural metastases can produce a bronchopleural fistula that results in a pneumothorax.

References

1. Hansell DM, Bankier AA, MacMahon H, McLoud TC, Muller NL, Remy J. Fleischner Society: Glossary of terms for thoracic imaging. *Radiology* 2008; 246: 697–722.
2. Zerhouni EA, Stitik FP, Siegelman SS et al. CT of the pulmonary nodule: A cooperative study. *Radiology* 1986; 160: 319–327.
3. Midthun DE, Swensen SJ, Jett JR. Approach to the solitary pulmonary nodule. *Mayo Clin Proc* 1993; 68: 378–385.
4. MacMahon H, Austin JH, Gamsu G et al. Guidelines for management of small pulmonary nodules detected on CT scans: A statement from the Fleischner Society. *Radiology* 2005; 237: 395–400.
5. Woodring JH, Fried AM. Significance of wall thickness in solitary cavities of the lung: A follow-up study. *AJR Am J Roentgenol* 1983; 140: 473–474.
6. Khan A. ACR Appropriateness Criteria on solitary pulmonary nodule. *J Am Coll Radiol* 2007; 4: 152–155.
7. Seo JB, Im JG, Goo JM, Chung MJ, Kim MY. Atypical pulmonary metastases: Spectrum of radiologic findings. *Radiographics* 2001; 21: 403–417.
8. Nathan MH, Collins VP, Adams RA. Differentiation of benign and malignant pulmonary nodules by growth rate. *Radiology* 1962; 79: 221–232.
9. Goo JM. A computer-aided diagnosis for evaluating lung nodules on chest CT: The current status and perspective. *Korean J Radiol* 2011; 12: 145–155.
10. Revel MP, Merlin A, Peyrard S et al. Software volumetric evaluation of doubling times for differentiating benign versus malignant pulmonary nodules. *AJR Am J Roentgenol* 2006; 187: 135–142.
11. van Klaveren RJ, Oudkerk M, Prokop M et al. Management of lung nodules detected by volume CT scanning. *N Engl J Med* 2009; 361: 2221–2229.
12. Swensen SJ, Viggiano RW, Midthun DE et al. Lung nodule enhancement at CT: Multicenter study. *Radiology* 2000; 214: 73–80.
13. Jeong YJ, Lee KS, Jeong SY et al. Solitary pulmonary nodule: Characterization with combined wash-in and wash-out features at dynamic multi-detector row CT. *Radiology* 2005; 237: 675–683.
14. Yi CA, Lee KS, Kim BT et al. Tissue characterization of solitary pulmonary nodule: Comparative study between helical dynamic CT and integrated PET/CT. *J Nucl Med* 2006; 47: 443–450.
15. Lee SM, Park CM, Goo JM et al. Transient part-solid nodules detected at screening thin-section CT for lung cancer: Comparison with persistent part-solid nodules. *Radiology* 2010; 255: 242–251.
16. Kim HY, Shim YM, Lee KS, Han J, Yi CA, Kim YK. Persistent pulmonary nodular ground-glass opacity at thin-section CT: Histopathologic comparisons. *Radiology* 2007; 245: 267–275.
17. Park CM, Goo JM, Lee HJ, Lee CH, Chun EJ, Im JG. Nodular ground-glass opacity at thin-section CT: Histologic correlation and evaluation of change at follow-up. *Radiographics* 2007; 27: 391–408.
18. Goo JM, Park CM, Lee HJ. Ground-glass nodules on chest CT as imaging biomarkers in the management of lung adenocarcinoma. *AJR Am J Roentgenol* 2011; 196: 533–543.
19. Henschke CI, Yankelevitz DF, Mirtcheva R, McGuinness G, McCauley D, Miettinen OS. CT screening for lung cancer: Frequency and significance of part-solid and nonsolid nodules. *AJR Am J Roentgenol* 2002; 178: 1053–1057.
20. UyBico SJ, Wu CC, Suh RD, Le NH, Brown K, Krishnam MS. Lung cancer staging essentials: The new TNM staging system and potential imaging pitfalls. *Radiographics* 2010; 30: 1163–1181.
21. Henschke CI, McCauley DI, Yankelevitz DF et al. Early Lung Cancer Action Project: Overall design and findings from baseline screening. *Lancet* 1999; 354: 99–105.
22. Aberle DR, Adams AM, Berg CD et al. Reduced lung-cancer mortality with low-dose computed tomographic screening. *N Engl J Med* 2011; 365: 395–409.
23. Flehinger BJ, Melamed MR, Zaman MB, Heelan RT, Perchick WB, Martini N. Early lung cancer detection: Results of the initial (prevalence) radiologic and cytologic screening in the Memorial Sloan-Kettering study. *Am Rev Respir Dis* 1984; 130: 555–560.
24. Frost JK, Ball WC, Jr, Levin ML et al. Early lung cancer detection: Results of the initial (prevalence) radiologic and cytologic screening in the Johns Hopkins study. *Am Rev Respir Dis* 1984; 130: 549–554.
25. Kubik A, Polak J. Lung cancer detection. Results of a randomized prospective study in Czechoslovakia. *Cancer* 1986; 57: 2427–2437.
26. Marcus PM, Bergstralh EJ, Fagerstrom RM et al. Lung cancer mortality in the Mayo Lung Project: Impact of extended follow-up. *J Natl Cancer Inst* 2000; 92: 1308–1316.
27. Melamed MR. Lung cancer screening results in the National Cancer Institute New York study. *Cancer* 2000; 89: 2356–2362.
28. Schaefer-Prokop C, Neitzel U, Venema HW, Uffmann M, Prokop M. Digital chest radiography: An update on modern technology, dose containment and control of image quality. *Eur Radiol* 2008; 18: 1818–1830.
29. Chern MS, Wu MH, Chang CY. CT and MRI for staging of locally advanced non-small cell lung cancer. *Lung Cancer* 2003; 42 Suppl 2:S5–S8.
30. Munden RF, Swisher SS, Stevens CW, Stewart DJ. Imaging of the patient with non-small cell lung cancer. *Radiology* 2005; 237: 803–818.
31. Glazer GM, Gross BH, Quint LE, Francis IR, Bookstein FL, Orringer MB. Normal mediastinal lymph nodes: Number and size according to American Thoracic Society mapping. *AJR Am J Roentgenol* 1985; 144: 261–265.

32. Boland GW, Lee MJ, Gazelle GS, Halpern EF, McNicholas MM, Mueller PR. Characterization of adrenal masses using unenhanced CT: An analysis of the CT literature. *AJR Am J Roentgenol* 1998; 171: 201–204.

33. Ohno Y, Adachi S, Motoyama A et al. Multiphase ECG-triggered 3D contrast-enhanced MR angiography: Utility for evaluation of hilar and mediastinal invasion of bronchogenic carcinoma. *J Magn Reson Imaging* 2001; 13: 215–224.

34. Seo JS, Kim YJ, Choi BW, Choe KO. Usefulness of magnetic resonance imaging for evaluation of cardiovascular invasion: Evaluation of sliding motion between thoracic mass and adjacent structures on cine MR images. *J Magn Reson Imaging* 2005; 22: 234–241.

35. Lee CH, Goo JM, Kim YT et al. The clinical feasibility of using non-breath-hold real-time MR-echo imaging for the evaluation of mediastinal and chest wall tumor invasion. *Korean J Radiol* 2010; 11: 37–45.

36. Ohno Y, Koyama H, Nogami M et al. STIR turbo SE MR imaging vs. coregistered FDG-PET/CT: Quantitative and qualitative assessment of N-stage in non-small-cell lung cancer patients. *J Magn Reson Imaging* 2007; 26: 1071–1080.

37. Lee HY, Lee KS, Kim BT et al. Diagnostic efficacy of PET/CT plus brain MR imaging for detection of extrathoracic metastases in patients with lung adenocarcinoma. *J Korean Med Sci* 2009; 24: 1132–1138.

38. Heyneman LE, Patz EF. PET imaging in patients with bronchioloalveolar cell carcinoma. *Lung Cancer* 2002; 38: 261–266.

39. Graeter TP, Hellwig D, Hoffmann K, Ukena D, Kirsch CM, Schafers HJ. Mediastinal lymph node staging in suspected lung cancer: Comparison of positron emission tomography with F-18-fluorodeoxyglucose and mediastinoscopy. *Ann Thorac Surg* 2003; 75: 231–235; discussion 235–236.

40. Bruzzi JF, Munden RF. PET/CT imaging of lung cancer. *J Thorac Imaging* 2006; 21: 123–136.

41. Detterbeck FC, Boffa DJ, Tanoue LT. The new lung cancer staging system. *Chest* 2009; 136: 260–271.

42. Goldstraw P, Crowley J, Chansky K et al. The IASLC Lung Cancer Staging Project: Proposals for the revision of the TNM stage groupings in the forthcoming (seventh) edition of the TNM Classification of malignant tumours. *J Thorac Oncol* 2007; 2: 706–714.

43. Postmus PE, Brambilla E, Chansky K et al. The IASLC Lung Cancer Staging Project: Proposals for revision of the M descriptors in the forthcoming (seventh) edition of the TNM classification of lung cancer. *J Thorac Oncol* 2007; 2: 686–693.

44. Rami-Porta R, Ball D, Crowley J et al. The IASLC Lung Cancer Staging Project: Proposals for the revision of the T descriptors in the forthcoming (seventh) edition of the TNM classification for lung cancer. *J Thorac Oncol* 2007; 2: 593–602.

45. Rusch VW, Asamura H, Watanabe H, Giroux DJ, Rami-Porta R, Goldstraw P. The IASLC lung cancer staging project: A proposal for a new international lymph node map in the forthcoming seventh edition of the TNM classification for lung cancer. *J Thorac Oncol* 2009; 4: 568–577.

46. Metintas M, Ak G, Akcayir IA et al. Detecting extrathoracic metastases in patients with non-small cell lung cancer: Is routine scanning necessary? *Lung Cancer* 2007; 58: 59–67.

47. Wynder EL, Muscat JE. The changing epidemiology of smoking and lung cancer histology. *Environ Health Perspect* 1995; 103(Suppl 8): 143–148.

48. Yang P, Allen MS, Aubry MC et al. Clinical features of 5,628 primary lung cancer patients: Experience at Mayo Clinic from 1997 to 2003. *Chest* 2005; 128: 452–462.

49. Noguchi M, Morikawa A, Kawasaki M et al. Small adenocarcinoma of the lung. Histologic characteristics and prognosis. *Cancer* 1995; 75: 2844–2852.

50. Aoki T, Tomoda Y, Watanabe H et al. Peripheral lung adenocarcinoma: Correlation of thin-section CT findings with histologic prognostic factors and survival. *Radiology* 2001; 220: 803–809.

51. Park CM, Goo JM, Lee HJ et al. CT findings of atypical adenomatous hyperplasia in the lung. *Korean J Radiol* 2006; 7: 80–86.

52. Travis WD, Brambilla E, Noguchi M et al. International association for the study of lung cancer/American Thoracic Society/European Respiratory Society international multidisciplinary classification of lung adenocarcinoma. *J Thorac Oncol* 2011; 6: 244–285.

53. Im JG, Han MC, Yu EJ et al. Lobar bronchioloalveolar carcinoma: "Angiogram sign" on CT scans. *Radiology* 1990; 176: 749–753.

54. Tomashefski JF, Jr, Connors AF, Jr, Rosenthal ES, Hsiue IL. Peripheral vs central squamous cell carcinoma of the lung. A comparison of clinical features, histopathology, and survival. *Arch Pathol Lab Med* 1990; 114: 468–474.

55. Saida Y, Kujiraoka Y, Akaogi E, Ogata T, Kurosaki Y, Itai Y. Early squamous cell carcinoma of the lung: CT and pathologic correlation. *Radiology* 1996; 201: 61–65.

56. Travis WD. Pathology of lung cancer. *Clin Chest Med* 2002; 23: 65–81, viii.

57. Oshiro Y, Kusumoto M, Matsuno Y et al. CT findings of surgically resected large cell neuroendocrine carcinoma of the lung in 38 patients. *AJR Am J Roentgenol* 2004; 182: 87–91.

58. Vallieres E, Shepherd FA, Crowley J et al. The IASLC Lung Cancer Staging Project: Proposals regarding the relevance of TNM in the pathologic staging of small cell lung cancer in the forthcoming (seventh) edition of the TNM classification for lung cancer. *J Thorac Oncol* 2009; 4: 1049–1059.

59. Sher T, Dy GK, Adjei AA. Small cell lung cancer. *Mayo Clin Proc* 2008; 83: 355–367.

60. Chong S, Lee KS, Chung MJ, Han J, Kwon OJ, Kim TS. Neuroendocrine tumors of the lung: Clinical, pathologic, and imaging findings. *Radiographics* 2006; 26: 41–57; discussion 57–48.

61. Rosado de Christenson ML, Abbott GF, Kirejczyk WM, Galvin JR, Travis WD. Thoracic carcinoids: Radiologic-pathologic correlation. *Radiographics* 1999; 19: 707–736.

62. Koo CW, Baliff JP, Torigian DA, Litzky LA, Gefter WB, Akers SR. Spectrum of pulmonary neuroendocrine cell proliferation: Diffuse idiopathic pulmonary neuroendocrine cell hyperplasia, tumorlet, and carcinoids. *AJR Am J Roentgenol* 2010; 195: 661–668.

63. Kazerooni EA, Bhalla M, Shepard JA, McLoud TC. Adenosquamous carcinoma of the lung: Radiologic appearance. *AJR Am J Roentgenol* 1994; 163: 301–306.

64. Yu JQ, Yang ZG, Austin JH, Guo YK, Zhang SF. Adenosquamous carcinoma of the lung: CT-pathological correlation. *Clin Radiol* 2005; 60: 364–369.

65. Kim TH, Kim SJ, Ryu YH et al. Pleomorphic carcinoma of lung: Comparison of CT features and pathologic findings. *Radiology* 2004; 232: 554–559.

66. Bruzzi JF, Komaki R, Walsh GL et al. Imaging of non-small cell lung cancer of the superior sulcus: Part 2: Initial staging and assessment of resectability and therapeutic response. *Radiographics* 2008; 28: 561–572.

67. Rice TW, Rodriguez RM, Light RW. The superior vena cava syndrome: Clinical characteristics and evolving etiology. *Medicine (Baltimore)* 2006; 85: 37–42.

68. Flehinger BJ, Melamed MR. Current status of screening for lung cancer. *Chest Surg Clin N Am* 1994; 4: 1–15.

69. Naidich DP, Marshall CH, Gribbin C, Arams RS, McCauley DI. Low-dose CT of the lungs: Preliminary observations. *Radiology* 1990; 175: 729–731.

70. Rusinek H, Naidich DP, McGuinness G et al. Pulmonary nodule detection: Low-dose versus conventional CT. *Radiology* 1998; 209: 243–249.

71. Sone S, Li F, Yang ZG et al. Results of three-year mass screening programme for lung cancer using mobile low-dose spiral computed tomography scanner. *Br J Cancer* 2001; 84: 25–32.

72. Nawa T, Nakagawa T, Kusano S, Kawasaki Y, Sugawara Y, Nakata H. Lung cancer screening using low-dose spiral CT: Results of baseline and 1-year follow-up studies. *Chest* 2002; 122: 15–20.

73. Swensen SJ, Jett JR, Sloan JA et al. Screening for lung cancer with low-dose spiral computed tomography. *Am J Respir Crit Care Med* 2002; 165: 508–513.

74. Diederich S, Wormanns D, Semik M et al. Screening for early lung cancer with low-dose spiral CT: Prevalence in 817 asymptomatic smokers. *Radiology* 2002; 222: 773–781.

75. Henschke CI, Yankelevitz DF, Libby DM, Pasmantier MW, Smith JP, Miettinen OS. Survival of patients with stage I lung cancer detected on CT screening. *N Engl J Med* 2006; 355: 1763–1771.

76. Lee WK, Duddalwar VA, Rouse HC, Lau EW, Bekhit E, Hennessy OF. Extranodal lymphoma in the thorax: Cross-sectional imaging findings. *Clin Radiol* 2009; 64: 542–549.

77. Lee DK, Im JG, Lee KS et al. B-cell lymphoma of bronchus-associated lymphoid tissue (BALT): CT features in 10 patients. *J Comput Assist Tomogr* 2000; 24: 30–34.

78. Cordier JF, Chailleux E, Lauque D et al. Primary pulmonary lymphomas. A clinical study of 70 cases in nonimmunocompromised patients. *Chest* 1993; 103: 201–208.

79. Lee JS, Tuder R, Lynch DA. Lymphomatoid granulomatosis: Radiologic features and pathologic correlations. *AJR Am J Roentgenol* 2000; 175: 1335–1339.

80. Logan PM, Finnegan MM. Pulmonary complications in AIDS: CT appearances. *Clin Radiol* 1998; 53: 567–573.

81. Whyte RI, Donington JS. Hamartomas of the lung. *Semin Thorac Cardiovasc Surg* 2003; 15: 301–304.

82. De Cicco C, Bellomi M, Bartolomei M et al. Imaging of lung hamartomas by multidetector computed tomography and positron emission tomography. *Ann Thorac Surg* 2008; 86: 1769–1772.

83. Khan AN, Al-Jahdali HH, Allen CM, Irion KL, Al Ghanem S, Koteyar SS. The calcified lung nodule: What does it mean? *Ann Thorac Med* 2010; 5: 67–79.

84. Cerfolio RJ, Allen MS, Nascimento AG et al. Inflammatory pseudotumors of the lung. *Ann Thorac Surg* 1999; 67: 933–936.

85. Gimenez A, Franquet T, Prats R, Estrada P, Villalba J, Bague S. Unusual primary lung tumors: A radiologic-pathologic overview. *Radiographics* 2002; 22: 601–619.

86. Im JG, Kim WH, Han MC et al. Sclerosing hemangiomas of the lung and interlobar fissures: CT findings. *J Comput Assist Tomogr* 1994; 18: 34–38.

87. Chung MJ, Lee KS, Han J, Sung YM, Chong S, Kwon OJ. Pulmonary sclerosing hemangioma presenting as solitary pulmonary nodule: Dynamic CT findings and histopathologic comparisons. *AJR Am J Roentgenol* 2006; 187: 430–437.

88. Lee E, Park CM, Kang KW et al. 18F-FDG PET/CT features of pulmonary sclerosing hemangioma. *Acta Radiol* 2013; 54: 24–29.

89. Kim EY, Kim TS, Han J, Choi JY, Kwon OJ, Kim J. Thoracic epithelioid hemangioendothelioma: Imaging and pathologic features. *Acta Radiol* 2011; 52: 161–166.

90. Crow J, Slavin G, Kreel L. Pulmonary metastasis: A pathologic and radiologic study. *Cancer* 1981; 47: 2595–2602.

91. Davis SD. CT evaluation for pulmonary metastases in patients with extrathoracic malignancy. *Radiology* 1991; 180: 1–12.

92. Stein MG, Mayo J, Muller N, Aberle DR, Webb WR, Gamsu G. Pulmonary lymphangitic spread of carcinoma: Appearance on CT scans. *Radiology* 1987; 162: 371–375.

93. Munk PL, Muller NL, Miller RR, Ostrow DN. Pulmonary lymphangitic carcinomatosis: CT and pathologic findings. *Radiology* 1988; 166: 705–709.

94. Grenier P, Chevret S, Beigelman C, Brauner MW, Chastang C, Valeyre D. Chronic diffuse infiltrative lung disease: Determination of the diagnostic value of clinical data, chest radiography, and CT and Bayesian analysis. *Radiology* 1994; 191: 383–390.

95. Maile CW, Rodan BA, Godwin JD, Chen JT, Ravin CE. Calcification in pulmonary metastases. *Br J Radiol* 1982; 55: 108–113.

96. Kiryu T, Hoshi H, Matsui E et al. Endotracheal/endobronchial metastases: Clinicopathologic study with special reference to developmental modes. *Chest* 2001; 119: 768–775.

97. Schriner RW, Ryu JH, Edwards WD. Microscopic pulmonary tumor embolism causing subacute cor pulmonale: A difficult antemortem diagnosis. *Mayo Clin Proc* 1991; 66: 143–148.

98. Shepard JA, Moore EH, Templeton PA, McLoud TC. Pulmonary intravascular tumor emboli: Dilated and beaded peripheral pulmonary arteries at CT. *Radiology* 1993; 187: 797–801.

24

Pathologies of the Mediastinum

Ahmed Abdel Khalek Abdel Razek

CONTENTS

24.1 Introduction

The mediastinum is bounded superiorly by thoracic inlet and inferiorly by diaphragm, posteriorly by thoracic spines, anteriorly by sternum, and laterally by parietal pleurae. The superior mediastinum begins at the root of the neck and ends caudally at a line drawn between T-4 vertebrae and the sternomanubrial junction. The area between this line and the diaphragm is further divided into three regions: anterior, middle, and posterior. Basically, the heart and pericardium form the middle section, everything anterior to the heart is the anterior mediastinum, and everything posterior to the heart back to the spine is the posterior mediastinum. The most common symptoms resulting from compression are chest pain, cough, and dispend. Superior vena cava syndrome, Horner's syndrome, hoarseness, and neurological deficits are more frequently associated with malignant disease. Anterior masses are best approached through a median sternotomy or an anterolateral thoracotomy, whereas middle and posterior lesions are best approached via a posterolateral thoracotomy. Mediastinal tumors are rare, and two-thirds of mediastinal tumors are benign. The incidence of primary mediastinal tumors is 25% for neurogenic tumors, 20% for thymoma, 15.3% for lymphomas, and 12.2% for germ cell tumors. The incidence varies with age [1–8]. Different studies discuss the role of imaging modalities, either computed tomography (CT) scan or magnetic resonance (MR) imaging, in different mediastinal masses [5–16].

We review the CT imaging appearance of mediastinal lesions including thymic tumors, germ cell tumors, malignant lymphoma, neurogenic tumors, mediastinal cysts, mesenchymal tumors, and mediastinitis.

24.2 Technique

Multi-detector CT scan is the imaging modality of choice in patients with mediastinal masses. Images of the CT scan are acquired using a narrow detector (0.5–1 mm) after an intravenous injection of nonionic contrast medium through the entire thorax and then reconstructed at 5 mm slice thickness using a mediastinal algorithm. An intravenous injection of nonionic contrast medium is given at a rate of 3 cm^3/s following a 30 second scan delay. The data are then transferred to a workstation to perform two-dimensional (2D) multiplanar reformatted imaging and three-dimensional (3D) imaging [5,6].

24.3 Interpretation

24.3.1 Clinical Presentation

With regard to clinical presentation, 75% of mediastinal masses in asymptomatic subjects are benign, whereas two-thirds of those in symptomatic patients are malignant; in addition, 85% of patients with a malignancy are symptomatic, whereas only 46% of cases of benign disease are associated with symptoms. Overall, 60% of expansile mediastinal lesions are associated with symptoms related to compression or direct invasion of neighboring structures or paraneoplastic syndromes such as myasthenia gravis (MG), Cushing syndrome, and multiple endocrine neoplasias [1–4].

24.3.2 Laboratory Tests

Testing of serum α-fetoprotein (α-FP) and β-human chorionic gonadotropin (β-HCG) is useful in the diagnosis of malignant germ cell tumor. These markers are singly or jointly increased in 80%–85% of nonseminomatous tumors [10–13]. Determination of the genetic markers by the application of new genomic methodologies has provided important insight into the pathogenesis of mediastinal disease. These new techniques have enabled scientists to uncover differential gene expression patterns between subtypes of thymomas and correlate tumor marker expression with germ cell tumors [4].

24.3.3 Age and Compartment

Mediastinal tumors are predominantly seen in the third to fourth decades. The incidence of mediastinal masses varies according to the anatomical compartment and the age of the patients. In the adult, 54% of mediastinal tumors develop in the anterior mediastinum, 20% in the middle mediastinum, and 26% in the posterior mediastinum. In children, percentages are 43%, 18%, and 39%, respectively [7–9].

24.3.4 Attenuation Value

Attenuation value of a mediastinal mass at CT scan may help in differential diagnosis of mediastinal masses. Fat-attenuation masses (–70 to –100 HU; HU denotes Hounsfield unit) are seen in benign fatty lesions such as lipoma and thymolipoma. Low-attenuation cystic masses (–20 to +20 HU) include congenital benign cysts (bronchogenic, esophageal duplication, pericardial, and thymic cysts), meningocele, mature cystic teratoma, and lymphangioma. Additionally, many tumors can undergo cystic degeneration and demonstrate mixed solid and cystic components at CT, including thymoma, lymphoma, germ cell tumors, and neurogenic tumors. Calcified masses (>100 HU) are seen in germ cell tumors, thymoma and neurogenic tumors, and calcified goiter [6].

24.3.5 Enhancement

Enhancing masses show a significant increase in attenuation following the injection of contrast. These lesions are highly vascular and include substernal thyroid, parathyroid glands, carcinoid tumor, paraganglioma, and hemangioma [6].

24.4 Thymic Tumors

24.4.1 Thymoma

Thymomas are the most common primary tumor in the mediastinum (20%). Thymomas most commonly arise in the upper part of the anterior mediastinum, but it may also occur in the inferior, middle, or posterior mediastinum. Thymomas usually occur in middle-aged adults (third to fourth decades) and equally in males and females. Patients are usually asymptomatic and may be associated with clinical symptoms due to its invasion. Toyotas are occasionally associated with paraneoplastic syndrome, and MG is the most common disease. Approximately 10%–23% of patients with MG have thymoma and 35%–40% of patients with thymoma have myasthenia. Thymoma is a benign or low-grade malignant tumor of the thymic epithelium. It can be of noninvasive type or invasive type (15%–40%) that has spread beyond the capsule. Invasive thymoma invades mediastinal fat, great vessels, pleura, and pericardium [17–27].

On CT, thymomas usually present as sharply demarcated round or oval soft-tissue masses in the region of the thymus. Tumors commonly reveal soft-tissue attenuation and mild to moderate contrast enhancement (Figure 24.1). Occasionally, focal low-attenuation areas are identified within the tumors, reflecting hemorrhage, necrosis, or cyst formation. Linear or ringlike calcifications are occasionally seen in thymoma. Invasive thymomas invade the mediastinum beyond the capsule and occasionally spread to the pleura and pericardium. CT may allow some distinction between invasive and noninvasive thymoma in some cases. Complete obliteration of the adjacent fat planes highly suggests mediastinal invasion (Figure 24.2), whereas partial obliteration

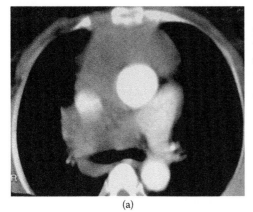
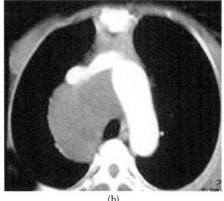

(a)   (b)

FIGURE 24.1
Noninvasive thymoma: (a, b) axial contrast computed tomography (CT) scans of the chest. A well-defined and sharply demarcated soft-tissue mass with mild homogeneous contrast enhancement is seen in the anterior mediastinum at the region of thymus, which extends into the middle mediastinum.

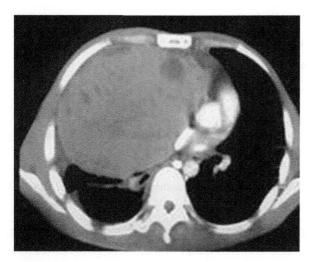

FIGURE 24.2
Invasive thymoma: axial contrast CT scan of the chest shows a large well-defined mass with nonenhanced regions. The mass is abutting the superior vena cava with no line of cleavage.

is indeterminate. Complete preservation of adjacent fat planes usually excludes extensive invasive disease but not minimal capsular invasion. Transpleural spread either as a sheet of tumor or as drop metastasis is a diagnostic finding of invasive thymoma [5,17,19,24].

24.4.2 Thymic Carcinoma

Thymic carcinomas are thymic epithelial tumors with a high degree of histological anaplasia. The most common histological variety is epidermoid or squamous cell carcinoma following lymphoepithelioma-like carcinoma, and anaplastic or undifferentiated carcinomas. Thymic carcinomas predominantly occur in adults. A paraneoplastic syndrome is uncommon in thymic carcinomas. Thymic carcinomas occasionally infiltrate adjacent tissue and mediastinal vascular structures or extend into the pleura, lungs, and pericardium. Distant metastases (lung, liver, brain, and bone) are found in 50%–65% of patients. On CT, thymic carcinomas usually show heterogeneous internal attenuation due to necrosis and hemorrhage and have poorly defined margins with invasion along the pleura, pericardium, or mediastinum (Figure 24.3). Intrathoracic lymphadenopathy, pleural effusion, and pericardial effusion are common [5,28].

24.4.3 World Health Organization Classification

Thymic epithelial tumors are divided into three groups, types A, B, and C, depending on the shape of the neoplastic epithelial cells and their nuclei. Type B tumors are subdivided into B1, B2, and B3 on the basis of proportional increases of epithelial competency. The World

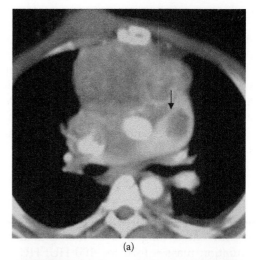

(a)

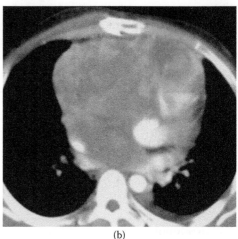

(b)

FIGURE 24.3
Thymic carcinoma: (a, b) axial contrast CT scan of the chest shows a soft-tissue mass with heterogeneous pattern of contrast enhancement. The mass lies in the anterior mediastinum that extends into the middle mediastinum. The mass infiltrates the pulmonary artery and cardiac chambers. Arrow (a) denotes thrombus in the left pulmonary artery.

Health Organization classification (2004) of thymic epithelial tumors are grouped into low-risk thymomas (types A, AB, and B1), high-risk thymomas (types B2 and B3), and thymic carcinomas (type C) [22]. On CT, Jeong et al. [26] found that lobular contour, calcification, and tumor necrosis are more often seen in high-risk than in low-risk thymomas. However, tumor shape, pattern, and degree of contrast enhancement; presence or absence of lymph node enlargement; and pleural or pericardial effusion were not different among the histological subtypes. Also, Priola et al. [21] added that invasive thymomas were more likely to be greater in size ($p < .01$) with lobulated or irregular contours ($p < .02$), a necrotic or cystic component ($p < .04$), the foci of calcification ($p < .05$), and heterogeneous contrast enhancement ($p < .01$) than noninvasive thymomas. On the other hand, Sadohara et al. [24] found no significant difference in visualization of the tumor capsule, internal tumor septation, calcification, hemorrhage, and pleural effusion on CT. CT can be very helpful in preoperative planning by the identification of important vascular structures, specifically thymic veins that may be avoided or ligated when resecting thymic tumors. Marom et al. [27] added that CT imaging features can differentiate between stage I/II and stage III/IV disease and, thus, help identify patients more likely to benefit from neoadjuvant therapy.

24.4.4 Thymic Lymphoma

Although thymic enlargement is seen in 30%–56% of patients with intrathoracic lymphoma, it is often impossible to differentiate the thymic enlargement from thymus infiltrated with tumor on CT. Posttherapeutic enlargement of the thymus may represent recurrent disease, thymic rebound (hyperplastic thymus), or development or persistence of thymic cysts. The hyperplastic thymus is usually triangular, whereas the infiltrated thymus is quadrilateral with a lobulated border. When thymic enlargement is present in adults, if the thymus is not the original site of disease or if there is no other evidence of disease relapse, it should be considered that this is due to hyperplasia rather than tumor infiltration. Thymic cysts may occur in Hodgkin lymphoma either at initial presentation (21%–50%) or after treatment [28,29].

24.4.5 Thymic Neuroendocrine Tumor (Carcinoid)

Thymic carcinoids are rare, well-differentiated neuroendocrine tumors. They occur in the fourth to fifth decades and occur three times as frequently in men as in women. Patients often present with endocrine disorders as Cushing syndrome (25%–40%) or multiple endocrine neoplasia types I and II (20%). Most thymic carcinoids are low-grade malignancy, and 50% of thymic carcinoid tumors are invasive. Thymic carcinoids are more aggressive than thymomas and cause more superior vena cava obstruction. On CT, the tumors appear as a lobulated thymic mass with homogeneous (Figure 24.4) and heterogeneous enhancement and central areas of low attenuation secondary to necrosis or hemorrhage and may show local invasion. Regional lymph node (LN) and distant metastasis develop in two-thirds of patients with thymic carcinoids. Bone metastases are typically osteoblastic [28–30].

24.4.6 Thymolipoma

Thymolipomas are rare, benign, well-encapsulated thymic tumors that account for 5% of thymic tumors. The average age of the patients is 22–26 years and has no sex predilection. Thymolipomas are often large, with a mean diameter of 20 cm. They may extend to cardiophrenic and costophrenic angles, and they do not invade neighboring structures. At CT, thymolipomas predominantly

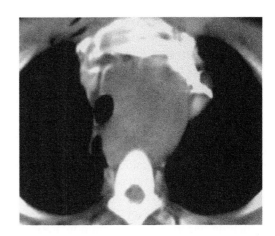

FIGURE 24.4
Thymic carcinoid: axial contrast CT scan of the chest shows a well-defined mass at the region of the thymus that shows homogeneous contrast enhancement.

show fat attenuation interspersed with fibrous septa and normal thymic tissue. CT should reveal a connection between the thymus and the tumor [28,29].

24.4.7 Thymic Hyperplasia

There are two types of thymic hyperplasia: true hyperplasia and lymphoid follicular hyperplasia. True thymic hyperplasia is less common than lymphoid follicular hyperplasia and is seen in association with thyrotoxicosis, Graves' disease, acromegaly, and red cell aplasia. True hyperplasia manifests as a diffuse, symmetric enlargement of the gland, involving both the cortex and the medulla. At CT, the gland is diffusely enlarged with preserved shape and has a homogeneous appearance similar to normal thymic tissue [6]. Thymic lymphoid follicular hyperplasia is characterized by the presence of a hyperplastic lymphoid germinal center in the thymic medulla that is associated with lymphocytic and plasma cell infiltration. Thymic lymphoid hyperplasia is commonly associated with autoimmune diseases such as MG, thyrotoxicosis, and connective tissue disease. At CT, thymic hyperplasia may appear normal (45%), enlarged (35%), or as a focal thymic mass (20%) [29].

24.5 Germ Cell Tumor

Germ cell tumors account for 10%–15% of anterior mediastinal masses in adults and 25% in children. They are thought to arise from mediastinal remnants left behind after embryonal cell migration. The mediastinum is the most common extragonadal site for germ cell tumors, and mediastinal lesions account for 60% of all germ cell tumors in adults. The vast majority of mediastinal germ cell tumors arise within the anterior mediastinum. Most germ cell tumors present during the second to fourth decades. Germ cell tumors consist of three categories: (1) teratoma (mature teratoma, immature teratoma, and teratoma with malignant transformation), (2) seminoma, and (3) nonseminomatous malignant germ cell tumors (embryonal carcinoma, endodermal sinus tumor, choriocarcinoma, and mixed type) [5,31].

Germ cell tumors are classified into benign (80%) and malignant forms. Benign tumors include mature teratomas and those mature teratomas with an immature component less than 50% of the volume. Malignant tumors include seminomas, nonseminomatous tumors, and some teratomas (immature teratomas in subjects older than 15 years and teratomas with malignant transformation). In adults, benign lesions are more frequent among women (teratomas) and malignant lesions among men (seminomas). In children, however, they are equally distributed between genders. A correlation has been reported between these tumors and Klinefelter's syndrome (karyotype 47, XXY) in 8% of cases. Hematological malignancies (commonly nonlymphoid leukemia and occasionally malignant histiocytosis) have also been found to be associated, in particular, with teratomas [5,31].

24.5.1 Teratoma

Teratomas are made up of tissues arising from one or all three of germ cell layers. The tumor is often diagnosed in adolescents and young adults. The tumor is almost exclusively seen in the anterior mediastinum. Teratomas may have solid or cystic appearance. The majority is cystic and benign; the solid forms are usually malignant. The histological types of teratoma are mature teratomas, immature teratomas, and teratomas with malignant transformation [5,32]:

1. Mature teratomas account for 70% of mediastinal germ cell tumors in children and 60% in adults. They are well delimited in relation to the surrounding mediastinal structures and may be uni- or multicystic. Mature teratomas are more commonly seen in children and young adults equally in males and females. These tumors may be of ectodermal (skin and adnexa such as teeth, hairs, and sweat and sebaceous glands), mesodermal (cartilage, bone, fat, and smooth-muscle tissue), and endodermal (bronchial and intestinal epithelium and pancreatic tissue) origins. The frequency of the most common components are 88% for fluid, 76% for fat, 53% for calcification, and 39% for a combination of the three elements. Pancreatic tissue may cause

spontaneous rupture (due to self-digestion by pancreatic juices) with leaks into neighboring hollow organs, such as bronchi, pleura, pericardium, or lung [5,32].

The appearance of teratoma depends on its content. On CT, teratoma most commonly appears as a well-defined unilocular or multilocular cystic lesion containing fluid (Figure 24.5), soft tissue, and fat attenuation. Calcifications of various morphological configurations also may be present (Figure 24.6) and a tooth is rarely seen. Common combinations of internal components of mature teratomas include soft tissue, fluid, fat, and calcification in 39%; soft tissue, fluid, and fat in 24%; and soft tissue and fluid in 15%. In 15% of cases, mature teratomas appear as cystic lesions with characteristic thick capsules [5,33].

2. Immature teratomas are made up of the same differentiated tissues as mature forms associated

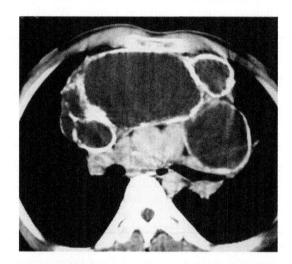

FIGURE 24.5
Mature teratoma: axial CT scan of the chest shows a large, well-defined, complex, thick-walled cystic mass with marginal calcification.

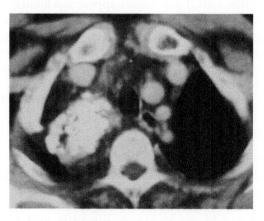

FIGURE 24.6
Teratoma: axial contrast CT scan of the chest shows a calcified mass of the teratoma in the anterior mediastinum.

with poorly organized fetal type tissue. Primitive neuroepithelial tissue is the most common. Their behavior varies with patient age. In childhood prognosis is good, whereas at any other age their behavior is often aggressive (locoregional or distant recurrence) and fatal [34].

3. Teratomas with malignant transformations, malignant teratomas, or teratocarcinomas contain malignant components, most commonly sarcoma (angiosarcoma, rhabdomyosarcoma), associated with fetal tissue or well-differentiated adult tissue. These tumors tend to be larger and invade adjacent structures than benign forms. They are aggressive tumors with local spread, distant metastasis, or both. On CT, the tumors show inhomogeneous soft-tissue density with areas of low attenuation representing cystic necrosis and hemorrhage (Figure 24.7) [5,33].

24.5.2 Seminoma (Germinoma)

Mediastinal seminomas occur exclusively in males during the second to fourth decades. Seminomas are symptomatic (2%–30%) with distant metastases (60%–70%). Gynecomastia and increased estradiol and β-HCG levels have been reported. On CT, the tumors typically have homogeneous internal attenuation and show minimal enhancement. Areas of degeneration due to hemorrhage and necrosis may present. They rarely show calcification. The most frequent sites for metastasis are lung, chest, lymph nodes, and bone [5,31].

24.5.3 Nonseminomatous Malignant Germ Cell Tumor

Nonseminomatous malignant germ cell tumors, including embryonal carcinoma, endodermal sinus (yolk sac)

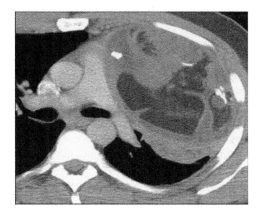

FIGURE 24.7
Malignant teratoma: axial contrast CT scan of the chest shows a large mediastinal mass with areas of calcification, fat, and soft-tissue density. (Courtesy of Dr. L. E. Quint.)

tumor, choriocarcinoma, and mixed types, are rare, highly malignant tumors that usually occur in young adults and are much more common in men. Their association with Klinefelter's syndrome (25%), hematological cancers, or solid cancers has been reported. Patients usually have elevated lactate dehydrogenase (LDH) and serum markers: α-FP (60%–80%) and β-HCG (30%–50%). On CT, the tumors show inhomogeneous soft-tissue density. Obliteration of adjacent fat planes and invasion of adjacent structures may be seen. Metastases to regional lymph nodes and distant sites are also common [5,6,33,35].

24.6 Mediasinal Lymphoma

Lymphomas are divided into Hodgkin lymphoma (HL) and non-Hodgkin lymphoma (NHL), and further subdivisions depend on histological types. The distribution of mediastinal involvement is important in tumor staging and treatment planning. Intrathoracic involvement is commoner in HL than NHL. Although HL represents only 10%–15% of lymphoma cases, 85% of patients with HL have intrathoracic disease. NHL represents 85%–90% of cases of lymphoma, and 40%–45% of patients with NHL have intrathoracic disease. Although HL and NHL may have overlapping imaging findings, there are some significant differences in their CT features [36,37].

HL is the most common lymphoma presenting with mediastinal lymphadenopathy and most frequently involves lymph nodes in anterior mediastinal and paratracheal areas in a contiguous manner, and thus it involves in decreasing order of frequency the nodes in the hilar, subcarinal, peridiaphragmatic, paraesophageal, and internal mammary areas. Nodular sclerosing HL, the commonest subtype, has a unique predilection for the nodes in the anterior mediastinum. On CT, HL is characterized by the presence of a discrete anterior mediastinal mass with a lobulated contour. The tumor most commonly demonstrates homogeneous soft-tissue attenuation, although large lymph node masses may demonstrate heterogeneity with complex low attenuation representing necrosis, hemorrhage, or cystic degeneration. Necrotic and cystic-appearing mediastinal lymph nodes were noticed at presentation in 21% of HL. Necrosis was observed most commonly in the nodular sclerosing and mixed cellularity cell types of HL and was not seen in the lymphocyte predominant variety (Figure 24.8). In NHL, thoracic involvement is present in 45% of cases and, most often, mediastinal lymphomatous involvement occurs as a disseminated or recurrent form of extrathoracic lymphoma. The involved lymph

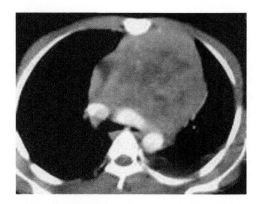

FIGURE 24.8
Hodgkin lymphoma: axial contrast CT scan of the chest shows an amalgamated mass of enlarged anterior mediastinal lymph nodes. The mass shows inhomogeneous pattern of enhancement.

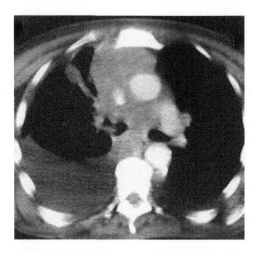

FIGURE 24.9
Non-Hodgkin's lymphoma (NHL): axial contrast CT scan of the chest shows anterior, middle, and posterior masses of enlarged mediastinal lymph nodes associated with right pleural effusion.

nodes tend to be larger compared with those in HL and have a predilection for noncontiguous or hematogenous spread to thoracic and distant nodal and extranodal sites. Unlike HL, in which anatomic sites of involvement are important, histological subtype and tumor bulk are more important prognostic factors in NHL. Nodes in the paratracheal and anterior mediastinal areas are still the most common sites for NHL followed by those in the subcarinal, hilar, posterior mediastinal (para-aortic, paravertebral, and retrocrural) (Figure 24.9), and pericardial areas [36–38].

Although lymphoma is one of the most common mediastinal tumors, it is uncommon for either NHL or HL to be limited to the mediastinum. The sole mediastinum involvement occurs in only 5% of lymphoma cases. On CT, the majority of tumors have a relatively homogeneous soft-tissue density; large tumors commonly contain areas of low attenuation due to hemorrhage or

necrosis. Enlarged nodes in contiguous lymph node groups are frequently present. Although there are many subtypes of NHL, large B-cell lymphoma and lymphoblastic lymphoma are the most common subtypes, primarily involving the anterior mediastinum. Primary mediastinal large B-cell lymphomas usually present with large and lobulated anterior mediastinal masses and occur predominantly in young adults. Low-attenuation areas of necrosis within the mass were seen in 50% and calcification in 5% of cases. Also, they often directly invade adjacent structures. Lymphoblastic lymphomas are highly aggressive and high-grade lymphomas, arising from thymic lymphocytes. They usually occur in patients in the first to second decades of life. The involvement of extrathoracic structures and bone marrow is more common in lymphoblastic lymphomas than in large B-cell lymphoma [36–39].

Recurrent disease is common in pericardial and internal mammary lymph nodes, since these nodes are usually not included in the radiation field. Dystrophic calcification may develop in involved lymph nodes following mediastinal radiation. The time interval between radiation and appearance of calcification may be 1–9 years. Lymph node calcification before treatment is unusual, but it has been associated with aggressive HL or NHL. A normal-sized lymph node may be involved in lymphoma. Conversely, a lymph node can remain enlarged after the successful treatment of lymphoma due to post-treatment changes [36–39].

24.7 Neurogenic Tumors

Neurogenic tumors represent 20% of adult and 35% of pediatric mediastinal tumors and are the most common cause of posterior mediastinal mass. Neurogenic tumors arise from peripheral, autonomic, or paraganglionic nervous systems. Neurogenic tumors are grouped into three categories: those arising from peripheral nerves, sympathetic ganglia, and rarely parasympathetic ganglia. Schwannoma, neurofibroma, and malignant tumors of nerve sheath origin arise from peripheral nerves, whereas ganglioneuroma, ganglioneuroblastoma, and neuroblastoma arise from sympathetic ganglia. Nerve sheath tumors are most common in adults, whereas sympathetic ganglia tumors are more common in children [40–42].

24.7.1 Schwannoma and Neurofibroma

They are benign, slow-growing tumors that frequently arise from a spinal nerve root but may involve any thoracic nerve. Both tumors are typically near the neural foramen. Schwannomas and neurofibromas are usually sharply marginated, spherical, and lobulated paraspinous masses that span one to two posterior rib interspaces, but they can attain large sizes [40].

24.7.1.1 Schwannoma

Schwannomas arise from the nerve sheath, extrinsically compress the nerve fibers, are typically located in the upper thorax, and present as a solitary lesion. They are divided histologically into two types. Antoni type A shows compactly packed nerve sheath cells, sometimes with palisading of tumor cells; Antoni type B shows scattered tumor cells within myxoid matrices. Both types may be present in a single schwannoma. They are encapsulated tumors composed of Schwann cells within a background of loose reticular tissue without nerve fibrils or collagen. Schwannomas appear as a well-defined paraspinal soft-tissue mass. The mass shows homogeneous or heterogeneous contrast enhancement with cystic degeneration (Figure 24.10) [42,43].

24.7.1.2 Neurofibroma

Neurofibromas are nonencapsulated or pseudoencapsulated, although they usually have discrete margins. It is noted that 10%–30% of neurofibromas are associated with von Recklinghausen neurofibromatosis (NF-1). In patients with neurofibromatosis (NF), the neurofibromas are frequently multiple and the presence of two or more neurofibromas is a criterion to diagnose NF-1. Neurofibromas show homogeneous paraspinal mass with contrast enhancement. A plexiform neurofibroma is a well-defined, nonencapsulated tumor that usually infiltrates along an entire nerve trunk (Figure 24.11) [42,43].

24.7.2 Malignant Peripheral Nerve Sheath Tumors

Malignant peripheral nerve sheath tumors (MPNSTs) are malignant variants of peripheral nerve sheath tumors that are derived from a peripheral nerve. They are rare tumors that arise from embryonic neural crest cells and are associated with NF and previous irradiation.

24.7.3 Tumors of the Autonomic Nervous System

Tumors of the autonomic nervous system include a spectrum of diseases ranging from purely benign encapsulated ganglioneuromas to malignant ganglioneuroblastomas to aggressively malignant neuroblastomas. The tumors arising from autonomic ganglia are more common in the pediatric patient population. Approximately two-thirds occur in patients less than 20 years old, and the majority of tumors are malignant. Sympathetic ganglia tumors collectively manifest as well-marginated, oblong masses with a broad base along the anterolateral aspect of the spine. They typically span three to five vertebrae, although larger sizes may be attained. Calcification can occur with sympathetic ganglia tumors and less commonly with nerve sheath tumors [43,44].

24.7.3.1 Ganglioneuroma

Posterior mediastinal ganglioneuromas frequently appear as an oblong-shaped mass in the craniocaudal direction and sometimes show calcification, fat components, internal whorled appearance, and extension to the intervertebral foramen. A tail-like extension might be a characteristic finding of posterior mediastinal ganglioneuromas (Figure 24.12) [43,44].

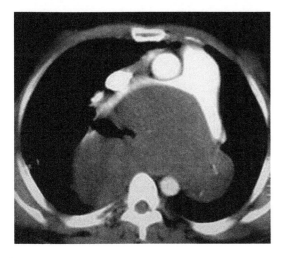

FIGURE 24.10
Schwannoma: axial contrast CT scan of the chest shows a large, well-defined posterior mediastinal mass with homogeneous pattern of contrast enhancement.

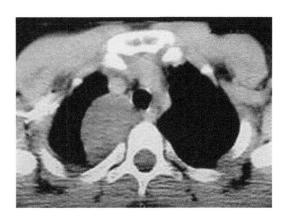

FIGURE 24.11
Schwannoma: axial contrast CT scan of the chest shows a well-defined right paraspinal mass.

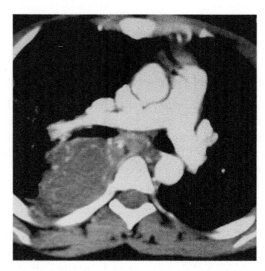

FIGURE 24.12
Ganglioneuroma: axial contrast CT scan of the chest shows a large, well-defined posterior mediastinal and right paraspinal soft-tissue mass with multiple discrete areas of calcification.

24.7.3.2 Ganglioneuroblastoma

Ganglioneuroblastomas occur with equal frequency in both genders and occur most commonly in babies and young children, with occurrence after 10 years of age being extremely rare. It is the third most common childhood malignancy after leukemia and brain tumors and is the commonest solid extracranial tumor among children. Ganglioneuroblastomas have intermediate malignancy potential, between that of neuroblastomas and ganglioneuromas. Histologically, they are considered malignant because they contain primitive neuroblasts along with mature ganglion cells. In contrast, their benign counterparts, ganglioneuromas, are fully differentiated tumors that contain all mature cell types but lack immature elements (such as neuroblasts), atypia, mitotic figures, intermediate cells, and necrosis [11].

24.7.3.3 Neuroblastoma

Neuroblastoma is composed of small round cells frequently arranged in sheets or pseudorosettes. Neuroblastoma is nonencapsulated; frequently contains extensive areas of hemorrhage, necrosis, and cystic degeneration; and may be locally invasive and widely metastatic. CT scans show tumors with homogeneous or heterogeneous texture and enhancement. Calcifications can be seen within the mass (Figure 24.13) [40–42].

24.7.4 Paraganglioma

Mediastinal paragangliomas are derived from neuroectodermal cells, which occur in two major clusters: aorticopulmonary (in the region of the aortic arch) and aorticosympathetic (in the posterior mediastinum). No

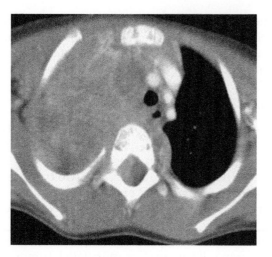

FIGURE 24.13
Neuroblastoma: axial contrast CT scan of the chest shows a large inhomogeneous soft-tissue mass with para- and intraspinal extension. (Courtesy of Dr. L. E. Quint.)

age or sex predilection has been reported. Mediastinal paragangliomas are rarely functional, and clinical presentation is often delayed until the compression of nearby structures causes pain or shortness of breath. Patients may be asymptomatic; however, dyspnea, hemoptysis, neurological symptoms, or occasionally superior vena cava syndrome may occur if the lesion reaches a size sufficient to compress contiguous structures. Aortic body paragangliomas are accompanied by other synchronous paragangliomas in about 10% of cases. Rarely, paragangliomas can occur as part of the syndrome known as Carney's triad in which they are associated with pulmonary chondroma and gastrointestinal stromal tumor. They can also occur as part of a familial disorder. Paragangliomas have typical imaging characteristics on CT. They are usually located in bifurcations of great vessels and show intense and homogeneous enhancement except for necrotic areas that are enhanced poorly [45].

24.8 Mediastinal Cyst

Most mediastinal cystic lesions are congenital (bronchogenic cysts, esophageal duplication cysts, neurenteric cysts, pericardial cysts, pleural cysts, and parathyroid cysts). Thymic cysts and thoracic duct cysts are either congenital or acquired in origin. Meningoceles, pancreatic pseudocysts, and solid lesions with cystic degeneration (i.e., schwannoma and germ cell tumor) also appear as cystic mediastinal masses. The incidence of each cystic lesion is 45% in bronchogenic, 28% in thymic, 11% in pericardial, 7% in pleural cysts, and 4% in esophageal duplication cysts. The features of mediastinal cysts at

CT are an encapsulated, smooth round or oval mass; homogeneous attenuation in the range of water attenuation (0–20 HU); and no enhancement of cyst contents. CT may reveal high attenuation due to a high level of protein and calcium in some mediastinal cysts [5,6,46,47].

24.8.1 Bronchogenic Cyst

Bronchogenic cysts are the most common foregut cyst, and they result from defective development (abnormal budding of the ventral foregut) during the fetal period. The cyst wall is lined by respiratory epithelium and contains cartilage, smooth muscle, and mucous gland. Cyst fluid is usually serous, but it can be hemorrhagic or highly viscous. Bronchogenic cysts are most commonly located in the near carina (52%) and the paratracheal region (19%), are less often adjacent to the esophagus or retrocardiac region, and are rarely in the anterior mediastinum. Bronchogenic cysts are typically stable in size or may enlarge over years. An abrupt increase in size indicates hemorrhage or infection and may result in the rupture of cysts (Figure 24.14) [5,48].

24.8.2 Thymic Cyst

Thymic cysts may be congenital in nature, arising from the remnants of the thymophargyngeal duct. Such lesions may occur anywhere along the course of thymic descent from the neck to the anterior mediastinum. Acquired thymic cysts are much more common than congenital cysts, and they arise in association with tumors such as thymomas, lymphomas, or germ cell tumors. Thymic cysts may also be seen after radiation therapy for Hodgkin's disease, and in patients with acquired immune deficiency syndrome related to an inflammatory process. Such lesions may contain cellular debris and cholesterol crystals and/or hemorrhage, leading to a complicated appearance on CT. On CT, thymic cysts have thin walls and no solid components and show no contrast enhancement. The cystic material may leak into surrounding mediastinal tissues, inciting an inflammatory response (Figure 24.15) [6,49].

24.8.3 Pericardial Cyst

Pericardial cysts are outpouchings of the parietal pericardium, which have no communication with the pericardial space and result from a defect in the embryogenesis of the celomic cavity. The majority of pericardial cysts are located in cardiophrenic angles, and they are more frequent on the right side. The cysts are also found in the higher mediastinum up to the level of pericardial reflection. Pericardial cysts in unusual locations, including upper mediastinum and anterior mediastinum, may be indistinguishable from bronchogenic or thymic cysts (Figure 24.16) [5,50].

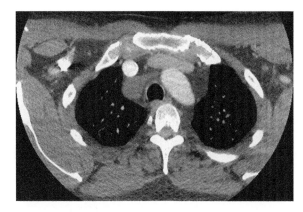

FIGURE 24.14
Bronchogenic cyst: axial contrast CT scan of the chest shows a well-defined cystic mass for which no areas of calcification could be detected. (Courtesy of Dr. D. J. Quint.)

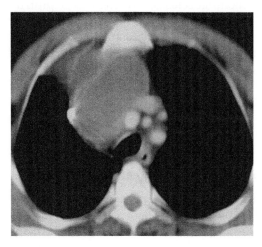

FIGURE 24.15
Thymic cyst: axial contrast CT scan of the chest shows a well-defined superior mediastinal mass at the region of thymus.

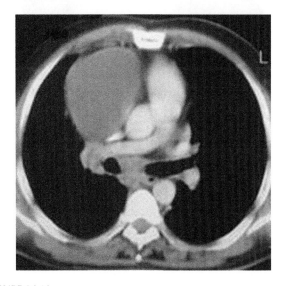

FIGURE 24.16
Pericardial cyst: axial contrast CT scan of the chest shows a well-defined, thin-walled, right-sided cyst, proved to be a pericardial cyst.

24.8.4 Esophageal Duplication Cysts

Esophageal duplication cysts are lined by gastrointestinal tract mucosa and have a double layer of smooth muscle. The cysts are commonly located in the lower mediastinum, adjacent to the esophagus. Imaging features of esophageal duplication cysts are similar to those of other mediastinal congenital cysts. However, the cyst walls may be thicker and the lesions may be more tubular in shape and be in more intimate contact with the esophagus [46,47].

24.8.5 Lateral Thoracic Meningocele

A lateral thoracic meningocele is a rare disorder that occurs frequently in association with NF type I. Spinal meningoceles are defined as a protrusion of the spinal meninges through a defect in the vertebral column or foramina usually in association with a congenitally dysraphic vertebrae, with the spinal cord remaining entirely confined to the vertebral canal. These lesions are frequently identified in a posterior location over the thoracic and sacral areas at birth and constitute about 10% of all patients with spina bifida (Figure 24.17) [51].

24.8.6 Mediastinal Pancreatic Pseudocysts

Mediastinal pancreatic pseudocysts are rare complications of acute or chronic pancreatitis and result from the extension of pancreatic juice through the diaphragm. Most mediastinal pseudocysts are retrocardiac, since

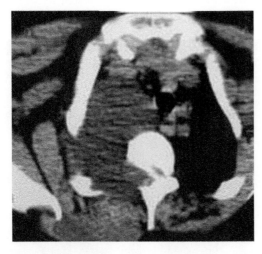

FIGURE 24.17
Lateral thoracic meningocele: axial contrast CT scan of the chest shows a large, well-defined posterior mediastinal mass that is associated with a defect in the right side of the spine with intraspinal extension of meningocele in a patient with neurofibromatosis type I. Subcutaneous schwannoma is seen along the posterior chest wall.

the inflammatory process extends through the esophageal or the aortic hiatus. Coronal CT scans assess the precise location and range of extension of the pseudocysts [52].

24.8.7 Thoracic Duct Cyst

The thoracic duct cyst is an extremely rare cystic lesion in the mediastinum. Such cysts occur anywhere along the course of the thoracic duct and occasionally communicate with the duct. The cysts may be associated with various conditions, including portal hypertension, liver cirrhosis, thoracic duct obstruction, and lymphangiomyomatosis [53].

24.9 Mediastinal Mesenchymal Tumors

Mediastinal mesenchymal tumors originate from the mediastinal connective tissue; account for 5% of mediastinal masses; and include benign and malignant lesions originating from fat, fibrous tissue, smooth and striated muscle, blood, and lymphatic vessels. Around 55% are malignant; there is no gender predilection. They may arise in any compartment, but the anterior mediastinum is most commonly involved. Adipose tissue is frequently found in the mediastinum. Adipose tissue may be seen in a wide spectrum of conditions—some nonpathological (lipomatosis, fat pads), others expressing local disease (lipomas, well-differentiated liposarcoma), and others expressing frankly progressive disease (undifferentiated liposarcoma). Vascular tumors of the mediastinum include hemangiomas, hemangioendotheliomas, and angiosarcoma. A total of 10%–30% of all vascular tumors is malignant. Mediastinal hemangiomas account for 0.5% of mediastinal tumors but represent the most common vascular tumor. They may have multiple localizations in the body; 60% are located in the anterior mediastinum and 25% in the posterior compartment. In 30% of cases, phleboliths are detected. Different types of soft-tissue sarcomas arising from mesenchymal soft tissue have been reported in the mediastinum [54,55].

24.10 Other Mediastinal Masses

24.10.1 Substernal Goiter

The incidence of substernal or mediastinal extension of goiter is 2.6%–30.4% in different studies. Symptoms caused by compression of the trachea, esophagus, or

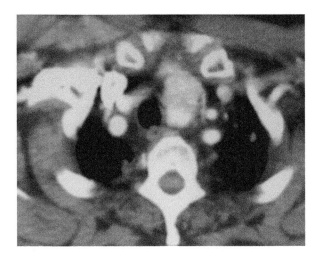

FIGURE 24.18
Substernal cancer thyroid: axial contrast CT scan of the chest shows the right thyroid nodule with substernal extension into the superior mediastinum.

vascular structures are related to the slow growth of goiter. Surgery is the treatment of choice for substernal goiter. Substernal goiter can be approached by cervical incision; however, some cases may require an extracervical approach. The CT classification system defines substernal goiter in the craniocaudal dimension as grade 1 (above aortic arch), grade 2 (level of aortic arch), and grade 3 (below aortic arch); in the anteroposterior dimension as type A (prevascular), type B (retrovascular–paratracheal), and type C (retrotracheal); and in the laterolateral dimension as monolateral and bilateral (Figure 24.18) [56].

24.10.2 Parathyroid Adenomas

Parathyroid adenomas usually occur adjacent to the thyroid gland; occasionally, they may be seen in ectopic locations such as within the thymus, tracheoesophageal groove, retroesophageal region, or posterosuperior mediastinum. They tend to be small, oval, well-defined soft-tissue attenuation structures that enhance strongly and may contain calcifications at CT. Sestamibi scanning and ultrasound of the neck are often the first imaging modalities used to search for a parathyroid adenoma in a patient with primary hyperparathyroidism; if these studies are inconclusive, then CT may be performed to look for an ectopic focus in the mediastinum [5,6].

24.10.3 Morgagni Hernia

Morgagni hernias contain omental fat that has herniated from the abdomen into the thorax via the foramen of Morgagni; the fat lies in a retrosternal or parasternal

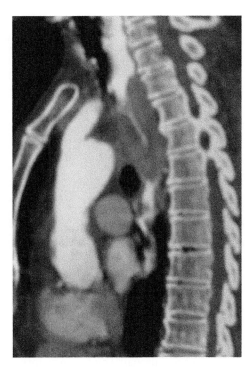

FIGURE 24.19
Esophageal cancer: sagittal contrast CT scan of the chest shows a diffuse infiltrative mass along the esophageal wall that extends into mediastinal structures.

location, usually on the right side. Occasionally, Morgagni hernias also contain small or large bowel or portions of the liver. On CT, a Morgagni hernia appears as a fat-containing mass in the lower, anterior mediastinum, usually large in size. The key to diagnosis on CT is the detection of linear-appearing soft-tissue opacities in the fat, which represent omental vessels; on close scrutiny, the vessels can be traced down into the upper abdomen [6].

24.10.4 Esophageal Lesions

Different esophageal lesions such as cancer esophagus, achalasia, and esophageal varices can be detected on CT scan as posterior mediastinal masses. Cancer esophagus may spread into the adjacent organs and posterior mediastinum. Evaluation for direct invasion by esophageal cancer into adjacent vital structures by CT is based on two criteria: mass effect and loss of fat planes. Coronal or sagittal reformatted images are best suited for this purpose and seem to be helpful (Figure 24.19). Most patients with liver cirrhosis develop esophageal varices (80%–90%). Approximately one-third of cirrhotic patients with esophageal varices develop an episode of esophageal hemorrhage. CT findings of esophageal

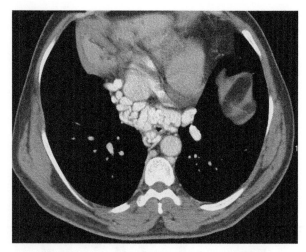

FIGURE 24.20
Esophageal varices: axial contrast CT scan of the chest shows multiple dilated tortuous serpiginous enhanced vascular structure are seen in the posterior mediastinum in the paraspinal region and paraesophageal region in a patient with portal venous hypertension.

varices are esophageal wall thickening, intraluminal protrusions or irregularities, and nodular enhancement within the wall. Paraesophageal varices may be seen as dilated veins closely juxtaposed to the outer wall of the esophagus (Figure 24.20) [57].

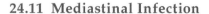

24.11 Mediastinal Infection

24.11.1 Acute Mediastinitis

Acute mediastinitis can be classified into three categories: diffuse mediastinitis, isolated mediastinal abscess, and mediastinitis or mediastinal abscess complicated by either empyema or subphrenic abscess [58].

24.11.2 Fibrosing Mediastinitis

CT of fibrosing mediastinitis shows a soft-tissue mass that infiltrates the mediastinum, sometimes invading the mediastinal structures. The middle mediastinum is the most common site of occurrence. CT is important for the identification of calcification within the lesion. Contrast CT is important in the assessment of extent of disease and helps to determine the compressive affect of fibrosis on mediastinal vessels. Airway involvement and parenchymal changes can be evaluated as well. CT may demonstrate pulmonary changes related to bronchial obstruction (such as pneumonia or atelectasis) or occlusion of major pulmonary vessels with resultant pulmonary infarction (Figure 24.21) [59–62].

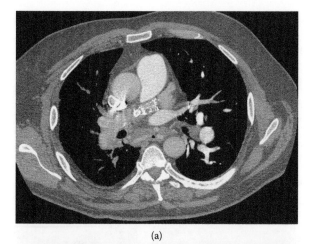

(a)

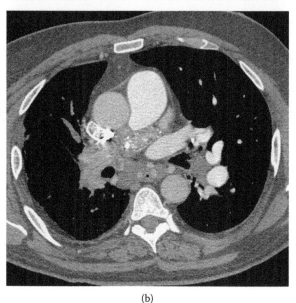

(b)

FIGURE 24.21
Chronic fibrosing mediastinitis: (a, b) axial contrast CT scan of the chest shows an ill-defined partially calcified lesion in the middle and posterior mediastinum that encases the mediastinal structures with the occlusion of the right pulmonary artery and multiple arterial collaterals. (Courtesy of Dr. L. E. Quint.)

24.12 Conclusion

The mediastinum is virtual space that may become the site of numerous pathological processes that arise from different complements of the mediastinum. CT facilitates precise assessment of location, pattern of extension, and anatomical relationship of mediastinal masses with the adjacent structures of disease. The exact location, morphology, and attenuation value of a mediastinal mass, in conjunction with clinical features and laboratory tests, can usually lead to a short list of possible etiologies.

Acknowledgments

The author thanks Dr. L. E. Quint and Dr. D. J. Quint, professors of radiology, Department of Radiology, University of Michigan Health System, Medical Center Drive, Ann Arbor, Michigan, for their help with some figures in this chapter.

References

1. Liu W, Deslauriers J. Mediastinal divisions and compartments. *Thorac Surg Clin* 2011; 21: 183–190.
2. Kim J, Hofstetter W. Tumors of the mediastinum and chest wall. *Surg Clin North Am* 2010; 90: 1019–1040.
3. Duwe B, Sterman D, Musani A. Tumors of the mediastinum. *Chest* 2005; 128: 2893–2909.
4. Taylor M, Jones D. Genetic markers of mediastinal tumors. *Thorac Surg Clin* 2009; 19: 17–27.
5. Takahashi K, Al-Janabi N. Computed tomography and magnetic resonance imaging of mediastinal tumors. *J Magn Reson Imaging* 2010; 32: 1325–1339.
6. Quint L. Imaging of anterior mediastinal masses. *Cancer Imaging* 2007; 7: S56–S62.
7. Gaubert JY, Cohen F, Vidal V et al. Imaging of mediastinal tumors. *Rev Pneumol Clin* 2010; 66: 17–27.
8. Moore S, Dave-Verma H, Singh A. Imaging of mediastinal tumors. *Cancer Treat Res* 2008; 143: 145–175.
9. Whitten C, Khan S, Munneke G, Grubnic S. A diagnostic approach to mediastinal abnormalities. *Radiographics* 2007; 27: 657–671.
10. Tomiyamaa N, Hondaa O, Tsubamoto M et al. Anterior mediastinal tumors: Diagnostic accuracy of CT and MRI. *Eur J Radiol* 2009; 69: 280–288.
11. Strollo D, Rosado de Christenson M, Jett J. Primary mediastinal tumors. Part I. Tumors of the anterior mediastinum. *Chest* 1997; 112: 511–522.
12. Priola A, Priola S, Cardinale L, Cataldi A, Fava C. The anterior mediastinum: Diseases. *Radiol Med* 2006; 111: 312–342.
13. Tecce P, Fishman E, Kuhlman J. CT evaluation of the anterior mediastinum: Spectrum of disease. *Radiographics* 1994; 14: 973–990.
14. Kim Y, Lee K, Yoo J et al. Middle mediastinal lesions: Imaging findings and pathologic correlation. *Eur J Radiol* 2000; 35: 30–38.
15. Strollo D, Rosado de Christenson M, Jett J. Primary mediastinal tumors. Part II. Tumors of the middle and posterior mediastinum. *Chest* 1997; 112: 1344–1357.
16. Kawashima A, Fishman E, Kuhlman J, Nixon M. CT of posterior mediastinal masses. *Radiographics* 1991; 11: 1045–1067.
17. Rosado-de-Christenson M, Strollo D, Marom E. Imaging of thymic epithelial tumors. *Hematol Oncol Clin North Am* 2008; 22: 409–431.

18. Benveniste M, Rosado-de-Christenson L, Sabloff B, Moran C, Swisher S, Marom E. Role of imaging in the diagnosis, staging, and treatment of thymoma. *Radiographics* 2011; 31: 1847–1861.
19. Marom EM. Imaging thymoma. *J Thorac Oncol* 2010; 5: S296–S303.
20. Maher M, Shepard J. Imaging of thymoma. *Semin Thorac Cardiovasc Surg* 2005; 17: 12–19.
21. Priola A, Priola S, Di Franco M, Cataldi A, Durando S, Fava C. Computed tomography and thymoma: Distinctive findings in invasive and noninvasive thymoma and predictive features of recurrence. *Radiol Med* 2010; 115: 1–21.
22. Müller-Hermelink HK, Ströbel P, Zettl A et al. Combined thymic epithelial tumours. In: Travis WD, Brambilla E, Müller-Hermelink HK, Harris CC, eds. *Pathology and Genetics of Tumours of the Lung, Pleura, Thymus and Heart* (WHO classification of tumours series). Lyon: IARC Press; 2004: 196–198.
23. Yanagawa M, Tomiyama N. Prediction of thymoma histology and stage by radiographic criteria. *Thorac Surg Clin* 2011; 21: 1–12.
24. Sadohara J, Fujimoto K, Muller N et al. Thymic epithelial tumors: Comparison of CT and MR imaging findings of low-risk thymomas, high-risk thymomas, and thymic carcinomas. *Eur J Radiol* 2006; 60: 70–79.
25. Yakushiji S, Tateishi U, Nagai S et al. Computed tomographic findings and prognosis in thymic epithelial tumor patients. *J Comput Assist Tomogr* 2008; 32: 799–805.
26. Jeong Y, Lee K, Kim J, Shim YM, Han J, Kwon OJ. Does CT of thymic epithelial tumors enable us to differentiate histologic subtypes and predict prognosis? *AJR Am J Roentgenol* 2004; 183: 283–289.
27. Marom E, Milito M, Moran C et al. Computed tomography findings predicting invasiveness of thymoma. *J Thorac Oncol* 2011; 6: 1274–1281.
28. Bogot N, Quint L. Imaging of thymic disorders. *Cancer Imaging* 2005; 5: 139–149.
29. Nishino M, Ashiku SK, Kocher O, Thurer R, Boiselle P, Hatabu H. The thymus: A comprehensive review. *Radiographics* 2006; 26: 335–348.
30. Schweigert M, Meyer C, Wolf F, Stein HJ. Peripheral primitive neuroectodermal tumor of the thymus. *Interact Cardiovasc Thorac Surg* 2011; 12: 303–305.
31. Drevelegas A, Palladas P, Scordalaki A. Mediastinal germ cell tumors: A radiologic–pathologic review. *Eur Radiol* 2001; 11: 1925–1932.
32. Hsu J, Kang W, Chou S, Chuang M. Mature cystic teratoma in the anterior mediastinum containing a carcinoid. *J Thorac Imaging* 2006; 21: 60–62.
33. Shimizu K, Nakata M, Hirami Y, Yamashina A, Nakano J, Kameyama K. Teratoma with malignant transformation in the anterior mediastinum. *J Thorac Cardiovasc Surg* 2008; 136: 225–227.
34. Sinclair D, Bolen M, King M. Mature teratoma within the posterior mediastinum. *J Thorac Imaging* 2003; 18: 53–55.
35. Tian L, Liu LZ, Cui CY, Zhang WD, Kuang YL. CT findings of primary non-teratomatous germ cell tumors of the mediastinum-A report of 15 cases. *Eur J Radiol* 2012; 81: 1057–1061

36. Bae Y, Lee K. Cross-sectional evaluation of thoracic lymphoma. *Thorac Surg Clin* 2010; 20: 175–186.

37. Bae Y, Lee K. Cross-sectional evaluation of thoracic lymphoma. *Radiol Clin North Am* 2008; 46: 253–264.

38. Hagtvedt T, Aaløkken TM, Smith HJ, Graff BA, Holte H, Kolbenstvedt A. Enhancement characteristics of lymphomatous lymph nodes of the mediastinum. *Acta Radiol* 2011; 52: 1113–1118.

39. Tateishi U, Muller NL, Johkoh T et al. Primary mediastinal lymphoma: Characteristic features of the various histological subtypes on CT. *J Comput Assist Tomogr* 2004; 28: 782–789.

40. Lee J, Lee K, Han J et al. Spectrum of neurogenic tumors in the thorax: CT and pathologic findings. *J Comput Assist Tomogr* 1999; 23: 399–406.

41. Ogino H, Hara M, Satake M et al. Malignant peripheral nerve sheath tumors of intrathoracic vagus nerve. *J Thorac Imag* 2001; 16: 181–184.

42. Lonergan G, Schwab C, Suarez E, Carlson C. Neuroblastoma, ganglioneuroblastoma, and ganglioneuroma: Radiologic-pathologic correlation. *Radiographics* 2002; 22: 911–934.

43. Kato M, Hara M, Ozawa Y, Shimizu S, Shibamato Y. Computed tomography and magnetic resonance imaging features of posterior mediastinal ganglioneuroma. *J Thorac Imaging* 2012; 27: 100–106.

44. Yam B, Walczyk K, Mohanty SK, Coren CV, Katz DS. Radiology-pathology conference: Incidental posterior mediastinal ganglioneuroma. *Clin Imaging* 2009; 33: 390–394.

45. Boulogianni G, Chourmouzi D, Sivitanidis E, Drevelegas A. An incidental nonfunctioning mediastinal paraganglioma. *Eur Radiol* 2010; 20: 506–509.

46. Kim J, Goo J, Lee H et al. Cystic tumors in the anterior mediastinum radiologic-pathological correlation. *J Comput Assist Tomogr* 2003; 27: 714–723.

47. Jeung M, Gasser B, Gangi A et al. Imaging of cystic masses of the mediastinum. *Radiographics* 2002; 22: S79–S93.

48. Cardinale L, Ardissone F, Cataldi A et al. Bronchogenic cysts in the adult: Diagnostic criteria derived from the correct use of standard radiography and computed tomography. *Radiol Med* 2008; 113: 385–394.

49. Choi YW, McAdams HP, Jeon SC` et al. Idiopathic multilocular thymic cyst: CT features with clinical and histopathologic correlation. *AJR Am J Roentgenol* 2001; 177: 881–885.

50. Agarwal P, Seely J, Matzinger F. Wandering pleuropericardial cyst. *J Comput Assist Tomogr* 2006; 30: 276–278.

51. Kaneda H, Saito T, Konobu T, Saito Y. Chest wall bleeding with giant intrathoracic meningocele in neurofibromatosis type 1. *Interact Cardiovasc Thorac Surg* 2011; 12: 328–330.

52. Visrutaratna P, Ukarapo N. Mediastinal pancreatic pseudocyst in chronic pancreatitis. *Pediatr Radiol* 2010; 40: 1298.

53. Gupta M, Lovelace T, Sukumar M, Gosselin M. Cervical thoracic duct cyst. *J Thorac Imaging* 2005; 20: 107–109.

54. Gladish G, Sabloff B, Munden R, Truong M, Erasmus J, Chasen M. Primary thoracic sarcomas. *Radiographics* 2002; 22: 621–637.

55. Sakurai K, Hara M, Ozawa Y, Nakagawa M, Shibamoto Y. Thoracic hemangiomas: Imaging via CT, MR, and PET along with pathologic correlation. *J Thorac Imaging* 2008; 23: 114–120.

56. Mercante G, Gabrielli E, Pedroni C et al. CT cross sectional imaging classification system for substernal goiter based on risk factors for an extracervical surgical approach. *Head Neck* 2011; 33: 792–799.

57. Ba-Ssalamah A, Zacherl J, Noebauer-Huhmann I et al. Dedicated multi-detector CT of the esophagus: Spectrum of diseases. *Abdom Imaging* 2009; 34: 3–18.

58. Aman C, Kantarci F, Cetinkaya S. Imaging in mediastinitis: A systematic review based on aetiology. *Clin Radiol* 2004; 59: 573–585.

59. Denlinger CE, Fernandez FG, Patterson GA, Kreisel D. Fibrosing mediastinitis associated with complete occlusion of the left main pulmonary artery. *Ann Thorac Surg* 2009; 87: 323.

60. Lee KY, Yi JG, Park JH, Kim YJ, So Y, Kim JS. Fibrosing mediastinitis manifesting as thoracic prevertebral thin band-like mass on MRI and PET-CT. *Br J Radiol* 2007; 80: e141–e144.

61. Worrell JA, Donnelly EF, Martin JB, Bastarache JA, Loyd JE. Computed tomography and the idiopathic form of proliferative fibrosing mediastinitis. *J Thorac Imaging* 2007; 22: 235–240.

62. Rossi SE, McAdams HP, Rosado-de-Christenson ML, Franks TJ, Galvin JR. Fibrosing mediastinitis. *Radiographics* 2001; 21: 737–757.

Index

Printed and bound by CPI Group (UK) Ltd, Croydon, CR0 4YY

18/10/2024

01776253-0017